FOURTH EDITION

Lippincott Essentials for Nursing Assistants

A HUMANISTIC APPROACH TO CAREGIVING

PAMELA J. CARTER, RN, BSN, MEd, CNOR

Pr_____ _____uctor
_____sions
Dav__ _____llege
_____Utah

Wolters Kluwer

Philadelphia • Baltimore • New York • London
Buenos Aires • Hong Kong • Sydney • Tokyo

Senior Acquisitions Editor: Kelley Squazzo
Development Editor: Helen Kogut
Associate Development Editor: Dan Reilly
Editorial Assistant: Leo Gray
Production Project Manager: Kim Cox
Design Coordinator: Stephen Druding
Illustration Coordinator: Holly McLaughlin/Jennifer Clements
Manufacturing Coordinator: Karin Duffield
Marketing Manager: Todd McKenzie
Prepress Vendor: Aptara, Inc.

4th edition

Library of Congress Cataloging-in-Publication Data

Names: Carter, Pamela J, author.
Title: Lippincott essentials for nursing assistants : a humanistic approach
    to caregiving / Pamela J Carter.
Other titles: Lippincott's essentials for nursing assistants.
Description: Fourth edition. | Philadelphia : Wolters Kluwer, [2017] |
    Preceded by Lippincott's essentials for nursing assistants / Pamela J.
    Carter. 3rd ed. c2013. | Includes index.
Identifiers: LCCN 2016032559 | ISBN 9781496339560 (paperback)
Subjects: | MESH: Nurses' Aides | Nursing Care–methods
Classification: LCC RT84 | NLM WY 193 | DDC 610.7306/98–dc23
LC record available at https://lccn.loc.gov/2016032559

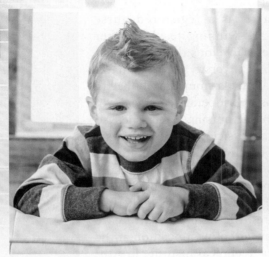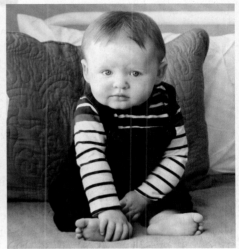

This book is dedicated to Granny's little buddies,

Carter and Kaysen, the loves of my life.

—Pam

ABOUT THE AUTHOR

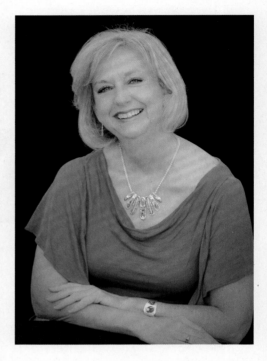

Pamela Carter is a registered nurse and an award-winning teacher. After receiving her bachelor's degree in nursing from the University of Alabama in Huntsville, Pamela immediately began her career as a perioperative nurse. Over the course of her nursing career, she also worked in a physician's office and as a staff nurse in an intensive care unit.

Pamela started teaching informally while serving as an officer in the United States Air Force Nurse Corps. She formally entered the field of health care education by accepting a position at the Athens Area Technical Institute in Athens, Georgia, where she taught surgical technology. After obtaining a master's degree in adult vocational education from the University of Georgia, Pamela moved to Florida and took a position teaching nursing assisting students. She continued teaching nursing assisting after accepting a position at Davis Applied Technology College in Kaysville, Utah. During her first year at Davis Applied Technology College, Pamela piloted a new "open-entry/open-exit" method of curriculum delivery for the nursing assistant program at the college and was awarded the Superintendent's Award for Outstanding Faculty for her work. She then opened a surgical technology program at the college and has obtained national accreditation from the Commission on Accreditation of Allied Health Education Programs (CAAHEP) for delivery of this program using the "open-entry/open-exit" method. In 2002, and again in 2014 and 2015, Pamela received a National Merit Award for having her program rank in the top 10% in the nation for students passing their national certification exam.

In addition to authoring this textbook, Pamela has also authored *Lippincott Textbook for Nursing Assistants*, *Lippincott Textbook for Long-Term Care Nursing Assistants*, as well as *Lippincott Advanced Skills for Nursing Assistants*. Pamela's writing style reflects her love of teaching, and of nursing. She is grateful for the opportunity teaching and writing have afforded her to share her experience and knowledge with those just entering the health care profession, and to help those who are new to the profession to see how they can have a profound effect on the lives of others.

Nursing assistants are increasingly being hired by health care facilities of all types as these facilities seek ways to provide top-quality nursing care in the most efficient manner. As a result, the need for qualified, well-trained nursing assistants is growing rapidly. Programs that train nursing assistants are tasked with preparing competent workers to meet this growing need as quickly as possible. Different regions of the United States have different requirements that govern the training of nursing assistants. Although different in the depth of training and the number of hours required, all nursing assistant educational programs must meet the minimum requirements established by the Omnibus Budget Reconciliation Act (OBRA) for the number of hours and specific areas of curriculum taught. Many nursing assistant educational programs focus on providing the student with the foundational concepts and facts that he or she will need to function competently in the workplace, whether that workplace is a long-term care facility, hospital, acute or extended care facility, hospice agency, or home health care agency. These *essential* requirements are the focus of this book.

Nursing assistant education is required to focus on skill competency. However, instilling in a new nursing assistant the confidence that he or she can perform the required skills properly is hardly enough. To function effectively in the health care setting, nursing assistants must also be able to recognize the person within the patient, resident, or client, and to understand that each person they are responsible for providing care for is unique and special, with individual needs that are very different from those of the person in the next bed. This textbook, *Lippincott Essentials for Nursing Assistants,* has been written not only to help students become competent in performing the skills that are the basis of the daily care they provide, but also to teach students to provide that care with compassion and humanism.

Guiding Principles

Three key beliefs guided the writing of this textbook:

1. Students need a textbook that provides foundational concepts and facts in a manner that is easy to comprehend and interesting to read.
2. Graduates of nursing assistant training programs must be able to provide competent, skilled care in a compassionate way.
3. The nursing assistant is a vital member of the health care team.

These beliefs form the basis for the textbook you hold in your hands.

Lippincott Essentials for Nursing Assistants, 4e, Is Written With the Student in Mind

Educators know that a student can easily understand complex information if it is explained in a way that the student can understand. I have worked hard to develop a conversational, yet professional, writing style that respects the student's intelligence. Concepts are presented in a straightforward, accessible way. Only the most basic, essential information is included, with the understanding that this foundational knowledge will be supplemented by classroom instruction and on-the-job training.

The structure of each chapter helps students in fast-paced, shorter nursing assistant programs learn and retain the information in the chapter. Each chapter is broken down into major sections, each with its own learning objectives ("**What Will You Learn?**"), vocabulary, and summary ("**Putting It All Together!**"). This approach allows the student to break up the reading assignment into smaller, more manageable parts.

Vocabulary words are highlighted in the text and defined in the margin. Illustrations are used as necessary to enhance and support the definitions.

Numerous photographs, both alone and in combination with line art, help the student to visualize and remember important concepts. Graphic elements, such as boxes and tables (many of which are illustrated), add visual interest and help to break up the monotony of large expanses of text.

Although the page count makes one think that this text is not short or concise, pages are set up in a "one-column" writing format so that information is spread out. The rationale behind this format style is to make the printed information look less intimidating to the student and easier to read and absorb.

New to This Edition!

We are excited to announce a major revision of this textbook! Not only have we updated the information contained in each chapter according to the changes that are constantly occurring in the health care industry, we have updated the look of the textbook and added new chapters, photos, and features. Updated information new to this edition is summarized as follows:

- All procedures have been reviewed and updated in accordance to current practice, infection control standards, and the NNAAP® Skills List for 2013. Updated photos showing the steps of procedures have been included. New procedures for tub and shower bathing and monitoring blood glucose have been added.

- Mnemonics for the "Getting Ready" (WEAVERS) and "Finishing Up" (ALSO Wash & Document) steps for procedures have been developed, along with new art to make it easier for students to remember these important steps.

- Photos and art have been updated throughout the text to show more modern equipment and techniques.

- A new unit, specific to long-term care and the people who reside in long-term care facilities has been added. Since dementia is so common in the LTC facilities, this chapter has been moved to this new unit.

- An exciting new feature, known as "Concerns for Long-Term Care," will appear throughout the text. This feature is intended to supply additional information specific to care of elderly residents in the LTC setting.

- Information specific to the use of electronic health records and computerized charting has been included in Chapter 4.

- Updated information related to nutrition and new dietary recommendations from the *2010 Dietary Guidelines for Americans* has been included, along with the related art and descriptions of MyPlate and MyPlate for Older Adults.

- Information related to developmental disabilities has been updated.
- Appendix B, Introduction to the Language of Health Care, has been revised to contain many new abbreviations that are currently in use in the health care setting.
- The instructor's test bank, power point slides, and lesson plans have been updated and revised.
- Along with the revision of this textbook all of the videos that accompany it have been updated and revised.

Lippincott Essentials for Nursing Assistants, 4e, Helps Prepare Students for Clinical Practice

It is my desire to help prepare students to enter the health care profession with the knowledge, skills, and confidence that education and training can provide. In addition, I want to help students develop the compassion and the critical thinking and communication skills they need to function effectively in the health care setting. Several of the textbook's features were designed specifically with these goals in mind:

- **Procedure boxes.** Certainly, a major objective of any nursing assistant training course is to ensure that graduates are able to provide care in a safe and correct manner. Each procedure in this text has been revised and updated in accordance to new infection control standards, current practice, and the National Nurse Aide Assessment Program (NNAAP®) Skills List for 2013. Those particular skills can be found in the following chapters:
  - **Hand Hygiene (Hand Washing):** Chapter 13
  - **Applies One Knee-High Elastic Stocking:** Chapter 32
  - **Assists to Ambulate Using Transfer Belt:** Chapter 18
  - **Assists with Use of Bedpan:** Chapter 25
  - **Cleans Upper of Lower Denture:** Chapter 21
  - **Counts and Records Radial Pulse/Respirations/Blood Pressure:** Chapter 20
  - **Donning and Removing PPE (Gown and Gloves):** Chapter 13
  - **Dresses Client with Affected (Weak) Right Arm:** Chapter 23
  - **Feeds Client Who Cannot Feed Self:** Chapter 24
  - **Gives Modified Bed Bath:** Chapter 21
  - **Measures and Records Urinary Output:** Chapter 25
  - **Measures and Records Weight of Ambulatory Client:** Chapter 20
  - **Performs Modified PROM for Knee and Ankle/Shoulder:** Chapter 18
  - **Positions on Side:** Chapter 17
  - **Provides Catheter Care for Female:** Chapter 25
  - **Provides Foot Care:** Chapter 23
  - **Provides Mouth Care:** Chapter 21
  - **Provides Perineal Care for Female:** Chapter 21
  - **Transfers from Bed to Wheelchair Using Transfer Belt:** Chapter 17

Seventy-three core procedures are presented in this text. The procedures for each chapter are grouped at the end of the chapter, to avoid breaking up the text with lengthy boxes. Each procedure box begins with a "Why You Do It" statement, to help students understand the "why behind the what," an understanding that is the foundation for the development of critical thinking skills. The concepts of privacy, safety, infection control, comfort, and communication are emphasized consistently in every procedure. *"Getting Ready"* and *"Finishing Up"* steps are included in every procedure box to help students remember these very important pre- and postprocedure actions. New, easy-to-remember mnemonics for the pre- and post-procedure actions have been developed to help students remember. The steps of the procedure are given using clear and concise language, and photograph and illustrations are provided as necessary. A "What You Document" section at the end of each procedure reminds students to document care given and what important observations should be noted. An icon (◉) identifies procedures that are demonstrated in *Lippincott Video Series for Nursing Assistants, 2nd edition.*

Procedure Box: Step-by-step instructions for key nursing assistant actions.

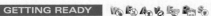

PROCEDURE 23-6
Combing a Person's Hair

Why you do it: Combing the hair helps to prevent tangles and gives the hair a neat appearance.

GETTING READY

1. Complete the "Getting Ready" steps.

SUPPLIES

- paper towels
- wide-toothed comb or pick
- brush
- mirror
- hair accessories (optional)
- detangler or leave-in conditioner (optional)
- towels

PROCEDURE

2. Make sure that the bed is positioned at a comfortable working height (to promote good body mechanics) and that the wheels are locked.
3. Clean the top of the over-bed table and cover it with paper towels. Place the hair care supplies and clean linens on the over-bed table.
4. Raise the head of the bed as tolerated. Gently lift the person's head and shoulders and cover the pillow with a towel. Drape another towel across the person's back and shoulders.
5. If the side rails are in use, lower the side rail on the working side of the bed. The side rail on the opposite side of the bed should remain up.
6. If the hair is tangled, work on the tangles first. Put a small amount of detangler or leave-in conditioner on the tangled hair. Begin at the ends of the hair and work toward the scalp. Hold the lock of hair just above the tangle (closest to the scalp) and use the wide-tooth comb to gently work through the tangle.
7. Using the brush and working with one 2-inch section at a time, gently brush the hair, moving from the roots of the hair toward the ends.

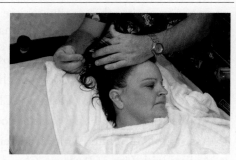

STEP 7 ■ Hold the lock of hair just above the tangle.

8. Secure the hair using barrettes, clips, or pins or braid the hair, as the person requests. Offer the person the mirror to check her appearance when you are finished. Remove the towels from the person's shoulders and the pillow.
9. Reposition the pillow under the person's head and straighten the bed linens. If the side rails are in use, return the side rails to the raised position. Lower the head of the bed as the person requests.
10. Gather the soiled linens and place them in the linen hamper or linen bag. Dispose of disposable items in a facility-approved waste container. Clean equipment and return it to the storage area.

FINISHING UP

11. Complete the "Finishing Up" steps.

WHAT YOU DOCUMENT

- Date and time
- Type of care provided
- Presence of excessive tangling or any unusual observations of the hair or scalp

- **Guidelines ("What You Do/Why You Do It") boxes.** These boxes summarize guidelines for carrying out key nursing assistant actions. The unique "What You Do/Why You Do It" format helps students to understand why things are done a certain way. I believe that if students understand why something is done a certain way, they will be more likely to remember to do it that way.

- **Tell the Nurse! notes.** A recurrent theme throughout the book is the important role the nursing assistant plays in making observations about the patient's or resident's condition and reporting these observations to the nurse. The *Tell the Nurse!* notes highlight and summarize signs and symptoms that a nursing assistant may observe that should be reported to the nurse. This information is presented within a context to help students remember and apply the information.

GUIDELINES BOX 13-1   Guidelines for Maintaining a Clean Environment

What you do	Why you do it
Wash your hands, instead of using an alcohol-based hand rub, after contact with any body fluid, whether it is your own or another person's. Examples of body fluids include blood, saliva, vomitus, urine, feces, vaginal discharge, semen, wound drainage, pus, mucus, and respiratory secretions.	*Pathogens often leave the body through the gastrointestinal tract, reproductive or urinary tract, respiratory tract, or breaks in the skin. In addition, some pathogens are transmitted in blood and other body secretions, such as breast milk.*
Handwashing, instead of hand hygiene with an alcohol-based rub, should be used when caring for a person who may have certain infections, such as *C. diff.*	*Alcohol-based hand rubs may not be effective against certain microorganisms.*
Wash your hands frequently, especially after using the bathroom, and before handling food, drink, or eating utensils. Perform hand hygiene before and after any contact with a patient or resident.	*Frequent hand hygiene eliminates a method of transmission for pathogens.*
Cough or sneeze into a tissue or into your sleeve at the elbow, and teach your patients and residents to do the same. Dispose of tissues properly by placing them in a waste container.	*Some pathogens are transmitted in particles of saliva or sputum. Coughing or sneezing into your sleeve or a tissue contains these particles and helps to prevent the spread of infection.*
Provide each patient or resident with individual personal care items, such as toothbrushes, drinking glasses, towels, washcloths, and soap. Disposable items are preferred when possible.	*If not properly cleaned after use, these items can spread pathogens. Therefore, it is better to limit their use to one person.*
Keep contaminated or dirty items, such as soiled linens, away from your uniform.	*Pathogens can be transferred from the dirty item to your uniform, which can then act as a fomite.*
When cleaning, take care not to stir up dust. For example, wiping dusty surfaces with a damp cloth or mop helps to prevent the movement of dust and lint into the air. Do not shake linens when making beds.	*Dust can carry pathogens from one area to another.*
Dispose of trash properly. Follow established procedures for preparing dirty linens and clothing for the laundry.	*If not disposed of properly, trash can provide an ideal environment for pathogens to grow, especially if the trash contains food or other materials that can rot. Soiled items and clothing can spread pathogens and must be handled in a way that will lessen the chance of someone else coming in contact with the dirty item.*
Maintain good personal hygiene, and help your patients or residents to do the same. Bathing, washing hair, brushing teeth, and wearing clean clothing are all grooming practices that help to prevent the spread of infection.	*Personal grooming practices help to reduce the number of pathogens present on the skin.*

Guidelines Box ("What You Do/Why You Do It"): Guidelines and rationales for key nursing assistant actions.

Tell the Nurse!

Signs of infection

- Fever (elderly people may only have a slight increase in body temperature, or even no increase at all)
- A rapid pulse, a rapid respiratory rate, or changes in blood pressure
- Pain or difficulty breathing
- Redness, swelling, or pain
- Foul-smelling or cloudy urine
- Pain or difficulty urinating
- Diarrhea or foul-smelling feces
- Nausea or vomiting
- Lack of appetite
- Skin rashes
- Fatigue
- Increased confusion or disorientation
- Any unusual discharge or drainage from the body

Tell the Nurse! Note: Observations that need to be reported to the nurse.

- **Stop and Think!** scenarios. Each chapter concludes with one or more *Stop and Think!* scenarios. These scenarios encourage students to critically solve problems, and help them to see that many situations they will encounter in the workplace do not have cut-and-dried answers.

Stop and Think! Scenario:
Situations to promote critical
thinking.

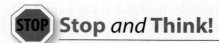 **Stop** *and* **Think!**

Mr. Lovell, one of the residents with dementia at the long-term care facility where you work, has become very agitated. He is prone to falling, and should not get up without help. However, today he is refusing to stay in his bed or his wheelchair. You get him situated, and then as soon as you leave the room, he tries to get up again. This has happened twice, and you are only in the first hour of your shift. You are very concerned that Mr. Lovell will fall and hurt himself, but you cannot stay with him all day because you have other residents to attend to. Describe some things that you could do to help protect Mr. Lovell.

- **Nurse Pam.** Nurse Pam, modeled and named after the author of this book, appears throughout the text in various scenarios to help students empathize with their patients or residents. Nurse Pam has been updated (because she is older now) and the information has been revised to remain consistent with current practice.

Nurse Pam: Highlights humanistic, holistic care.

Having to help another person with perineal care may seem unpleasant or embarrassing to you. But think of it this way—what if you were sick or injured to the point that you had wet yourself or had a bowel movement in the bed? Think of how wonderful it would feel to have someone clean you up, help you change your clothes, and give you fresh bed linens. You would feel clean and cared for.

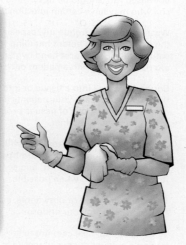

Lippincott Essentials for Nursing Assistants, 4e, Promotes Pride in the Profession

It is my desire to impress upon students entering the health care profession that no one is "just" a nursing assistant. Nursing assistants are often the members of the health care team with the most day-to-day contact with patients, residents, and clients. As such, they bear a large part of the responsibility for the well-being of those in their care. Nursing assistants who feel that they can and do make a difference in the lives of others will go the "extra mile" to ensure that the care they provide is holistic.

An Overview of *Lippincott Essentials for Nursing Assistants, 4e*

This textbook consists of six units. The following is a brief survey of these units and the information they contain.

Unit 1: Introduction to Health Care

The six chapters that make up Unit 1 provide the student with basic background knowledge. Chapter 1 introduces the student to the health care setting and the governmental regulations that play a role in establishing standards and funding for health care. The nursing home survey process is introduced so that students become better informed of how regulatory organizations determine a facility's ability to provide quality care to the residents. Chapter 1 also introduces the holistic approach to health care. Chapter 2 focuses on the nursing assistant's responsibilities as a member of the health care team. The concepts of delegation and the nursing process are introduced. In addition, Chapter 2 explores legal and ethical issues related to the nursing assistant's job, including patient and resident rights, the Health Insurance Portability and Accountability Act (HIPAA), advance directives, and abuse. New information, specific to abuse and defining "vulnerable adults" who are often victims of abuse, has been added. Professionalism, job-seeking skills, and the concept of work ethic are thoroughly discussed in Chapter 3, introducing students to the idea that a professional attitude promotes respect and is necessary for career advancement. Communication, one of the most essential responsibilities of the nursing assistant, is discussed in Chapter 4. Chapter 5 focuses on the central member of the health care team—the patient, resident, or client. This chapter introduces the concept of human needs and explains how the person being cared for in a health setting has many needs other than those specifically associated with illness or disability. The impact that illness and disability have on a patient's or resident's family members and their need to be involved in the person's plan of care are also addressed. The unit concludes with Chapter 6, which focuses on the person's environment in a health care setting. OBRA requirements related to the physical environment of a long-term care setting are listed and explained.

Unit 2: The Human Body in Health and Disease

Having a basic understanding of how each of the body's organ systems functions in health is essential to understanding how failure of an organ system to work properly leads to disease and disability. Chapter 7 gives a basic description of the structure and function of each of the body's organ systems. In addition, for each organ system, the effects of the normal aging process on that organ system's function are described. Chapter 8 discusses disorders that frequently create the need for a person to be cared for in a health care setting. Rehabilitation and restorative care are discussed in Chapter 9, with an emphasis on the role that the nursing assistant plays in this important aspect of patient and resident care.

Unit 3: Long-Term Care

This is a new unit for this textbook, comprised of two new chapters and an additional chapter that was moved here to accompany this information. Chapter 10, Overview of Long-Term Care, introduces the students to the long-term care setting and includes a discussion about the past, present, and future of long-term care. Chapter 11, The Long-Term Care Resident, helps students understand the factors that can lead to admission to a long-term care facility, and the special needs that residents of long-term care facilities, and their families, may have. Chapter 12 continues the discussion by providing information about dementia, a condition that affects many long-term care residents.

Unit 4: Safety

The four chapters in this unit are concerned with measures taken to ensure safety, both for the patient or resident and for the nursing assistant. Chapter 13 covers communicable disease and how the spread of communicable disease is prevented in the health care setting. Updated guidelines related to hand hygiene from the CDC have been included. Chapter 14 deals with workplace safety, and includes an extensive discussion about the importance of using proper body mechanics and ergonomics to prevent work-related injuries. Information related to workplace violence and tips on how to avoid and remain safe at the workplace has been included. Also in Chapter 13, the student is introduced to the "Getting Ready" and "Finishing Up" steps that are taken before and after each procedure. New mnemonics help students to easily remember each of these important pre- and postprocedure steps. Chapter 15 explores some of the conditions that put patients and residents at risk for injury, followed by a discussion about methods used to prevent accidents from occurring. Restraints, with a focus on methods that can be used as alternatives to restraints, are discussed in-depth. Information and guidelines to help prevent "entrapment" has been included in this chapter. This unit concludes with Chapter 16, which contains information related to recognizing emergencies and responding to them. Chapter 16 also includes the updated 2010 AHA Guidelines for BLS and updated procedures for clearing an obstructed airway.

Unit 5: Basic Patient and Resident Care

The eleven chapters in this unit focus on the skills and equipment used to provide basic daily care to people in a health care setting. In Chapter 17, the techniques used to safely assist patients and residents with repositioning and transferring are explained. Chapter 18 discusses the complications that can result from immobility and explains how to safely assist a person in a health care setting with ambulation and exercise. Chapter 19 describes bedmaking skills. Chapter 20 covers vital signs, height, and weight. Because many students find the procedures related to taking vital signs intimidating and difficult to master at first, encouragement and practical tips are included throughout. Chapter 21 covers bathing and routine skin care. Chapter 22 focuses on the prevention and treatment of pressure ulcers and other types of wound care. Updated information about the staging of pressure ulcers has been added. Chapter 23 covers routine grooming. In Chapter 24, New dietary recommendations from the *2010 Dietary Guidelines for Americans* introduces MyPlate and MyPlate for Older

Adults, along with basic nutrition is presented in a factual, useful manner without undue emphasis on specific diets, as these continue to change as research dictates. Information about preparing and serving thickened liquids is included. Chapters 25 and 26 cover urinary and bowel elimination, respectively. Unit 5 concludes with Chapter 27, which discusses how the nursing assistant helps to promote comfort, including a discussion about the importance of recognizing and reporting signs of pain.

Unit 6: Special Care Concerns

The final unit in this text contains five chapters that cover special care situations that the nursing assistant will most likely encounter during a career in health care. Chapter 28 describes how a person and his or her loved ones cope with a terminal illness and impending death. The care provided to the dying person in the hours leading up to, and following, death is also discussed. In Chapter 29, some of the major types of developmental disabilities are reviewed, along with updated information related to each disability. Chapters 30 and 31 cover the special care needs of people who have cancer and HIV/AIDS, respectively. Chapter 32 discusses the special care required by patients and residents before and after a surgical procedure.

Chapter 33 introduces the student to the home health care setting. Building on basic knowledge and skills presented in previous units, this chapter explores some of the concerns and issues that are unique to the home health care setting. Chapter 33 provides students with an overview of what home health care is and who might require it, and explores some of the qualities that a person must have to succeed as a home health aide. Specific issues related to safety and infection control within the home are also covered.

Appendices and Glossary

The textbook concludes with two appendices and a comprehensive glossary.

- Appendix A consists of the answers to the **What Did You Learn?** exercises that appear at the end of each chapter.

- Appendix B introduces the student to the language of health care. This discussion about medical terminology is included as an appendix so that it can be introduced at any point during the training course, and referred to frequently. The tables containing common roots, prefixes and suffixes, and abbreviations are in close physical proximity to the glossary for easy and quick reference. Also included in Appendix B is the Joint Commission's "Do Not Use" abbreviations list.

- The glossary is an alphabetical compilation of the vocabulary words from each chapter.

A Comprehensive Package for Teaching and Learning

To further facilitate teaching and learning, a carefully designed ancillary package is available. In addition to the usual print resources, multimedia tools have been developed in conjunction with the text.

Resources for Students

- **Student Resources at http://thePoint.lww.com/CarterEssentials4e** include *Watch and Learn!* 🔲 (a series of video clips that support information given in the text) and *Listen and Learn!* 🔲 (an interactive glossary that enables students to hear the vocabulary words pronounced, defined, and used in a sentence, and then to quiz themselves using the flashcard feature). In addition, the *Nursing Assistants Make A Difference!* feature allows the student to listen to first-person accounts of how nursing assistants have made a difference in the lives of patients, residents, clients, and family members. Certification-style review questions help students prepare to face exams armed with confidence and knowledge.

- **Workbook to Accompany** *Lippincott Essentials for Nursing Assistants, 4e.* This illustrated workbook provides the student with a fun and engaging way of reviewing important concepts and vocabulary. Each part of the student workbook has been updated and revised alongside the changes made in the fourth edition of the textbook. Its multiple-choice questions, matching exercises, true–false exercises, word finds, crossword puzzles, coloring and labeling exercises, and other types of active-learning tools will appeal to many different learning styles. The workbook also contains procedure checklists for each procedure in the textbook.

Resources for Instructors

This fourth edition comes with an updated collection of ancillary materials designed to help you organize your class, effectively teach the material, and evaluate your students' progress and comprehension. Resources that can be found online at *thePoint*—http://thepoint.lww.com/CarterEssentials4e—include:

- **PowerPoint Presentations** and **Guided Lecture Notes**
- Sample **Syllabus**
- **Test Generator** with more than 700 multiple-choice questions
- **Pre-Lecture Quizzes**
- **Assignments, Discussion Topics,** and **Case Studies**
- **Image Bank**

Additional Resources

- *Lippincott Video Series for Nursing Assistants,* 2nd edition. Procedure-based modules provide step-by-step demonstrations of the core skills that form the basis of the daily care the nursing assistant provides. As in the textbook, all procedures have been reviewed and updated in accordance to current practice, infection control and the NNAAP Skills List for 2013. *Getting Ready and Finishing Up* actions are reviewed on every procedure-based module, and the themes of privacy, safety, infection control, comfort, and communication are emphasized throughout. Four non–procedure-based modules, on the topics of preparing for entry into the workforce, caring for people with dementia, death and dying, and communication and patient and resident rights, are also available.

- **Copper Ridge *Dementia Care Modules.*** Developed by the esteemed Copper Ridge Institute in affiliation with Johns Hopkins University School of Medicine, this two-CD set consists of nine interactive modules designed to teach students how to care for people with dementia. The causes and types of dementia are reviewed, along with dementia-related behaviors and the best way to manage them. Communication and compassion are emphasized throughout. Learning is enhanced through video clips, interactive exercises, and short multiple-choice quizzes at the conclusion of each module.

It is with great pleasure that my colleagues and I introduce these resources to you. One of our primary goals in creating these resources has been to share with those just entering the health care field our sense of excitement about the health care profession, and our commitment to the idea that being a nursing assistant involves much more than just "bedpans and blood pressures." I hope we have succeeded in that goal, and I welcome feedback from our readers.

PAMELA J. CARTER

How to Use This Book to Prepare for Class and Study

Learning is an active process. You need to read, make notes, and ask questions about anything you are having trouble understanding. Most students who are successful learners take a three-step approach to learning:

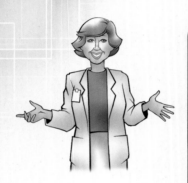

Welcome! Health care is an exciting, yet demanding, field. During your training course, you will be expected to learn and apply a lot of new information. My name is Pam Carter, and I am the author of the book you hold in your hands. It is my pleasure and my honor to assist you on your journey toward becoming a health care professional. Let me begin by explaining to you a little bit about how you can use this book to prepare for class and study.

Preview

During the *preview* stage of learning, you focus on preparing yourself for class. Most likely, your instructor will give you reading assignments that must be completed before each class. The course *syllabus* that you will receive at the beginning of the course will tell you when each reading assignment must be completed. The reading assignments give you the chance to get a general idea of what is going to be discussed in the next class.

To prepare for class, just read the assignment as if you were reading a novel or a newspaper for enjoyment. During the preview, you do not need to take notes or try to memorize facts—just read through the material to get the "big picture" of the information you are about to learn. Some people find it helpful to read the chapter out loud to themselves (or into a tape recorder, so that they can listen to the chapter again later). Others like to highlight parts of the chapter using a highlighting pen, or make notes in the margin. Learning becomes much easier when you discover what methods work best for you.

To assist you with previewing, each section in each chapter begins with a *What Will You Learn?* section. This section contains a list of specific goals for

What will you learn?

When you are finished with this section, you will be able to:

1. List changes that occur in a person's feet as a result of aging or illness.
2. State observations that you may make when assisting a patient or resident with foot care that should be reported to the nurse.
3. Demonstrate proper technique for assisting with foot care.
4. Define the word **podiatrist**.

What Will You Learn?: Specific goals for the section.

that section, called *learning objectives*. Learning objectives tell you what you will be expected to know or be able to do to demonstrate complete understanding of the material in that section of the chapter. During the preview stage, the learning objectives can be very useful in giving you an overview of the key goals of that section.

The *What Will You Learn?* section also contains a list of the new vocabulary words you will need to learn. The vocabulary words, which appear in **bold type** throughout the chapter, are listed in the order that they appear. The definition of each vocabulary word is found in the margin near where the word appears in the text. The *Listen and Learn!* icon next to the vocabulary words lets you know that you can visit thePoint to hear the words in each vocabulary list pronounced, defined, and used in a sentence. This is an effective and fun way to preview vocabulary words! Familiarizing yourself with the chapter's vocabulary words before class puts you one step ahead, because when you hear those words in class, they will not sound strange to you, and you may already know what they mean.

As you read the chapter, look for the *Watch and Learn!* icon too. This symbol lets you know that you can visit thePoint to watch a video clip that supports the information you are reading about.

View

The *viewing* stage is when you get down to business and really work to understand the material. During the classroom lecture or discussion, highlight important points and take notes as you need to. Ask questions about any of the material that you do not fully understand. Remember, there are no "stupid" questions! If you do not fully understand something, you need to speak up so that the instructor can help you. This is your instructor's job.

Review

After class, go back over the notes you took in class, and reread the chapter in your book. Some students like to read the entire chapter over again. Others just skim the chapter, paying close attention to the topics they still have questions about. Each section in the chapter closes with a short summary called *Putting It All Together!* which repeats and summarizes the key concepts of that section.

When you feel comfortable with your understanding of the material, test yourself! Go back to the learning objectives in the *What Will You Learn?* section at the beginning of each section in the chapter and pretend they are questions. Try to answer them. If you have trouble answering them, then you know that you need to review those sections of the chapter again. You can also test yourself using the *What Did You Learn?* section

Putting it all together!

- Clean, dry, wrinkle-free linens promote comfort and rest.
- Clean, dry, wrinkle-free linens help to prevent complications, such as pressure ulcers. Dampness contributes to skin breakdown, and wrinkled sheets can cause friction, both of which are factors in the development of pressure ulcers.
- Clean, dry linens are important for odor and infection control.
- Bed linens are changed according to facility policy and as often as necessary to ensure that the patient or resident has a clean, dry, wrinkle-free bed at all times.

Putting It All Together!: A review of key points from the section.

WHAT DID YOU LEARN?

Multiple Choice

Select the single best answer for each of the following questions.

1. A person with an airway obstruction will usually:
   a. Have a seizure
   b. Vomit
   c. Be able to speak and breathe normally
   d. Clutch at his/her throat

2. In the Guidelines for BLS, the "C" stands for:
   a. Cardiac
   b. Consciousness
   c. Compressions
   d. Check for bleeding

3. Where do you place your fist while clearing an obstructed airway in a conscious adult?
   a. On the person's back
   b. Above the person's navel
   c. On the person's chest
   d. Below the person's navel

4. If a person with an obstructed airway is coughing but able to breathe, you should:
   a. Administer oxygen
   b. Use a finger sweep to remove the object that is obstructing the person's airway
   c. Perform abdominal thrusts
   d. Stay with the person and allow him to continue coughing

5. Which is a sign or symptom of shock?
   a. Low blood pressure
   b. A weak, rapid pulse
   c. Cool, clammy, pale skin
   d. All of the above

6. Which of the following actions should you take to assist a person who is having a seizure?
   a. Protect the person's head by placing a pillow underneath it
   b. Clear the area by moving furniture out of the way
   c. Avoid placing anything in the person's mouth
   d. All of the above

7. Which of the following best describes the recovery position?
   a. Positioned on the back
   b. Positioned on the abdomen
   c. Sitting with the head between the knees
   d. Lying on the side

What Did You Learn?: A tool for self-assessment.

at the end of each chapter. The answers to the questions in the *What Did You Learn?* section are in Appendix A in the back of the book, so that you can see how well you understood the material you just studied. Again, if you have trouble answering these questions, then you will know that your studying is not quite finished! You may need to read certain parts of the chapter again, or ask your instructor for help.

Try to set aside short periods of time for studying each day. For example, you might study for 30 to 45 minutes, take a break to do other activities or chores, and then come back and study for another 30 to 45 minutes. After 30 to 45 minutes of studying, most people become tired and lose their ability to concentrate. Studying in short bursts will help keep you focused on the material you are trying to learn.

How to Prepare for Tests

Did you learn the material or not? This is what instructors want to know when they give tests, quizzes, and exams. Not doing well on a test does not mean that you are a failure. It just means that you need to figure out what went wrong, and make an effort to improve the next time. Perhaps you did not study as well as you could have for the test. Or maybe you got so nervous, you forgot everything you learned when it came time to take the test!

The course syllabus will tell you when a test is scheduled to be given, and what material it will cover. Mark these dates on your calendar, so you are not surprised! Preparing for a test should not be a major event. If you use the preview–view–review approach and study each day, when the time comes to prepare for the test, you will be very well prepared. In the days leading up to the test, all you will need to do is review the material that will be covered on the test one more time, by skimming the chapters in the book and reviewing the notes you took in class.

When it comes time to actually take the test, remember the following tips:

- Relax! You have prepared for this test, and you know the answers to these questions!

- Take a deep breath and make sure you read the directions carefully. The directions will tell you whether there is only one correct answer for each question, or whether it is possible for a question to have more than one correct answer.

- Read each question completely and carefully. Many students answer questions incorrectly simply because they are in a hurry and miss important words, like "except" or "not."

- If the question is a multiple-choice question, try to state the answer in your head before looking at the answer choices. Then read each answer choice before choosing the one that best matches the answer you have in your head. This will increase your confidence that the answer you have selected is the correct one.

- After selecting an answer, avoid second-guessing yourself. Research has shown that your first choice is most likely to be correct, if you studied the material well. Sometimes, however, you will come across a question later in the test that makes you realize that you answered an earlier question incorrectly. In this case, when you are sure that you have made a mistake, it is all right to go back and change your answer. But if you do not have a clear idea of what the correct answer is, doubting your first choice will most likely result in changing a correct answer to an incorrect one!

- If you cannot answer a question, go on to the next. Often, another question on the test will jog your memory and help you to remember the answer to the question you skipped earlier. Just remember to go back over your answer sheet before you hand in your test to make sure you have answered all of the questions.

Many people think that the goal of studying is to pass a test. It is true that as you work through your training course, you will have to pass many tests. And most states require people who want to be nursing assistants to pass a certification exam at the end of the training course. But passing the test is a short-term goal. It is more important for you to be able to remember and use the information that you learned during your training course long after you complete the course and pass the certification exam. The people you will be caring for are depending on you to be knowledgeable and good at what you do. They will be trusting you with their health and well-being. Study hard, ask questions, and remember that each and every person you care for throughout your career deserves the same type of competent, compassionate care that you would expect to be given to your own mother, father, spouse, sibling, or child. As a nursing assistant, you will have the chance to have a positive effect on the lives of many people.

Caring for those in need is very important work. Let me be among the first to thank you for your interest in pursuing a career in health care, and to wish you luck on your journey.

Sincerely,
PAM

REVIEWERS

I would like to extend my heartfelt thanks to my fellow instructors across the country who took the time to review the text and provide me with such valuable suggestions for improvement.

Cheryl Ballantyne, BSN
Program Coordinator
Black Hawk Community College
Moline, Illinois

Ruth Belec-Olander, MSN, RN
Nursing Faculty
College of Lake County
Grayslake, Illinois

Alice Bream, BSN, RN
Educator
Harrisburg Area Community College
Harrisburg, Pennsylvania

Sally Christiansen, BSN, MS
Coordinator Basic
Nursing Assistant Program
Waukesha County Technical College
Pewaukee, Wisconsin

Sheila F. Douglas-Collins, MSN, RN
Associate Dean of Nursing
Wayne County Community College District
Detroit, Michigan

Sherril Ehlert-Longmuir, RN, BSN
Program Director for the NA/MA Training
Programs
University of Wisconsin-Oshkosh
Oshkosh, Wisconsin

Laurie Ellefson, BSN
Faculty
Western Technical College
La Crosse, Wisconsin

Mary Joyce Fain, ADN
Allied Health Instructor
West Georgia Technical College
LaGrange, Georgia

Joanmarie Fantozzi, RN, CPP
BNAT Coordinator/Instructor
Wilbur Wright College
Chicago, Illinois

Pamela Foy, ADN
NATP Coordinator
Kellogg Community College
Battle Creek, Michigan

Mary Garcia, BSN
Lead Instructor, CNA Program
City Colleges of Chicago
Chicago, Illinois

Lana Gordineer, MSN, RN, CDE
HLH 130 Lead Instructor
Delaware Technical Community College
Dover, Delaware

Karen Grove, RN, BSN, MEd
Associate Professor, Program Head
J. Sargeant Reynolds Community College
Richmond, Virginia

Jo Hart, BSN, RN
Nursing Assistant Instructor
Gateway Technical College
Elkhorn, Wisconsin

Donna Nielson, MSN, RN
Assistant Professor
Pasadena City College
Pasadena, California

Elizabeth Pagenkopf, MSN
CAN Coordinator
Harper College
Palatine, Illinois

Linda Sulkowski, RN, BSN
Program Director of Nurse Aide Training
Lorain County Community College
Elyria, Ohio

Donna Walsworth, BSN, RN
Instructor/Coordinator
Genesee Valley Educational Partnership
Mt. Morris, New York

Kelly M. Winters, MSN, RN
Director of Workforce Development
College of Southern Maryland
La Plata, Maryland

ACKNOWLEDGMENTS

Change is a necessity of life, especially in the health care profession. Sometimes change happens so rapidly in health care that it is difficult for textbook authors and instructors to keep up with it. But major changes happened as we worked to update and improve this textbook. Not only did we update the book, but the entire video series that accompanies our nursing assisting textbooks was revised. There were many new people who worked with me on the project and I appreciate the efforts of all who were involved.

I would especially like to thank Kelley Squazzo, Senior Acquisitions Editor, for your support and guidance in this project. Thanks also to Helen Kogut, Senior Product Development Editor, for joining us mid-way through the project, and to Dan Reilly for keeping me on track and for helping Nurse Pam age gracefully. As always, I want to extend thanks to all of the sales representatives at Wolters Kluwer who share my vision and passion and offer such great support to the faculty members who use this text.

CONTENTS

UNIT 3

LONG-TERM CARE   219

UNIT 4

SAFETY   265

UNIT 5

BASIC PATIENT AND RESIDENT CARE 357

Introduction to Health Care

Welcome to the health care field! Today, working in the health care field offers more opportunities than ever before. The health care field is the focus of Unit 1.

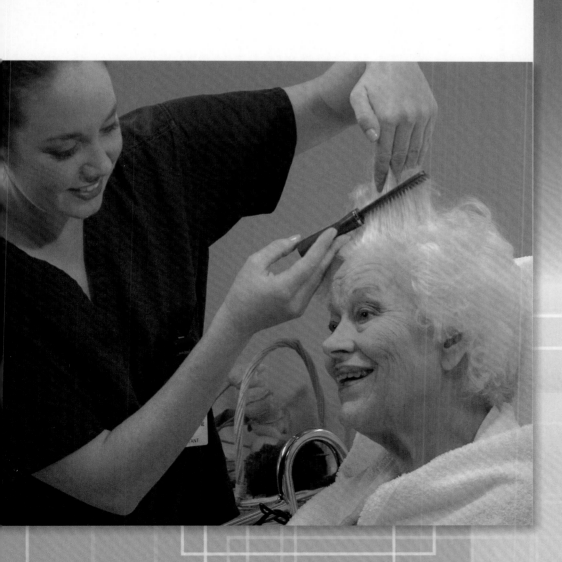

The Health Care System

As a nursing assistant, you will be part of the health care system. In this chapter, you will learn about how we approach health care delivery in the United States today, as well as about the many different settings in which health care is provided. You will learn about how this system groups people in need of health care. We will also discuss how health care is paid for and some of the government regulations that people working in the health care field need to be aware of.

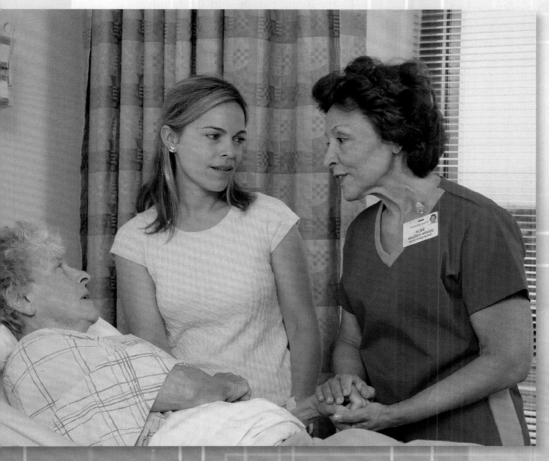

Photo: Health care is a people-oriented business.

A Holistic Approach to Health Care

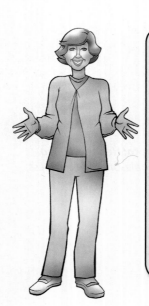

Providing holistic care means recognizing that each person you care for is unique and special, with individual needs that are very different from those of the person in the next bed. While you carry out your daily duties, you will have plenty of chances to get to know your patients or residents as individuals. You will help to take care of your patients' or residents' emotional needs, as well as their physical ones. This is the essence of holistic care.

Holistic care of the whole person, physically and emotionally

Health care team group of people with different types of knowledge and skill levels who work together to provide holistic care to the patient or resident

In the past in the United States, health care delivery focused mainly around the home and family. Most health care was provided by a family doctor, who would come to the person's home (Fig. 1-1). Because people did not move much and towns were small, the family doctor would get to know each of his or her patients well. The family doctor took care of all of the person's health care needs: for example, he would deliver the babies, attend to wounds and broken bones, and provide comfort to both the dying person and the family.

By the 1940s, this started to change. New medications were being discovered, and new equipment was being developed. Hospitals were becoming more modern. Now, instead of being cared for in their homes, people would go to the hospital when they were sick. As researchers learned more about what causes disease and how to treat it, health care became more complex. Slowly, the family doctor who took care of all of a person's health care needs began to be replaced by a team of doctors, each with a specific type of knowledge.

Although the advances in knowledge and technology helped people to live longer lives, an interesting thing started to happen. The focus started to shift from the patient to the technology—from *caring* to *curing*. Fortunately, we are now seeing a return to a more **holistic** approach to health care. The best aspect of the care provided by the old-fashioned "family doctor"—the doctor's familiarity with the person as an individual—is combined with modern-day availability of specialized care when needed.

Today, holistic care is provided by a **health care team** made up of many people with different types of knowledge and skill levels (Fig. 1-2). The person receiving the care is always the focus of the health care team's efforts. As a nursing assistant, you will be a member of this team. The job of each member of the team is as important as that of any other member. Think of the members of the health care team as links in the chain of care. Because a chain is only as strong as its weakest link, each member of the health care team must provide care to the best of his or her ability.

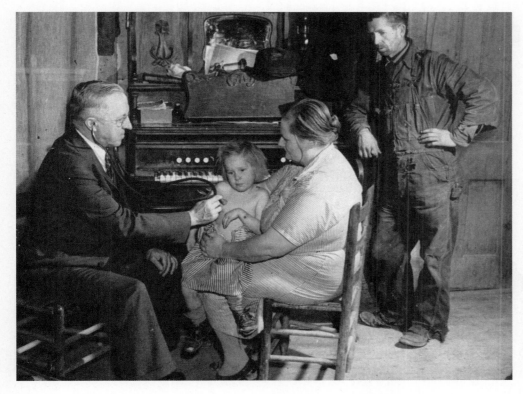

■ **FIGURE 1-1**

In the past, health care was delivered in the home, usually by a "family doctor."

Library of Congress, Prints & Photographs Division, FSA/OWI Collection, [LC-USF346-064221-D (b&w film transparency)].

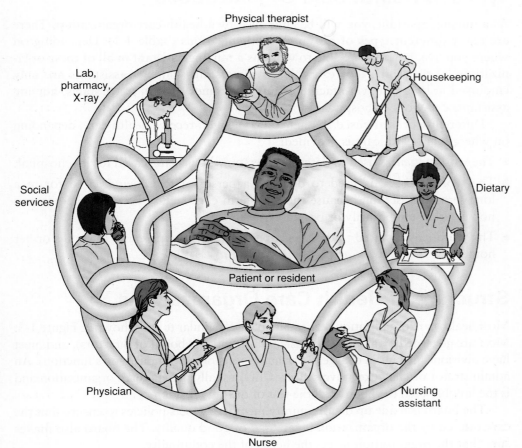

■ **FIGURE 1-2**

Care is provided by the health care team. The patient or resident is the primary focus of the team's efforts. Because a chain is only as strong as its weakest link, each member of the health care team must provide care to the best of his or her ability.

Putting it all together!

- Today, we take a holistic approach to health care. That is, we take into consideration the person's emotional as well as physical needs.
- Health care is provided by a team of people, each with different areas of expertise and job responsibilities. The patient or resident is the focus of the health care team's efforts.
- As a nursing assistant, you are a critical part of the health care team.

Health Care Organizations

What will you learn?

When you are finished with this section, you will be able to:
1. Describe the different types of health care organizations.
2. Briefly explain the structure of a health care organization.

Types of Health Care Organizations

As a nursing assistant, you will be employed by a health care organization. There are many different types of health care organizations (Table 1-1). Depending on where you live, you may be able to work as a nursing assistant in all of these organizations or just some. For example, in some states, nursing assistants are only employed in long-term care facilities (nursing homes), but in other states, nursing assistants can work in hospitals.

Different words are used to refer to people who receive health care, depending on where that health care is provided:

- The word *patient* is used to describe a person who is being cared for in a hospital.
- The word *resident* is used to describe a person who is being cared for in a long-term care setting because the long-term care facility becomes the person's home, either temporarily or permanently.
- The word *client* is used to describe a person who is being cared for in his or her home.

Structure of Health Care Organizations

Most health care organizations are set up in a way similar to that shown in Figure 1-3. Most are governed by a board of trustees (also called a board of directors), and most have divisions (groups in charge of certain aspects of the organization's function). An administrator or chief executive officer (CEO) usually manages the organization and is the link between the board and the rest of the organization.

The board is made up of community members. It sets policies to ensure that the care offered by the organization is safe and of good quality. The board also makes sure that the organization meets the needs of the community.

TABLE 1-1 Types of Health Care Organizations

	Type of Organization	Description
	Hospital	Provides care for people with acute medical or surgical conditions Provides inpatient care (the person stays for one or more nights) or outpatient care (the person comes to the hospital for a scheduled treatment and then goes home the same day) May provide care for specific groups of people (for example, cancer patients, children) or for all people
	Subacute care unit (skilled nursing unit, skilled nursing facility)	Provides care for people who have been discharged from the hospital but still need care from a skilled health care professional Care is focused on rehabilitation and helping the person move from hospital care to home care; examples of services provided include intravenous drug therapy, physical therapy, respiratory care or ventilator services, and wound management May be a unit within a hospital or long-term care facility, or a separate facility
	Long-term care facility (nursing home)	Provides care for people who are unable to care for themselves at home but do not need to be hospitalized May become the person's permanent home May provide care for specific groups of people (for example, people with Alzheimer's disease) or for all people
	Assisted-living facility	Provides care for people who are able to provide most of their own care but need limited help with medications, transportation, meals, and housekeeping; a type of long-term care facility Residents usually live in private apartments but have access to help 24 hours a day if they need it

Catrina Genovese/Index Stock Imagery, Inc.

(*table continues on page 8*)

TABLE 1-1	Types of Health Care Organizations (continued)	
	Type of Organization	**Description**
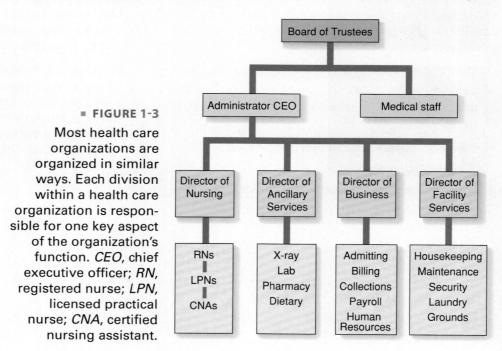	Home health care agency	Provides skilled care in a person's home Provides services for people of all ages with any number of different medical needs
	Hospice organization	Provides care for people who are dying and their families Care is focused on relieving pain and providing emotional and spiritual support for both the dying person and the family Care may be provided in the home, hospital, or long-term care facility or in a facility devoted exclusively to providing care to the dying

Each division within a health care organization is responsible for one key aspect of the organization's function. Each division is managed by a division director or division manager. The medical services division is led by a medical director, and is responsible for the doctors on staff. Nursing services is headed by a director of nursing (DON) or chief nursing officer (CNO), and is responsible for all aspects

■ FIGURE 1-3

Most health care organizations are organized in similar ways. Each division within a health care organization is responsible for one key aspect of the organization's function. *CEO*, chief executive officer; *RN*, registered nurse; *LPN*, licensed practical nurse; *CNA*, certified nursing assistant.

Board of Trustees

Administrator CEO — Medical staff

Director of Nursing — Director of Ancillary Services — Director of Business — Director of Facility Services

RNs
LPNs
CNAs

X-ray
Lab
Pharmacy
Dietary

Admitting
Billing
Collections
Payroll
Human Resources

Housekeeping
Maintenance
Security
Laundry
Grounds

of the organization that have to do with patient or resident care. Business services is led by a business director, and usually oversees admissions, billing, and payroll. The business division may also oversee maintenance and housekeeping. The ancillary services division typically contains the departments in the organization that provide patient or resident services, such as social services and dietary services.

 Putting it all together!

- Today, health care is delivered in the home through home health care agencies and hospice organizations. In addition, people can go to health care facilities, such as hospitals, subacute care units, long-term care facilities ("nursing homes"), and assisted-living facilities to receive health care.
- Health care organizations are governed by a board of directors and have divisions that manage certain aspects of the organization's function.

Patients, Residents, and Clients

What will you learn?

When you are finished with this section, you will be able to:
1. Discuss why people need health care.
2. Describe how the health care industry classifies people in need of its services.

Generally speaking, a person needing health care has some sort of illness, injury, or disability. These conditions can be either temporary or permanent. To make providing care more efficient, the health care industry groups people according to their age, illness or medical condition, or special health care needs:

- *Surgical patients* have illnesses or conditions, such as appendicitis or certain types of injuries, that are treated by surgery.
- *Medical patients* have an illness or a condition that is treated with methods other than surgery, such as medication, physical therapy, or radiation.
- *Obstetric patients* are those who are pregnant or have just given birth.
- *Pediatric patients* are children and adolescents.
- *Geriatric patients* are older adults, more than 65 years of age.
- *Psychiatric patients* are people with mental health disorders.
- *Rehabilitation patients* are those who are receiving therapy to restore their highest level of functioning.
- *Subacute or extended-care patients* do not need the total care provided by a hospital but are not quite ready to return home. They may need intravenous medications, physical therapy, or other treatments that cannot be provided by untrained caretakers.
- *Intensive care patients* are people who are critically ill and require highly skilled monitoring and care.

Putting it all together!

- Patients, residents, and clients are people who need the services of the health care industry because they are sick, injured, or unable to care for themselves.
- People in health care settings are grouped according to their age, illness or medical condition, or special health care needs.

Oversight of the Health Care System

What will you learn?

When you are finished with this section, you will be able to:

1. List some of the agencies that provide oversight of the health care system.
2. Describe how the survey process is used to monitor the quality of care given by health care organizations.
3. Discuss how government agencies help protect health care workers.
4. Define the words **United States Department of Health and Human Services (DHHS), Omnibus Budget Reconciliation Act (OBRA), The Joint Commission, Accreditation, Survey**, and **Occupational Safety and Health Administration (OSHA)**.

United States Department of Health and Human Services (DHHS) the primary government agency responsible for protecting this nation's health; includes organizations, such as the Food and Drug Administration (FDA), the Centers for Disease Control and Prevention (CDC), the National Institutes of Health (NIH), and the Centers for Medicare and Medicaid Services (CMS)

Omnibus Budget Reconciliation Act (OBRA) of 1987 an act passed in 1987 to improve the quality of life for people who live in long-term care facilities by making sure that residents receive a certain standard of care

Today in the United States, many agencies exist to protect both the recipients and the providers of health care. Health care facilities must follow regulations set by the federal, state, and local governments. These regulations help to protect the entire community by making sure of the following:

- Providers of health care are properly trained and able to do their jobs.
- Health care facilities meet standards of cleanliness and quality.
- All products used in the delivery of health care are safe.
- Providers of health care are protected from on-the-job injuries.
- Quality health care is available to everyone.

The government monitors the activity of health care organizations and makes sure that organizations provide the type of care they say they provide. The government inspects health care organizations regularly to make sure that the standards are being followed. Any problems are addressed; and if the problems are serious, the organization faces being fined or closed.

The **United States Department of Health and Human Services (DHHS)** is the primary government agency that is responsible for protecting this nation's health. The DHHS oversees many different agencies that are concerned with ensuring that quality health care is provided.

An in-depth investigation of long-term care facilities was carried out by the DHHS in response to complaints of neglect and abuse from people who had family members in long-term care facilities. This investigation resulted in a law known as the **Omnibus Budget Reconciliation Act (OBRA) of 1987**. OBRA improves the quality of life for people who live in long-term care facilities by making sure that residents receive a certain standard of care. This care must take into account the residents' physical, emotional, spiritual, and social needs. OBRA also sets standards for the training and evaluation of nursing assistants who work in long-term care facilities. OBRA legislation is reviewed and passed by Congress each year. As you read this book, look for the OBRA icon, which highlights key information related to this law.

Several independent, nonprofit organizations also exist to help ensure that facilities provide quality health care. The largest and best known of these independent organizations is **The Joint Commission,** which sets national standards of all types of health care organizations and establishes expectations for how the organization carries out certain activities, especially activities that affect patient and resident safety and the quality of patient and resident care. Health care organizations request and pay for inspections by The Joint Commission. Those organizations that meet the standards receive **accreditation** by The Joint Commission and are permitted to display The Joint Commission's Gold Seal of Approval, which is recognized nationwide as a symbol of quality (Fig. 1-4).

To ensure that a health care organization is meeting the established regulations, standards, or requirements set by the government agency or private organization that accredits or approves it, a survey process is utilized. A **survey** is an actual inspection and evaluation of a health care organization or facility. A *survey team* visits the facility and directly observes the care and services provided there. Afterward, a report is written up to show if there are any deficiencies that the facility must correct in order to maintain its accreditation status. If you work in an accredited health care facility, you will no doubt hear a lot about the survey process. In fact, many people will actually fear the survey process. However, if you are providing the type of quality care that you have been trained to do and are following the policies and procedures that have been established by your facility, you have nothing to be nervous about. Guidelines Box 1-1 lists ways that you can both excel in your job and help your facility do well during a survey regardless of the type of facility you work at.

The **Occupational Safety and Health Administration (OSHA)** is a government agency that is responsible for protecting the health and safety of American workers by enforcing standards and providing education to improve standards in the workplace. OSHA seeks to protect workers across all industries, not just the health

The Joint Commission an independent, nonprofit organization that sets national standards for all types of health care organizations and officially recognizes (accredits) organizations that meet these standards

Accreditation official recognition that the organization meets certain standards of quality

Survey an inspection of a nursing home carried out by the government to ensure that care is being provided according to standards and regulations

Occupational Safety and Health Administration (OSHA) an agency within the Department of Labor that establishes safety and health standards for the workplace to protect the safety and health of employees

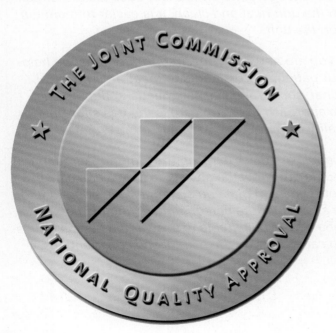

■ **FIGURE 1-4**

Health care facilities that comply with the standards set by The Joint Commission are allowed to display The Joint Commission's Gold Seal of Approval.

GUIDELINES BOX 1-1 Guidelines for Excelling at Your Job and Helping Your Facility Do Well During a Survey

What you do	Why you do it
Always act within your scope of practice, as defined by facility policy, your job description, and your state's regulations.	*This is the best way to ensure that the care you are providing is within the legal limits of your job.*
Always behave like the professional that you are. Be courteous and respectful toward others. Offer your assistance to patients or residents and co-workers readily. Have a positive attitude.	*Having a professional attitude and displaying a solid work ethic indicates to others that you take pride in your job and are interested in doing it to the best of your ability.*
Make sure that your conversations with co-workers are appropriate for the workplace. Be aware of the volume of your voice.	*You would not want anyone to overhear anything that would reflect poorly on you or your work ethic. Gossiping about others or going into great detail about your personal life is inappropriate in the workplace. Speaking in a loud voice adds to the noise level on the unit.*
When discussing a patient's or a resident's care with a co-worker, be mindful of where the discussion is taking place and the volume of your voice.	*Discussions that involve a patient's or a resident's care need to be held in private areas to protect the resident's right to confidentiality.*
Do your part to maintain a neat and clean environment. Put items away after you use them. Dispose of trash properly. If you notice a spill or other mess, clean it up promptly.	*A cluttered, messy environment is unpleasant for everyone, patients or residents and staff alike. It may even present safety issues. It is difficult to work efficiently if you cannot locate something you need because it was not put away properly after the last person used it. If everyone on the unit does his or her part to keep the unit neat and clean, it is easier to maintain order on the unit.*
Always put your patients' or residents' needs first. Strive to provide humanistic, holistic care.	*When you are at work, your first priority must be helping your patients or residents to meet their physical, emotional, social, and spiritual needs. A humanistic, holistic approach to health care is the basis for providing quality care.*
Answer questions honestly and to the best of your ability. If you do not know the answer to a question, simply say that you do not know and offer your help in getting the person the answer he needs.	*Most people are quick to recognize bluffing. Admitting that you do not know the answer to a question conveys to the other person that you are honest. Offering to find out the answer for the person or directing the person to someone who is better able to answer the person's question indicates that you are helpful and conscientious.*

care industry. You will see OSHA standards referenced frequently throughout this text. These standards protect you while you care for others.

Putting it all together!

- Government agencies set and enforce regulations and standards that help to protect both the people receiving health care and the people providing the care.
- The United States Department of Health and Human Services (DHHS) is the primary government agency that is responsible for protecting this nation's health and oversees many different aspects of health care.
- The Omnibus Budget Reconciliation Act (OBRA) ensures that people in long-term care facilities receive a certain standard of care.
- The Joint Commission sets national standards of all types of health care organizations and accredits those that meet these standards.
- The survey process is an actual on-site inspection of a health care organization by an accrediting organization.
- The Occupational Safety and Health Administration (OSHA) helps to protect workers from on-the-job injuries.

Paying for Health Care

What will you learn?

When you are finished with this section, you will be able to:

1. Discuss how health care is paid for.
2. Describe the difference between Medicare and Medicaid.
3. Explain how a Minimum Data Set (MDS) is used to justify Medicare reimbursement.
4. Define the words **Medicare, Minimum Data Set (MDS),** and **Medicaid.**

Health care can be expensive. Insurance can help to reduce these costs to the individual. As a nursing assistant, you should know how health care is paid for in the United States.

Private and Group Insurance

Although people can pay for health insurance privately using their own funds, many people participate in group insurance plans. *Group insurance* is insurance that is purchased at group rates by an employer or corporation. The employee may be covered in full as a benefit of employment or may pay for part of the coverage.

To reduce costs, many insurance companies use a *managed care system* to provide group insurance. Managed care systems help to deliver health care to people who need it by arranging contracts with various health care providers that agree to provide services for a standard, reduced cost. Examples of managed care systems you might be familiar with include *preferred provider organizations (PPOs)* and *health maintenance organizations (HMOs).*

Medicare

Medicare a type of insurance plan that is federally funded by Social Security and which all people aged 65 years and older, and some younger disabled people, are eligible to participate in

Medicare is a type of insurance plan that is funded by the federal government. People who are 65 years or older are eligible for Medicare, regardless of their financial situation. Some younger people who are disabled also qualify for Medicare.

Health care facilities that are eligible to receive Medicare reimbursements must follow strict rules to receive payment. For example, to receive Medicare reimbursements, long-term care facilities must complete a **Minimum Data Set (MDS)** report for each resident in their care (Fig. 1-5). Information such as the person's weight, bowel and bladder habits, and ability to care for himself or herself is recorded regularly as part of the MDS report. Changes in these areas could indicate that a higher level of care is needed or that the person is not receiving the necessary care and, as a result, his or her condition is getting worse. One of your duties as a nursing assistant will be to accurately record the care that you give to patients and residents. Proper recording of the care you provide is necessary to ensure that the health care facility continues to receive Medicare reimbursements for the care provided.

Minimum Data Set (MDS) a report that focuses on the degree of assistance or skilled care that each resident of a long-term care facility needs

Like insurance companies that insure the general public, the Medicare program is faced with the problem of controlling increasing health care costs. To help control these costs, Medicare has started a reimbursement program based on *diagnosis-related groups (DRGs)*. Under this system, payment for hospitalization, surgery, or other treatment is specified according to the diagnosis. Lengths of hospital stays are also determined by the diagnosis, and are typically short. Since being introduced by Medicare, the DRG system has been adopted by insurance companies in the private and group sectors as well, resulting in industry-wide changes. As a result of the DRG system, patients are discharged from the hospital sooner and sicker, a situation that has created an increased need for subacute care and home health care.

Medicaid

Medicaid a federally funded and state-regulated plan designed to help people with low incomes to pay for health care

Medicaid is another type of insurance plan that is funded by the federal government. Medicaid helps people with low incomes to pay for health care. Elderly people, as well as those who are disabled, may also be eligible, especially if they have limited incomes. To receive Medicaid reimbursement, a facility must be approved by the state agency. Not all facilities or health care providers choose to participate in the Medicaid plan.

 Putting it all together!

- Private and group insurance policies are one way that individuals pay for health care. Many group insurance policies rely on managed care systems, such as preferred provider organizations (PPOs) and health maintenance organizations (HMOs), to keep costs down.

- Medicare is a federally funded insurance plan for people who are 65 years of age and older and for some people with disabilities who are younger. Health care facilities must meet government regulations to receive Medicare reimbursement for services provided.

- Medicaid is a federally funded insurance plan for people with low incomes.

Section G Functional Status

G1. Activities of Daily Living (ADL) Assistance

Code for most dependent episode in last 5 days:

Coding:

0. **Independent**—resident completes activity with no help or oversight

1. **Set up assistance**

2. **Supervision**—oversight, encouragement or cueing provided throughout the activity

3. **Limited assistance**—guided maneuvering of limbs or other non-weight bearing assistance provided at least once

4. **Extensive assistance, 1 person assist**—resident performed part of the activity while one staff member provided weight-bearing support or completed part of the activity at least once

5. **Extensive assistance, 2 + person assist**—resident performed part of the activity while two or more staff members provided weight-bearing support or completed part of the activity at least once

6. **Total dependence, 1 person assist**—full staff performance of activity (requiring only 1 person assistance) at least once. The resident must be unable or unwilling to perform any part of the activity.

7. **Total dependence, 2 + person assist**—full staff performance of activity (requiring 2 or more person assistance) at least once. The resident must be unable or unwilling to perform any part of the activity.

8. **Activity did not occur** during entire period

→ Enter Codes in Boxes →

Enter Code

a. **Bed mobility**—moving to and from lying position, turning side to side and positioning body while in bed.

Enter Code

b. **Transfer**—moving between surfaces including to or from: bed, chair, wheelchair, standing position (**excludes** to/from bath/toilet).

Enter Code

c. **Toilet transfer**—how resident gets to and moves on and off toilet or commode.

Enter Code

d. **Toileting**—using the toilet room (or commode, bedpan, urinal); cleaning self after toileting or incontinent episode(s), changing pad, managing ostomy or catheter, adjusting clothes (**excludes** toilet transfer).

Enter Code

e. **Walk in room**—walking between locations in his/her room.

Enter Code

f. **Walk in facility**—walking in corridor or other places in facility.

Enter Code

g. **Locomotion**—moving about facility, with wheelchair if used.

Enter Code

h. **Dressing upper body**—dressing and undressing above the waist, includes prostheses, orthotics, fasteners, pullovers.

Enter Code

i. **Dressing lower body**—dressing and undressing from the waist down, includes prostheses, orthotics, fasteners, pullovers.

Enter Code

j. **Eating**—includes eating, drinking (regardless of skill) or intake of nourishment by other means (for example, tube feeding, total parenteral nutrition, IV fluids for hydration).

Enter Code

k. **Grooming/personal hygiene**—includes combing hair, brushing teeth, shaving, applying makeup, washing/drying face and hands (**excludes** bath and shower).

Enter Code

l. **Bathing**—how resident takes full-body bath/shower, sponge bath and transfers in/out of tub/shower (**excludes** washing of back and hair).

G2. Mobility Prior to Admission—complete only on admission assessment (A10a = 01)

Enter Code

a. Did resident have a **hip fracture, hip replacement, or knee replacement** in the 30 days prior to this admission?

0. **No** → Skip to G3, Balance During Transitions and Walking
1. **Yes** → Continue to G2b

Check all that apply.

b. **If yes, check all that apply for tasks in which the resident was independent prior to fracture/replacement.**

☐ 1. **Transfer**

☐ 2. **Walk across room**

☐ 3. **Walk 1 block on a level surface**

☐ 4. **Resident was not independent in any of these activities**

☐ 9. **Unable to determine**

Recommended MDS 3.0

■ **FIGURE 1-5** (*Continues on the next page*)

Nurses in long-term care facilities that receive Medicare funding must complete a Minimum Data Set (MDS) report for each resident in their care. This report is used to assess the degree of assistance that each resident needs. The form is broken down into Sections A–T and addresses all aspects related to a resident's care needs. The MDS report helps to ensure that the resident receives quality care that is directed toward his or her specific needs by requiring the nursing staff to evaluate these needs at regular intervals.

Section G Functional Status

G3. Balance During Transitions and Walking

After observing the resident, **code the following walking and transition items for most dependent** over the last 5 days:

Coding:

0. **Steady at all times**
1. **Not steady, but <u>able</u> to stabilize without human assistance**
2. **Not steady, <u>only able</u> to stabilize with human assistance**
8. **Activity did not occur**

→ Enter Codes in Boxes →

Enter Code		
☐	a.	**Moving from seated to standing position**
☐	b.	**Walking** (with assistive device if used)
☐	c.	**Turning around** and facing the opposite direction while walking
☐	d.	**Moving on and off toilet**
☐	e.	**Surface-to-surface transfer** (transfer between bed and chair or wheelchair)

G4. Functional Limitation in Range of Motion

Code for limitation during last 5 days that interfered with daily functions or placed resident at risk of injury.

Coding:

0. **No impairment**
1. **Impairment on one side**
2. **Impairment on both sides**

→ Enter Codes in Boxes →

Enter Code		
☐	a.	**Upper extremity** (shoulder, elbow, wrist, hand)
☐	b.	**Lower extremity** (hip, knee, ankle, foot)

G5. Mobility Devices

Check all that were normally used in the past 5 days:

Check all that apply.

- ☐ a. **Cane/crutch**
- ☐ b. **Walker**
- ☐ c. **Wheelchair (manual or electric)**
- ☐ d. **Lower extremity limb prosthesis**
- ☐ e. **None of the above** were used

G6. Bedfast

Enter Code ☐

Has the resident been in bed or in recliner in room for more than 22 hours on at least three of the past 5 days?

    0. **No**
    1. **Yes**

G7. Functional Rehabilitation Potential—complete only on full assessment (A10a = 01)

Enter Code ☐

a. **Resident believes he or she is capable of increased independence** in at least some ADL's.
    0. **No**
    1. **Yes**
    9. **Unable to determine**

Enter Code ☐

b. **Direct care staff believe resident is capable of increased independence** in at least some ADL's.
    0. **No**
    1. **Yes**

Recommended MDS 3.0

■ **FIGURE 1-5** (*Continued*)

WHAT DID YOU LEARN?

Multiple Choice

Select the single best answer for each of the following questions.

1. Who is the focus of the health care team's efforts?
   a. The doctor
   b. The director of nursing
   c. The organization's board of trustees
   d. The patient or resident

2. What does OSHA do?
   a. Sets standards for the education of nursing assistants
   b. Ensures that the rights of patients and residents are upheld
   c. Makes sure that organizations follow safety and health standards designed to keep workers safe
   d. Sets policies to ensure that the care offered by the organization is safe and of good quality

3. The inspection of a nursing home carried out by the government to ensure that care is being provided according to standards and regulations is called a/an:
   a. OBRA requirement
   b. survey
   c. sentinel event
   d. MDS report

Matching

Match each type of health care facility with its description.

_____ 1. Assisted-living facility

_____ 2. Long-term care facility (nursing home)

_____ 3. Hospice organization

_____ 4. Home health care agency

_____ 5. Subacute care unit (skilled nursing unit, skilled nursing facility)

a. Place where people who can provide for most of their own care but who need limited assistance can live

b. Provides skilled care in a person's home

c. Provides care for people who cannot care for themselves but are not ill enough to be hospitalized

d. Provides care for people who are dying and their families

e. Provides care that is focused on rehabilitation; assists patients in making the transition from hospital care to home care

Match each vocabulary word with its definition.

_____ **1.** Holistic

_____ **2.** Minimum Data Set

_____ **3.** Omnibus Budget Reconciliation Act

_____ **4.** Medicare

_____ **5.** Medicaid

a. Improves the quality of life for people who live in long-term care facilities by making sure that they receive a certain standard of care

b. A federally funded and state-regulated insurance plan designed to help people with low incomes pay for health care

c. Care of the whole person, physically and emotionally

d. A federally funded insurance plan in which all people aged 65 years or older and some younger people with disabilities are eligible to participate

e. A report that focuses on the degree of assistance or skilled care that each resident of a long-term care facility needs

 Stop *and* **Think!**

Think about what health care was like in the United States 100 years ago. How has health care delivery changed in the United States since the early 1900s? What aspects of the "old-fashioned" way of delivering health care were good? Not so good? What aspects of modern health care delivery are good? Not so good?

The Nursing Assistant's Job

As a nursing assistant, you will be responsible for providing safe, quality care to your patients or residents. In this chapter, you will learn about the education that is needed to work as a nursing assistant. You will also learn about how the nursing assistant works as a member of the nursing team, and about some of the legal and ethical aspects of the nursing assistant's job.

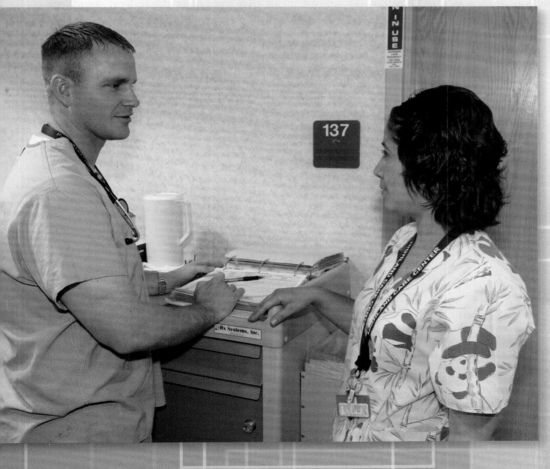

Photo: Nurses and nursing assistants work together to provide safe, competent patient or resident care.

Education of the Nursing Assistant

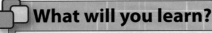

What will you learn?

When you are finished with this section, you will be able to:

1. Discuss the Omnibus Budget Reconciliation Act (OBRA) requirements for nursing assistant training.
2. Describe the certification process.
3. Describe the contents of the registry.
4. Define the words **competency evaluation**, **reciprocity**, and **registry**.

Training and Certification

The Omnibus Budget Reconciliation Act (OBRA) requires all nursing assistants who want to be employed in long-term care facilities to complete a training program and to pass a test that evaluates their knowledge and skills. A minimum of 75 hours of training is required by OBRA, but many states require more hours. Although the minimum training and competency evaluation requirements for nursing assistant training programs are set by OBRA, each state must create and regulate its own training programs following the education and certification requirements specified by OBRA. These state training programs, known as nursing assistant training and competency evaluation programs (NATCEP), must submit proof that they meet the federal standards as well as any state-specific standards. This training must include classroom lectures and hands-on practice of skills, as well as supervised experience in an actual health care setting (Fig. 2-1). Topics that are included as part of the required training include:

- Basic nursing skills, such as how to measure vital signs
- Personal care skills, such as assisting with bathing and grooming
- Safety and emergency procedures
- Infection control procedures
- Communication skills
- Patient and resident rights

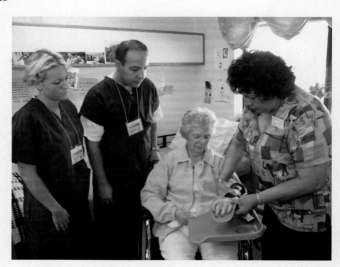

■ **FIGURE 2-1**

Part of a nursing assistant's training involves working with patients or residents in an actual health care setting.

The training ends with a **competency evaluation**. During the written portion of the competency evaluation, you will have to answer approximately 75 multiple-choice questions. During the skills portion, you will be asked to perform selected nursing skills. The actual number of test questions that you must answer and the skills that you must perform are determined by your state. OBRA specifies that you will have three chances to complete the evaluation successfully. The score that you must get to pass the evaluation varies from state to state.

In some cases, a person who has worked in a health care setting and already knows how to perform the duties required of a nursing assistant may be allowed to take the competency evaluation without completing the training program first. However, the person must pass both the written and the skills portions of the test on the first try. If he does not, then he must complete the course before taking the competency evaluation again.

When you complete your training program and pass the competency evaluation, you will be certified to work as a nursing assistant in the state where you completed your training and passed your competency evaluation. In many cases, you will be able to work in other states as well, due to the principle of **reciprocity**. Some states accept the OBRA minimum of 75 hours of training, while others require more hours. If you want to work in a state that requires more hours of training than you have, additional training can be obtained.

If you stop working as a nursing assistant for 2 or more years and then decide that you want to return to the profession, you will need to retake your training course and pass the competency evaluation again before you will be allowed to work.

Competency evaluation an exam consisting of a written portion and a skills portion that must be passed at the end of the nursing assistant training course to obtain certification

Reciprocity the principle by which one state recognizes the validity of a license or certification granted by another state

Registry

OBRA requires every state to maintain a **registry** that contains the following information about each nursing assistant:

Registry an official record, maintained by the state, of the people who have successfully completed the nursing assistant training program

- Full name, including maiden name and any married names
- Last known home address
- Registry number and the date of expiration
- Date of birth
- Date the competency evaluation was passed
- Reported incidents of resident abuse or neglect, or theft of resident property

Registry information can be requested by any long-term care facility needing the information. Information about performance concerns, such as resident abuse, must remain in the registry for at least 5 years.

The knowledge, skills, and responsibilities of the nursing assistant have grown over the years. The very first nursing assistants usually did not have training in the health care field, which led to poor care in many cases. Today's nursing assistants, however, are well-trained members of the health care team with many important responsibilities.

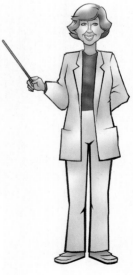

Continuing Education

Regular in-service education and performance reviews are also mandated by OBRA. Long-term care facilities must provide a minimum of 12 hours of in-service training per year to nursing assistants. During in-service training, new skills may be taught or existing skills reviewed, depending on the needs of the facility.

Putting it all together!

- Educational standards, such as those set by OBRA, help to ensure that nursing assistants have the skills and knowledge they need to perform their jobs safely and competently.
- All states must meet the minimum training and competency evaluation requirements set by OBRA. State training programs are known as nursing assistant training and competency evaluation programs (NATCEP).

The Nursing Assistant as a Member of the Nursing Team

What will you learn?

When you are finished with this section, you will be able to:

1. List the members of the nursing team, and describe the role of each team member.
2. Describe various ways that nursing teams work together in a health care setting.
3. List the steps of the nursing process, and describe how the nursing team uses the nursing process to plan the patient's or resident's care.
4. Discuss the delegation process as it relates to the nursing assistant.
5. List the five rights of delegation.
6. Define the words **interdisciplinary care plan**, **nursing care plan**, **nursing process**, **delegate**, and **scope of practice**.

How the Nursing Team Works Together

The nursing team, part of the health care team, is responsible for providing care to the patient or resident (Table 2-1). At a minimum, the nursing team consists of a nurse and a nursing assistant. The nursing assistant assists the nurse in giving care to patients or residents by performing basic nursing functions, also called *nursing tasks*. The nurse may be either a *registered nurse (RN)* or *a licensed practical nurse (LPN)*. In some states, LPNs are called *licensed vocational nurses*, or *LVNs*. Other members of the nursing team may include a *charge nurse*, an RN or LPN/LVN who supervises the other nurses for a particular shift, and a *unit manager*, an RN who is in charge of a department or section. Each health care organization has an RN who directs all of the nursing care within that facility. This person is the *director of nursing (DON)*.

There are many different ways the members of the nursing team can work together:

- In **primary nursing,** one nurse (an RN or LPN/LVN) is assigned several patients or residents and is responsible for planning and carrying out all aspects of care

TABLE 2-1 The Nursing Team

Team Member	Requirements to Practice	Contribution to Team
Registered nurse (RN)	A baccalaureate degree from a liberal arts college or university (4 years) OR An associate degree from a junior or community college (2 years) PLUS A license obtained by passing a state board examination	Develops nursing care plans and coordinates all aspects of patient or resident care Provides nursing care to patients or residents Delegates selected aspects of patient or resident care to other team members and supervises these team members as they carry out the delegated tasks
Licensed practical nurse (LPN) OR Licensed vocational nurse (LVN)	A certificate from a 12- to 18-month training program offered by a vocational school, community college, or hospital PLUS A license obtained by passing a state board examination	Under the supervision of an RN, provides nursing care to patients or residents Delegates selected aspects of patient or resident care to other team members and supervises these team members as they carry out the delegated tasks
Nursing assistant OR Patient care attendant Patient care technician (PCT) Nursing technician Nurse's aide Home health aide	A certificate from a 75- to 200-hour training program offered by a vocational school, community college, or health care facility, obtained by completing the training and passing a state-administered competency evaluation	Assists the RN or LPN with providing nursing care to patients or residents; responsibilities include basic nursing tasks related to meeting hygiene, safety, comfort, nutrition, exercise, and elimination needs

for those people. The nurse performs all of the nursing duties for his or her patients, from feeding and bathing to giving medications and other treatments. Other nurses and nursing assistants are responsible for the primary nurse's patients or residents when the primary nurse is not on duty, but all nursing efforts on behalf of those patients or residents are directed and coordinated by the primary nurse.

- In **functional (modular) nursing,** each member of the nursing team carries out the same assigned task for all patients or residents. For example, for a particular group of patients or residents, one nurse may give all medications and another nurse may do assessments and special treatments. One nursing assistant may be assigned to take vital signs and assist with meals, while another nursing assistant may be assigned bathing and bedmaking tasks.

- In **team nursing,** a team leader (an RN) determines all of the nursing needs for the patients or residents assigned to the team and assigns tasks according to each team member's skills and level of responsibility. For example, the nurse may assist the nursing assistant with bathing a patient or resident and then give that person his or her medication, or two nursing assistants may work together to complete the tasks usually handled by nursing assistants, such as bathing and bedmaking.

- A recent trend being utilized in many health care facilities is known as "**patient-centered** or **patient-focused care.**" This method of nursing care is designed around the needs of the patient or resident and works to meet that person's needs more efficiently. Members of the nursing team are cross-trained to perform tasks that have in the past been done by other departments. For example, a nursing assistant may be trained to draw blood for laboratory tests or to do an EKG instead of relying on technicians from another department to come and perform those tasks.

The Nursing Process

Interdisciplinary care plan a specific plan of care for each patient or resident developed with input from all members of the health care team

Nursing care plan a specific plan of care for each patient or resident developed by the nursing team

Nursing process a process that allows members of the nursing team to communicate with each other regarding the patient's or resident's specific needs (in regard to nursing care), what steps will be taken to meet those needs, and whether or not the steps were effective in meeting the person's needs; it consists of five parts: assessment, diagnosis, planning, implementation, and evaluation

The doctor is responsible for diagnosing a person's medical problems and ordering medication or other therapies to correct those problems. However, the actual coordination, planning, and implementation of that care require the efforts of other members of the health care team. Those members involved with the patient's or the resident's care may include nurses, nursing assistants, dietitians, social workers, and physical therapists. The patient or resident and his or her family members also play an important role in this process, especially in the long-term care setting. All health team members meet with the patient or the resident and family members to develop a specific, individualized plan of care called an **interdisciplinary care plan**. As part of the interdisciplinary care plan, the nursing team will then develop a specific plan of care for each patient or resident called the "**nursing care plan**."

The **nursing process** is used to create the nursing care plan. The five steps of the nursing process are described in Box 2-1. As a nursing assistant, you will be involved in the implementation step of the nursing process. You will also help

BOX 2-1 The Nursing Process

1. **Assessment.** During this step, the nurse gathers information about the patient or resident. As part of the assessment process, the nurse examines the patient or resident and asks questions about his or her abilities, level of discomfort, eating and toileting habits, and specific needs.

2. **Diagnosis.** Using the information gathered during the assessment step, the nurse then develops a *nursing diagnosis*, or a statement that describes a problem the person is having, as well as the cause of the problem. Unlike a medical diagnosis, which identifies a medical problem that must be managed by a doctor, a nursing diagnosis identifies a problem that the nursing staff can manage independently.

3. **Planning.** The next step in the nursing process involves making a plan for the person's care. Using information obtained from the nursing diagnosis, the nurse develops *interventions* (actions that will be taken to help the person) and *goals* (descriptions of what the interventions are meant to achieve). The interventions and goals that have been set for the patient or resident are written down in a formal way. This document is the nursing care plan.

4. **Implementation.** During the implementation step, the interventions that were detailed in the nursing care plan are carried out. (The nursing care plan specifies the team members who are responsible for doing each intervention.)

5. **Evaluation.** During the evaluation step, the nursing team checks the effectiveness of the nursing care plan and revises it as necessary. Is the care plan working? Are the goals being met? What needs to be improved or changed to meet the goals? Has the patient's or resident's status changed? Is the existing nursing care plan still appropriate for the patient or resident? If certain interventions are not working or if the goals have been met, the nursing care plan will change.

the nurse with the assessment and evaluation steps of the nursing process by observing how your patients or residents are doing and reporting this information to the nurse.

Delegation

To ensure that the nursing team functions efficiently, an RN or LPN has the authority to **delegate** selected tasks to a nursing assistant. Typically, the nurse will delegate nursing tasks related to routine care (hygiene, comfort, exercise) to nursing assistants. An RN can also delegate certain nursing tasks, such as data collection and documentation, to a nursing assistant. However, nursing tasks that require professional judgment, such as assessment, planning, or evaluating, cannot be delegated to a nursing assistant. For example, a nursing assistant can take a person's vital signs and record this information on the person's chart, but the assistant is not qualified to interpret the data.

    To help nurses make good decisions about which tasks to delegate and to whom, the National Council of State Boards of Nursing (NCSBN) has developed guidelines called the *five rights of delegation* (Table 2-2). You and the nurse share the responsibility for making sure that delegated tasks are carried out without causing harm to the patient or resident. The nurse is responsible for making good decisions about which tasks to delegate and for providing adequate supervision. You are responsible for recognizing which delegated tasks are within your **scope of practice** (also known as *range of functions*) and range of abilities and using this knowledge as the basis for either accepting or refusing the assignment. Just as a

Delegate to authorize another person to perform a task on your behalf

Scope of practice the range of tasks that a nursing assistant is legally permitted to do

TABLE 2-2   Five Rights of Delegation

	Questions the Nurse Must Consider	Questions the Nursing Assistant Must Consider
The right task	Is this a task that can be delegated? Does the nurse's practice act in this state allow me to delegate the task? Is the task in the job description for the nursing assistant?	Does the state allow me to perform this task? Have I been trained to do this task? Do I have experience performing this task? Is this task in my job description?
The right circumstance	What is the patient's or resident's condition? Is he or she stable? What are the needs of the patient or resident at this time?	Can I perform this task safely, given the patient's or resident's condition?
The right person	Does the nursing assistant have the right training and experience to safely complete the task?	Am I confident that I can perform this task safely? Do I have any reservations about performing this task; and if so, what are they?
The right direction	Am I able to give the nursing assistant clear direction regarding how to perform this task? Am I able to explain to the nursing assistant what is expected?	Did the nurse give me clear instructions? Do I understand what the nurse expects?
The right supervision	Will I be available to supervise and answer questions?	Will the nurse be available to supervise and answer questions?

BOX 2-2   Tasks That Are Generally Beyond the Nursing Assistant's Scope of Practice

Giving medications (including oxygen). Some states allow nursing assistants to give medications to residents in assisted-living facilities if the nursing assistant has received specialized training to do so. Generally, only a licensed nurse (RN or LPN) or doctor is allowed to give medications. Nursing assistants may assist patients in taking medication by bringing water or helping to open the medicine bottle.

Receiving verbal orders (in person or over the telephone) from doctors. Licensed nurses (RNs or LPNs) are the only personnel authorized to receive doctors' orders.

Diagnosing illness and prescribing treatments. Only doctors can diagnose illness and prescribe medical or surgical treatment.

Supervising other nursing assistants. Licensed nurses (RNs or LPNs) are responsible for supervising nursing assistants.

Performing procedures that require sterile technique. Nursing assistants are permitted to assist a nurse in performing a sterile procedure, but they are not trained to do these procedures themselves.

Inserting or removing tubes from a person's body (bladder, esophagus, trachea, nose, ears). Nursing assistants generally are not trained in procedures that involve inserting or removing tubes from a patient's or resident's body. Exceptions may be made if the nursing assistant has had the opportunity to practice a procedure under an instructor's supervision.

nurse uses the five rights of delegation to decide which tasks to delegate and to whom, you can use the five rights of delegation to help you decide whether to accept or decline a delegated task (see Table 2-2).

You should never refuse an assignment simply because you do not want to do it. You must have a good reason for refusing to carry out an assignment, or you could lose your job. Valid reasons for refusing an assignment include the following:

- The task is outside of your scope of practice. Box 2-2 summarizes tasks that are generally outside of the scope of practice of a nursing assistant.
- The task is illegal or unethical or could cause harm to the patient or resident.
- The nurse is not available to supervise your efforts.
- You do not have the proper equipment.
- The directions are not clear.
- You have not received adequate training about the task or the equipment used.

General guidelines for accepting or declining an assignment are given in Guidelines Box 2-1. A good general rule to keep in mind is that you should not perform any task that is not listed in your job description (Fig. 2-2). Make sure that you are familiar with your employer's policies and with your duties and obligations as listed in your job description. Be aware of the limits of practice for nursing assistants in your state. Ask your supervisor about anything you do not understand. Keeping yourself informed is critical to ensuring that the care you give is within the legal limits of your job and to protecting yourself as well as your patients or residents (Fig. 2-3).

If you must decline a task that you have been assigned to do, it is your responsibility to state clearly that you are not going to do the task and your reason why. Failure to communicate your refusal to complete a task to the person requesting your help can jeopardize the care or safety of the patient or resident. The person

GUIDELINES BOX 2-1   Guidelines for Accepting or Declining an Assignment

What you do	Why you do it
Always ask the nurse for clarification if there is something you do not understand.	*It is your responsibility to make sure that you know what is to be done and how it is to be done before going to the patient or resident.*
Never perform a task that you have not been taught to do, or that you feel uncomfortable doing, unless you are supervised by a nurse.	*The nurse is ultimately responsible for ensuring the patient's or resident's safety. This means that it is the nurse's responsibility to ensure that whoever is performing the task on his or her behalf is qualified to do so and capable. It is irresponsible for you to misrepresent your abilities or to proceed unsupervised with a task that you are not fully capable of doing well.*
Never ignore an assignment because you do not know how to perform the task or the task is beyond your scope of practice.	*The patient's or resident's needs must be attended to, either by you or by someone else. If you feel that you cannot perform the task that you are being asked to do, explain your concerns to the nurse so that he or she can either help you with the task or reassign it.*

requesting your help assumes that you are doing the task, unless he or she hears otherwise. Declining a task is a discussion that you should have privately with the person requesting the task of you. Do not discuss the issue in front of the resident, patient, or visitors.

When you agree to perform a task, you accept responsibility for your actions. If the task is within your scope of practice and you fail to perform the task properly, then you are responsible for any injury to the patient or resident that occurs. You must ask for help when you have questions or are unsure about how to proceed, and you must communicate with the nurse by reporting what you have done and what you observed.

 Putting it all together!

- Nursing assistants are key members of the nursing team. Nursing assistants assist the nurse by performing basic functions, such as those related to hygiene, safety, comfort, nutrition, exercise, and elimination.
- The nursing team may organize their work according to the primary nursing model, the functional (modular) nursing model, the team nursing model, or use a patient-centered care approach.

(text continues on p. 29)

JOB DESCRIPTION

JOB TITLE: Certified Nursing Assistant (Class 1)   (Non-Exempt Employee)

DEPARTMENT NAME: Nursing Services

OVERALL RESPONSIBILITIES

Responsible for the hands on delivery of care and assistance with activities of daily living for all residents. Provides care in a manner that meets or exceeds Western States Senior Communities expectations.

WORKING RELATIONSHIPS

Reports to: Assistant Living Administrator

Supervises: None

Interfaces with: Resident Care Coordinator Residents, Families, Visitors, and Associates

PRIMARY JOB DUTIES

Provide assistance to residents with activities of daily living (ADL).

Maintain the dignity and privacy of all residents. Protect all resident rights.

Assist residents with personal needs as requested, while helping to maintain the resident's independence and well-being.

Document appropriately services delivered to residents and any significant changes in condition.

Report any concerns with the health and well-being to the Assistant Living Administrator.

Maintain and protect the confidentiality of resident information at all times.

Meet or exceed Western States Senior Communities standards of appearance; comply with Western States Senior Communities sanitation, hygiene, and health standards of community personnel.

Serve meals in a fine and gracious manner, ensuring the dignity and nutritional needs of the resident.

Perform other reasonable tasks as assigned by supervisor.

JOB QUALIFICATIONS

Completion of state of Utah approved Certified Nursing Assistants Course.

Must possess a current Nursing Assistant certificate or be able to obtain one within 4 months of employment.

Must possess a current Food Handlers permit.

Ability to effectively communicate with residents, families, supervisor, and employees.

Willingness to work with the older people.

OSHA OCCUPATIONAL EXPOSURE CATEGORY

After careful analysis, it has been determined that this position falls into the OSHA Occupational Exposure Category _____ and requires the following protective equipment to be worn by anyone filling this position: Gloves and eye protection.

I have read and agree that the contents of this job description accurately reflect what is expected of me in my current position.

Associate's Signature   _Date_

Associate's Printed Name

Immediate Supervisor's Signature   _Date_

■ **FIGURE 2-2**

Because a nursing assistant's duties can vary from state to state and also from facility to facility, it is always a good idea to be very familiar with your formal job description. Here is an example of a typical job description for a nursing assistant.

(Courtesy of Legacy Village of Layton—A Continuing Care Senior Living Community, Layton, Utah)

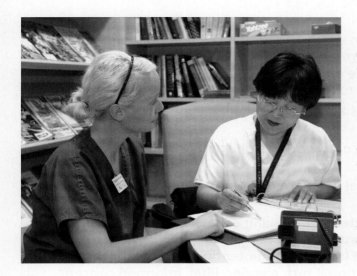

■ **FIGURE 2-3**

To stay within the legal limits of your job, know your scope of practice (as defined by the state and your job description), familiarize yourself with your employer's "policies and procedures" manual, and always seek clarification from your supervisor if there is something you do not understand.

■ The nursing process is used by the nursing team to develop a plan of care for each patient or resident. The nursing process is ongoing, and the nursing care plan is adjusted as the patient's or resident's needs change. Nursing assistants participate in the nursing process by carrying out interventions and communicating information about the person's condition to the nurse.

■ To ensure that the nursing team operates smoothly and efficiently, a "chain of command" exists. This means that licensed nurses (RNs or LPNs) are able to assign (delegate) certain tasks to nursing assistants.

■ The delegation of tasks cannot be taken lightly by either the nurse or the nursing assistant. Both share the responsibility for ensuring that the procedure is carried out without harm to the patient or resident.

■ The nursing assistant must know which tasks are within his or her scope of practice and which tasks are not.

Legal and Ethical Aspects of the Nursing Assistant's Job

What will you learn?

When you are finished with this section, you will be able to:

1. List and discuss patients' rights as set forth in *A Patient's Bill of Rights.*

2. List and discuss residents' rights as set forth by the Omnibus Budget Reconciliation Act (OBRA).

3. Describe two major types of advance directives and explain why advance directives play an important role in health care.

4. Describe the seven violations of civil law that nursing assistants are at risk for committing in the workplace (defamation, assault, battery, fraud, false imprisonment, invasion of privacy, and larceny), and how to avoid each.

5. Define the types of abuse and describe signs that indicate abuse.

6. Discuss the health care worker's obligations in the reporting of suspected abuse.

7. Describe the ethical standards that govern the nursing profession.

8. Define the words **decision-making capacity**, **advance directive**, **durable power of attorney for health care**, **living will**, **laws**, **civil laws**, **criminal laws**, **tort**, **unintentional tort**, **negligent**, **malpractice**, **intentional tort**, **slander**, **libel**, **informed consent**, **confidentiality**, **Health Insurance Portability and Accountability Act (HIPAA)**, **abuse**, **vulnerable adult**, **ethics**, and **value**.

Patients' and Residents' Rights

All of the people in our care have certain rights. In the hospital setting, these rights are listed in a document called *A Patient's Bill of Rights*, created by the American Hospital Association (AHA) in 1973 (Box 2-3). Since 1973, the health care industry has changed dramatically, and "A Patient's Bill of Rights" has been revised to reflect those changes and is now called "The Patient Care Partnership." In a long-term care setting, these rights are included as part of the *Resident Rights* portion of OBRA (Box 2-4). Long-term care facilities that receive federal payments from Medicare must follow the *Resident Rights* portion of OBRA to be eligible to receive these payments. In respecting the rights of patients and residents, health care workers behave according to legal and ethical standards.

Advance Directives

Many patients and residents in health care facilities are not able to make their preferences for health care known, or they will become unable to make their preferences known in the future. For example, if a person has dementia or (a medical condition that results in the permanent and progressive loss of the ability to think and remember) experiences a loss of consciousness, the person will lose his or her **decision-making capacity**.

For these situations, state laws allow a person to make his or her wishes known through an **advance directive**. Examples of advance directives include a **living will** and **durable power of attorney for health care**.

A patient or resident may wish to give instructions about the type of care he or she wishes to receive in an effort to save his or her life, which may mean choosing to avoid "heroic measures" that will prolong life. The living will allows the person to ask that no life-sustaining treatments—such as cardiopulmonary resuscitation (CPR), mechanical ventilation, feeding tubes, or intravenous (IV) lines—be used to prolong his or her life.

Decision-making capacity the ability to make a thoughtful decision based on an understanding of the potential risks and benefits of taking a certain course of action

Advance directive a document that allows a person to make his or her wishes regarding health care known to family members and health care workers, in case the time comes when the person is no longer able to make those wishes known himself or herself

Living will a type of advance directive that states a person's wish that death not be artificially postponed

Durable power of attorney for health care a type of advance directive that transfers the responsibility for handling a person's affairs and making medical decisions to a family member, friend, or other trusted individual, in the event that the person is no longer able to make these decisions on his or her own behalf

BOX 2-3 The Patient Care Partnership (formerly known as A Patient's Bill of Rights)

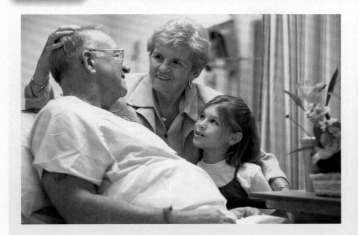

The patient has the right to:

1. Receive considerate and respectful care.

2. Have information about his diagnosis, treatment, and prognosis.

3. Make decisions about his plan of care and to refuse a recommended treatment.

4. Specify his wishes regarding his health care in advance in case the time comes when he can no longer make his wishes known himself.

5. Have privacy.

6. Expect that all communication (written and oral) related to his care will be treated with confidentiality.

7. Review the records related to his medical care and have the information they contain explained or interpreted as necessary.

8. Suggest alternatives to his planned care or transfer to another facility if he so desires.

9. Be informed of any business relationships between parties that influence the care he receives (for example, the hospital and an insurance provider).

10. Participate in, or decline to participate in, experimental studies.

11. Be informed of his options for care when he is discharged from the hospital.

12. Know how the hospital settles disputes, what the hospital charges for its services, and what options for payment are available.

In addition to having rights, the patient has responsibilities. The patient is responsible for:

1. Cooperating with health care providers.

2. Respecting the property, comfort, environment, and privacy of other patients.

3. Making an effort to understand and follow instructions concerning treatment.

4. Providing accurate and complete information about his health status by answering questions as truthfully and completely as possible.

5. Ensuring payment for services received (including providing insurance information in a cooperative and timely manner).

6. Informing the health care staff of any medications brought from home.

7. Accepting responsibility for the consequences of refused treatment or disregarded instructions.

BOX 2-4   Residents' Rights

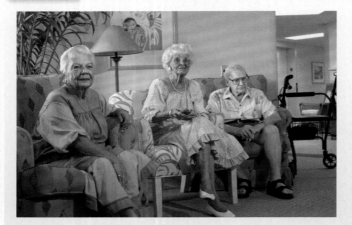

The resident has the right to:

1. Know what rights and responsibilities he has, in language that he can understand.
2. Exercise his rights, as a resident of the facility and as a citizen of the United States. This includes the freedom to make choices about how to live his life (subject to the facility's rules), the freedom to vote, and freedom from discrimination.
3. A dignified existence.
4. Make decisions regarding his care, including choosing his own doctor, participating in planning and implementing his own care, and having his individual needs and preferences accommodated. The resident has the right to refuse treatment and participate in experimental research.
5. Privacy, including privacy while receiving treatments and nursing care, making and receiving telephone calls, sending and receiving mail, and receiving visitors. The resident has the right to confidentiality of personal and medical records.
6. Be free from physical or psychological abuse, including the improper use of restraints.
7. Receive visitors and to share a room with a spouse if both partners are residents in the same facility.
8. Communicate with and have access to people and services both inside and outside of the facility, including advocacy groups. The resident has the right to organize and participate in groups organized by other residents, or the families of residents. For example, residents or their families may organize groups dedicated to improving life for residents, by suggesting changes that could be made at the facility or by planning group outings and activities. The resident also has the right to participate in social, religious, and community activities of his choosing.
9. Keep and use personal possessions (as space and safety permit).
10. Control his own finances (or, if he wishes, have the facility manage personal funds).
11. Information about eligibility for Medicare or Medicaid funds, and to be protected from Medicaid discrimination.
12. Information about the facility's compliance with regulations, planned changes in living arrangements, and available services (and the fees for those services).
13. Remain in the facility unless transfer or discharge is required by a change in the resident's health, the resident is unable to pay for the services he is receiving, or the facility is closed. The resident has the right to refuse transfer from a distinct unit (for example, the certified skilled unit) of the facility.
14. Choose to work at the facility, either as a volunteer or as a paid employee. Working or helping others gives many people a sense of purpose. However, under no circumstances is a resident obligated to work (for example, in exchange for services).
15. Self-administer medications, if the health care team determines that the resident can do so safely.
16. Voice grievances, and to have the facility respond to those grievances.

A durable power of attorney for health care allows the patient or resident to name someone else to make medical decisions on his or her behalf in case the person is no longer able to make these decisions on his or her own. The designated person can be a family member, friend, or other trusted individual and may be called the person's *health care agent*.

Advance directives play a very important role in the health care setting, because many patients and residents have conditions that may result in either the temporary or permanent loss of their decision-making capacity. The *Patient Self-Determination Act of 1990* requires health care facilities to educate patients and residents about advance directives and to offer them the opportunity to establish a living will, a durable power of attorney for health care, or both.

Concerns for Long-Term Care

Advocacy is the process of making a plea or providing support on another's behalf. Because many of the residents of long-term care facilities are vulnerable, federal laws provide advocacy programs for their benefit. An example of a federally funded advocacy program is the Long-Term Care Ombudsman Program. An *ombudsman* (a Swedish word that means "one who speaks on behalf of another") is a person from a state or local Office on Aging who regularly visits residents of long-term care facilities to check on their welfare and overall satisfaction with their care. Ombudsmen gather information from residents and work on their behalf to negotiate solutions to their concerns. These concerns could be related to care issues, misunderstandings between residents and staff, violations of resident rights, or suspected abuse and neglect. While an ombudsman does not have the authority to force a facility to take action, the ombudsman can work with the appropriate people and agencies to ensure that resident issues are addressed.

OBRA requires nursing homes to post information notifying residents of their right to file complaints, and listing the contact information for agencies that can assist them (for example, the state agencies that handle licensure of long-term care facilities, Medicare and Medicaid certification, and reports of Medicare or Medicaid fraud). In addition, the contact information for the ombudsman program must also be posted for resident use. As a nursing assistant, you should know where this information is posted in your facility and be able to assist a resident or visitor who asks you how to contact one of these agencies. If a resident or visitor asks you for this information, you should report the person's request to the nurse. The person's request may indicate that he or she is unhappy about something that has happened in the facility. By alerting the nurse to the person's request, the nurse may be able to talk with the person about the issue, and perhaps resolve it without involving the state agency.

Laws

One way the government works to protect its citizens' basic human rights is by making and enforcing **laws**. There are two types of laws: **civil laws** and **criminal laws**. People found guilty of violating civil laws usually must pay a fine or make a financial settlement to the party that was wronged. Those who violate criminal laws are often sentenced to prison.

Laws rules that are made by a governing authority, such as the local, state, or federal government, with the intent of preserving basic human rights

Civil laws laws concerned with relationships between individuals

Criminal laws laws concerned with the relationship between the individual and society

Violations of Civil Law

When a patient or resident is admitted to a health care facility, he or she signs a form giving the facility permission to provide medical care. A health care worker employed by that facility likewise agrees to provide that care to the patient or resident. This arrangement is a contractual agreement. Contracts, such as the contract that exists between a nursing assistant and the person she or he cares for, are covered by civil law. When this civil law is violated, a *tort*, or wrong, is committed.

An **unintentional tort** occurs when someone causes harm or injury to another person or that person's property by accident. A person who commits an unintentional tort is considered **negligent**. For example, in each of the following scenarios, the nursing assistant would be considered negligent:

- A nursing assistant becomes distracted by another resident's needs and forgets to lock the wheels on the wheelchair she has just placed by the resident's bed. As the resident moves from the bed to the wheelchair, the wheelchair rolls, causing the resident to fall (Fig. 2-4).
- While changing a resident's bed, a new nursing assistant forgets to check the linens for personal objects. As a result, the resident's dentures are sent to the laundry

Unintentional tort a violation of civil law that occurs when someone causes harm or injury to another person or that person's property without the intent to cause harm

Negligent word used to describe a person who fails to do what a "careful and reasonable" person would do in any given situation

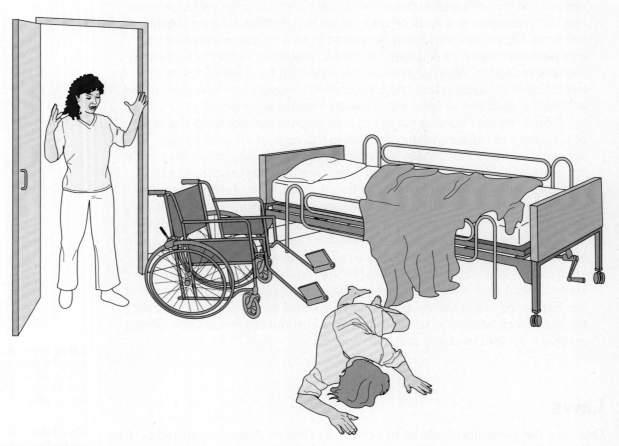

■ **FIGURE 2-4**

The nursing assistant who was responsible for this resident has committed an unintentional tort and would be considered negligent for failing to lock the wheels on the wheelchair, an action that would have prevented the resident from falling.

with the soiled linens, and the dentures are damaged when they go through the washing machine.

- A nursing assistant who is caring for a resident with a reputation for complaining fails to report the resident's complaints of pain to the nurse. It turns out that this time the resident's complaints were valid.

Negligence committed by people who hold licenses to practice their profession, such as doctors, nurses, lawyers, dentists, and pharmacists, is considered **malpractice**. Nursing assistants (who receive certification, but not licensure) are not charged with malpractice.

A violation of civil law committed by a person with the intent to do harm is considered an **intentional tort**. Intentional torts that nursing assistants are particularly at risk for committing in the workplace include the following:

- **Defamation** is making untrue statements that hurt another person's reputation. Defamation may take the form of **slander** or **libel**.
- **Assault** is threatening or attempting to touch a person without his or her consent, causing that person to fear bodily harm.
- **Battery** is touching a person without her consent. To avoid being charged with battery, health care providers must obtain **informed consent** from patients and residents before starting a treatment or procedure.
- **Fraud** is deception that could cause harm to another person.
- **False imprisonment** is confining another person against his or her will. In the health care setting, it is sometimes necessary to confine a person to a chair, a bed, or a room to maintain that person's safety (or the safety of others). However, the use of restraints can be considered false imprisonment if the restraints are not needed for the safety of the patient, the resident, or the staff (see Chapter 15).
- **Invasion of privacy** is violating another person's right to keep certain information away from the examination of others (that is, violating the person's right to **confidentiality**). Confidentiality applies not only to spoken and observed information, but also to written information. The **Health Insurance Portability and Accountability Act (HIPAA)** of 1996 regulates who has the right to view a person's medical records and sets standards for how a person's protected health information is to be stored and transmitted from one place to another.
- **Larceny** is theft (the act of stealing another person's property).

Violations of Criminal Law—Abuse

Abuse is a criminal act and is punishable by a court of law. A person can commit abuse by *actively doing something* to another person or by *failing to do something for* another person. Abuse takes many forms. The injury that results from the abuse may be physical or emotional. Table 2-3 lists the types of abuse and gives examples of signs that abuse may be occurring.

RISK FACTORS FOR BECOMING A VICTIM OF ABUSE. Anyone can become the victim of abuse, but those who depend on others for their care (the very young, the disabled, and the elderly) are particularly at risk. *Elder abuse* is the physical, emotional, or sexual abuse of an older person. *Child abuse* is the physical, emotional, or sexual abuse of a child. The more dependent the person is on others for care, the more at risk the person is for abuse or neglect.

Abuse victims can be any age, sex, race, culture, or religion. Abuse occurs without respect to the level of education, employment status, or marital status. *Domestic*

Malpractice negligence committed by people who hold licenses to practice their profession, such as doctors, nurses, lawyers, dentists, and pharmacists

Intentional tort a violation of civil law committed by a person with the intent to do harm

Slander spoken statements that injure someone's reputation; a form of defamation

Libel written statements that injure someone's reputation; a form of defamation

Informed consent permission granted by a patient or resident to begin treatment or perform a procedure after receiving a full explanation of the treatment or procedure from the health care provider

Confidentiality keeping personal information that someone shares with you to yourself

Health Insurance Portability and Accountability Act (HIPAA) a federal privacy regulation that helps to keep a person's protected health information private and secure

Abuse the repetitive and deliberate infliction of injury on another person

TABLE 2-3 Types of Abuse

Type of Abuse	Examples	Signs That Abuse May Be Occurring
Physical abuse: Causing pain or injury to the person's body through the use of force	■ Hitting and slapping ■ Pushing and shoving ■ Pinching and kicking ■ Shaking ■ Burning ■ Force feeding ■ The inappropriate use of medications ■ The inappropriate use of physical restraints	■ Red marks, welts, or bruises, particularly on the face or torso ■ Broken bones ■ Broken or bent eyeglasses ■ Patches of missing hair ■ Laboratory work that indicates under- or overdosing of medications ■ Person displays fearful or anxious behavior, especially in the presence of the abuser ■ Person reports physical abuse
Neglect: Failing or refusing to provide for the person's basic human needs	■ Failing to provide food, water, clothing, shelter, or ordered medications ■ Failing to help the person meet hygiene and toileting needs ■ Withdrawing support or help from another person, in spite of duty or responsibility (abandonment)	■ Unusual weight loss ■ Dehydration ■ Pressure ulcers ■ Poor personal hygiene; unkempt appearance ■ Incontinence, dried feces on the skin, or skin irritation ■ Inadequate or inappropriate clothing for environment ■ Pain ■ Contractures ■ Uncontrolled medical conditions (possibly the result of a lack of prescribed medication or treatment) ■ Person reports improper care
Psychological (emotional) abuse: Causing emotional pain or injury through the use of words or actions	■ Insulting or threatening a person ■ Bullying, humiliating, or harassing a person ■ Treating a person in an undignified or childlike way ■ Giving a person the silent treatment ■ Isolating the person from others (involuntary seclusion)	■ Person appears emotionally upset (for example, the person cries frequently) ■ Person appears withdrawn or apathetic (does not seem to care about anything), or person stops responding ■ Changes in the person's behavior, or unusual behavior (such as rocking or biting) ■ Person reports psychological abuse

Type of Abuse	Examples	Signs That Abuse May Be Occurring
Sexual abuse: Subjecting the person to unwanted attention of a sexual nature, forcing the person to engage in unwanted sexual activity, or sexually exploiting the person (for example, by taking nude photographs of the person)	■ Touching personal body parts in an inappropriate way ■ Making inappropriate, sexually suggestive comments or gestures ■ Committing sexual assault or battery (for example, forced nudity, inappropriate photography, rape)	■ Bruising on breasts or in genital area ■ Torn or stained underwear ■ Unexplained bleeding from the vagina or rectum ■ Person reports sexual abuse or harassment
Financial abuse: Misusing or stealing another person's money or property	■ Stealing money or belongings ■ Withholding a person's Social Security checks or other sources of income ■ Making withdrawals from a person's bank account or cashing checks without the person's permission ■ Forging the person's signature on checks or legal documents ■ Tricking or blackmailing a person into giving away money or property ■ Tricking or blackmailing a person into signing a legal document or making changes to an existing legal document	■ Unexplained disappearance of money or belongings ■ Sudden change in bank account activity, such as unauthorized withdrawals from the person's account ■ Unexplained money or property transfers, or changes to the person's will ■ The inclusion of additional names on the person's bank account ■ The discovery of forged documents ■ Person reports mishandling or loss of money or property

violence and abuse occur within a relationship by one person's attempts to control the other. Another population at high risk for being abused is known as **vulnerable adults.**

RISK FACTORS FOR BECOMING ABUSIVE. There are many reasons why a person may become abusive toward another. Sometimes, abuse is rooted in the desire of one person to overpower and dominate another. Many abusers were victims of abuse themselves. Other times, in a situation in which a person requires a great deal of care, the caregiver may become tired, frustrated, and overwhelmed by the responsibility of providing care, leading to abuse and neglect. This is often the case with an adult child who has to care for an ill and demanding elderly parent, without the proper training or support system.

Even people who are trained to give care may become overwhelmed by their responsibilities or by a particular situation. A health care worker is particularly at risk for becoming abusive when the patient or resident is "difficult" or hard to manage and the relationship is long term rather than short term. Regardless of the reason abuse occurs, abuse is never an acceptable form of behavior! Be very careful not to place yourself in the position of potentially abusing a patient or resident. Being found guilty of abuse could destroy your potential for future employment in the health care field.

Vulnerable adult a person who is 18 years of age or older who may be in need of community care services because he has an intellectual or other disability, an illness, or is at an age (elderly) that causes him to be unable to care for or protect himself against significant harm or exploitation

Elder Abuse

Many older people can be considered vulnerable adults and become victims of abuse. Elder abuse can take any of the forms described in Table 2-3. Most cases of elder abuse occur in private homes, but elder abuse can and does occur in health care settings as well.

Many factors can place an older person at risk for abuse:

- **Multiple health conditions.** Multiple health conditions may cause an older person to require a great deal of care and overwhelm caregivers.
- **An inability to defend oneself.** Physical disabilities, intellectual disabilities, or both can make an older person unable to defend herself if abuse occurs.
- **"Difficult" behavior.** Medical conditions (for example, dementia), emotional distress, fear, and feelings of resentment and anger that an older person may have about needing care may cause him to behave in a manner that is "difficult" or take out his feelings on a caregiver.
- **The caregiver's perception of the person needing care.** Sometimes, the caregiver does not realize the extent of disability caused by a person's health problem and thinks the person is being purposefully difficult to care for.
- **Social isolation.** Many older people are isolated from the rest of society making it more difficult for them to report abuse or for others to detect signs of abuse.
- **A reluctance to report abuse.** Older people are often reluctant to report those who mistreat them for fear of getting the abuser in trouble or having the abuser turn against them and refuse to provide further care.

ROLE OF THE NURSING ASSISTANT IN REPORTING ABUSE. As a nursing assistant, you may find yourself in a situation in which you suspect that one of your patients or residents is being abused (Table 2-3). When this is the case, you are required by law to report your suspicions to the proper person in your facility. This person may be your supervisor or someone else. Follow your facility's policy. It is not your responsibility to investigate whether or not abuse has actually occurred or who has caused it. Your responsibility is to simply report your suspicions to the proper person.

Ethics

Ethics moral principles or standards that govern conduct

Like laws, **ethics** guide our behavior in the workplace. The word "ethics" is derived from the Greek word *ethos*, which means "beliefs that guide life." Ethics helps us to determine the difference between right and wrong when there is no clear law or policy to tell us what to do. Each profession has a code of ethics. The code of ethics for nursing assistants is given in Box 2-5.

Value a cherished belief or principle

In addition, each person has a code of ethics that is derived from that person's **values**. Factors that influence a person's values include his or her religious or spiritual beliefs, level and type of education, culture and heritage, and life experiences. As a nursing assistant, you need to think about how you feel about certain moral and ethical issues. Only then will you be able to understand that although another person's values may differ from yours, that person's values are as important to him or her as yours are to you. Ethical dilemmas can arise when we attempt to judge other people by our own ethical standards.

BOX 2-5 **Code of Ethics for Nursing Assistants**

- Treat patients and residents with respect for their individual needs and values.
- Respect the patient's or resident's right to choice in regard to the individual's right to control his or her own care.
- Hold confidential all information about patients and residents learned in the health care setting.
- Be guided by consideration for the dignity of patients and residents.
- Fulfill the obligation to provide competent care to patients and residents.

 ## Putting it all together!

- Both the AHA's *Patient's Bill of Rights* and the *Resident Rights* portion of OBRA protect the people who receive our care. Health care workers are legally and ethically responsible for respecting the rights of patients and residents.

- Advance directives help to ensure that a person's wishes regarding end-of-life care are honored, even if the person is no longer able to express those wishes verbally.

- A living will states that the person does not want the health care team to take extreme measures to prolong his or her life.

- A durable power of attorney for health care allows the person to designate someone else to make medical decisions on his or her behalf.

- Laws and ethics guide our behavior in the workplace. Laws are rules established by a governing authority. Failing to obey these rules can result in punishment. Ethics refers to moral principles or standards that govern conduct. When we act according to ethical standards, we act in a certain way because we believe it is the right way to act, not because we risk punishment if we do not behave in that way.

- Civil laws are concerned with relationships between individuals. Violations of civil law are called torts. Torts may be intentional or unintentional.

- An unintentional tort occurs when someone causes harm or injury to another person or that person's property without the intent to do harm. A nursing assistant who commits an unintentional tort is considered negligent for failing to do what a careful and reasonable person would do.

- An intentional tort occurs when someone causes harm or injury to another person with the intent to do harm. Intentional torts that nursing assistants are particularly at risk for committing in the workplace include defamation, assault, battery, fraud, false imprisonment, invasion of privacy, and larceny.

- Abuse is a violation of criminal law. A nursing assistant who abuses a patient or resident could lose his or her job, as well as the potential for future employment in the health care field.
- Abuse can be physical, emotional, or sexual. Anyone can be a victim of abuse, but people who depend on others for their care (such as children, elderly people, and people with disabilities) are at high risk for abuse.
- Laws require any health care worker who suspects the abuse of a child or vulnerable adult to report his or her suspicions to the proper authorities.

WHAT DID YOU LEARN?

Multiple Choice

Select the single best answer for each of the following questions.

1. Nursing assistants who work in the long-term care setting must complete a course of training and undergo a competency evaluation. These requirements are set by the:
   a. Centers for Disease Control and Prevention (CDC)
   b. Food and Drug Administration (FDA)
   c. Omnibus Budget Reconciliation Act (OBRA)
   d. Occupational Safety and Health Administration (OSHA)

2. As a nursing assistant, it is your responsibility to:
   a. Plan the patient's or resident's care
   b. Perform the tasks your supervisor assigns to you
   c. Do the best you can without asking for help
   d. Compare assignments with your co-workers

3. If you do not know how to do a delegated task, you should:
   a. Call another nursing assistant for help
   b. Ask the patient or resident how he or she prefers to have it done
   c. Decline to do the task
   d. Follow the instructions in the procedure manual

4. Nursing assistants work under the supervision of:
   a. A doctor
   b. A registered nurse (RN) or licensed practical nurse (LPN)
   c. Other nursing assistants
   d. The long-term care facility administrator

5. Which step of the nursing process involves gathering information about a patient or a resident?
   a. Implementation
   b. Assessment
   c. Planning
   d. Evaluation

6. To "delegate" means to:
   a. Do what you are told to do
   b. Give another person permission to perform a task on your behalf
   c. Transfer your duties to another assistant
   d. Have the charge nurse take your assignment

7. What information is included in the registry?
   a. The nursing assistant's full name
   b. The nursing assistant's Registry number and date of expiration
   c. Any reported incidents of abuse or theft
   d. All of the above

8. All of the following are legal terms that relate to making false statements that injure another person's reputation except:
   a. Defamation
   b. Assault
   c. Slander
   d. Libel

9. If a registered nurse (RN) fails to raise the side rails on the bed of a confused patient and the patient falls out of bed and is injured, the nurse may be charged with:
   a. Malpractice
   b. Negligence
   c. An intentional tort
   d. Assault

10. *Resident Rights* are a part of which legislation?
    a. American Medical Association (AMA)
    b. Omnibus Budget Reconciliation Act (OBRA)
    c. Federal Emergency Management Agency (FEMA)
    d. Social Security Act

11. Which of the following is a basic right of residents?
    a. Right to choice
    b. Right to privacy and confidentiality
    c. Right to be free from verbal abuse, or any other abuse
    d. All of the above

12. Confidentiality means:
    a. Only sharing information with those directly involved in a patient's or resident's care
    b. Respecting a patient's or resident's right to privacy
    c. Never sharing information with anyone
    d. Both a and b

13. You are a nursing assistant working in a home health care setting. You suspect that one of your clients is being emotionally and physically abused by her husband. What should you do first?
    a. Call the police
    b. Keep your suspicions to yourself but continue to observe the situation
    c. Immediately report your suspicions to the case manager
    d. Tell another nursing assistant at the agency

14. One of your co-workers has been having a very hard time with one of her residents. The resident is confused and, as a result, is being uncooperative. In a moment of complete frustration, your co-worker says to the resident, "If you don't shut up and behave yourself right now, I'm going to slap you!" What kind of an intentional tort has this nursing assistant committed?
    a. Assault
    b. Battery
    c. Negligence
    d. Malpractice

15. A nursing assistant answers the telephone at the nursing station. The doctor who is calling wants to give a verbal order, and the nursing assistant tells the doctor that she is a nurse and can take the order. What intentional tort has the nursing assistant committed?
    a. Slander
    b. Fraud
    c. Libel
    d. Informed consent

16. What does the Health Insurance Portability and Accountability Act (HIPAA) protect?
    a. The patient's or resident's right to privacy
    b. The patient's or resident's right to sue negligent health care workers
    c. The patient's or resident's right to be free from abuse
    d. The patient's or resident's right to choose who will provide his or her care

17. A legal document that transfers the responsibility for handling a person's medical decisions to a family member, friend, or other trusted individual is known as a:
    a. Living will
    b. HIPAA agreement
    c. Form of consent
    d. Durable power of attorney for health care

 Stop *and* **Think!**

A licensed practical nurse (LPN) who works with you in a long-term care facility stops in Mrs. Taylor's room to give Mrs. Taylor her daily medications. Mrs. Taylor is in the bathroom and you are changing the linens on her bed. The nurse hands you the medication cup, which contains three pills, and asks you to have Mrs. Taylor take the pills as soon as she comes out of the bathroom. You are aware that in your state, nursing assistants who work in long-term care facilities are not allowed to give medications. When you mention your concern about giving Mrs. Taylor her medication to the nurse, she says, "It's okay; the other nursing assistants do this for me all of the time." What should you do?

 Stop *and* **Think!**

You have just received your assignment for the shift. Another assistant does not like her assignment and asks to switch residents with you. This makes you uncomfortable because you have just started at the facility and do not know if switching assignments is permitted. What should you do?

Professionalism and Job-Seeking Skills

The health care field relies on all types of professionals, including nursing assistants, to provide quality care to patients and residents. In this chapter, you will learn about what it means to be a "professional" and what personal qualities you will need to succeed in the health care field. You will also learn about the skills you will need to find a job that is both rewarding and enjoyable.

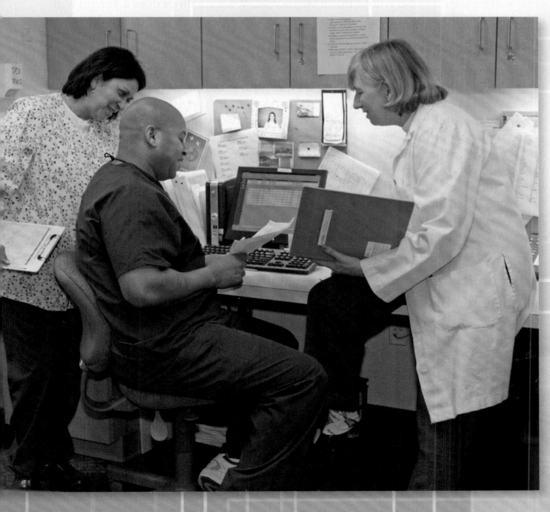

Photo: *The health care industry relies on all types of professionals to provide quality care to patients and residents.*

Working as a Professional

What will you learn?

When you are finished with this section, you will be able to:

1. Discuss the qualities that contribute to a strong work ethic.
2. Describe what a "professional" looks like and how a professional behaves.
3. Understand the importance of taking proper care of yourself, and describe ways to keep yourself healthy, both physically and emotionally.
4. Define the words **work ethic**, **professional**, **attitude**, and **hygiene**.

Having a Strong Work Ethic

Work ethic a person's attitude toward his or her work

A strong **work ethic** is what distinguishes an average employee from a great employee (Fig. 3-1). Two nursing assistants can have solid skills and be very good at getting their work done on time, but the nursing assistant with the strongest work ethic will be the one who enjoys the most success. What qualities does a person with a strong work ethic have, and how can one go about developing these qualities?

A Professional Attitude

Professional a person who has credentials, obtained through education and training, that enable him to become licensed or certified to practice a certain profession; also, a person who demonstrates a professional attitude

Attitude the side of ourselves that we display to the world, communicating outwardly how we feel about things

One definition of a **professional** is a person who has training that allows him or her to become licensed or certified to do a certain job. But even people who have jobs that do not require licensure or certification can behave in a professional manner. Being a professional also means having a positive **attitude**. A person's attitude is apparent from things he says (and the way he says them), the way he behaves, and the way he looks. Having a professional, positive attitude means that you are caring and compassionate toward your patients or residents and that you are committed to doing your job to the best of your ability at all times.

Professionalism is a choice you make and requires effort. Members of the health care team are often held to higher standards for professional behavior than other professional groups. As a nursing assistant, you become a very visible representative of that team. What attitude will you choose to show?

Punctuality

Being punctual means that you are on time or a little bit early. Many people are relying on you! Your patients or residents need you to help them. The staff members working the shift before yours need to go home so that they can attend to their families and other responsibilities, just as you need to attend to yours when you are at home.

Being late is sometimes unavoidable. But you can increase your chances of being on time by knowing how long it will take you to get to work and then adding 15 minutes to that travel time. Preparing ahead of time (for example, by packing your lunch and making sure that your uniform is clean and ready to wear before you go to bed) can also make getting out the door easier when it is time to leave for work. Remember, chronic lateness is one of the main reasons employers take corrective action against nursing assistants.

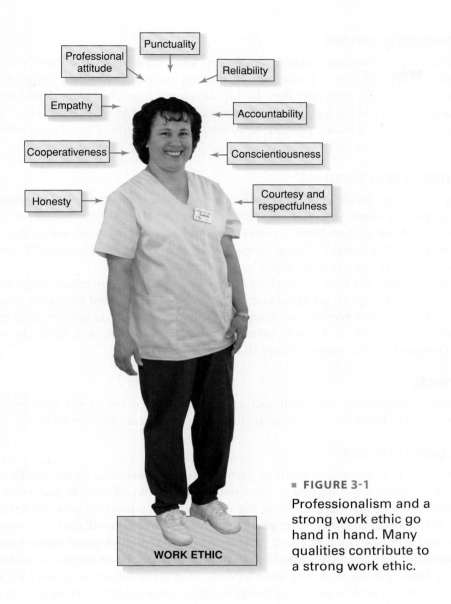

Professional attitude

Punctuality

Reliability

Empathy

Accountability

Cooperativeness

Conscientiousness

Honesty

Courtesy and respectfulness

WORK ETHIC

■ **FIGURE 3-1**

Professionalism and a strong work ethic go hand in hand. Many qualities contribute to a strong work ethic.

Reliability

Reliability means that others can count on you to come to work every day as scheduled and to remain there during your entire shift. Have an emergency plan in place for transportation and childcare before the need arises, and try to keep yourself healthy to decrease your need to take sick days. Poor attendance is another major reason people lose their jobs.

Reliability also means that others can count on you to do your job well with minimal supervision. Your supervisor should not feel the need to look over your shoulder or check up on you to make sure that your work has been finished.

Accountability

An accountable person accepts responsibility for his or her actions and the results of those actions. Being accountable means that you can accept criticism that is intended to help you improve, admit a mistake, and work to correct the situation.

Conscientiousness

A conscientious nursing assistant attends to details and goes the extra mile to complete a task with care. Conscientious nursing assistants take their assignments seriously and make sure that they follow directions carefully. They demonstrate responsibility by asking for additional explanation or clarification when necessary, seeking help with difficult tasks, and admitting that they may not know how to perform a particular task.

Courtesy and Respect

Being polite and having good manners are correct in any situation. Use phrases such as *please, thank you,* and *excuse me.* Show respect for your patients or residents by addressing them as they prefer to be addressed. If in doubt, err on the side of formality ("Dr. Smith," "Mrs. Jones," "Mr. Davis," "Miss Thomson"). Avoid using "baby talk" or "talking down" to patients or residents.

Show respect for your co-workers by not saying anything negative about them to others. Do not speak poorly about your place of employment to others, even if there are things that you are not happy with. If the person you are speaking to is a patient or resident (or a family member of a patient or resident), he or she may begin to question the quality of care that is being given.

Honesty

An honest person tells the truth and acts with integrity. He or she does not lie, cheat, or steal. Honesty is a critical quality for a health care worker to have.

Cooperativeness

Being able to cooperate, or work as part of a team, is essential in the health care field. Remember how important your part of the chain of care is and what an essential role you play in providing for the care and comfort of your patients or residents. Making an effort to get along with your co-workers will make your work easier and will ease the burden on your co-workers as well. A good nursing assistant does not wait for a co-worker to ask for help. Rather, he or she sees a need and offers a helping hand. You may have to work with a person you may not like, but a professional is able to put his or her personal feelings aside for the benefit of the patient or resident.

Empathy

Empathy means that you are able to try to imagine what it would feel like to be in another person's situation. There are times when other people will really try your patience, but if you think of how you would feel if you were in a similar situation, you may find that you are able to understand the offending behavior better. Empathy gives us another perspective and helps us to be kinder and more tolerant.

Maintaining a Professional Appearance

Hygiene personal cleanliness

Others often judge us based on our appearance. To be considered a professional, you need to look the part! That means practicing good personal **hygiene** and dressing neatly and professionally (Guidelines Box 3-1). Good personal hygiene helps to

GUIDELINES BOX 3-1 Guidelines for a Professional Appearance

What you do	Why you do it
Style your hair neatly and away from your face.	*Securing your hair away from your face keeps it away from equipment, out of your eyes, and out of your work. If your hair is not secured back, when you move your hair out of your eyes, any germs on your hands will be transferred to your hair and face.*
Keep your nails short and clean, with smoothly filed edges.	*Germs can hide under the tips of long nails. Long nails can also scratch a person's skin. Frequent hand washing can cause acrylic and false nails to lift, allowing water to become trapped underneath and can lead to a fungal infection in the nailbed.*
Leave bracelets, necklaces, rings, and dangling earrings at home.	*A child or confused person might pull dangling earrings through your earlobes. Necklaces and bracelets get in the way and can get caught in equipment and broken. If you wear rings, germs can become trapped underneath them, which makes hand hygiene less effective. Rings can also scratch a person's skin when you are providing care.*
If you wear make-up, apply it lightly and tastefully.	*Wearing too much make-up or make-up that is too bright or too dark does not contribute to a professional appearance.*
If you wear cologne or perfume, it should be of a light fragrance and lightly applied.	*Many people are sensitive to fragrances and may find perfume or cologne that is of a strong scent or heavily applied offensive.*
Wear a clean, pressed uniform each day. Make sure that your shoes are polished.	*Attention to details, such as making sure that your uniform is wrinkle-free and your shoes are polished, says to others that you care about your appearance. A clean uniform is also essential for limiting the spread of infection.*
If you have a tattoo, try to select a uniform style that will conceal it. If you are thinking about getting a tattoo or body piercing, consider its location carefully.	*Many people feel that tattoos and body piercings make a person look less professional. Many employers now have dress code policies that require tattoos to be covered and limit the number of piercings an employee is allowed to have exposed.*
Practice good personal hygiene and grooming daily.	*Good personal hygiene helps to prevent breath and body odors and limits the spread of infection. In addition, if you care enough about yourself to keep yourself clean and neat, the people in your care will feel that you will do the same for them.*

prevent the spread of infection and promotes a neat, clean appearance. To practice good personal hygiene:

- Bathe daily and use a deodorant.
- Shampoo your hair regularly and treat dandruff or other scalp conditions.
- Keep your nails short and clean, with smoothly filed edges.
- Brush and floss your teeth, and use mouthwash. Visit a dentist regularly. Poor dental health can cause breath odors.
- If you are a man, shave daily, or keep facial hair neatly groomed and trimmed.
- Wear a clean, pressed uniform each day.
- Wash your hands often.

Staying Healthy

To care for your patients or residents to the best of your ability, you must first care for yourself, both physically and emotionally. By taking proper care of yourself, you demonstrate that you are a professional who takes his or her responsibilities seriously.

Maintaining Your Physical Health

The duties of a nursing assistant require much physical effort. You will be constantly lifting, bending, walking, and reaching as you perform your daily tasks at work. Your employer, your co-workers, your family, and especially your patients or residents rely on you to be able to do your duties. In addition to giving you more energy, staying physically fit keeps your body strong and allows you to avoid many types of job-related injuries. Guidelines for keeping your body in good physical condition are given in Guidelines Box 3-2.

Even the healthiest people occasionally get sick. If you are sick (especially if you have a fever), do not go to work. If you go to work with a contagious illness, you could give the illness to the people in your care. Many of the people in your care will have conditions that make it harder for them to fight off an infection if they are exposed to one (for example, they may be older people or in poor general health). In this situation, the responsible thing to do is to notify your supervisor that you are ill and unable to come to work. Follow your facility's policy for calling in sick. This will allow your supervisor to find someone else to cover your shift.

Maintaining Your Emotional Health

Caring for others is an emotionally demanding job, as well as a physically demanding one, for many reasons:

- Because of the shortage of health care workers, as well as a need to cut costs, many facilities are understaffed, which means that employees are often overworked.
- Not all patients or residents are happy, or grateful for the care they are receiving. Many people in need of care do not feel well and, as a result, may be difficult or hard to manage.

GUIDELINES BOX 3-2   Guidelines for Staying Physically Healthy

What you do	Why you do it
Get enough sleep.	*Most people need an average of 7 to 8 hours of sleep to function properly. Not only does rest relax the muscles, it also relaxes the mind and allows you to think clearly. Too little rest can weaken your immune system, making you more likely to get infections, such as cold and flu viruses.*
Eat well-balanced, nutritious meals.	*A working body needs good nutrition. You need fuel for your muscles and your brain.*
Exercise regularly.	*Regular exercise gives you more strength and energy and keeps your heart and lungs healthy. In addition, regular exercise helps reduce the mental stress that sometimes goes along with intensely emotional jobs, such as those in the health care field.*
Do not smoke.	*Smoking causes the blood vessels in the body to narrow, reducing the flow of oxygen-carrying blood to the body's cells. Smoking is associated with serious diseases, such as lung cancer, emphysema, and heart disease.*
Do not take recreational drugs. Limit the amount of alcohol you drink.	*Using recreational drugs or drinking too much alcohol can have many negative effects on your health. In addition, these substances can impair your ability to make good decisions, both on and off the job.*
Have a routine physical examination.	*Many chronic illnesses, such as high blood pressure and diabetes, go undetected until they have caused permanent damage to your body. Many types of cancers can be cured if detected early enough. Routine physical examinations can help you detect problems early so that actions can be taken to correct them.*

■ As a health care worker, you will have to face the death of some of your patients or residents. This can be difficult, especially in situations where you have had a chance to develop a relationship with the person and his or her family members.

Fortunately, there are actions you can take to help keep your emotions in check while you are on the job and prevent emotional burnout. Some of these actions are listed in Guidelines Box 3-3.

GUIDELINES BOX 3-3 Guidelines for Staying Emotionally Healthy

What you do	Why you do it
Maintain your physical health.	*Physical activity relieves mental and emotional stress.*
Schedule time for yourself.	*Most of us are not just caregivers in the workplace; we are caregivers at home as well. It is important to make time for yourself, to do what you like to do, in order to avoid feeling overwhelmed by your responsibilities at home and at work.*
Take advantage of counseling services offered by your employer or confide in a clergy member.	*Talking to a professional can help you to manage work-related stress and define your feelings and beliefs about difficult subjects, such as death and dying.*
When a situation becomes particularly "heated" at work, take a physical and emotional break. Ask someone to relieve you, and take a walk outside to calm down.	*When we reach our limits, we may say or do something we regret later. Acting in frustration or anger can put your professional relationships at risk and may even cause you to harm a patient or resident. Physically removing yourself from the situation can give you a new perspective and the opportunity to calm down before going back to work.*
Ask to be assigned to different work areas or to different patients or residents occasionally.	*New situations and challenges help to prevent boredom and burnout.*

 Putting it all together!

- Regardless of the level of education, certification, or experience a health care professional has, professionalism is all about exhibiting the right attitude, to co-workers, patients or residents, and visitors.

- A person with a strong work ethic can be depended on and trusted; treats others with kindness, respect, and compassion; and is committed to doing his or her job to the best of his or her ability at all times.

- Personal hygiene promotes a professional image and helps to prevent the spread of infection. In the health care field, many of the traits we have come to associate with a professional image are related to maintaining safety and health.

- To care for your patients or residents to the best of your ability, you must first care for yourself. Staying physically fit keeps your body strong and helps to prevent many types of job-related injuries. Taking steps to maintain your emotional health helps to prevent emotional burnout.

Finding a Job

What will you learn?

When you are finished with this section, you will be able to:

1. Describe questions a person should consider before beginning a job search.
2. List places to search for job openings.
3. Describe how to complete a job application.
4. Describe ways to make a good first impression during an interview.
5. Define the words **résumé**, **reference list**, and **interview**.

The health care field is one of the most rapidly growing areas in industry, and the trend is expected to continue. People who are trained to work as nursing assistants are in great demand. Your goal is to find a job situation in which you will be happy and professionally fulfilled. To do that, you need to take a methodical approach to looking for a job.

Think About Your Ideal Job

Before you begin the process of searching for job openings, completing applications, and going on interviews, it is important that you take time to explore what you really want from your employment and what you will be able to offer to your employer. Some questions to consider are shown in Figure 3-2.

Search for Job Openings

Once you have some specific goals in mind, there are many places to search for job openings. Some examples are:

- Classified ads in the local newspaper
- Telephone directories (look under listings such as "retirement communities and homes," "home health services," and "hospitals" for names of local places that might hire nursing assistants)
- Internet sites dedicated to helping people find jobs
- Your school's job placement service
- Bulletin boards in the facility where you are receiving clinical training
- Friends and colleagues

Prepare Your Paperwork

Before applying for a job, you should prepare two key documents: a **résumé** and a **reference list**. You may also wish to prepare a cover letter.

Résumé a brief document that gives a possible employer general information about a job candidate's education and work experience

Reference list a list of three or four people who would be willing to talk to a potential employer about a job candidate's abilities

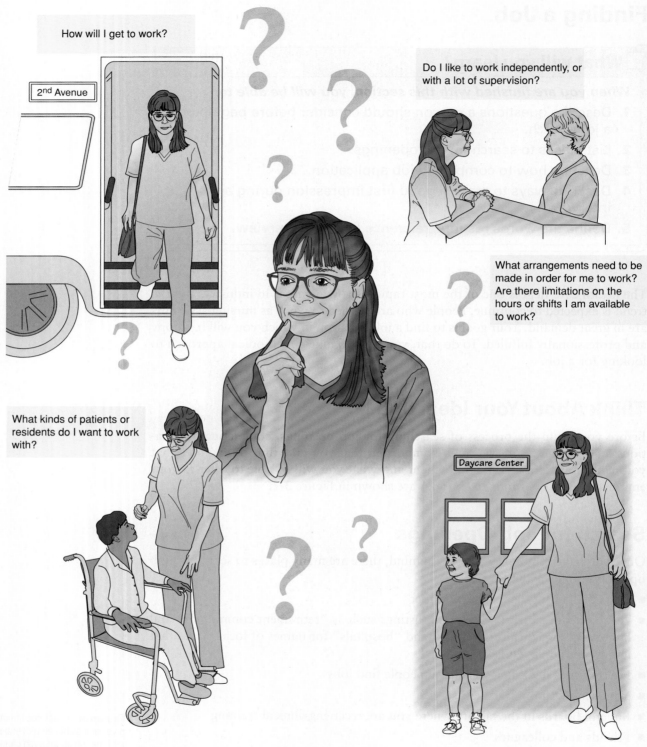

■ **FIGURE 3-2**

The first step to finding a job is thinking about what sort of situation best fits your personality, lifestyle, and interests.

Résumés

Type or print your résumé using a computer on white or off-white paper. Include only facts, and try to keep your résumé to one page, if at all possible. Your résumé should include:

- Your full name, mailing address, telephone number, and, if you have one, e-mail address.
- A short objective or career goal.
- A history of your education (list the schools you attended most recently first, and for each school, include the dates you attended the school and the degree you graduated with).
- An employment history (list each of your previous employers, and for each employer, include the dates that you worked, your job title, and your primary job duties). List your most recent job first.

There is some information that should never be included on a résumé, including your age, marital status, weight, religion, sexual preference, and whether or not you have children (or are planning to have them). This information should not matter to an employer who is considering you as an employee.

Reference Lists

When considering people to include on your reference list, think about people who know you well and have worked with you in a professional capacity, such as your teachers, co-workers, and previous supervisors. Before listing a person as a reference, make sure that you have the person's permission to do so. After a person has agreed to be your reference, make sure that you have accurate contact information for that person, including his or her full name and title (if any), a current and complete address, an e-mail address, and a telephone number. Type your reference list on a sheet of paper that matches your résumé.

Cover Letters

You may also want to prepare a cover letter to send out with your résumé and reference list. A cover letter is written as a way of introducing yourself to a potential employer. Your résumé contains information about your education, training, and experience, but a cover letter goes beyond the straight facts. A cover letter says, "Hello, this is why I want to work for your organization, and this is why I am the best person for the job." Your cover letter should be fairly short and typed or printed using a computer on white or off-white paper. Pay special attention to your grammar and spelling.

Put in Applications

The next step is to apply for jobs that you are interested in. You can visit facilities where you are interested in working and ask to complete a job application. A job application is a form that employers use to obtain basic information about you, such as which position you are applying for, how you can be reached, and what shifts you can work. The application form will also require you to provide information about your education, your work history, and the reasons you left your previous job. The job application is a legal document, and your signature at the bottom states that all the information is true and accurate. Always be honest when filling out a job application. An employer who finds out that you lied about any information on the application form has grounds to fire you without notice.

Usually, when you go to an organization to complete a job application, the receptionist at the main desk will give you the application to complete. When completing the job application, use blue or black ink and write clearly. Have your résumé and reference list with you. Many employers request copies of these along with your completed job application. In addition, having these documents with you will make it easier to fill out the job application accurately.

Many facilities now have prospective employees complete the application process online. As with filling out a paper application form, make sure that you are careful to fill out each space and use correct spelling and grammar. There is usually also the ability to upload copies of your résumé and cover letter that you have saved on your computer.

When you go to complete your job application, dress appropriately. Some facilities may choose to interview you at that time, especially if there is an opening. Appropriate dress means "clean and neat." Even if you do not interview, this will be the first impression you make on a possible employer.

Ask for an appointment for an interview when you submit your résumé, reference list, and completed application. Some facilities will make the appointment at this time. Others may want to review your résumé and application and call you for an appointment at a later date. If you have not heard from a potential employer in 1 week's time, it is appropriate to call and ask about the status of your application. A follow-up call shows a potential employer that you have initiative and are interested in the job.

Go on Interviews

Interview a meeting between an employer and a potential employee during which information is exchanged regarding the organization, the job, and the potential employee's qualifications for the job

During the **interview**, the interviewer will be trying to determine whether you are the right person for the job. The interview is also a chance for *you* to learn more about the employer and the position in an effort to determine whether they are right for you. Being properly prepared for the interview will allow you to gather as much information about the organization and the job as possible during the interview so that you can make a decision about the job if it is offered to you. In addition, being properly prepared can make all the difference in how a potential employer views your potential! Your résumé and application contain all of the "hard" facts about your education and experience, but you are the one responsible for persuading the interviewer of your interest in the job, dedication to your profession, and abilities.

Before going to the interview, make a list of questions you would like answers to, and refer to this list during the interview. This shows that you are interested in the position and are taking the opportunity to interview seriously. Some questions you might want to ask are shown in Box 3-1. You should also think about the answers to questions the interviewer might ask you so that you can be prepared to answer them. Some of these questions are shown in Box 3-2.

You are interviewing for a job in the health care setting, so help the interviewer see you as a part of his or her staff. Present yourself as a well-groomed professional (see Guidelines Box 3-1). Make sure that your clothing is pressed and that all repairs, such as replacing missing buttons or fixing loose seams, have been taken care of before the interview. Your shoes should be clean and polished. If you are a man, wear slacks (not jeans), a button-down shirt or a polo shirt, and a belt, and possibly a sport jacket if the weather is cool. A tie is optional. If you are a woman, wear a skirt (or dress slacks) and a blouse or a simple dress. Wear stockings, and make sure that the hem length of your skirt or dress is modest.

BOX 3-1 Questions You Might Want to Ask the Interviewer

- "What are the major responsibilities or duties of the position? May I have a copy of the job description?"
- "May I see the unit where I will be working and meet the person who will be supervising me?"
- "What do you think nursing assistants like best about working here? Least?"
- "How many nursing assistants staff each unit?"
- "When would I be eligible for a performance evaluation, and what are the standards I will be evaluated against?"
- "What qualities are you looking for in a nursing assistant?"
- "What opportunities exist for career growth and furthering my education?"

BOX 3-2 Questions That an Interviewer Might Want to Ask You

- "Tell me about yourself. Why did you become a nursing assistant?"
- "What part of your last job did you like the most? The least?"
- "Why are you leaving your current job?" (or, "Why did you leave your last job?")
- "What are you looking for in a manager?"
- "How do you describe your work habits?"
- "How do you set priorities?"
- "How do you handle yourself under stress?"
- "How do you handle problems with patients or co-workers?"
- "Tell me about a specific situation that interfered with your ability to do your job, and how you handled it."
- "What is the most satisfying workday you have had this year? Why?"
- "Do you have a mentor? What have you learned from this person?"
- "Who in your life would you consider to be 'successful'? Why?"
- "What do you consider to be your greatest strength? Your greatest weakness?"
- "Where do you want to go with your career? What steps have you taken to achieve your goal?"
- "What is it about our organization that appeals to you?"

Carrying a small notebook containing the questions you want to ask during the interview and a copy of your résumé, reference list, and your certified nursing assistant certification or registration looks very professional. Do not chew gum during the interview, and make sure that your cellular phone is turned off. You only have one chance to make a first impression, so make it a good one!

Give yourself adequate time to get to the interview. Ideally, you will arrive a few minutes early. After being introduced to the interviewer, shake his or her hand and take a seat when you are invited to do so. Do not address the interviewer by his or her first name unless the interviewer specifically asks you to. Thank the person for the opportunity to interview at the beginning of the interview.

During the interview process, sit up straight and try not to fidget. You might be nervous, but try to appear as confident and comfortable as you can. Maintain good eye contact during the interview and speak clearly. Try to answer questions concisely yet completely; it is best if you can strike a balance between listening and talking. If you do not know the answer to a question, simply say that you do not know—most interviewers are quick to recognize bluffing.

At the end of the interview, the interviewer will usually give you an opportunity to ask any questions that you may have. Now is the time to refer to your list! Asking questions of your own indicates that you have an active interest in making sure that you are a good fit for the job and the organization. When the interview is over, thank the interviewer again for his or her time and for considering you for the position. If the interviewer did not mention when you can expect to hear from him or her regarding the position, ask. Then leave! The interview is over, and there is nothing left to do but write a thank-you note.

You should write a short thank-you note within 1 day of interviewing for the position, thanking the interviewer for considering you for the position and briefly explaining why you are excited about the possibility of working for his or her organization. You may hand write your thank-you note on a plain note card or type it.

> Getting the perfect job is just the beginning. Keeping the job and growing professionally are just as important. Remember the qualities that a person with a strong work ethic possesses? By demonstrating these qualities daily at work, you will quickly become a valuable member of the health care team. You will be open to learning new information and skills, and your patients or residents will certainly benefit from your professional growth and dedication to providing quality care.

Accept an Offer

When someone calls to offer you a job, you may be ready to accept it right away. Or, you might need time to think about it. If so, it is acceptable to ask the person if you can call him or her back with an answer within a day or so. If you have not heard from the organization you interviewed with within the amount of time specified at the close of the interview, it is appropriate to follow up with a telephone call. Even if this job did not work out, another one will. Just keep trying!

Chances are, you will accept many different jobs over the course of your career. You may need to leave a job when a better opportunity comes along or because of a change in your personal circumstances (such as a move to a new area). You may leave a job to stay at home with your children or go back to school. When leaving a job, give your employer at least 2 weeks' notice so that arrangements can be made to cover your shifts. Write a letter stating your desire to leave the job and thanking your present employer for the opportunity to work at the organization. Make sure that you leave in good standing because you never know when you may need a good job reference from that employer or actually find that you really want your old job back!

Putting it all together!

- Thinking about the type of job you want helps to give direction to your job search.
- Applying and interviewing for jobs can be a time-consuming process that requires a lot of effort. However, by taking the time to prepare, you increase your chances of finding a situation in which you will be happy and satisfied with your work.

WHAT DID YOU LEARN?

Multiple Choice

Select the single best answer for each of the following questions.

1. A short, precise document with information about you, your work experience, and your education is called a:
   a. Minimum Data Set (MDS)
   b. Résumé
   c. Reference
   d. Cover letter

2. All of the following information should be included on your résumé, except for your:
   a. Name
   b. Address
   c. Employment history
   d. Religion

3. Which one of the following is a legal document used when applying for a job?
   a. Résumé
   b. Cover letter
   c. Reference list
   d. Application

4. The chance for a potential employer to meet you personally occurs during the:
   a. Application process
   b. Interview process
   c. Job posting process
   d. Reference checking process

5. A nursing assistant can promote his or her physical health by doing all of the following except:
   a. Eating well-balanced meals
   b. Getting plenty of rest
   c. Smoking and drinking socially
   d. Attending aerobics classes

6. A nursing assistant's personal cleanliness is referred to as:
   a. Sanitization
   b. Neatness
   c. Hygiene
   d. Fashion

7. Qualities that characterize a good work ethic include all of the following except:
   a. Reliability
   b. Punctuality
   c. Honesty
   d. Tardiness

8. What type of a nursing assistant accepts responsibility for his or her actions?
   a. An accountable nursing assistant
   b. A respectful nursing assistant
   c. A courteous nursing assistant
   d. A punctual nursing assistant

9. What type of a nursing assistant is able to imagine what it would feel like to be in another person's situation?
   a. A creative nursing assistant
   b. An empathetic nursing assistant
   c. An experienced nursing assistant
   d. An honest nursing assistant

10. What type of a nursing assistant can be counted on to come to work every day?
    a. A punctual nursing assistant
    b. A nursing assistant with access to public transportation
    c. A reliable nursing assistant
    d. An ethical nursing assistant

11. What type of nursing assistant has a professional attitude?
    a. A nursing assistant who acts smarter than the other nursing assistants
    b. A nursing assistant who is certified
    c. A nursing assistant who is committed to doing his or her best at all times
    d. A nursing assistant who is always late to work

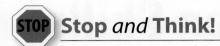

Imagine that you have just completed your nursing assistant training and taken the state test. While you are waiting for your test results, you decide to begin reading job postings to see what opportunities are available. At this point, you are considering several options. You are excited about beginning your career in the health care field, and you are anxious to get into the workforce and put your new skills to use. However, you think that you might also want to continue your education and become either a licensed practical nurse (LPN) or a registered nurse (RN) someday. What sorts of organizations may be looking for nursing assistants in your community? How could working as a nursing assistant now help you to further define your career goals?

 Stop *and* Think!

Your best friend Martha is also a nursing assistant at the long-term care facility where you work. She has a very difficult time managing her personal life and her professional life. Many times, Martha has asked you to clock her in when you get to work so that your supervisors will not see that she is late. This makes you uncomfortable, but you do not want to lose Martha's friendship. What should you do?

Communication Skills

Communicating—that is, sharing and receiving information—is something that you have to do every day. In this chapter, you will learn skills and tactics that you can use to enhance your ability to communicate. We will also review some of the tools that are used by members of the health care team to ensure that important information is available to all who are involved with the care of a patient or resident.

Photo: *A nursing assistant talks with one of her residents.*

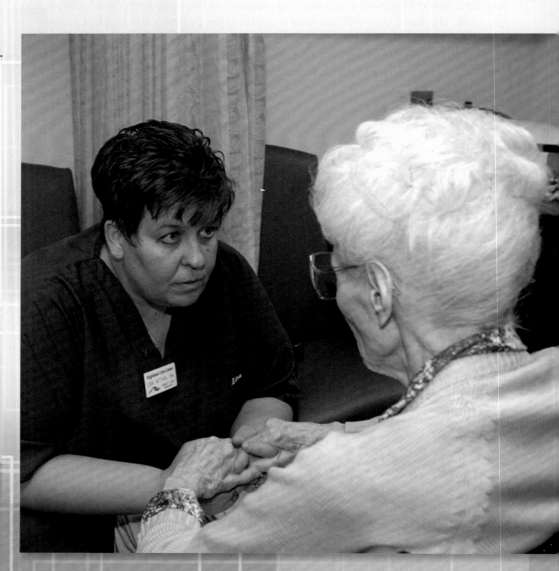

Introduction to Communication

What will you learn?

When you are finished with this section, you will be able to:

1. Understand what communication is.
2. Discuss why it is important for a nursing assistant to be able to communicate effectively.
3. Describe the two major forms of communication and give examples of each.
4. Discuss techniques that promote effective communication.
5. Define the words **communication**, **verbal communication**, and **nonverbal communication**.

The key to understanding what **communication** is lies within the word "exchange." If you exchange gifts with another person, you give that person a gift, and, in return, you receive one back. Communicating is not just about telling someone something (giving information). It is also about listening and observing (receiving information). For communication to be effective, all of the people who are involved must actively participate in the exchange of information (Fig. 4-1).

There are two major forms of communication, **verbal communication** and **nonverbal communication**. Verbal communication uses words, either spoken or written, to exchange information. Examples of verbal communication include telephone conversations, written notes and memos, e-mail and text messages, and ASL (American Sign Language) that is used to communicate with people who are deaf. Verbal communication tends to be more direct—when we use language to express

Communication the exchange of information

Verbal communication a way of communicating that uses written or spoken language

Nonverbal communication a way of communicating that uses facial expressions, gestures, and body language, instead of written or spoken language

■ **FIGURE 4-1**

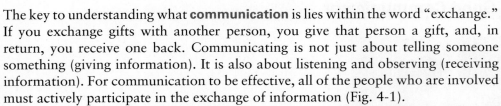
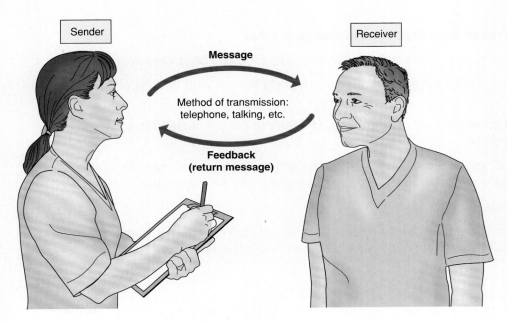

Communication involves at least two people, a *sender* and a *receiver*. The sender is the person with information to share, and the receiver is the person for whom the information is intended. The sender delivers the information in the form of a *message*, which the receiver may or may not understand. Through *feedback*, or a return message, the receiver lets the sender know whether the message was received and understood. Note that as information is transmitted back and forth, the sender and the receiver switch roles.

a thought, it is usually with the intent of giving specific information to another person. Nonverbal communication, on the other hand, tends to be more indirect. Being aware of nonverbal cues can give you a better understanding of what other people are truly feeling and thinking.

As a nursing assistant, you must be a successful communicator, both as a sender and a receiver of information, with both those you care for and your co-workers. You will use your communication skills to:

- Comfort, reassure, and teach your patients or residents
- Share information about changes in your patients' or residents' health status with other members of the health care team
- Accept or decline assigned tasks and seek additional clarification about how to do those tasks as necessary

Tips on how to be a good communicator are given in Box 4-1.

BOX 4-1   ## How to Be a Good Communicator

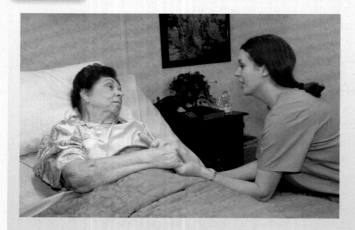

When you are the sender, make sure that your message is clear

- Think about what you want to say. Present the information in a logical, organized way.

- If your message is written, make sure that your handwriting is neat and your spelling is accurate.

- Speak clearly at a normal pace, and avoid mumbling. Unless the person is hearing impaired, there is no reason to raise your voice.

- Use words that the person you are speaking to understands. When appropriate, use simple, common words in place of more technical words. If necessary, use an interpreter.

- Face the person you are speaking to.

- Make sure that the person you are speaking to is able to physically receive the message. For example, if the person wears a hearing aid, make sure that it is turned on.

When you are the receiver, be a good listener

- Focus your attention on the speaker.

- Sit down and do not appear rushed or in a hurry.

- Make eye contact with the speaker.

- Do not interrupt or try to finish the speaker's sentences.

Learn techniques for encouraging people to talk

- Ask open-ended questions instead of "yes/no" questions. For example, instead of asking "Did you have breakfast this morning?," ask "What did you have for breakfast this morning?"

- Rephrase what the person says to you. For example, if a resident says that she feels sad and lonely, instead of asking "Why?," say "You're feeling sad and lonely?" This invites the person to talk more about what she is feeling.

- Observe for and ask questions about nonverbal signals the person may be sending.

- Remember the value of silence and a comforting touch.

Provide and seek feedback

- When you are the receiver, ask questions and repeat information back to the sender so that he or she knows that his or her message was received and understood.

- When you are the sender, seek feedback from the receiver to make sure that he or she understood your message. This is always important, but especially so when the person may be embarrassed about an inability to understand you (for example, if the person has hearing loss or speaks a language that is different from yours).

- Observe for nonverbal cues that indicate that the receiver did not understand your message. For example, the person may be nodding his or her head but looking confused.

Avoid behaviors that block effective communication

- Avoid being judgmental. A person who is judgmental forms quick opinions about whether or not another person is right or wrong. A judgmental attitude can be revealed through body language or comments you make and indicates to the other person that you do not respect his or her thoughts, beliefs, or feelings.

- Avoid assuming that another person knows what you are thinking. Instead, keep others informed about what you have done and what you expect them to do.

- Avoid "tuning out" others. Always listen carefully.

- Avoid negative body language, such as tapping your fingers or foot impatiently, constantly looking at your watch or toward the door, crossing your arms, and rolling your eyes.

- Avoid using slang or foul language.

Putting it all together!

- For communication to be effective, all of the people who are involved must actively participate in the exchange of information.

- The two major forms of communication are verbal and nonverbal. Verbal communication involves the use of language, either spoken or written. Nonverbal communication gives information through the use of facial expressions, gestures, or body language.

- Nursing assistants must be effective communicators, both as senders and receivers of information, with both co-workers and people who are receiving care.

- Listening is one of the most important communication skills, especially in the health care field. Speaking clearly, asking open-ended questions, and using appropriate body language are other ways to ensure effective communication.

Communicating With People With Special Needs

What will you learn?

When you are finished with this section, you will be able to:

1. Discuss situations that might affect a person's ability to communicate effectively.

2. Describe how a nursing assistant can assist with communication in these situations.

Communicating With a Person Who Speaks a Language Different From Yours

Some of your patients or residents may not speak the same language that you do. When caring for a person who speaks a foreign language:

- Use hand gestures or a picture board (Fig. 4-2) to communicate very basic ideas.

- You may need to use an interpreter to avoid misunderstandings.

Communicating With a Person Who Has Hearing Loss

You may care for patients or residents who have been deaf since birth or who have become completely or partially deaf as a result of a disorder that affects the ear. In addition, many older people gradually lose the ability to hear high-pitched sounds as part of the normal aging process. When this occurs, the older person has trouble

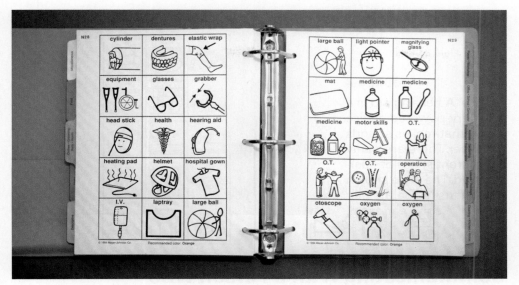

■ **FIGURE 4-2**
A picture board is often useful when trying to communicate on a basic level with someone who speaks a different language, is hearing impaired, or has a developmental disability.

telling the difference between similar-sounding high-pitched sounds like *th* and *s*. This can lead to frequent misunderstandings. When caring for a person with hearing loss:

- Face the person when you are speaking to him or her. This gives the person a clear view of your mouth, which is helpful if the person lip-reads. Avoid chewing gum or speaking unusually fast because these actions can make it hard for the person to read your lips. If the person needs glasses, make sure that he or she is wearing them so that your lips can be seen clearly.

- Use a note pad to write down important questions or directions so that the person can read them.

- Consider learning sign language or using a sign language interpreter (Fig. 4-3).

- If a person who uses a hearing aid (Fig. 4-4) seems unable to hear you, make sure that the hearing aid is turned on and that the volume is turned up high enough. If the hearing aid still does not seem to be working, check the batteries to see whether they need to be replaced. You will learn more about how to care for and operate hearing aids in Chapter 23.

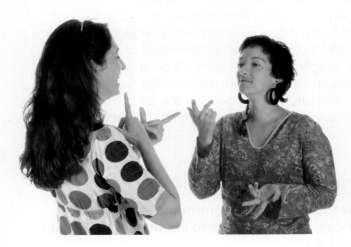

■ **FIGURE 4-3**
Sign language is a form of verbal communication used by many people with significant hearing loss.

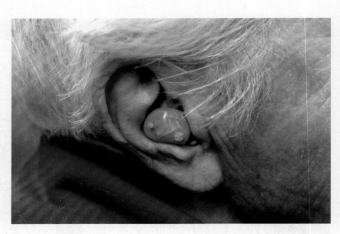

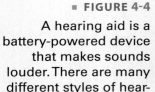

■ **FIGURE 4-4**

A hearing aid is a battery-powered device that makes sounds louder. There are many different styles of hearing aid. The style shown here fits inside the person's ear canal.

Communicating With a Person Who Has Speech Difficulties

There are many reasons why a person might have trouble speaking clearly. People who are completely deaf often do not speak clearly. A person who has had a stroke may lose the ability to form sounds into meaningful words. Surgical procedures affecting the mouth or vocal cords can make it difficult or impossible for a person to speak. So can medical devices, such as breathing tubes. When caring for a person who has trouble speaking:

■ Ask "yes/no" questions when all you need is basic information.

■ If you cannot understand what the person is saying, please tell the person that you did not understand and look for other ways to help the person communicate. For example, you might offer the person a note pad so that she can write down what she needs to tell you or a picture board so that she can point to what she needs.

> **Concerns for Long-Term Care**
>
> The majority of your residents in the long-term care setting are older people and may experience difficulty with communication due to hearing problems, aphasia, or dementia. Unfortunately, many people think of the older people as people who are "going through their second childhood" and speak to them accordingly. When speaking with your elderly residents, avoid the use of "baby talk" or calling them all "sweetie" or "honey". Your elderly residents, like all people needing health care services, deserve to be spoken to with respect and as the adults they are. If a resident has a specific communication difficulty, learn about why the person has the difficulty and use communication techniques specific for that problem.

 Putting it all together!

■ Special situations that may affect communication include language differences, hearing loss, and conditions that affect a person's ability to speak.

- When communicating with a person who has special needs, it is especially important to practice the good communication techniques described in Box 4-1. If the person has trouble hearing or understanding the language, always seek feedback so that you know the person received your message. If the person has trouble speaking, always provide feedback so that the person knows that you received his or her message.

Resolving Conflicts

What will you learn?

When you are finished with this section, you will be able to:
1. Identify causes of conflict and discuss ways of resolving conflicts.
2. Define the word **conflict**.

Conflict is common in the health care field because health care is a people-oriented, emotional business. Patients and residents are sick, hurting, confused, and frightened. Family members feel helpless and sad. Staff members are often stressed by the emotional and physical demands of their work. As a result, conflicts may arise between a member of the health care team and a patient or resident, between two patients or residents, or between two members of the health care team. Conflict makes the people directly involved, as well as those around them, uncomfortable. If you find yourself involved in a conflict, take steps to resolve the problem quickly and professionally (Box 4-2).

Conflict discord resulting from differences between people; can occur when one person is unable to understand or accept another's ideas or beliefs

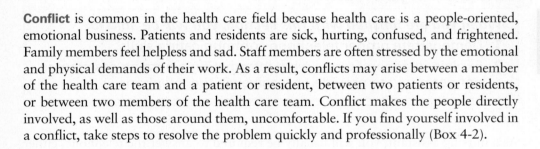

BOX 4-2 How to Resolve a Conflict

- Ask to speak privately with the person you have a conflict with. Because the two of you may be able to resolve your disagreement on your own, try this approach before involving a supervisor. Remain polite and professional, and thank the person for his or her time.

- During your conversation, focus on the specific area of conflict. Do not focus on how you feel about the other person or how you think he or she should have acted under the circumstances.

- Be specific about what you understand the problem to be. Express why you are upset, but avoid being accusatory. For example, instead of saying "You really hurt my feelings by what you said the other day," say "I am bothered by what you said the other day." This allows you to take responsibility for your emotions while allowing the other person to explain his or her side of the story.

- Be prepared to hear how the other person may feel toward you or the problem, even if it is not pleasant. Perhaps you were the one who was initially misunderstood.

- Be gracious enough to apologize for misunderstanding the other person or for being the one who was misunderstood.

- Ask the other person for ideas about how to resolve the conflict. His or her suggestions might surprise you!

- Sometimes it is necessary to "agree to disagree." People with differing opinions and beliefs can focus on things they have in common, such as caring about the patient's or resident's well-being, and still disagree on certain issues. Learning to respect others' beliefs is part of being professional.

- If you cannot resolve a conflict on your own, seek the advice of your supervisor.

Putting it all together!

- Getting along with other people, although it is a very important part of your job, can sometimes be the hardest part of your job.
- Good communication is essential to preventing conflict, as well as helping to resolve it.
- A conflict that affects the quality of the care you provide must not be allowed to continue! If you find yourself involved in a conflict, remember what it means to be a professional and take appropriate steps to resolve the issue.

Using the Telephone

What will you learn?

When you are finished with this section, you will be able to:

1. Demonstrate proper telephone communication skills.
2. Explain in general terms what information a nursing assistant is not permitted to provide or receive via the telephone.

As a nursing assistant, you will usually be required to answer the telephone, either at the nursing station or in a patient's or resident's room. The way you handle yourself on the telephone reflects directly on your facility. General policies for how to use the telephone properly are given in Box 4-3.

BOX 4-3 **How to Use the Telephone**

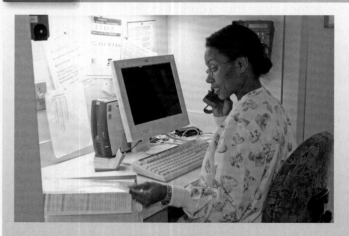

- Answer the telephone promptly, within the first three rings.
- Answer with a pleasant greeting, such as "Good morning" or "Good afternoon."
- Identify yourself by name and title and by your unit or floor according to facility policy: "3 West; Mary Smith, CNA, speaking."
- Because the caller obviously needs something (otherwise, he or she would not be calling), ask "How may I help you?"
- Know how to perform basic functions using your facility's telephone system, such as how to transfer a call or place a caller on hold.

- If you must place a caller on hold, ask his or her permission first ("May I put you on hold for a minute?"). Be aware of the length of time a caller has been on hold; if the time becomes excessive (more than 5 minutes), ask the caller if he or she wants to continue to hold, leave a message, or call back later.

- If the person the caller wants to speak to is unavailable, offer to take a message. When taking a telephone message, be sure to write down the date and time of the call, the name of the caller, a telephone number where the caller can be reached, and your name. Write clearly, and ask the caller to spell his or her name if you are not sure how to spell it. Be sure to deliver the message to the person for whom it was intended.

- A nursing assistant is not to take doctor's orders or receive or give results of diagnostic tests. Calls of this nature should be handled by a nurse.

- Know your facility's policy regarding what information can be provided over the telephone and to whom. The Health Insurance Portability and Accountability Act (HIPAA), discussed in Chapter 2, specifically regulates who may be given information about a person in a health care facility. In general, callers seeking information about a patient or resident should be referred to the nurse.

- Do not use the telephone at the nurse's station to make or receive personal calls. Personal calls should be made from a pay phone or your own cellular phone, while you are on break or at lunch. Never tie up a telephone used for health care communication by using it for personal business.

 Putting it all together!

- Using proper telephone etiquette improves communication and promotes a professional image.

- Confidentiality is of concern when the telephone is used as a means of communication. Protect yourself, your employer, and your patients or residents by being aware of your facility's policies with regard to telephone use.

> *Nursing assistants are an important link between the patient or resident and other members of the health care team. The nursing assistant is often the first member of the health care team to become aware of a change in a patient's or resident's condition that could be a sign of something serious.*

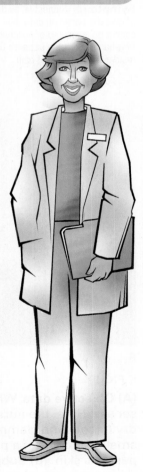

Communication Among Members of the Health Care Team

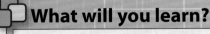 **What will you learn?**

When you are finished with this section, you will be able to:

1. Explain why a nursing assistant is often considered the "eyes and ears" of the health care team.

2. Discuss the methods of reporting and recording information in a health care setting.

Observation something that you notice about the patient or resident, typically related to a change in the person's physical or mental condition

Objective information that is obtained directly, through measurements or by using one of the five senses (sight, smell, taste, hearing, touch)

Subjective information that cannot be objectively measured or assessed

Signs Objective evidence of disease, based on data that are obtained directly, through measurements or by using one of the five senses

Symptoms Subjective evidence of disease, based on data that cannot be measured or observed first-hand, such as a patient's or resident's complaint of pain

3. Describe communication technologies that are being used in the health care field today.
4. Define the words **observations**, **objective data**, **signs**, **subjective data**, **symptom**, **reporting**, **recording**, **medical record (chart)**, **electronic health record (EHR)**, and **Kardex**.

Making Observations

The amount of time you will spend with your patients or residents, combined with the duties you are responsible for performing daily (for example, bathing, feeding, ambulating, toileting), means that you may notice things about your patients or residents that other health care team members may overlook. These things you notice are called **observations**. Your observations may be based on either **objective** data or **subjective** data (Fig. 4-5). Objective data—such as an elevated temperature, a rash, or a low urine output—are called **signs**. Subjective data—such as pain, nausea, or dizziness—are called **symptoms**.

Reporting and Recording

Nursing assistants use two methods of communicating observations about their patients or residents and documenting the care provided so that other health

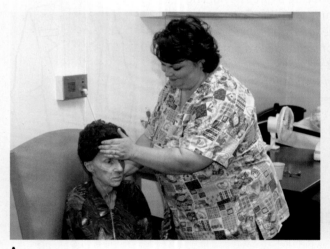
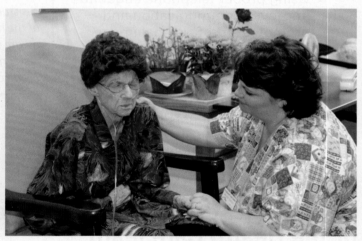

A   **B**

■ **FIGURE 4-5**

(A) Objective data. When you collect objective data, you obtain information by using one of your five senses. Here, the nursing assistant is feeling the resident's forehead to find out whether the skin is hot and dry or cool and clammy. Other examples of objective data include a person's vital sign measurements, the smell and color of a person's urine, the sound of a person's breathing, and the color and condition of a person's skin. **(B) Subjective data.** Subjective data are information that you get second-hand. This nursing assistant knows that her resident is experiencing stomach pain because the resident is describing it to her, not because she detected the resident's pain using one of her five senses. Other examples of subjective data include a person's complaint of a headache, feeling nauseated, or feeling dizzy.

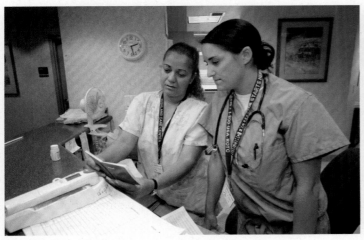
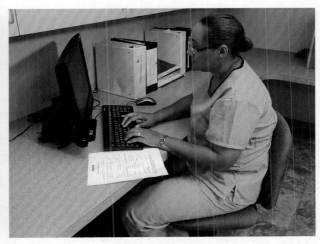

A   **B**

■ **FIGURE 4-6**

(A) Reporting is the spoken exchange of information between health care team members. Here, a nursing assistant is reporting a change in one of her resident's vital signs to the nurse. **(B) Recording** is communicating information about a patient or resident to other health care team members in written form. Here, a nursing assistant checks a resident's medical record.

care team members are kept "in-the-know." These methods are **reporting** and **recording** (Fig. 4-6).

Reporting

Nursing assistants use reporting to communicate information to the nurse throughout the shift. Reporting is also used when shifts change to keep the staff members who are just arriving at work aware of all the information that is necessary to ensure a smooth continuation of care for the patient or resident. Throughout this text, specific observations that need to be reported to the nurse immediately are highlighted as "Tell the Nurse!" notes.

When reporting, remember to be a good communicator (see Box 4-1). Make sure the information that you are reporting is accurate—refer to the patient or resident by name and room number, and if you are reporting measurements, such as vital signs, write the numbers down so that you do not forget them or report them incorrectly. Report your observations in an orderly, concise manner. Avoid adding information that is not relevant to what you are trying to communicate. Use correct terminology when reporting, and make sure that the person you are reporting to gives you feedback so that you know he or she received the information and will act on it.

Recording

MEDICAL RECORD (CHART). The **medical record** is usually organized in sections with specific forms contained in each section. Some of these forms provide general information about the patient or resident. Others are specific to a particular health care department. The forms used may vary depending on the type of facility or health care agency. Table 4-1 describes some of the forms that are typically found in a medical record.

Your employer will have specific policies about whether or not nursing assistants are allowed to record information in the medical record. If you are allowed

Reporting the spoken exchange of information between health care team members

Recording communicating information about a patient or resident to other health care team members in written form; sometimes called *charting or documenting*

Medical record a legal document where information about a patient's or resident's current condition, the measures that have been taken by the medical and nursing staff to diagnose and treat the condition, and the patient's or resident's response to the treatment and care provided is recorded; also called a *medical chart*

TABLE 4-1 — Forms Found in a Typical Medical Record (Chart)

Form	Purpose
Admission sheet	Contains standard information about the person, such as the person's name, address, age, gender, insurance information, emergency notification information, and advance directive information
Medical history	Lists a person's previous surgeries and medical conditions, current medications, allergies, and current medical diagnosis
Nursing history	Contains information about the person's needs as they relate to nursing care
Physician's order sheet	Used to order diagnostic tests and treatments and to specify dietary orders or activity status
Medication administration record (MAR)	Lists the medications ordered for the patient or resident, as well as the dose and time at which they are to be given; also used to record when medications were given and by whom. The electronic version of the MAR, sometimes referred to as the eMAR, is used by the person administering the medication at the person's bedside. The recorded information is then immediately saved to the person's electronic health record.
Physician's progress notes	Contains observations about the person's responses to treatments
Narrative nurse's notes	Used to document the person's complaints (symptoms) and the actions taken by the nursing staff in response to them
Graphic sheet	Contains information that is gathered routinely, such as vital signs, the frequency of urination and bowel movements, and food and fluid intake

Tell the Nurse!

In general, you need to report the following types of observations to the nurse immediately:

- Observations that suggest a change in the patient's or resident's condition
- Observations regarding the patient's or resident's response to a new treatment or therapy
- A patient's or resident's complaints of pain or discomfort
- A patient's or resident's refusal of treatment
- A patient's or resident's request for clergy

Electronic health record (EHR) a computer information system that stores and saves a person's medical information

to record information in the medical record, remember that the medical record is a formal record of the care the person received from the health care facility, and it can be retrieved at any time and used in a court of law as evidence in a lawsuit. For this reason, it is important to follow the guidelines in Guidelines Box 4-1 for recording.

The information contained in a person's medical record is considered confidential and is only to be read by members of the health care team who are directly involved in the care of that person and need access to the information in the record to provide that care. For example, although a custodial worker is part of the health care team, he or she does not need access to the information in the medical record to perform his or her duties. Therefore, custodial workers generally do not have access to patients' or residents' charts.

Most health care settings are managing patient's and resident's records electronically using computers. An **electronic health record (EHR)** maintains a person's medical record by having data entered into a computer in response to the computer's prompts, rather than filling out a paper form. Medical records created in this way tend to be more accurate and legible because they are typed rather than handwritten. The advantages to using electronic health record systems are:

- The patient's or resident's health record is easily and quickly accessible to the health care team members involved in the person's care.
- The patient's or resident's admission information, such as address or next of kin, can be updated quickly and the changes are immediately accessible to all of the people involved in that person's care.

GUIDELINES BOX 4-1   Guidelines for Recording

What you do	Why you do it
Write legibly, using dark blue or black ink, according to facility policy.	*It is important to write legibly to avoid miscommunication. A pen is used instead of a pencil because pencil can be erased, allowing someone to change the person's medical record. Dark blue and black ink reproduce best when a document is photocopied.*
Always sign or initial your entry, according to facility policy.	*By signing or initialing your entry, you indicate that you are the person who needs to be consulted if further clarification of the information you have entered is necessary. In addition, signing or initialing your entry indicates that you accept legal responsibility for what you have written.*
Only record observations that you have made, or care that you have given. Do not make entries for another person.	*By making an entry in a medical record, you accept legal responsibility for that entry. Therefore, it is best to record only information that you, personally, can vouch for.*
Date and time your entries correctly (see below).	*The date and time that actions occurred or observations were made are extremely important elements of the medical record, which is a legal account of care provided.*
Check the patient's or resident's name on the medical record and on the form where you are recording.	*By verifying the patient's or resident's identification information, you will ensure that you are recording the person's information in the correct medical record.*
Use appropriate medical terminology and facility-approved abbreviations when recording.	*Using correct terminology and abbreviations will prevent others from having to second-guess your meaning.*
Do not record care as given or procedures as performed before you have provided the care or performed the procedure. Only document after the fact.	*You may become distracted or involved in another situation that prevents you from carrying out the duties you have already charted. If you record duties as "completed" in the medical record, but then do not actually complete these duties, you will have committed fraud.*
Record information in a timely manner. If you must wait to record something, keep notes about your observations and care so that the information you record in the medical record will be accurate.	*If you wait until the end of your shift to record, you may forget important information.*
If you make an error, do not erase, use correction fluid to cover, or scribble through the mistaken entry. Simply draw a line through the mistake and initial it according to facility policy.	*Striking through an error is the only legal way to indicate a change in the medical record. Erasing or using correction fluid to correct an error could be seen as an attempt to hide or change existing information.*

(*box continues on page 74*)

GUIDELINES BOX 4-1 Guidelines for Recording (continued)

What you do

Remember that in a liability situation, care not recorded was care not provided.

If your facility uses computerized recording, never give anyone else your password or leave the computer active after you have used it.

Why you do it

Proper and conscientious recording of patient or resident information protects the patient or resident, your employer, and you.

If you fail to log off after using the computer, the information on the screen may be accessible to people who are not authorized to have access to it. In addition, if you fail to log off when you are finished with the computer, someone else could enter information under your password, and it will appear that you have entered it.

How to Record Time

Most facilities use the 24-hour time clock ("military time") to record the time in a person's medical record. With the 24-hour time clock, it is not necessary to note whether the time is in the morning (AM) or evening (PM) because each hour has its own specific number.

When time is stated according to the 24-hour time clock, the first two numbers indicate the hour and the last two numbers indicate the minute. On the 24-hour time clock, the hours from 1:00 AM to 12:00 PM (noon) are the same as on a regular clock. To indicate a time between 1:00 PM and 12:00 AM (midnight), add "12" to the time on the regular clock.

Examples are as follows:

Regular Clock Time	24-Hour Time
2:00 AM	0200
2:00 PM	1400
2:24 AM	0224
2:24 PM	1424

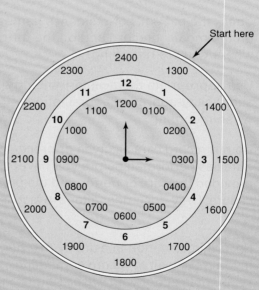

Regular Clock Time	24-Hour Time
1:00 AM	0100
2:00 AM	0200
3:00 AM	0300
4:00 AM	0400
5:00 AM	0500
6:00 AM	0600
7:00 AM	0700
8:00 AM	0800
9:00 AM	0900
10:00 AM	1000
11:00 AM	1100
12:00 PM (noon)	1200
1:00 PM	1300
2:00 PM	1400
3:00 PM	1500
4:00 PM	1600
5:00 PM	1700
6:00 PM	1800
7:00 PM	1900
8:00 PM	2000
9:00 PM	2100
10:00 PM	2200
11:00 PM	2300
12:00 AM (midnight)	2400

- Information such as a person's vital signs and intake and output can be recorded at the person's bedside using portable tablets or bedside computer terminals.
- Doctor's orders for dietary changes, medications, lab requests, and treatments are immediately sent to the appropriate departments.

To protect the patient's or resident's confidentiality, each user of the computer or EHR system is assigned a password, which permits the user to have access to certain patients' or residents' medical records. Your facility will have specific policies—mandated by the Health Insurance Portability and Accountability Act (HIPAA)—regarding computer use and confidentiality. Make sure that you are familiar with these policies, and follow them carefully.

KARDEX. The **Kardex** card provides a one-page summary of the patient's or resident's condition and care needs. The Kardex may be available either in a printed paper format or in an electronic format in the person's EHR. Members of the health care team can check the Kardex card instead of searching through the entire record every time they need information about the person's status and care plan.

Kardex a card file that contains condensed versions of each patient's or resident's medical record

Putting it all together!

- Reporting and recording are two methods of communication used by the health care team to make sure that everyone involved in the care of a patient or resident has current, reliable information about that person. Reporting is the spoken exchange of information between members of the health care team. Recording is the written exchange of information between members of the health care team.
- Observations may be subjective or objective. Observations are reported, recorded, or both. Observations about a change in a person's condition must be reported to the nurse immediately.
- As the member of the health care team with the most opportunity to interact with the patients or residents, you will be in a unique position to observe changes in your patients' or residents' physical or emotional status and report these observations to the nurse.

WHAT DID YOU LEARN?

Multiple Choice

Select the single best answer for each of the following questions.

1. Which one of the following is an open-ended question?
   a. "Are you Mrs. Brown?"
   b. "Mr. Jones, when you were growing up, what was your favorite meal?"
   c. "Are you feeling okay, Mrs. Smith?"
   d. "It's beautiful outside today, Mrs. Murphy! Do you want to go for a walk?"

2. Which one of the following is an example of positive body language?
   a. Nodding encouragingly as someone speaks
   b. Crossing your arms across your chest
   c. Tapping your feet or fingers
   d. Rolling your eyes

3. An example of an action that blocks effective communication is:
   a. Interrupting
   b. Not listening carefully
   c. Being judgmental
   d. All of the above

4. Which one of the following is an example of objective data?
   a. "Mr. Wohl says that his back hurts when he coughs."
   b. "Ms. O'Connell's urine is cloudy, and has a strong odor."
   c. "Mr. McAndrews is complaining of a headache."
   d. "The resident in room 201B is complaining of a stomachache."

5. Which one of the following is an example of nonverbal communication?
   a. Using sign language to communicate with a deaf person
   b. Recording vital sign measurements in a patient's or resident's chart
   c. Gently touching a patient or resident on the shoulder to reassure her
   d. Making a telephone call

6. What usually forms the basis for subjective data?
   a. A symptom or a patient or resident complaint
   b. A measurement
   c. A doctor's order
   d. All of the above

7. Michael is taking care of Miss Jordan, who has a hearing loss. Miss Jordan is wearing her hearing aid, but it does not seem to be working. What should Michael do first?
   a. He should raise his voice.
   b. He should make sure that the hearing aid is turned on and that the volume is high enough.
   c. He should remove the hearing aid and replace its batteries.
   d. He should report the problem to the nurse immediately.

8. With regard to telephone communication, nursing assistants are responsible for all of the following except:
   a. Writing down the caller's name and telephone number if the person the caller wants to speak to is not available, and delivering this message to the intended recipient
   b. Answering the telephone promptly, with a pleasant greeting
   c. Taking down doctor's orders if the nurse is not available and a doctor calls
   d. Identifying themselves to the caller by name and title, per facility policy

9. When recording information in a person's medical chart, what should you remember to do?
   a. Use pencil so that errors can be corrected neatly
   b. Sign or initial and date and time your entry, per facility policy
   c. Update all of your patients' or residents' charts at one time at the end of each shift
   d. All of the above

10. What is it called when people have differences and they are unable to come to an agreement?
   a. Communication
   b. Conflict
   c. Culture
   d. Personality difference

11. Mr. Campi, one of your elderly residents, is very hard of hearing. What should you remember when you are talking to Mr. Campi?
   a. You should sit or stand so that Mr. Campi has a clear view of your face, and you should avoid chewing gum or speaking quickly.
   b. If you think that Mr. Campi has not completely understood what you are saying, you should demand that he repeat it back to you so that you can correct his mistakes.
   c. If you do not understand what Mr. Campi has said, you should just let it pass. Letting him know that you did not understand might embarrass or frustrate him.
   d. There is no point in talking to Mr. Campi. He cannot hear you anyway. It is better to just write everything down.

Matching

Match each form typically found in a medical record with its description.

_____ **1.** Admission sheet

_____ **2.** Narrative nurse's notes

_____ **3.** Medical history

_____ **4.** Physician's order sheet

_____ **5.** Graphic sheet

a. Used to document the person's complaints and the actions that were taken by the nursing team in response to them

b. Used to record routine data, such as vital signs, frequency of urination and bowel movements, and food and fluid intake

c. Used to order diagnostic tests and treatments and to specify dietary orders or activity status

d. Lists a person's previous surgeries and medical conditions, current medications, allergies, and current medical diagnosis

e. Contains standard information about the patient or resident, such as his or her name and address

Stop *and* Think!

■ You are caring for Mr. Thompson today and notice that he seems distracted and is having difficulty speaking clearly. You know that you should report this to the nurse immediately. What other subjective and objective data should you gather to report to the nurse? How can you make sure that the nurse receives the information from you?

■ You work in the rehabilitation unit of a long-term care facility and have become quite comfortable with the electronic health record computer system that it has recently started using. You like that you can use the bedside computer terminals to record your resident's vital signs and other information on the nurse's progress notes. One of your co-workers has struggled with the new computerized charting system and keeps telling you that she would rather keep using the "old fashioned" method of writing her notes in the person's records. Today, your co-worker comes to you asking to use your user name and password because she cannot remember hers, and she really needs to get her vital signs and care procedures recorded. What should you do?

Those We Care For

As you are probably beginning to realize, there is much more to being a nursing assistant than blood pressures and bedpans. Those in need of health care services are not merely defined by their illnesses and disabilities. First and foremost, patients, residents, and clients are *people*. In this chapter, we will take a closer look at some of the things that all people have in common, as well as some of the things that make us different.

Photo: *Throughout the course of our lives, we pass through a series of stages. Here, members from the same family represent the stages of school age, adolescence, young adulthood, and middle adulthood. (©Jupiter Images)*

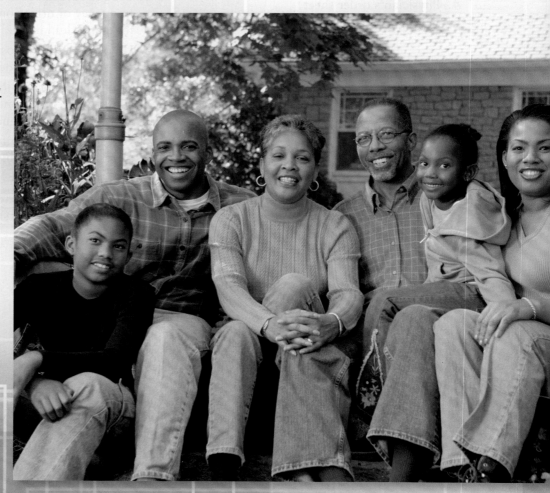

Growth and Development

What will you learn?

When you are finished with this section, you will be able to:
1. List and briefly describe the stages of human growth and development.
2. Define the words **growth**, **development**, and **tasks**.

Throughout our lives, we are constantly changing, from the moment our life begins until the moment it ends. This process of change is called **growth** and **development**. Growth is shown by changes in height and weight and by physical changes in the body's organ systems. Development is shown by changes in a person's behavior and way of thinking.

The process of growth and development is divided into stages of normal progression (Table 5-1). Although the stages of growth and development can be generalized by age, it is important to note that each person progresses through the stages at his or her own pace. A person cannot progress to the next stage without successfully completing the **tasks** associated with the stage he or she is currently in. With young children and teenagers, it is quite common to see some overlap in the stages. This is because growth and development occur unevenly or in spurts, with one part occurring faster than the other.

Growth changes that occur physically as a person passes through life

Development changes that occur psychologically or socially as a person passes through life

Tasks growth and development milestones that must be completed before a person can move on to the next stage of growth and development

TABLE 5-1 Stages of Growth and Development

	Name of Stage	Approximate Age	Major Growth Tasks	Major Development Tasks
	Infancy	Birth to 1 year	New tasks are accomplished on a weekly and monthly basis; by his first birthday, an infant will typically weigh three times what he did when he was born, and he will have progressed from a totally helpless newborn to a child learning how to walk and feed himself	The infant begins to smile, laugh, recognize parents and siblings, and say simple words

(*table continues on page 80*)

TABLE 5-1 **Stages of Growth and Development** (continued)

	Name of Stage	Approximate Age	Major Growth Tasks	Major Development Tasks
	Toddlerhood	1 to 3 years	Growth of the muscular and nervous systems allows the toddler to become quite active Toilet training begins as control over bladder and bowel function becomes physically possible	The toddler is able to express himself in short, complete sentences and becomes quite expressive of his emotions
	Preschool	3 to 5 years	Physical coordination continues to improve, allowing the preschooler to dress himself and tie his own shoes Toileting becomes more independent	The preschooler likes to play with other children and uses his active imagination to create detailed play stories and scenes Curiosity about the differences between boys and girls develops
	School age	5 to 12 years	Several major growth spurts lead to increases in both height and weight As fine motor skills develop, the ability to write and draw improves	Play usually involves groups of same-sex friends Logical thinking patterns develop, and the school-age child is able to incorporate other people's perspectives into her own thinking
	Adolescence	12 to 20 years	Secondary sex characteristics develop and reproductive organs begin to function (puberty occurs)	The adolescent is likely to question authority Many adolescents take jobs, learn to drive, and begin to make plans for the future

	Name of Stage	Approximate Age	Major Growth Tasks	Major Development Tasks
	Young adulthood	20 to 40 years	Physical changes during this stage are usually minor, with the exception of pregnancy in women	The young adult focuses on completing his education, starting a career, and possibly, finding a life partner
	Middle adulthood	40 to 65 years	Early signs of aging, such as wrinkles or a few gray hairs, may start to appear Although good health is usually still enjoyed, some chronic illnesses, such as hypertension and diabetes, may be diagnosed during this stage Menopause occurs in women	Many middle adults have raised their families and now have more time to reconnect as a couple and pursue their own interests and hobbies; however, many middle adults find themselves caring for their own children as well as their aging parents Many people become grandparents during this stage
	Later adulthood	65 to 75 years	Physical signs of aging become more obvious, and the development of chronic illnesses becomes more common Strength diminishes, as do many senses, such as hearing and sight	Retirement gives the person an opportunity to travel and pursue hobbies Many people must cope with the death of a friend or a spouse
	Older adulthood	75 years +	Chronic illnesses may become more severe. Falls resulting in broken bones are common. The older adult may need assistance with routine activities, such as eating, bathing, and toileting	Many older adults enjoy sharing the wisdom of their years with younger people Although some older adults continue to be healthy and independent, many must adjust to failing health and a growing dependency on others A primary task during this stage is preparing for one's own death

Putting it all together!

- The process of growth and development is divided into stages of normal progression: infancy, toddlerhood, preschool, school age, adolescence, young adulthood, middle adulthood, later adulthood, and older adulthood.

- As a person moves through life, the growth and development changes that occur affect the type of care the person needs and the way we communicate with him or her. Becoming familiar with the various stages of growth and development will help you become a better caregiver.

Basic Human Needs

What will you learn?

When you have finished with this section, you will be able to:

1. Draw Maslow's hierarchy of human needs and explain each level.
2. Describe ways that a nursing assistant helps patients and residents to meet their needs.
3. Define the word **needs**.

Need something that is essential for a person's physical and mental health

The primary focus of health care is to help provide for patients' or residents' physical and emotional **needs**. Abraham Maslow (1908–1970), an American psychologist, defined what he thought to be the basic human needs, and then arranged them in a pyramid to show that some needs are more basic than other needs (Fig. 5-1). Maslow's pyramid, called *Maslow's hierarchy of human needs*, reflects Maslow's belief that the more basic, lower-level needs must be met before the higher-level needs can be met. Many people can meet their needs with little or no outside help. But people who are ill, injured, or disabled must rely on the health care team to make sure that their needs are met.

Physiologic Needs

At the most basic level, we need oxygen, water, food, sleep, exercise, and shelter to survive (see Fig. 5-1). We also need the ability to remove waste products from our bodies. Meeting these physiologic, or physical, needs is of the highest priority because unless these needs are met, we will die. Assisting with meals, toileting, and ambulating and providing a relaxing environment in which to sleep are just some of the many ways you will help people to meet their most basic needs.

Safety and Security Needs

As a nursing assistant, you will follow many policies and procedures that are designed to keep your patients or residents safe, such as making sure that a resident who needs a walker to walk always has the walker nearby (see Fig. 5-1). Safety and security needs are both physical and emotional. When you help your patients

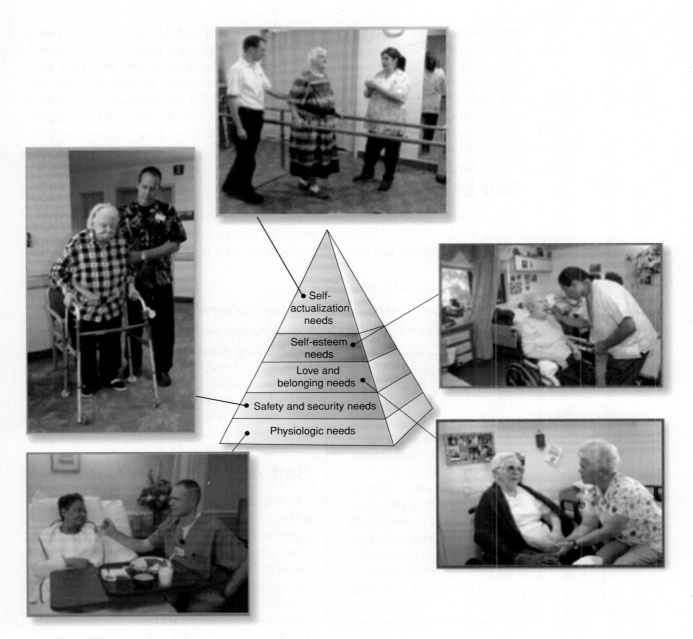

■ **FIGURE 5-1**

Maslow's pyramid. Basic needs (the needs at the bottom of the pyramid) must be met before more complex needs (the ones toward the top of the pyramid) can be met. Patients and residents who are not able to meet their needs on their own rely on members of the health care team to recognize and help meet these needs for them.

or residents to *be* safe, they also *feel* safe. They are able to relax and trust that you will take good care of them.

Love and Belonging Needs

All people need to feel loved, accepted, and appreciated by others. We need to feel that we are part of an accepting group. People meet this need for one another by showing affection and forming close (intimate) relationships. When our love and belonging need is unmet, feelings of loneliness and isolation develop. Being a patient or a resident in a health care facility can cause a person to feel isolated, unlovable, and unappreciated. Patients and residents often feel that they have become a medical condition instead of a person. By taking an interest in the person and showing respect for the person's specific likes and dislikes, you can help to meet that person's love and belonging needs. A smile, a kind word, or a gentle touch can go a long way toward making someone feel loved, appreciated, and like he or she "belongs" (see Fig. 5-1).

Self-Esteem Needs

Self-esteem is influenced by how people think of themselves and how they think others think of them. Everyone wants to be respected and thought well of by others. Many things can affect the self-esteem of a person who is receiving health care, such as:

- Having to wear a hospital gown
- Having surgery that might cause the person's appearance to change
- Having to depend on others for something one used to be able to do for oneself

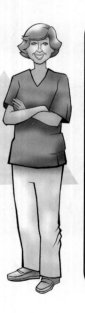

The needs of the people you care for will change as their conditions get better or worse. By helping people to meet their most basic needs first, you will help them to meet their higher-level needs. For example, it is difficult to work on a person's self-esteem if he is struggling to breathe! Recognizing needs that people have difficulty meeting on their own and helping them to meet these needs is one of the most valuable contributions you will make as a nursing assistant.

Nursing assistants help to preserve their patients' and residents' self-esteem by providing for privacy when it is necessary to expose someone's body, by allowing people to wear their own clothing whenever possible, and by assisting people with basic grooming (see Fig. 5-1).

Self-Actualization Needs

The highest level on the hierarchy of needs is self-actualization. To achieve self-actualization, a person must reach his or her fullest potential. Most of us try throughout life to meet this need because we are constantly setting new goals for ourselves. As a nursing assistant, you will have the chance to help the people you care for achieve self-actualization by helping them to set small, realistic goals for a positive outcome. For example, when you encourage a person who has had a stroke to practice exercises learned in physical therapy, you are helping that person to get one step closer to his or her goal of being able to be independent again (see Fig. 5-1).

Putting it all together!

- People in health care settings have many different physical and emotional needs. Basic needs must be met before higher-level needs can be met.
- As a nursing assistant, you will help your patients or residents to meet their physiologic needs, their safety and security needs, their love and belonging needs, their self-esteem needs, and their self-actualization needs.

Human Sexuality and Intimacy

What will you learn?

When you have finished with this section, you will be able to:

1. Understand the difference between sex and sexuality.
2. Discuss ways in which nursing assistants help patients and residents to fulfill their need to be thought of as sexual beings and engage in intimate relationships with others.
3. Define the words **sexuality**, **intimacy**, **sex**, and **masturbation**.

Sexuality and **intimacy** are basic human needs, common to all people, young and old. Sexuality and intimacy are not the same as **sex**, although a person's sexuality does influence who he or she is sexually attracted to, and sex is a part of some intimate relationships.

Sexuality is an inborn part of our personalities. A person's sexuality can be influenced by many factors, including the person's culture and religious beliefs. From birth, we are surrounded by symbols of our sexuality—little boys receive baseball mitts and miniature toolboxes "just like Dad's"; little girls receive dolls and tea sets (Fig. 5-2). We grow up being taught by our parents and peers what is appropriate behavior for a "little girl" or for a "big boy." As we progress through the developmental stages of life, we develop personal ideas and beliefs about our own sexuality.

As a nursing assistant, you will meet people whose feelings about their sexuality and the ways in which they express these feelings might be very different from your feelings about your sexuality and the way you express those feelings. You must avoid being judgmental or critical of how another person chooses to express his or her sexuality. Acceptance of another person's views does not mean that you approve of that person's beliefs and practices. It only means that you respect that person's right to make his or her own decisions.

There are many ways that, as a nursing assistant, you can help patients and residents to fulfill their need to be thought of as sexual beings and to engage in intimate relationships with others:

- Avoid being judgmental.
- Help your patients and residents with rituals that make them feel either feminine or masculine, such as dressing and applying make-up, perfume, or aftershave lotion.

Sexuality how a person perceives his or her maleness or femaleness

Intimacy a feeling of emotional closeness to another human being

Sex the physical activity one engages in to obtain sexual pleasure and reproduce

■ **FIGURE 5-2**
Society influences our ideas about our sexuality from an early age.

Masturbation stimulation of the genitals for sexual pleasure or release by a means other than sexual intercourse

Concerns for Long-Term Care

Sexuality and intimacy are basic human needs for *all* people, including elderly people. Many elderly people are involved in, or will begin, intimate relationships, which may or may not involve sexual activity (Fig. 5-3). As we age, we still maintain an image of how we feel about our own sexuality and sexual intimacy. The desire to be clean, well groomed, and dressed attractively remains. An older person who enjoyed sexual intimacy when he or she was younger will still have those needs. Many elderly people have health problems and reduced mobility or movement of the joints that can make sexual intercourse uncomfortable. As a result, sexual intimacy does not always involve sexual intercourse. An elderly person may take great comfort in being intimate in ways such as cuddling, touching, or caressing. **Masturbation**, either mutual or alone, is another way that elderly people can help to meet their sexual needs.

If you work in a long-term care facility, you must take into consideration your residents' needs for sexuality and intimacy. The Omnibus Budget Reconciliation Act (OBRA) requires that long-term care facilities allow married residents to share the same room and the same bed if their health allows. But what about unmarried residents? If two unmarried residents wish to begin a sexually intimate relationship, then this must be allowed and privacy provided. However, both residents must enter the relationship willingly. If you suspect that one resident is taking advantage of another resident, then you should report this to the nurse.

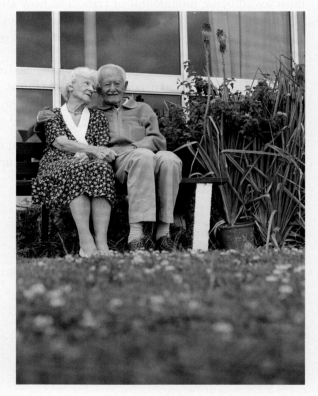

■ **FIGURE 5-3**

Sexuality and intimacy are basic human needs for everyone, young and old.

■ Allow for privacy. If the person is in a private room, close the door and use a "do not disturb" sign as the person requests. If the person has a roommate, suggest to the roommate that the two of you take a walk or participate in another activity outside of the room. Privacy is necessary for people in intimate relationships, whether or not the relationship involves sex. It is also necessary for people who want to engage in masturbation.

■ If a person is masturbating in a public room (some confused patients or residents will do this), take the person to his or her room and provide for safety and privacy.

■ Always knock before entering a person's room. If you do interrupt a sexual encounter, excuse yourself quietly and say you will return later.

Some people become sexually aggressive and will behave in an unwelcome way toward you or another patient or resident. It is important for you to be able to recognize situations that could be considered sexual abuse or assault. Although it is inappropriate for you to attend to the sexual needs of your patients or residents, it is important to avoid being unkind or hateful in your response. Depending on the situation, tell the patient or resident kindly, yet firmly, that you are not going to do what he or she is asking you to do, or that he or she must not touch you in that manner. Avoid giggling or teasing the patient or resident. This will only reinforce the inappropriate behavior. If the behavior does not stop, or if the behavior is directed at another patient or resident, discuss the matter with your supervisor.

Putting it all together!

■ Sexuality is how a person feels about his or her maleness or femaleness. Sexuality differs from intimacy (the need to feel close to another person) and from sex (a physical act engaged in for pleasure and reproduction). Sexuality and intimacy are basic human needs.

■ As a nursing assistant, you must avoid being judgmental or critical of how another person chooses to express his or her sexuality.

■ A person's feelings of sexuality and the need for intimacy continue through the older years.

■ Assisting with grooming routines and providing for privacy are two ways nursing assistants help patients or residents fulfill their sexuality and intimacy needs.

Culture and Religion

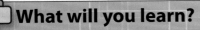

What will you learn?

When you are finished with this section, you will be able to:

1. Discuss how culture and religion can affect how a person views illness and health care.

2. Understand why it is important for health care workers to recognize their patients' and residents' cultural and religious differences.

3. Define the words **culture**, **race**, and **religion**.

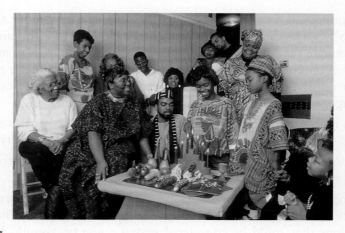

■ **FIGURE 5-4**

This African-American family is celebrating Kwanzaa, a holiday celebrated by Africans and people of African descent throughout the world. Kwanzaa, a celebration of African history and culture, with a special emphasis on family life, occurs from December 26 through January 1. Kwanzaa is a cultural holiday, not a religious one. Celebrants are united by their African heritage, not their religion.
©Lawrence Migdale.

Culture the beliefs (including religious or spiritual beliefs), values, and traditions that are customary to a group of people; a view of the world that is handed down from generation to generation

Race a general characterization that describes skin color, body stature, facial features, and hair texture

Religion a person's spiritual beliefs

All people have a **culture**, although everyone's culture is not the same. A culture can be shared by people of the same **race** or ethnicity, by people who live within the same geographic area or speak the same language, or by a combination of these two (Fig. 5-4).

Many different cultures are represented here in the United States. As a health care worker, it is important for you to learn as much as possible about the characteristics of other cultural or ethnic groups of people because your patients or residents will have cultural differences that may affect their preferences regarding health care. In addition, a primary goal of the nursing team is to provide for the comfort of those we care for. A person who feels that his culture is not understood or respected by the people who are caring for him will feel uncomfortable.

There are many ways in which a health care worker can accidentally be disrespectful of a patient's or resident's culture, which can lead to conflict. Sometimes, misunderstandings occur simply because a health care worker is not aware of how a certain person's culture influences his behavior. Although it is difficult to make generalizations about culture—not everyone from the same geographic region, or with the same skin tone, necessarily has the same beliefs or value system—being aware of what a patient or resident is telling you can help you to know when cultural differences need to be taken into account. Areas in which culture and health care often intersect include beliefs and practices associated with food and meals; religious beliefs and practices; and attitudes toward health, sickness, and death.

A person's **religion** is often very closely linked with his or her culture. Many people are very spiritual and find comfort and solace in prayer, reading scriptures or spiritual books, singing, and praying. You may care for patients or residents whose religious beliefs are very different from yours, but you can be certain that their beliefs are as important to them as yours are to you. Helping a person to be comforted by his spiritual beliefs does not mean that you need to share those beliefs. It only means that you respect the person's right to have those beliefs and to seek comfort from them (Fig. 5-5). If a patient or resident asks to see a spiritual

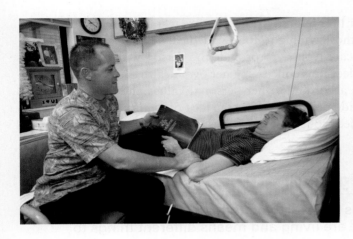

■ **FIGURE 5-5**
A nursing assistant can help people to obtain comfort from their religious beliefs, even if he does not share those same beliefs.

leader or clergy member, communicate the request promptly and according to your facility's policy, and allow for privacy during the visit.

 Putting it all together!

- Culture is made up of the beliefs, values, and traditions that are customary to a group of people.
- Problems can arise when people are not sensitive to, or respectful of, the cultural uniqueness of each person.

Quality of Life

What will you learn?

When you are finished with this section, you will be able to:
1. Explain the concept of "quality of life."
2. Explain why it is important for health care workers to respect patients' and residents' decisions regarding their own quality of life.

A holistic approach to health care takes into consideration a person's emotional needs as well as his or her physical ones. To provide holistic care for your patients or residents, you must respect their decisions related to maintaining their quality of life. Quality of life has to do with getting satisfaction and comfort from the way we are living. The idea of what quality of life means is different for each person and may change as a person's situation changes.

As a nursing assistant, you will learn that a person who has diabetes must control his or her diet carefully. You will learn that a person with heart disease should stop smoking. But what if your patient or resident does not follow the recommendations of the health care team? Is a woman with diabetes a bad person if she truly loves sweets and does not want to give them up? Is a man with heart disease a bad person if he continues to smoke? What if a person refuses a treatment or surgery that may prolong his or her life? Should the health care team simply write that person off and focus only on those willing to follow medical advice?

The role of the health care team is to provide the person with all of the information she needs to make decisions concerning her own health. But then the person must make these decisions according to her personal values and sense of what is best for herself, as an individual. This is where the idea of *quality of life* comes into play. It is important to respect your patients' or residents' decisions, even if you do not agree with them.

Putting it all together!

- Quality of life has to do with getting satisfaction and comfort from the way we are living and means different things to different people.
- Allowing patients and residents to make decisions related to their quality of life is an important part of providing holistic care.

What Is It Like to Be a Patient or Resident?

What will you learn?

When you are finished with this section, you will be able to:

1. Understand how being a patient or resident can affect how a person acts toward others.
2. Understand how it might feel to be a patient or a resident.
3. Discuss how family members may be affected by a person's illness or disability.

What is it like to be a patient? Patients feel scared and lonely. They feel sick. They are unsure about their health, now and in the future. Some patients worry about whether they will be able to return to work, and they may be concerned about how the cost of their medical care will affect their family finances. Others worry about how their illness (or its treatment) will affect their physical appearance. Patients worry about spouses, children, and pets at home and whether they are being cared for properly. They worry about the emotional effects of their illness on their family members. The hospital environment itself can be frightening and uncomfortable, full of strange noises and smells. If you were in this circumstance, how would you feel and how might this affect your behavior?

Similarly, what is it like to be a resident? Imagine what it would be like to have to move from a home you loved to a long-term care facility. You really liked your house with your cat and the shady back porch where you could sit on hot summer evenings. Now, you are not managing as well as you once did—you have fallen twice, and left the stove on a few times and forgotten about it. Even though you know that it makes sense to move to a place where there is always someone around to "take care of you," when you gave up your home, you gave up a certain amount of your independence along with it. You cannot take all of your furniture, and you must find a new home for your pet cat. You have a roommate (at your age!) and you have to eat the meals that are prepared for you, when they are served to you. Gone are the lazy summer evenings eating peaches on the porch for dinner and relaxing in the bathtub with a glass of wine. How would you feel about this loss of independence, and how might this affect your behavior?

Although some patients and residents are pleasant and grateful, others may be depressed, angry, anxious, or just mean. When you must care for a patient or resident who makes you wish you had never chosen to be a nursing assistant (and you can be certain you *will* encounter patients or residents like this), stop and think for a moment about the reasons that person may be acting out of sorts. When you look into that person's eyes, you will find your reason for choosing to be a nursing assistant . . . a person who needs you very much.

When you are providing care for a person in a health care setting, you must always remember to consider the impact that person's illness or disability can have on his or her family members and loved ones. Families, just like patients and residents, are very diverse and deal with illness and disability in many different ways. Most family members experience a sense of helplessness when someone they care for is sick. Family members may feel guilty that they are no longer able to care for an aging parent at home and now have to place him or her in a long-term care facility. These feelings may cause them to behave in ways you think are unusual. They may act angry or overly protective, and it will be important that you do not take their actions personally.

If the patient or resident consents, it is very important for family members to be included in their care decisions. If the person is a resident of a long-term care facility, family members are encouraged to participate in the interdisciplinary care planning meetings and to be involved in helping to develop the resident's care plan. If you are able to allow family members to participate in the patient's or the resident's care as much as possible, it can help them to regain some sense of usefulness and control. Make sure that you listen to a family member's suggestions, especially when it concerns the patient's or resident's personal preferences. In reality, you do not just provide care for the patient or resident, you also must consider the needs of the person's family.

 ## Putting it all together!

- Adjusting to a new role—that of someone who needs the services of the health care industry—can be very difficult. Illness, disability, pain, fear, and loss of independence can cause some patients or residents to act unpleasantly toward you.

- Try to practice empathy by imagining yourself in the patient's or resident's situation. This might help you understand behavior that is not fair or appropriate.

- It is important for you to recognize the impact that illness or disability has on a patient's or a resident's family members.

WHAT DID YOU LEARN?

Multiple Choice

Select the single best answer for each of the following questions.

1. Sally is caring for Mrs. Norville, who lives in a long-term care facility. Sally encourages Mrs. Norville to make her own decisions about what to do each day. She helps her with dressing and grooming, but lets her do as much as she can for herself. These activities help fulfill Mrs. Norville's need for:
   a. Security
   b. Shelter
   c. Spirituality
   d. Self-esteem

2. When caring for people from different cultures, you should try to:
   a. Understand and respect their special needs
   b. Encourage them to change their beliefs while in your facility
   c. Pretend that the cultural differences do not exist
   d. Avoid talking to them

3. A resident's religion forbids him from eating pork. Pork chops are being served for dinner. What should you do?
   a. Tell the resident that religious restrictions on diet do not count in times of illness
   b. Ask the nurse to call the dietary department
   c. Insist that the resident eat the pork because it contains protein, an essential nutrient
   d. Reassure the resident by telling him that the doctor ordered this diet

4. A resident in a long-term care facility may show her sexuality by doing all of the following except:
   a. Desiring sexual intercourse
   b. Engaging in public fondling
   c. Giving her granddaughter a doll for her birthday
   d. Applying make-up and scented powder before receiving a male visitor

5. Which one of the following is a basic physical need?
   a. Fear
   b. Self-actualization
   c. Self-esteem
   d. Water

6. Which one of the following is a basic social need?
   a. Food
   b. Water
   c. Air
   d. Love

Matching

Match each person with his or her stage of growth and development.

_____	**1.** A 16-year-old girl going to the junior prom	**a.** Infancy
_____	**2.** A 42-year-old executive running his own company	**b.** Toddlerhood
_____	**3.** A 2-year-old boy starting toilet training	**c.** Preschool
_____	**4.** A 6-month-old girl learning to sit up	**d.** School age
_____	**5.** A 92-year-old great-grandmother moving to a long-term care facility	**e.** Adolescence
_____	**6.** A 4-year-old boy learning to tie his shoes	**f.** Middle adulthood
_____	**7.** An 11-year-old Boy Scout participating in his troop's annual canned food drive	**g.** Older adulthood

 Stop *and* **Think!**

You are caring for Mr. Spencer, whose wife passed away several years ago. When you enter his room, after knocking to announce yourself, you find Mr. Spencer being fondled by Miss Rich, another resident. You are embarrassed, as well as somewhat disgusted—you were raised to believe that sex is something that only married people engage in. What should you do?

The Patient's or Resident's Environment

In this chapter, we will take a closer look at the physical environment in a health care setting and how that environment can affect a person's well-being. We will also provide an overview of the standard equipment and furniture that are typically found in a patient's or resident's room.

Photo: *The patient's or resident's room is considered the person's home.*

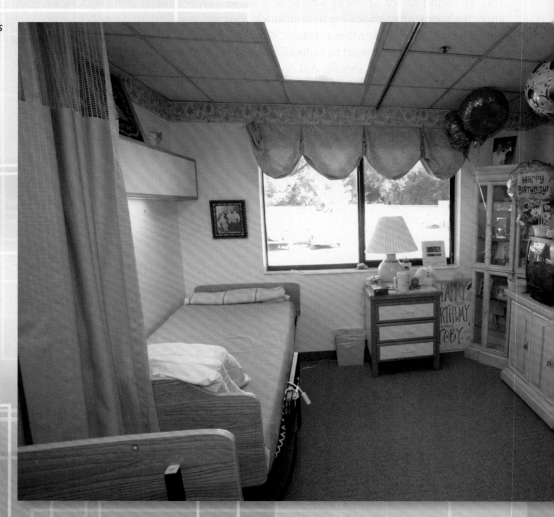

The Physical Environment

What will you learn?

When you are finished with this section, you will be able to:

1. Discuss aspects of the physical environment that affect safety and comfort.
2. Understand your role in helping to keep the patient's or resident's environment safe and comfortable.
3. Discuss the Omnibus Budget Reconciliation Act (OBRA) regulations relating to the physical environment in long-term care facilities.

Environmental conditions, such as a facility's cleanliness, temperature, lighting, and noise level, affect safety and comfort. To ensure the safety and comfort of patients and residents, health care facilities set policies that regulate the physical environment. In long-term care facilities, standards for the resident's environment are set by the Omnibus Budget Reconciliation Act (OBRA) (Box 6-1).

Cleanliness

A health care facility must be clean and neat. Cleanliness is essential for controlling the spread of infection. In addition, one standard people use to judge the care provided by a facility is the facility's cleanliness.

BOX 6-1 **Aspects of the Resident's Environment Regulated by OBRA**

- The size of the room.
- The lighting that must be available.
- The temperature at which the facility must be maintained (between 71°F and 81°F).
- The measures that must be taken to maintain air quality.
- The measures that must be taken to control noise.
- The types of furnishings and equipment that must be present.
- The types of modifications to the room that must be present to ensure safety (such as handrails and a call light or intercom system in the bathroom).
- The minimal amount of personal space for storage of belongings that each resident is allowed to have.
- The ability to provide privacy for each resident.
- The measures that must be taken to keep each resident's unit safe, clean, orderly, and free of obstacles where people must walk.

Members of the housekeeping (custodial) staff are responsible for routine cleaning. However, each member of the health care team also has responsibilities related to keeping the facility clean. Nursing assistants help to keep the facility clean by:

- Changing bed linens according to facility policy
- Helping patients and residents to keep their belongings neat and clean
- Wiping up spills on floors and counters promptly
- Picking up and disposing of stray pieces of trash
- Reporting problems with major housekeeping duties to the nurse

Odor Control

In a health care setting, vomit (emesis), urine, feces, and wound drainage can cause unpleasant odors. Nursing assistants help to minimize odors by:

- Handling trash and soiled linens according to facility policy
- Keeping the lids on linen hampers and waste containers closed
- Emptying and cleaning emesis basins, urinals, bedside commodes, and bedpans promptly
- Using a facility-approved air freshener when appropriate
- Assisting patients and residents with routine personal care
- Paying attention to your own personal hygiene

Temperature

Most people prefer a room temperature that is between 68°F and 74°F. However, people who are ill, elderly, or relatively inactive may prefer a warmer room temperature.

Fresh Air

The health care facility's ventilation system provides fresh air and keeps air circulating throughout the building. Proper ventilation is essential for carrying away unpleasant odors and preventing rooms from feeling stuffy.

Ventilation systems can create drafts (air currents), which can feel cold. Provide your patients or residents with an extra blanket, a sweater, or a lap robe as needed, and be sure to position people away from drafts created by the ventilation system.

Lighting

Good lighting is necessary for safety.

- **General lighting** provides overall light that allows people to see and move around safely. Sunlight and light from ceiling fixtures are examples of general lighting.
- **Task lighting** directs bright light toward a specific area. In a patient's or resident's room, task lighting is usually provided by a fixture mounted at the head of the bed. Task lighting helps people to see clearly when doing detailed work, such as reading or providing patient or resident care.

Lighting can also affect a person's comfort level. Some people prefer a brightly lit room, while others prefer a darker room. Some people like sunlight, while others prefer light from a lamp or ceiling fixture instead. Ask each of your patients or residents what he or she prefers.

Lighting helps us to orient ourselves to the time of day. During the evening and night hours, overhead lights should be dimmed, and the use of bright task lighting should be kept to a minimum. These measures help patients and residents maintain orientation to the time of day.

Noise Control

Places that are busy tend to be noisy. In a health care facility, ringing telephones, people talking, loud television sets and radios, and equipment can all add to the noise level. Too much noise can affect the patient's or resident's ability to rest and relax. Nursing assistants help to minimize noise by:

- Answering phones promptly
- Keeping their voices down when talking to co-workers
- Reporting noisy equipment that needs to be oiled or adjusted
- Closing the person's door when the person is trying to rest
- Encouraging patients or residents to use headphones when listening to TV or music in their rooms.

Putting it all together!

- Environmental conditions, such as a room's cleanliness, temperature, noise level, and quality of light, affect how we feel.
- To enhance the comfort and safety of patients and residents, health care facilities set policies that regulate the environment within the health care facility. In long-term care facilities, these policies are designed to meet standards set by OBRA.

Furniture and Equipment

What will you learn?

When you are finished with this section, you will be able to:

1. List the work areas that are common in a patient or resident unit in a health care facility.
2. Describe the standard equipment and furniture found in a person's room in a health care facility.
3. Explain how to change the height and mattress position of an adjustable bed.
4. Discuss the importance of allowing a person to have and display personal items.
5. Define the words **unit**, **hopper**, and **gatches**.

The patient or resident **unit** is set up according to the type of care that the person needs and with the person's safety and comfort in mind.

Unit a patient's or resident's room

In addition to patient and resident rooms, both acute care and long-term care facilities have similar work areas for staff use:

- The *nurses' station* serves as the central base of operations for the nursing staff. Staff members use the nurses' station to complete documentation and other paperwork, receive and make telephone calls, and monitor activity in that particular care area.
- The *medication room* is used to store medications and the supplies for administering medications.
- The *clean utility room* is used to store clean and sterile supplies, such as packaged personal care products and supplies used for medical treatments and procedures.
- The *soiled utility room* is where dirty items are handled or stored. Bins for trash and soiled linens are usually found here. This is also the room where used equipment (such as a bedside commode) is placed until it can be cleaned and disinfected. Soiled utility rooms often have a **hopper** that is used for tasks, such as cleaning bedpans and rinsing clothing or linens that have been soiled with feces.
- The *nourishment room* is where snacks and beverages are stored and prepared for patients and residents.

To ensure your own safety, as well as that of your patients or residents, you must make sure that you know how to operate and adjust any furniture and equipment that are considered standard in the facility where you work.

Hopper a sink-like fixture that flushes like a toilet and is connected to a sewer line

Beds

An adjustable bed, commonly referred to as a *hospital bed*, is used in most health care settings. Adjustable beds have a crank system or electrical control device that allows the position of the bed to be adjusted. Adjustable beds also have side rails and wheels.

Manual Crank System/Electrical Control Device

Adjustable beds allow you to adjust the height of the bed and the position of the mattress. Most health care facilities use adjustable beds that are adjusted electrically, using control buttons located on or near the side rails (Fig. 6-1). When using an electrical control device, appropriate safety precautions should be taken to avoid electrical shock (see Chapter 14). However, some long-term care facilities may still use beds that are adjusted manually, using a system of cranks located at the foot of the bed. When using the crank system, remember to fold the cranks down and away under the bed after you are finished using them so that people who are walking near the foot of the bed do not bump into them.

MOVING THE BED FRAME UP AND DOWN. The frame of an adjustable bed can be raised or lowered, moving the entire bed either further from or closer to the floor (Fig. 6-2). Raising the bed prevents health care workers from having to bend over so far when performing care procedures on a person who is in bed. Lowering the bed helps the patient or resident to get into or out of the bed safely.

A "low bed" (that is, a bed that is specially designed to lower to a height that is very close to the floor) is often found in the long-term care environment. A low bed is very useful for residents who may roll out of bed or get out of bed without calling for assistance when needed.

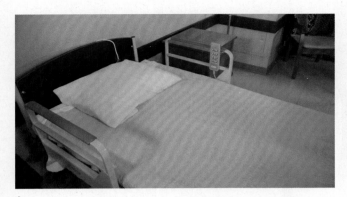

A

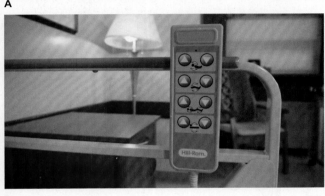

B

■ **FIGURE 6-1**
Adjustable beds may be adjusted using electrical controls.

CHANGING THE POSITION OF THE MATTRESS. The mattress platform on an adjustable bed can also be positioned in a variety of ways (see Fig. 6-2). Different mattress positions may be used for different activities, or the doctor may order a specific mattress position for a patient or resident.

- Most adjustable beds permit the mattress to be "tilted" without bending the person at the waist (see Fig. 6-2). In *Trendelenburg's position*, the foot of the mattress is raised so that the person's head is lower than his or her feet. In the *reverse Trendelenburg's position*, the head of the mattress is raised so the person's head is higher than his or her feet.

- **Gatches** allow the bed to bend at certain points (see Fig. 6-2). The hip gatch raises the person's upper body to a semisitting position. The knee gatch raises the person's knees to help prevent the person from sliding toward the end of the bed while sitting up.

Gatches the joints at the hips and knees of the mattresses of most adjustable beds that allow the mattress to "break" or bend so that the person's head can be elevated or his knees bent

Side Rails

Adjustable beds usually have side rails that can be raised to help prevent a person from falling out of the bed. The patient or resident may also use a raised side rail as an assistive device for repositioning himself or herself in bed. Side rails are positioned according to your facility's policies and the person's individual care plan.

Wheels (Casters)

Wheels make the bed easier to move from place to place, which is sometimes necessary when a person needs to be moved from one part of the facility to another without leaving his or her bed. Wheels are also useful when it is necessary to move the bed to clean underneath it. The wheels have locking devices that are used to

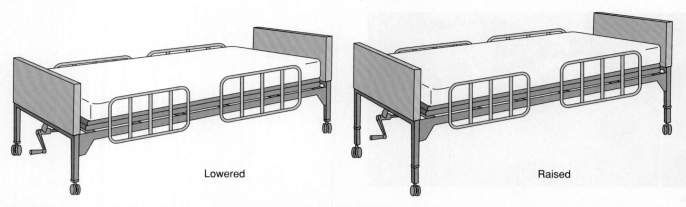

Lowered   Raised

The bed can be moved up or down in terms of distance from the floor.

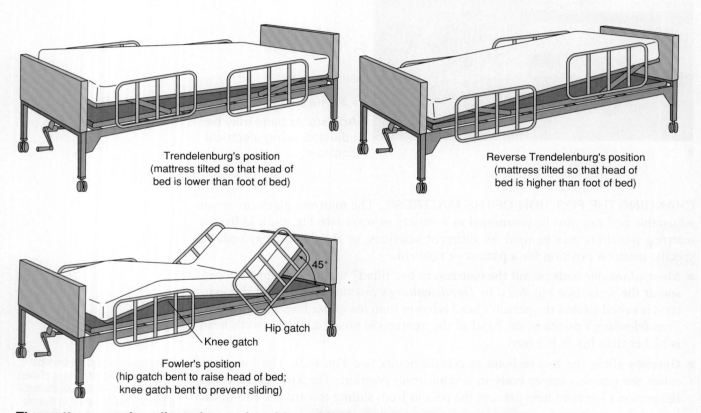

Trendelenburg's position
(mattress tilted so that head of
bed is lower than foot of bed)

Reverse Trendelenburg's position
(mattress tilted so that head of
bed is higher than foot of bed)

45°

Hip gatch

Knee gatch

Fowler's position
(hip gatch bent to raise head of bed;
knee gatch bent to prevent sliding)

The mattress can be adjusted to assist with positioning of the patient or resident.

■ **FIGURE 6-2**

Adjustable beds allow you to adjust the height of the bed from the floor and the position of the mattress.

keep the bed steady and prevent it from rolling (Fig. 6-3). Always make sure that the bed's wheels are locked unless you are moving it!

Chairs

A person's room should be furnished with one or two chairs that are comfortable for the person and any visitors.

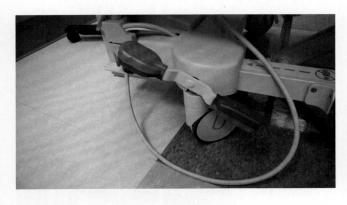

■ **FIGURE 6-3**

Wheel locks are used for safety. In the type of wheel lock shown here, the red pedal locks the wheel and the green pedal unlocks it.

Over-Bed Tables

The over-bed table fits over the bed or a chair and can be raised or lowered as needed (Fig. 6-4). The over-bed table provides a work surface for both the patient or resident and the health care worker. Because the over-bed table is considered a "clean" area, items placed there should be either sterile or clean. One way to help remember this is to consider the over-bed table the person's dining room table—you would never place dirty items, such as bedpans or soiled linens, there.

Bedside Tables

The bedside table is used to store personal care items (Fig. 6-5). The person's toothpaste and toothbrush, lotion, soap, deodorant, and other personal hygiene items are usually stored in the top drawer. Basins, bedpans, and other care equipment are stored underneath in the lower drawers or shelves. The telephone, a flower arrangement, and other personal items may be placed on top of the bedside table.

 ## Closets and Dressers

OBRA regulations require long-term care facilities to provide each resident with enough storage space for his or her clothing and other personal items. The resident must have free access to this storage space and the items it contains. Because the

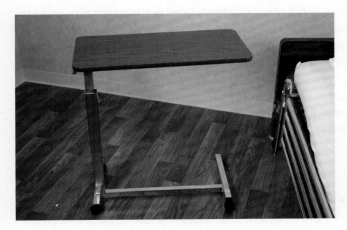

■ **FIGURE 6-4**

An over-bed table fits over a person's bed or chair to provide a work surface. The over-bed table is considered a "clean" area.

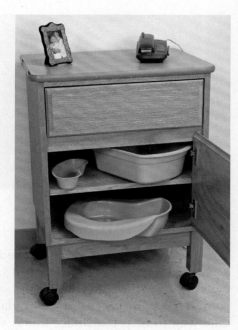

■ **FIGURE 6-5**
Personal care items are usually stored in the bedside table.

resident's closet, wardrobe, or chest of drawers is considered private, personal property, you must have the person's permission to remove items from it.

Call Light and Intercom Systems

Call light and intercom systems are used for communication (Fig. 6-6). The call light system allows patients or residents to signal that they need help. The intercom system allows members of the health care team to communicate with patients or residents from the nurses' station. Remember, however, that a person with hearing loss may not be able to understand what you are saying over the intercom.

Answer all requests for assistance promptly. Always leave the call light control within the person's reach, whether the person is in the bed or in a chair. An unconscious or comatose person will be unable to call for help and should be checked on frequently.

Privacy Curtains and Room Dividers

OBRA regulations require long-term care facilities to use privacy curtains or room dividers to protect the privacy of each resident. The privacy curtain should be closed or a room divider used when you are providing care for your patients or residents. The door to the room should also be closed because the privacy curtains do little to keep voices and other sounds private.

Pay attention to the cleanliness of privacy curtains or room dividers. Report any stains to the proper person so that the privacy curtain or room divider can be cleaned or replaced, as needed.

Personal Items

When a person enters a health care facility, he or she may bring personal items along to add a "touch of home." Usually the number and type of personal items

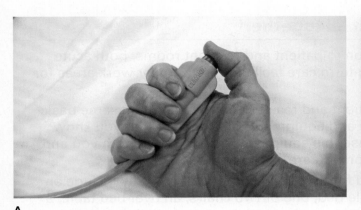

A

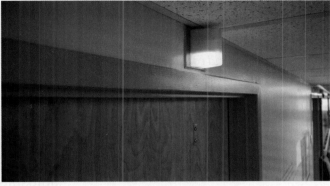

B

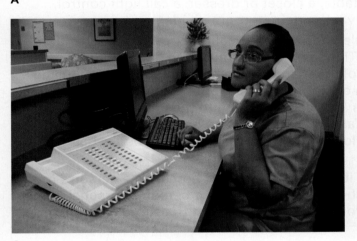

C

■ **FIGURE 6-6**

Call light and intercom systems allow patients and residents to communicate with members of the health care team. (**A**) The resident pushes a call light control button or pulls a cord, (**B**) the light above the person's door and the corresponding light on the panel at the nurses' station light up, and (**C**) a nurse or nursing assistant can use the intercom system to communicate with the person before going to the person's room.

depend on whether the stay at the health care facility is temporary or permanent. You should help your patients and residents to decorate their rooms according to their own individual taste and preference while making sure that they stay within the safety standards established by your facility and OBRA.

> *Concerns for Long-Term Care*
>
> Although the long-term care facility is a health care facility, it is also the resident's home. OBRA requires that the facility provide a home-like environment that reflects the individuality of each resident and minimizes the institutional nature of the setting to the best extent possible. OBRA regulations protect each resident's right to personalize his or her living space, and to have and to use personal items. Personal items help to create a living space that is as home-like as possible for the resident, and foster the resident's sense of independence and individuality. You should help your residents to decorate their rooms according to their own individual taste and preference, while making sure that they stay within the safety standards established by OBRA and your facility.

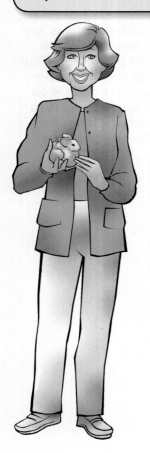

> Always respect and care for a person's personal items as if they belonged to you. Although you may consider a resident's personal things quite a bit of clutter, especially if you have to help keep them neat, just remember that each one of those items represents a piece of that person's life. When you show respect for, and take an interest in, a patient's or resident's personal belongings, you are letting the person know that you truly care for him or her.

Putting it all together!

- In addition to patient and resident rooms, both acute and long-term care facilities have similar work areas for the staff.
- Most patient and resident units contain the same basic furniture and equipment. Making sure that you know how to use this equipment helps to keep both you and the person you are caring for safe.
- Standard furniture and equipment typically include an adjustable bed, one or two chairs, an over-bed table, a bedside table, a closet or dresser, a call light control, and a privacy curtain or room divider.
- Adjustable beds have special features for safety and comfort. The height of an adjustable bed and the position of the mattress can be changed by hand (using a system of cranks) or using an electrical control device. Side rails are used according to the person's care plan to prevent falls. Wheels allow the bed to be moved easily but should always be locked unless the bed is being moved.
- Personal items add a "touch of home" to a person's room. Always show as much care for a person's personal items as you would for your own most treasured belongings.

Adapting the Environment to the Individual

What will you learn?

When you are finished with this section, you will be able to:

1. Explain why adapting the environment to meet the individual patient's or resident's needs is important.
2. Give examples of modifications that can be used in the health care setting.

Overall, the basic furniture and equipment in each patient's or resident's room will be the same depending on the particular type of unit within the health care facility. Per OSHA regulations, long-term care facilities are expected to provide care in a manner that promotes residents' independence. Environmental factors can get in the way of the person functioning at his or her best. The health care environment can and should be adapted as necessary to suit the person's individual needs and to promote independence.

Examples of environmental adaptations commonly found in the health care setting include:

- Lowering the hanging rod in a closet will allow a person in a wheelchair to independently remove clothing from the closet.

- Installing an elevated seat on a toilet will make easier for a person who has difficulty sitting down and standing up to use the toilet independently.
- Installing a toilet seat in a color that contrasts with the bathroom floor and walls can help a person with visual problems identify the toilet more easily.
- Placing signs with words or pictures on dresser drawers or doorways can help a person with dementia find what he is looking for.
- Using low beds, lower chairs, and pediatric wheelchairs can help a very petite person get in and out of bed and chairs safely.
- Providing special furniture and equipment for large or obese people will help to promote comfort and safety. For example, bariatric beds and wheelchairs are designed and constructed to meet the comfort and safety needs of an obese person. (*Bariatrics* is the branch of medicine that specializes in the treatment of obesity.)

As you are helping your patients and residents with their care, it is important for you to report any environmental barriers to their comfort and independence. Share your observations with the nurse and other team members. Together, you may be able to find a creative solution to the person's challenges!

 Putting it all together!

- **The environment should be adapted as necessary to help each patient or resident remain as independent as possible and to ensure comfort and safety.**

WHAT DID YOU LEARN?

Multiple Choice

Select the single best answer for each of the following questions.

1. How should a resident's room look?
   a. Functional and sparsely decorated
   b. Like a hospital room
   c. As home-like as possible
   d. Like a hotel room

2. You show respect to a patient or resident when you:
   a. Knock before entering his or her room
   b. Close the door and pull the privacy curtain when you are providing care
   c. Handle the person's personal belongings with care
   d. All of the above

3. Which regulations state that a resident's unit must be clean, safe, orderly, and free of obstacles in the pathway?
   a. Occupational Safety and Health Administration (OSHA) regulations
   b. Omnibus Budget Reconciliation Act (OBRA) regulations
   c. Medicare regulations
   d. Medicaid regulations

4. One of your patients has had back surgery, and the nurse asks you to position his bed so that the head of the bed is elevated. The patient's body needs to remain flat against the mattress. What position would the nurse tell you to put the patient in?
   a. Reverse Trendelenburg's position
   b. Fowler's position
   c. Prone position
   d. Trendelenburg's position

5. How can you help to control unpleasant odors in the workplace?
   a. Empty emesis basins promptly
   b. Assist your patients or residents with skin care and oral hygiene
   c. Use facility-approved air fresheners as necessary
   d. All of the above

(STOP) Stop *and* Think!

- One of your residents, Mrs. Grant, is complaining that she is cold even though you are feeling a bit too warm. What are some measures that you can take to help make Mrs. Grant more comfortable?

- Mrs. Tinetti is a new resident at the long-term care facility where you work. She is 86 years old and still able to walk on her own with the help of her walker. Mrs. Tinetti is only 4'9" tall and weighs 96 pounds. You notice that she seems to be having a great deal of difficulty getting out of her bed and chair. When she is seated on either one, her feet do not touch the floor. You see her struggling to get out of bed and go over to offer her assistance. She accepts the assistance, but snaps that this just should not be. She has always prided herself at being able to do things for herself, despite her age. She does not want to lose that just because she has moved to this facility! What can be done to help Mrs. Tinetti maintain the independence that she is so proud of?

The Human Body in Health and Disease

In this unit, we will explore how each organ system functions normally, as well as how aging, disease, and injury can affect the function of the organ system. We will also explore the measures that are taken to help the body return to its best level of functioning after injury or illness. Knowing how the body works when it is healthy helps us to understand how to help the body heal and function more effectively during illness.

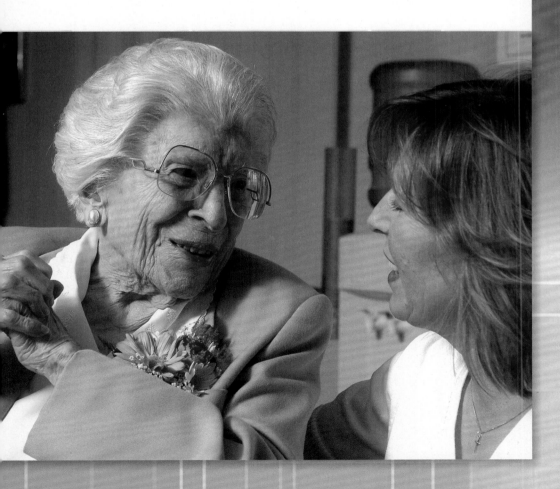

The Human Body in Health and Disease

In this unit, we will explore how each organ system functions normally, as well as how aging, disease, and injury can affect the function of the organ system. We will also explore the measures that are taken to help the body return to its best level of functioning after injury or illness. Knowing how the body works when it is healthy helps us to understand how to help the body heal and function more effectively during illness.

Basic Body Structure and Function

Anatomy is the study of what body parts look like, where they are located, how big they are, and how they connect to other body parts. *Physiology* is the study of how the body parts work. Learning about the parts of the body and how they work normally will help you to better understand how aging, disability, and disease can affect a person's abilities. This knowledge will help you to provide the type of care that each patient or resident needs from you.

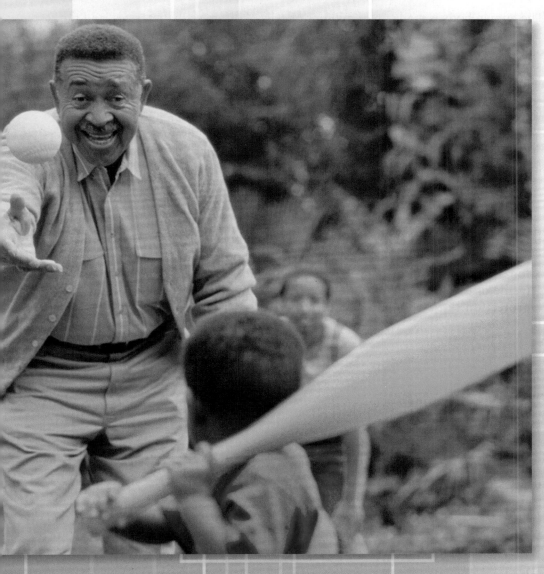

Photo: *When we are healthy, our bodies allow us to do the things we like to do.*

How the Body Is Organized

What will you learn?

When you are finished with this section, you will be able to:

1. List and describe the basic organizational levels of the body.
2. Define the words **cell**, **tissue**, **organ**, **organ system**, **nutrients**, **metabolism**, and **homeostasis**.

Cell the basic unit of life

Tissue a group of cells similar in structure and specialized to perform a specific function

Organ a group of tissues functioning together for a similar purpose

Organ system a group of organs that work together to perform a specific function for the body

Nutrients substances in food and fluids that the body uses to grow, to repair itself, and to carry out processes essential for living

Metabolism the physical and chemical changes that occur when the cells of the body change the food that we eat into energy

All living things share the same general organization (Fig. 7-1). **Cells** group together to form **tissues**. Tissues group together to form **organs**, and organs group together to form **organ systems**. A living thing, such as a human being, is made up of several organ systems, all of which work together to maintain life.

Cells

The human body is made up of millions of cells of different shapes, sizes, and functions. Each type of cell in the body has a specific duty. Our overall health depends on the ability of the cells of the body to do their jobs.

To function properly, cells need oxygen, water, **nutrients**, and the ability to eliminate waste products that result from **metabolism**. Structures inside of the cell called *organelles* help the cell to make the energy it needs to stay alive and to rid itself of waste products (Fig. 7-2). The organelles float in a jelly-like substance called *cytoplasm*. The *nucleus* of the cell is like the cell's "brain." It contains all of the information the cell needs to do its job, grow, and reproduce. A *cell membrane* surrounds the cytoplasm and gives the cell its shape.

Tissues

There are four main types of tissue in the human body:

- **Epithelial tissue** covers the outside of the body. It also lines the respiratory, digestive, and urinary systems; the inside of the blood vessels; and the inside of the chest and abdominal cavities. The purpose of epithelial tissue is protection.

■ **FIGURE 7-1**

All living things (organisms) share the same basic levels of organization. Cells form tissues, tissues form organs, and organs form organ systems.

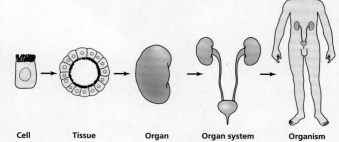

Cell   Tissue   Organ   Organ system   Organism

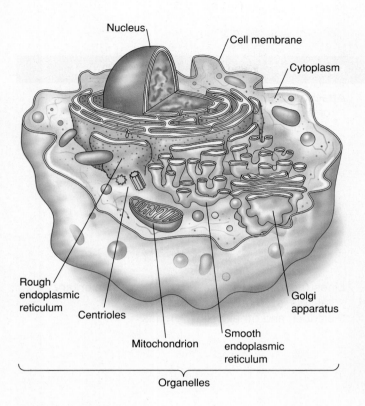

Nucleus

Cell membrane

Cytoplasm

Rough
endoplasmic
reticulum

Centrioles

Mitochondrion

Smooth
endoplasmic
reticulum

Golgi
apparatus

Organelles

■ **FIGURE 7-2**

A cell contains organelles and a nucleus, which float in a jelly-like substance called cytoplasm. A cell membrane surrounds the cytoplasm and gives the cell its shape.

- ■ **Connective tissue** supports and forms the framework for all of the parts of the body. Examples of connective tissue are bone, cartilage, ligaments, tendons, and fatty tissues. Blood is also considered a form of connective tissue.
- ■ **Muscle tissue** produces movement. There are three types of muscle tissue found in the body (Table 7-1). Muscle tissue is either *voluntary* (under the person's control) or *involuntary* (not under the person's control).
- ■ **Nervous tissue** allows one part of the body to "talk" to another part. The brain, spinal cord, and nerves are made of nervous tissue.

Organs

A group of tissues working together for a similar purpose form an organ. For example, the heart is made of all four tissue types, and its main function is to pump blood throughout the body. Other examples of organs are the stomach, liver, kidneys, and lungs. An organ may have one function or it may have several.

Organ Systems

For an organ system to work properly, each organ within the system must function well. All of the organ systems are constantly working together to maintain **homeostasis.** For a person to stay alive, certain conditions within the body must remain the same, within a range of normal limits. For example, the body temperature must remain within a certain range. When the external or internal

Homeostasis a state of balance

TABLE 7-1   Types of Muscle Tissue

Type	Function	Control
 Skeletal muscle	Attaches to the bones and allows for movement of the various parts of the body	Voluntary
 Smooth muscle	Lines the walls of the blood vessels, stomach, intestines, bladder, and other hollow organs	Involuntary
 Cardiac muscle	Forms the heart; contraction and relaxation of this muscle pumps blood throughout the body	Involuntary

environment changes, the organ systems must make adjustments to make up for the change. Most of the time, you are not even aware of the adjustments your body is making to keep everything within the normal range. The body's ability to maintain balance is a sign of good health. Diseases and disorders can negatively affect the body's ability to maintain balance.

As we age, changes occur in all of our organ systems. These changes are not related to illness. Rather, they are normal changes that occur in everyone who reaches a certain age. However, in a person who has a disease or disorder, the physical effects of aging on the body can be increased.

Putting it all together!

- All living things are organized in the same way. Cells group together to form tissues. Tissues group together to form organs. Organs work together to form organ systems. Organ systems work together to keep the body alive.

- The body's organ systems work together to maintain homeostasis, or balance. The body's ability to maintain balance is a sign of good health.

- Because there is a good chance that many of the people you will be caring for will be elderly, it is important for you to know about the changes that normally occur in each body system with aging. Knowing about normal age-related changes will allow you to provide better care for your elderly patients or residents because you will be aware of their special needs.

> *Many people associate old age with poor physical health, disability, and a loss of mental function. But many things affect how we age—our genes, our outlook on life, and our overall health, for example. You may care for a 60-year-old who seems much older than he or she really is, while the 80-year-old down the hall may get around better than you do! Be sure to notice the real differences in all of the people you care for.*

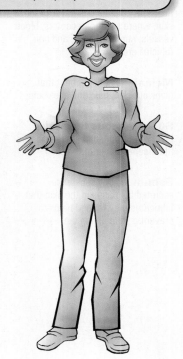

The Integumentary System

What will you learn?

When you are finished with this section, you will be able to:

1. List and describe the main parts of the integumentary system.
2. Discuss the major functions of the integumentary system.
3. List the layers of the skin.
4. Describe the normal changes related to aging that occur in the integumentary system.
5. Define the words **epidermis, dermis, melanin, subcutaneous tissue,** and **sebum**.

Structure and Function of the Integumentary System

The integumentary system gets its name from the Latin word *integumentum*, which means "a covering." The integumentary system includes the skin and its glands, the hair, and the nails.

The integumentary system helps to maintain the body's homeostasis in three important ways:

- It protects us against germs, chemicals, and other agents that could harm the body if they were able to reach the delicate organs inside. It also helps to protect us by allowing us to sense pain, pressure, temperature, and touch.

- It helps to maintain the body's fluid balance by preventing excessive loss or absorption of water.

- It helps to regulate the temperature of the body. When we are hot, the blood vessels in the skin dilate (widen), allowing more blood to flow close to the surface of the skin. As the blood passes beneath the surface of the skin, the heat in the blood leaves the body, lowering the temperature of the blood. Similarly, when we are cold, the blood vessels in the skin constrict (become narrower), limiting the amount of blood that passes close to the surface of the body and limiting the amount of heat lost to the outside environment.

Of all the body's organ systems, the integumentary system is the most easily observed. Healthy skin is glowing and vibrant, and may range in color from very light to very dark. The condition of a person's hair and nails can also provide clues to the person's overall health.

Skin

The skin is the body's largest organ. The skin has two layers, the **epidermis** and the **dermis** (Fig. 7-3). **Melanin** in the epidermis helps to protect the skin from exposure to sunlight. The dermis consists of elastic connective tissue that allows it to stretch and move without damage. The dermis rests on a layer of fat called the **subcutaneous tissue** (see Fig. 7-3). The blood vessels and nerves that supply the skin begin in the subcutaneous tissue and extend into the dermis. Nerves, glands, and hair follicles are also found in the dermis.

Accessory Structures

The accessory structures of the skin include the following:

- **Sebaceous (oil) glands.** These glands secrete **sebum**.
- **Sweat glands.** These glands produce a thin, watery liquid that helps to cool the body through the process of evaporation.
- **Hair.** The entire body (except for the soles of the feet and the palms of the hands) is covered in hair. Hair, especially that covering the scalp, helps to keep us warm. Hair around the eyes, such as the eyelashes and eyebrows, and in the lining of the nose helps to protect us from foreign materials and dust.
- **Nails.** Nails are made of special skin cells that have been hardened by a protein called *keratin*. Nails help to protect the ends of our fingers and toes.

Epidermis the outer layer of the skin

Dermis the deepest layer of the skin, where sensory receptors, blood vessels, nerves, glands, and hair follicles are found

Melanin a dark pigment that gives our skin, hair, and eyes color

Subcutaneous tissue the layer of fat that supports the dermis (the deepest layer of the skin)

Sebum an oily substance secreted by glands in the skin that lubricates the skin and helps to prevent it from drying out

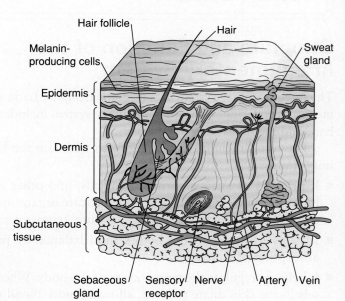

■ **FIGURE 7-3**

The skin has two layers, the dermis and epidermis. The skin rests on a layer of subcutaneous tissue.

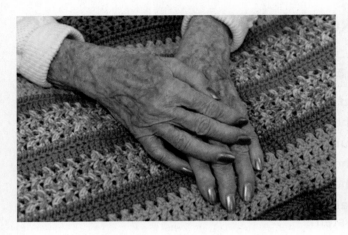

■ **FIGURE 7-4**
As skin ages, it becomes more delicate and prone to injury.

The Effects of Aging on the Integumentary System

The effects of aging on the integumentary system include the following:

- The skin becomes thin, fragile, and dry, putting the person at risk for skin injury (Fig. 7-4).
- Blood flow to the skin decreases, resulting in slower healing if injury occurs and putting the person at increased risk for infection.
- Decreased blood flow to the skin and decreased sweat production make it harder for the body to cool itself, putting the person at risk for heat-related injuries, such as heat stroke.
- The nails become thick, tough, and yellow.
- Loss of melanin causes the hair to turn gray.
- Deposits of melanin in certain areas, such as the backs of the hands and the face, lead to the formation of "age spots" (also called "liver spots").

 ## Putting it all together!

- The integumentary system consists of the skin and its accessory structures (hair, nails, sweat glands, and sebaceous glands).
- As the body's most visible organ system, the integumentary system can provide clues to a person's overall health. As a nursing assistant, you will observe for changes in the integumentary system when you assist patients or residents with bathing, hair care, and hand and foot care.
- The integumentary system helps to maintain the body's homeostasis by offering us physical protection from germs and other harmful agents, helping us to maintain our internal fluid balance, and playing a role in temperature regulation.
- When caring for an elderly person, keep the delicate nature of older skin in mind. It is very easy to tear or scratch an older person's skin, causing it to bleed.

The Musculoskeletal System

What will you learn?

When you are finished with this section, you will be able to:

1. List and describe the main parts of the musculoskeletal system.
2. Discuss the main functions of the musculoskeletal system.
3. List and describe the four general types of bones.
4. List and describe the three general types of joints.
5. Describe the normal changes related to aging that occur in the musculoskeletal system.
6. Define the words **skeleton**, **joint**, **cartilage**, **ligaments**, **tendons**, and **atrophy**.

Structure and Function of the Musculoskeletal System

The musculoskeletal system consists of the bones, joints, and muscles. The musculoskeletal system gives structure to the body and allows us to move.

Bones

Skeleton the framework for the body formed by the bones

The 206 bones in the human body form the **skeleton** (Fig. 7-5). The skeleton gives structure and shape to the body and protects key vital organs, such as the heart and the brain, from injury. The skeleton also serves as a storage site for calcium, an important mineral that keeps the bone tissue hard and is necessary for the proper functioning of skeletal and cardiac muscle. In addition, blood cells are produced in the bone marrow.

The bones of the skeleton vary in size and shape. Bones can be put in general categories according to their shape (Fig. 7-6).

Bones must be strong enough to support and protect the body, yet light enough to allow us to move. Therefore, bones have two layers. The outside of the bone is hard and solid. The inside of the bone is sponge-like and airy. Thin strands of bone form a net-like structure, and the spaces in between the thin strands of bone are filled with bone marrow. This combination of a solid, hard outside and a sponge-like inside results in bones that are strong and able to resist a great amount of force, yet lightweight.

The cells that form the bones are constantly broken down and replaced with new bone cells throughout a person's lifetime. A complex network of blood vessels supplies the bone cells with the oxygen and nutrients they need.

Joints

Joint the area where two bones join together

Cartilage a tough, fibrous substance found in joints and other parts of the body; in slightly movable joints, the cartilage acts as a "shock absorber"; in freely movable joints, the cartilage provides a smooth surface for the bones of the joint to move against

Joints can be classified according to the amount of movement they allow (Fig. 7-7):

- **Fixed joints** do not permit any movement at all. The joints between the bones of the skull are examples of fixed joints.

- **Slightly movable joints** allow for limited movement. Slightly movable joints are found between the bones in the spine and where the ribs attach to the sternum (breastbone). **Cartilage** fills in the space between the bones in the slightly

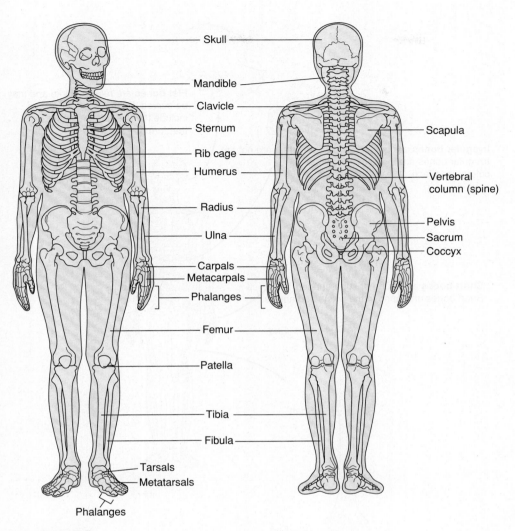

Skull

Mandible

Clavicle

Sternum

Scapula

Rib cage

Humerus

Vertebral column (spine)

Radius

Pelvis

Ulna

Sacrum

Coccyx

Carpals
Metacarpals

Phalanges

Femur

Patella

Tibia

Fibula

Tarsals
Metatarsals

Phalanges

■ **FIGURE 7-5**

The human skeleton contains 206 bones. Some of the major bones are labeled here.

movable joint. The cartilage permits limited movement and acts as a "shock absorber" between the bones.

■ **Freely movable joints** allow for a wide range of movement. Examples of freely movable joints include the knees, elbows, finger and toe joints, and hip joints. The ends of the bones that form the freely movable joint are covered with cartilage, which provides a smooth surface for the other bones to move against. A capsule formed of connective tissue encloses the ends of the bones, forming a *joint cavity*. The lining of the capsule secretes a thick fluid called *synovial fluid* into the joint cavity. The synovial fluid lubricates the joint, which helps the joint to move smoothly. **Ligaments** stabilize the joint. If the ligament is torn or weak, the joint may be able to move too much in any one direction.

Ligaments very strong bands of fibrous tissue that cross over the joint capsule, attaching one bone to another and stabilizing the joint

Muscles

Skeletal muscle (see Table 7-1) is the type of muscle tissue found in the musculoskeletal system (Fig. 7-8). Skeletal muscles vary in shape. Some are long, thick, and

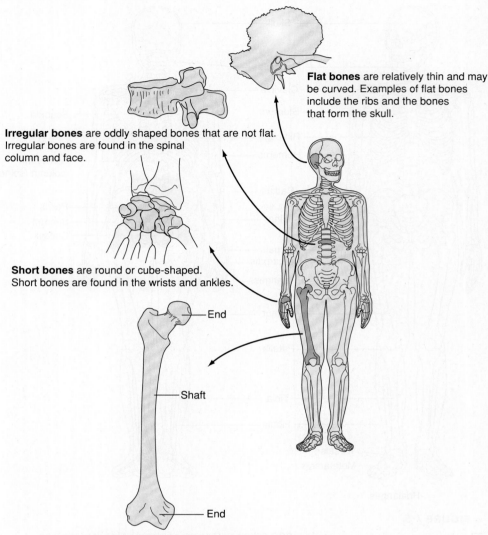

Flat bones are relatively thin and may be curved. Examples of flat bones include the ribs and the bones that form the skull.

Irregular bones are oddly shaped bones that are not flat. Irregular bones are found in the spinal column and face.

Short bones are round or cube-shaped. Short bones are found in the wrists and ankles.

End

Shaft

End

Long bones are found in the arms and the legs. Long bones have a shaft and two rounded ends.

■ **FIGURE 7-6**

Bones can be classified by their shape. General types of bones include long bones, short bones, flat bones, and irregular bones.

band-like. Others are flat or fan-like. Muscles are named according to their location, their shape, or their function.

The skeletal muscles perform three important functions for the body:

- The skeletal muscles allow us to move. **Tendons** attach the skeletal muscles to the bones. In freely movable joints, each skeletal muscle attaches to the bone at two points. The two points are on opposite sides of the joint. When the muscle contracts, the muscle shortens and the two points are drawn closer to each other, causing the part of the body to move.

- Contraction of the skeletal muscles produces heat and helps to maintain a constant body temperature. This is why when we are cold, we may start to shiver.

- Contraction of the skeletal muscles helps us to maintain an upright posture, such as sitting or standing.

Tendons bands of connective tissue that attach the skeletal muscles to the bones

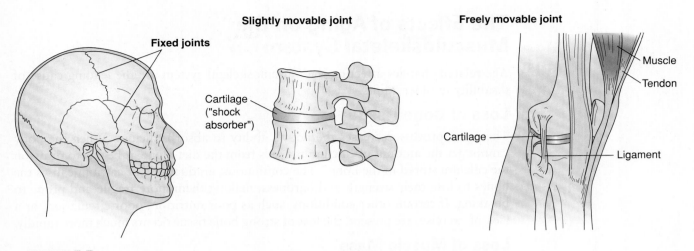

■ **FIGURE 7-7**

Joints can be classified by the amount of motion they permit.

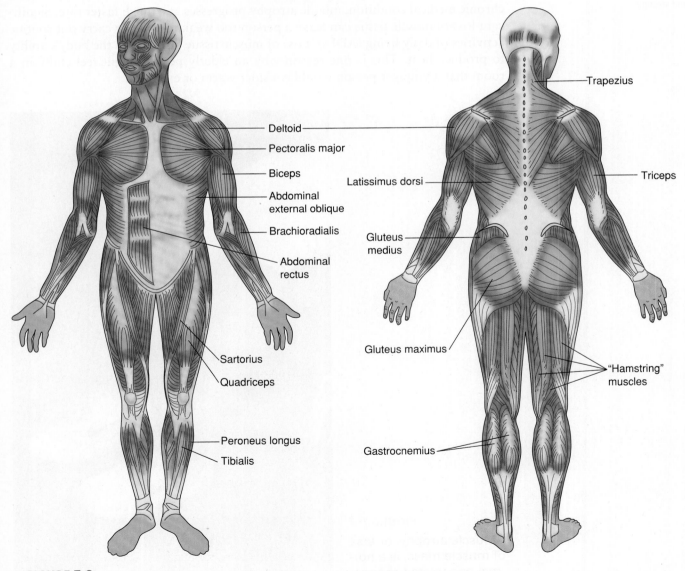

■ **FIGURE 7-8**

There are more than 700 skeletal muscles in the body! Some of the more familiar ones are labeled here.

The Effects of Aging on the Musculoskeletal System

Age-related changes affecting the musculoskeletal system are the leading cause of disability in older adults.

Loss of Bone Tissue

The aging process decreases the body's ability to absorb calcium. When the body cannot get the amount of calcium it needs from the diet alone, it begins to draw on the calcium stored in the bones. The continuous, gradual loss of calcium causes the bones to lose their strength and hardness, making them more fragile and prone to breaking. If certain other conditions, such as poor nutrition, poor circulation, or a lack of exercise, are present, the loss of strong bone tissue occurs much more rapidly.

Loss of Muscle Mass

Atrophy the loss of muscle size and strength

As we age, the number of muscle cells gradually decreases, resulting in muscle **atrophy** (Fig. 7-9). If a person is poorly nourished, is not physically active, or has a chronic medical condition, muscle atrophy progresses at a much faster rate. Significant loss of muscle tissue can leave a person too weak to walk or carry out routine activities of daily living (ADLs). Loss of muscle tissue also affects the body's ability to produce heat. This is one reason why an elderly person might feel chilly in a room that a younger person would consider warm or even hot.

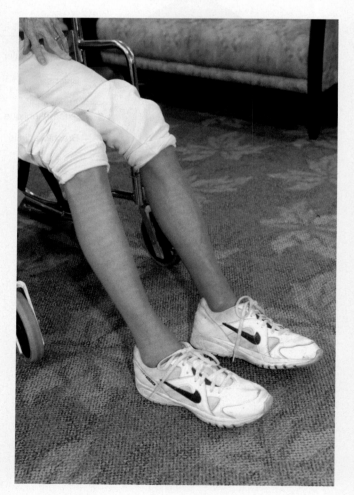

■ **FIGURE 7-9**

Muscle atrophy, or loss of muscle mass, is a normal age-related change.

Wear and Tear on the Joints

As we age, we lose the proteins that make the ligaments, tendons, and cartilage elastic (stretchy) and flexible, which can lead to stiffness and pain in the joints. The normal demands of daily life also cause a lot of wear and tear on the joints, which can, over time, lead to stiffness and pain. Overuse or injury of a joint, or being overweight, places extra strain on certain joints and will make the normal changes associated with aging more severe. Joint pain and stiffness can make simple activities, such as walking or getting out of a chair, difficult. Joint stiffness can also make a person more likely to fall.

Putting it all together!

- The musculoskeletal system consists of the bones, joints, and muscles.
- The primary function of the musculoskeletal system is movement. Other functions of the musculoskeletal system include protection, support, heat production, calcium storage, and blood cell production.
- Bones can be categorized by their shape. General categories include long bones, short bones, flat bones, and irregular bones.
- Joints are areas where two bones join together. Joints can be categorized by the amount of movement they permit. General categories include fixed joints, slightly movable joints, and freely movable joints.
- Skeletal muscle is the type of muscle tissue found in the musculoskeletal system. Skeletal muscle is under voluntary control. Tendons attach the skeletal muscle to the bones.
- As we age, we lose bone tissue and muscle mass, and our joints begin to show the effects of a lifetime of wear and tear. Eating a nutritious diet and exercising regularly throughout life can help to delay or decrease the effects of aging on the musculoskeletal system.

The Respiratory System

What will you learn?

When you are finished with this section, you will be able to:

1. List and describe the main parts of the respiratory system.
2. Discuss the main functions of the respiratory system.
3. Describe the normal changes related to aging that occur in the respiratory system.
4. Define the words **mucous membrane**, **mucus**, **respiration**, **gas exchange**, and **diaphragm**.

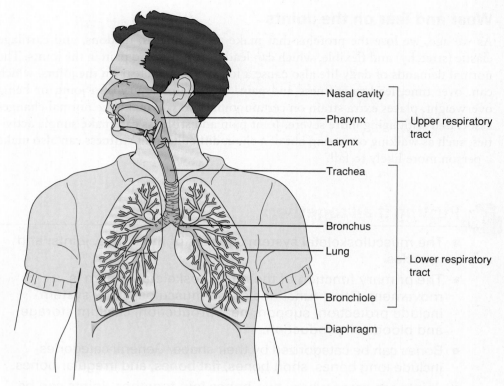

■ **FIGURE 7-10**

The respiratory system consists of the lungs and a series of passages called the "airway." The structures that form the airway include the nasal cavity, pharynx, larynx, trachea, bronchi, and bronchioles.

Nasal cavity
Pharynx
Larynx
— Upper respiratory tract

Trachea
Bronchus
Lung
Bronchiole
Diaphragm
— Lower respiratory tract

The respiratory system consists of the airway and the lungs (Fig. 7-10). The respiratory system allows us to take in oxygen, which we need to live, and get rid of carbon dioxide, a waste product of cellular metabolism.

Structure and Function of the Respiratory System

Airway

The purpose of the airway is to move air from the outside of the body to the lungs and from the lungs to the outside of the body. The airway consists of a series of passages that become narrower as they approach the lungs. These passages are lined with a **mucous membrane**. The surface of the membrane is kept moist by **mucus**.

NASAL CAVITY. Air enters the body through the nostrils and passes into the nasal cavity, which is lined by a mucous membrane and coarse hairs. The coarse hairs and the mucous membrane help to trap dirt, dust, and germs, preventing them from entering the delicate lungs. The warm, moist mucous membrane also heats and moistens the air. Warm, moist air is less likely than cold, dry air to damage the delicate lung tissue.

PHARYNX. The pharynx is the throat. Both the nose and the mouth open into the pharynx, which means that both air and food pass through the pharynx.

LARYNX. From the pharynx, air passes into the larynx. The opening of the larynx is covered by a flap of cartilage called the *epiglottis*, which snaps shut when you swallow, closing off the opening and preventing food from passing into the

Mucous membrane a special type of epithelial tissue that lines many of the organ systems in the body and is coated with mucus

Mucus a slippery, sticky substance that is secreted by special cells and serves to keep the surfaces of mucous membranes moist

lower respiratory tract. In addition to serving as part of the airway, the larynx (also known as the "voice box") is the organ responsible for speech.

TRACHEA AND BRONCHI. The trachea, also called the "windpipe," is the passage that carries air from the larynx down into the chest toward the lungs. "C"-shaped rings of cartilage give the trachea a ridged appearance. These cartilage rings support the trachea and keep it open. At its lower end, the trachea divides into two separate passages called the bronchi. One bronchus goes to the right lung and the other goes to the left lung.

The mucous membrane lining of the trachea and bronchi contains millions of tiny hair-like structures called *cilia*. The cilia move back and forth, moving mucus upward toward the pharynx so that it can be coughed up and removed from the respiratory tract along with any trapped particles or germs.

Lungs

The lungs are the main organs of **respiration**. Once inside the lungs, the bronchi divide into smaller and smaller branches called bronchioles. At the end of each bronchiole, there is a grape-like cluster of tiny air sacs called *alveoli*. Each alveolus is surrounded by a network of tiny blood vessels. **Gas exchange** occurs in the alveoli (Box 7-1).

The tissue of healthy lungs is very elastic and sponge-like because of all of the air-filled alveoli. The many blood vessels that surround the alveoli give healthy lung tissue its bright pink color.

The lungs are located in the chest cavity. The inside of the chest cavity is lined with a membrane called the *pleura*, which also covers the outside of the lungs. Because the lungs almost fill the chest cavity, the pleura on the outside of the lungs almost touches the pleura on the inside of the chest cavity. The pleura secretes a thin fluid that allows the lungs to slide easily against the chest cavity walls during the process of breathing.

Breathing has two phases: *inhalation* and *exhalation*. When we inhale, the **diaphragm** contracts, moving downward and making the chest cavity bigger. Air flows into the lungs, filling the alveoli and causing them to expand. When we exhale, the diaphragm relaxes, moving upward and pushing the air in the alveoli out of the lungs. The *intercostal muscles*, located between the ribs, also help us to breathe.

The rate and depth of breathing are controlled mainly by the brain. Special cells, called *chemoreceptors*, are located in the brain and in some of the major arteries. The chemoreceptors monitor the amount of carbon dioxide and oxygen in the blood and adjust the rate and depth of breathing as necessary. Although the brain ensures that breathing occurs automatically, you also have some voluntary control over breathing (for example, when you hold your breath while swimming).

The Effects of Aging on the Respiratory System

Exercising regularly and avoiding tobacco smoke and other pollutants help to keep the respiratory system functioning properly well into old age. However, as a person ages, there are two changes that are likely to occur to the respiratory system, even if the person is otherwise healthy:

- The lung tissue loses some of its ability to expand and bounce back.
- The diaphragm and intercostal muscles become weaker.

These changes mean that the amount of air taken in and let out with each breath is smaller.

Respiration the process the body uses to obtain oxygen from the environment and remove carbon dioxide (a waste gas) from the body

Gas exchange the transfer of oxygen into the blood, and carbon dioxide out of it

Diaphragm the strong, dome-shaped muscle that separates the chest cavity from the abdominal cavity and assists in breathing

BOX 7-1   Gas Exchange

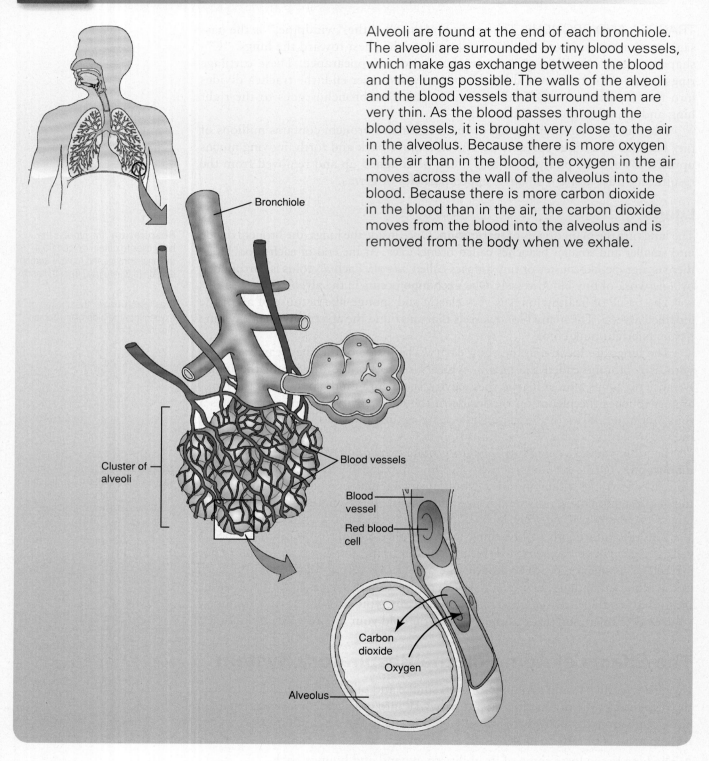

Bronchiole

Cluster of alveoli

Blood vessels

Blood vessel

Red blood cell

Carbon dioxide

Oxygen

Alveolus

Alveoli are found at the end of each bronchiole. The alveoli are surrounded by tiny blood vessels, which make gas exchange between the blood and the lungs possible. The walls of the alveoli and the blood vessels that surround them are very thin. As the blood passes through the blood vessels, it is brought very close to the air in the alveolus. Because there is more oxygen in the air than in the blood, the oxygen in the air moves across the wall of the alveolus into the blood. Because there is more carbon dioxide in the blood than in the air, the carbon dioxide moves from the blood into the alveolus and is removed from the body when we exhale.

In healthy older people who do not smoke, these changes do not usually cause any problems. Often, the person will not be aware of any change, except possibly during exercise, when the body needs more oxygen. However, when the processes of aging are combined with chronic illness, immobility, or a lifetime of exposure to toxic chemicals (such as those in pollution and tobacco smoke), the respiratory system's ability to function properly is significantly reduced. The person may have trouble breathing even at rest and be at increased risk for respiratory infections.

Putting it all together!

- The function of the respiratory system is to provide the body with oxygen and rid the body of carbon dioxide. We can live for days without food and water, but only for a few minutes without oxygen.

- Air passes through the airway on its way to and from the lungs. The structures that make up the airway are the nasal cavity, the pharynx, the larynx, the trachea, and the bronchi.

- The lungs are the main organs of respiration and gas exchange. When we inhale, the diaphragm contracts and the lungs fill with air. Once in the lungs, the oxygen in the air passes from the alveoli into the blood in the blood vessels that surround the alveoli. Each time the heart beats, the oxygen-rich blood is sent to all of the cells in the body. At the same time, carbon dioxide, a waste gas, moves from the blood into the alveoli. When we exhale, the diaphragm relaxes, pushing the air and carbon dioxide out of the lungs.

- The rate and depth of breathing are controlled mainly by the brain.

- As a person ages, the lung tissue becomes less elastic and the muscles used for breathing become weaker. These changes mean that the amount of air that is taken in with each breath is smaller. When the processes of aging are combined with chronic illness, immobility, or a lifetime exposure to toxic chemicals, the respiratory system's ability to function properly is significantly reduced.

The Cardiovascular System

What will you learn?

When you are finished with this section, you will be able to:

1. List and describe the main parts of the cardiovascular system.
2. Discuss the main functions of the cardiovascular system.
3. Describe the normal changes related to aging that occur in the cardiovascular system.
4. Define the words **plasma, erythrocytes, hemoglobin, leukocytes, thrombocytes, circulation, cardiac cycle, systole, diastole,** and **varicose veins.**

Structure and Function of the Cardiovascular System

The cardiovascular system is made up of the blood, the blood vessels, and the heart. The cardiovascular system transports oxygen, nutrients, and other important substances (for example, hormones) to the cells of the body and carries waste products away. The cardiovascular system also helps the body to fight off infection.

Blood

Blood is the life-giving fluid of our bodies. Blood consists of **plasma** and blood cells:

- **Plasma** is about 90% water. The other 10% is made up of substances that are dissolved in the water (such as glucose, amino acids, fats, and salts) and proteins.
- **Red blood cells** (**erythrocytes**) are disc-shaped cells that contain **hemoglobin**. When combined with oxygen, hemoglobin is bright red. As the blood circulates through the body, giving off oxygen and taking on carbon dioxide, the amount of oxygen on the hemoglobin decreases, and the blood becomes darker red in color.
- **White blood cells** (**leukocytes**) fight infection. There are five different types of white blood cells. Some destroy germs by surrounding them and "eating" them in a process called *phagocytosis*. Others secrete substances that cause germs to die. Still others make proteins called *antibodies*, which prevent us from getting some diseases twice.
- **Platelets** (**thrombocytes**) are responsible for clotting of the blood. This process, known as *hemostasis*, stops the loss of blood from the circulatory system.

Blood Vessels

The blood vessels carry blood to and from all of the tissues in the body. The walls of the blood vessels have three layers: a smooth inner layer, a muscular middle layer, and a tough outer layer. The smooth muscle in the middle layer is what allows the blood vessels to constrict (narrow) or dilate (widen) according to the body's needs. Constriction slows the flow of blood, and dilation allows blood to flow more rapidly.

- **Arteries** carry blood away from the heart. As the arteries get further away from the heart, they branch into a network, becoming more and more narrow (Fig. 7-11). The smallest arteries are called *arterioles*. Arterioles send off branches called *capillaries,* which form a network in the tissues called the *capillary bed.* As blood passes through the capillary bed, the oxygen and nutrients in the blood pass into the tissues, and carbon dioxide and other waste materials from the tissues pass into the blood.
- Veins carry blood back to the heart. After the blood passes through the capillary bed, it starts its journey back to the heart by way of very tiny veins called *venules.* Venules drain into small veins, which become wider as they approach the heart (see Fig. 7-11).

Heart

The heart is a hollow, muscular organ about the size of a fist that lies in the center of the chest, tilted a bit toward the left, behind the sternum (breastbone). Like the walls of the arteries and veins, the walls of the heart are made of three layers of

---

Plasma the liquid part of the blood

Erythrocytes red blood cells; responsible for carrying oxygen to all of the tissues of the body

Hemoglobin a protein found in red blood cells that combines with oxygen to carry it to the tissues of the body

Leukocytes white blood cells; responsible for fighting infection

Neutrophil   Monocyte

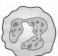

Eosinophil   Lymphocyte

Basophil

Thrombocytes pinched-off pieces of larger cells that are found in the red bone marrow and are responsible for clotting of the blood; also called *platelets*

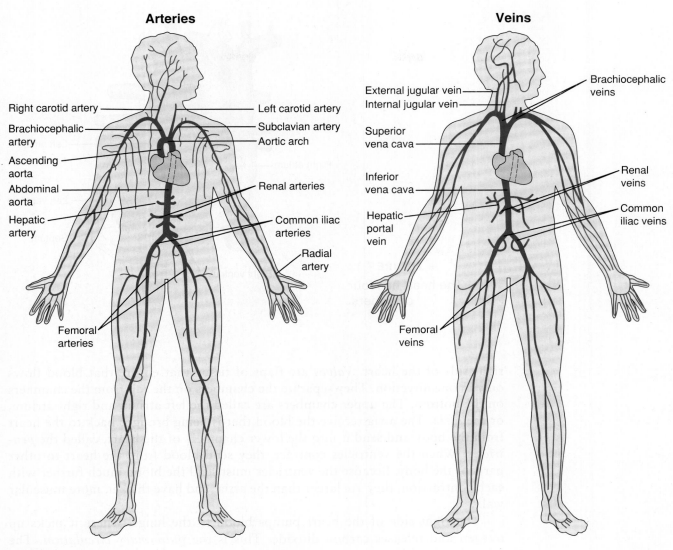

Arteries

Right carotid artery
Brachiocephalic artery
Ascending aorta
Abdominal aorta
Hepatic artery

Left carotid artery
Subclavian artery
Aortic arch
Renal arteries
Common iliac arteries
Radial artery

Femoral arteries

Veins

External jugular vein
Internal jugular vein
Superior vena cava
Inferior vena cava
Hepatic portal vein

Brachiocephalic veins
Renal veins
Common iliac veins

Femoral veins

■ **FIGURE 7-11**

Arteries carry blood away from the heart. Veins carry blood back to the heart. Some of the major arteries and veins are shown here.

tissue. The *endocardium* is the smooth inner layer of the heart. The *myocardium*, the middle layer, is formed of cardiac muscle. Coordinated contraction and relaxation of the myocardium is what causes the heart to pump, powering **circulation**. The *epicardium* is the smooth outermost layer of the heart. The epicardium forms part of the *pericardium*, a double-layered protective sac that surrounds the heart. A thin film of fluid between the epicardium and the outer layer of the pericardium allows the pericardial layers to slide smoothly against each other each time the heart pumps.

The heart muscle contracts in two phases, called the **cardiac cycle**. During **systole** the myocardium contracts, sending blood out of the heart. During **diastole** the myocardium relaxes, allowing the heart to fill with blood.

ATRIA AND VENTRICLES. The heart has four chambers (Fig. 7-12). A thick wall of muscle, called the *septum*, separates the left side of the heart from the

Circulation the continuous movement of the blood through the blood vessels; powered by the pumping action of the heart

Cardiac cycle the pumping action of the heart in an organized pattern (all of the events associated with one heartbeat)

Systole the active phase of the cardiac cycle, during which the myocardium contracts, sending blood out of the heart

Diastole the resting phase of the cardiac cycle, during which the myocardium relaxes, allowing the chambers to fill with blood

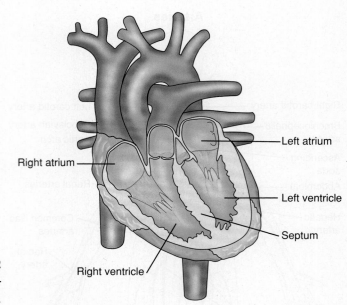

Right atrium
Left atrium
Left ventricle
Septum
Right ventricle

■ **FIGURE 7-12**

The heart has four chambers.

right side of the heart. *Valves* are flaps of tissue that ensure that blood flows only in one direction. They separate the chambers on the top from the chambers on the bottom. The upper chambers are called the left atrium and right atrium, or the *atria*. The atria receive the blood that is being brought back to the heart from the body and send it into the lower chambers of the heart, called the *ventricles*. When the ventricles contract, they send blood from the heart to other parts of the body. Because the ventricles must send the blood much further with each contraction, they are larger than the atria, and have thicker, more muscular walls.

The right side of the heart pumps blood to the lungs, where it picks up oxygen and releases carbon dioxide. This is the *pulmonary circulation*. The left side of the heart pumps the newly oxygenated blood to the body. This is the *systemic circulation*. You can learn more about the pattern of circulation in Box 7-2.

CONDUCTION SYSTEM. The muscle cells that make up the myocardium are very specialized, so that they contract as a unit. This unified contraction is what allows the heart to work efficiently as a pump, moving blood continuously through the body. A small mass of special tissue in the heart, called the *sinoatrial node*, sets the pace for contraction by generating an electrical impulse. The electrical impulse travels through the myocardium via a special pathway called the *conduction system*. As it passes through, the electrical energy causes the cardiac muscle cells in the myocardium to contract. First the atria contract, there is a pause, and then the ventricles contract.

CORONARY CIRCULATION. The tissues of the heart have their own special network of arteries and veins, just like all of the other organs in the body. The arteries and veins that supply the heart with oxygen and nutrients are called the *coronary circulation*. Coronary arteries carry oxygen-rich blood into the heart tissue. Coronary veins remove carbon dioxide and other waste products.

BOX 7-2 · Circulation

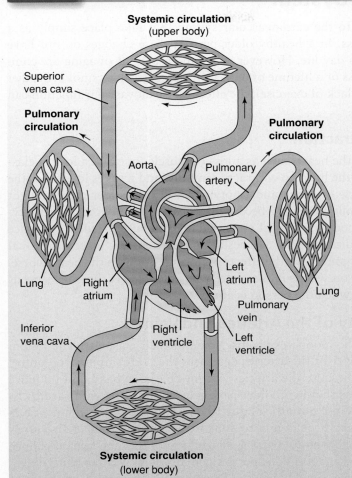

Systemic circulation
(upper body)

Superior
vena cava

**Pulmonary
circulation**

**Pulmonary
circulation**

Aorta

Pulmonary
artery

Lung

Right
atrium

Left
atrium

Lung

Pulmonary
vein

Inferior
vena cava

Right
ventricle

Left
ventricle

Systemic circulation
(lower body)

The pattern of circulation actually involves two circuits, the pulmonary circulation and the systemic circulation. Follow along on the figure. (*Red* stands for oxygen-rich blood and *blue* stands for oxygen-poor blood.)

Pulmonary Circulation

■ The largest veins in the body, the superior vena cava and the inferior vena cava, empty into the right atrium of the heart. The blood in these veins is returning from its journey to the tissues, so it has given up most of its oxygen and taken on a load of carbon dioxide.

■ The right atrium pumps the oxygen-poor blood into the right ventricle.

■ The right ventricle pumps the oxygen-poor blood into the pulmonary artery. The pulmonary artery branches into the right pulmonary artery, which goes to the right lung, and the left pulmonary artery, which goes to the left lung.

■ Once in the lungs, the pulmonary arteries quickly branch into smaller arteries and arterioles to carry the oxygen-poor blood to the capillary beds surrounding the alveoli. The oxygen in the alveolus moves into the blood, and the carbon dioxide in the blood moves into the alveolus, to be exhaled from the body.

■ The blood, which now contains fresh oxygen, is carried by the network of venules, then veins, to the pulmonary veins (right and left), which empty into the left atrium of the heart.

Systemic Circulation

■ The left atrium pumps the oxygen-rich blood into the left ventricle.

■ The left ventricle pumps the oxygen-rich blood into the largest artery of the body, the aorta.

■ The aorta branches very quickly into arteries that carry oxygen-rich blood to the rest of the body.

■ The arteries branch into arterioles and then into capillaries, which join together to form a capillary bed. In the capillary bed, oxygen and nutrients move out of the blood and into the tissues, and carbon dioxide moves out of the tissues and into the blood.

■ The blood, which now contains less oxygen, is carried by the network of venules, then veins, back to the right atrium, where the process begins again.

The Effects of Aging on the Cardiovascular System

There are some changes to the cardiovascular system that take place simply as a result of the aging process. In a healthy older person, these changes do not have a major impact on day-to-day life. However, when the processes of aging are combined with a chronic illness or a lifetime of unhealthy habits (such as smoking, a diet high in "bad" fats, and a lack of exercise), the effect on cardiovascular function can be major.

Less Efficient Contraction

Changes in the tissues of the heart, such as a loss of muscle tone and a loss of elasticity, affect the ability of the heart to contract forcefully, and it takes longer for the heart to complete the cycle of filling and emptying. A healthy older person might find that he tires faster while exercising because the heart is not able to deliver oxygen and nutrients to the body in times of increased demand as efficiently as it once did. Certain medical conditions, such as obesity or hypertension, place additional strain on the heart muscle and make the effects of normal aging on the heart worse. The heart of an older person who is ill may barely be able to meet the body's needs for oxygen and nutrients when the person is at rest.

Decreased Elasticity of the Arteries and Veins

As we age, the walls of the blood vessels lose some of their elasticity. The loss of elasticity in the muscle layer of the arteries decreases the body's ability to control blood pressure and flow because the arteries are not able to expand and "bounce back" as easily. This means that in an older person (especially one with cardiovascular disease), the arteries lose both the ability to dilate to allow for an increase in blood flow when needed and the ability to constrict back to a smaller size afterward. The "stretch" is gone from the vessel. The effects of this age-related change are especially noticeable when an older person gets up quickly after lying down. The arteries do not constrict quickly enough to maintain adequate blood flow to the brain, and the person feels dizzy or light-headed as a result.

The loss of elasticity in the walls of the veins causes them to "stretch out," slowing the flow of blood back to the heart. Pooling of blood in the veins in the legs can cause **varicose veins**. Immobility and bed rest can make the effects of aging on the veins worse.

Varicose veins a condition that results from pooling of blood in the veins just underneath the skin, causing them to become swollen and "knotty" in appearance

Decreased Numbers of Blood Cells

The production of blood cells slows as a person ages. A decreased number of red blood cells affect the blood's ability to deliver oxygen to the tissues. A decreased number of white blood cells put the older person at higher risk for developing infections because the body's ability to fight them off is reduced.

Putting it all together!

- The cardiovascular system is made up of the blood, the blood vessels, and the heart.
- Blood consists of plasma and blood cells.
- The blood vessels include the arteries, which carry blood away from the heart, and the veins, which carry blood back to the heart.

- The heart, a hollow, muscular organ, pumps blood through the blood vessels. The pattern of circulation involves the pulmonary circulation and the systemic circulation. The right side of the heart (pulmonary circulation) pumps blood to the lungs to pick up oxygen. The left side of the heart (systemic circulation) pumps the oxygenated blood to the rest of the body.

- During systole, the heart contracts, sending blood out of the heart. During diastole, the heart relaxes, allowing the chambers to fill.

- As we age, changes in the tissue of the heart decrease the heart's ability to contract forcefully, which decreases the heart's ability to deliver oxygen and nutrients to the body. In a healthy older person, the effect of these age-related changes on the person's cardiovascular function may go unnoticed. But when combined with a chronic illness or a lifetime of unhealthy habits, the effect on the person's cardiovascular function can be major.

- A loss of elasticity in the muscle layer of the body's blood vessels decreases the body's ability to control blood pressure and blood flow. This is why many older people feel dizzy or light-headed when they get up quickly after lying down.

The Nervous System

> ## What will you learn?
>
> *When you are finished with this section, you will be able to:*
> 1. List and describe the main parts of the nervous system.
> 2. Discuss the main functions of the nervous system.
> 3. Describe the normal changes related to aging that occur in the nervous system.
> 4. Define the words **central nervous system**, **peripheral nervous system**, **neuron**, **myelin**, **synapse**, **sensory nerves**, and **motor nerves**.

Structure and Function of the Nervous System

The nervous system includes the brain, spinal cord, and nerves. The nervous system controls the other organ systems. In this way, it helps to maintain the body's homeostasis by constantly monitoring what is going on inside and outside of the body and making adjustments to keep things within the range of normal. It also allows us to interact with our environment through the special senses (sight, hearing, smell, taste, and touch). The nervous system has two main divisions, the **central nervous system** and the **peripheral nervous system** (Fig. 7-13).

Central nervous system (CNS) the brain and spinal cord; responsible for receiving information, processing it, and issuing instructions

Peripheral nervous system (PNS) the nerves outside of the brain and spinal cord; receives information from the environment and carries commands from the brain and spinal cord to the other organs of the body, such as the muscles

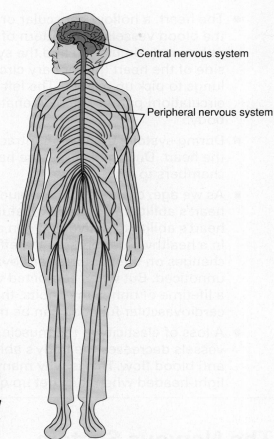

■ FIGURE 7-13

The nervous system has two main divisions, the central nervous system (CNS) and the peripheral nervous system (PNS). *Peripheral* means "along the edge" or "away from the center."

Central nervous system

Peripheral nervous system

Neuron a cell that can send and receive information

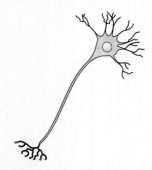

Myelin a fatty, white substance that protects the axon and helps to speed the conduction of nerve impulses along the axon

Synapse the gap between the axon of one neuron and the dendrites of the next

Cerebrospinal fluid (CSF) a clear fluid that circulates around the brain and spinal cord and acts as a "shock absorber" to protect these structures

Nervous tissue, which forms the organs of the nervous system, is made up of a special kind of cell called a **neuron**. A neuron has dendrites, a cell body, and an axon (Fig. 7-14). *Dendrites* are short extensions from the cell body that *receive* information. The *axon* is a long extension from the cell body that sends information. The *axons* of some neurons are wrapped in **myelin**.

An electrical signal, called a *nerve impulse*, enters the neuron at the dendrites. It passes through the cell body and travels down the axon and then on to the dendrites of the next neuron in line. The axon of one neuron does not actually connect with the dendrites of the next. Instead, chemicals called *neurotransmitters* carry the nerve impulse across the **synapse**.

The Central Nervous System

The central nervous system is protected by three layers of connective tissue called *meninges* and the bony skull and vertebrae (Fig. 7-15). The three meninges are, from the inside out:

■ The *pia mater*, a thin, delicate layer of tissue rich in blood vessels that is attached to the surface of the brain and spinal cord.

■ The *arachnoid mater*, the web-like middle layer.

■ The *dura mater*, a thick, tough outer layer that is attached to the inside of the skull and the vertebrae.

The space between the pia mater and the arachnoid mater contains **cerebro-spinal fluid (CSF)**.

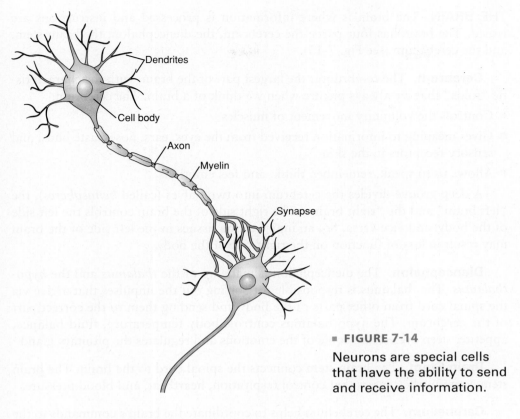

■ FIGURE 7-14

Neurons are special cells that have the ability to send and receive information.

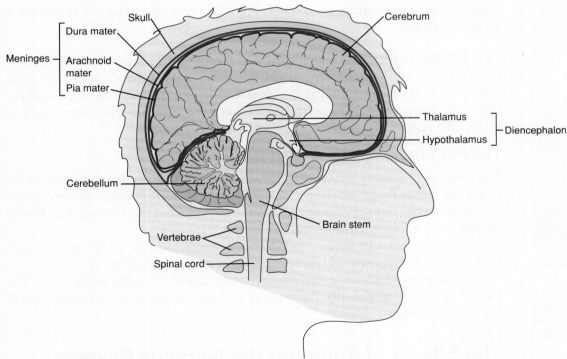

■ FIGURE 7-15

The brain and the spinal cord make up the central nervous system (CNS). The brain has four parts: the cerebrum, the diencephalon, the brain stem, and the cerebellum. Three layers of connective tissue, called the dura mater, the arachnoid mater, and the pia mater, help to cushion and protect the brain and spinal cord. Additional protection is provided by the bony skull and vertebrae.

THE BRAIN. The brain is where information is processed and instructions are issued. The brain has four parts: the cerebrum, the diencephalon, the brain stem, and the cerebellum (see Fig. 7-15).

Cerebrum. The cerebrum is the largest part of the brain, with the characteristic "folds" that we always picture when we think of a brain. The cerebrum:

- Controls the voluntary movement of muscles
- Gives meaning to information received from the eyes, ears, nose, taste buds, and sensory receptors in the skin
- Allows us to speak, remember, think, and feel emotions

A deep groove divides the cerebrum into two halves (called *hemispheres*), the "left brain" and the "right brain." The right side of the brain controls the left side of the body, and vice versa. So, an injury to the tissues in the left side of the brain may result in loss of function on the right side of the body.

Diencephalon. The diencephalon is made up of the *thalamus* and the *hypothalamus*. The thalamus is responsible for sorting out the impulses that arrive via the spinal cord from other parts of the body and sending them to the correct part of the cerebrum. The hypothalamus controls body temperature, fluid balance, appetite, sleep cycles, and some of the emotions and regulates the pituitary gland.

Brain Stem. The brain stem connects the spinal cord to the brain. The brain stem contains the centers that control respiration, heartbeat, and blood pressure.

Cerebellum. The cerebellum helps to coordinate the brain's commands to the muscles so that the muscles move smoothly and in an orderly fashion. It also plays a role in balance.

THE SPINAL CORD. The spinal cord is a "cord" of nervous tissue that extends from the base of the brain downward to a point approximately even with your belly button. The spinal cord is the main connection between the brain and the rest of the body. The *vertebrae* (the bones that make up your spine) surround and protect the spinal cord.

The Peripheral Nervous System

The peripheral nervous system consists of the nerves that supply every part of the body. The nerves that form the peripheral nervous system are either sensory nerves or motor nerves. **Sensory nerves** carry information from the "outside in." **Motor nerves** carry information from the "inside out."

Thirty-one pairs of nerves, called *spinal nerves*, connect to the spinal cord. Each spinal nerve consists of one sensory nerve and one motor nerve.

Twelve pairs of nerves, called *cranial nerves*, connect directly to the brain. The cranial nerves are responsible for many of our special senses, such as sight, smell, hearing, and taste.

Sensory nerves nerves that carry information from the internal organs and the outside world to the spinal cord and up into the brain so that the brain can analyze the information

Motor nerves nerves that carry commands from the brain down the spinal cord and out to the muscles and organs of the body

The Effects of Aging on the Nervous System

Slower Reaction Times

You may notice that some of your elderly patients or residents are not as quick to react to things as they used to be. As we age, the amount of myelin surrounding the axons decreases, reducing the speed of nerve conduction by approximately 10%.

In addition, chemical imbalances can interfere with the ability of a nerve impulse to travel across a synapse, slowing conduction. These changes are a normal part of the aging process, and they occur gradually over time. Slowed conduction times can increase an elderly person's risk for falling and having other household accidents.

Memory Changes

Memory and thought processes usually remain intact with normal aging. It may take an older person slightly longer to remember names, dates, or other information from the past, but given enough time, the person will eventually remember. Many older people experience a mild loss of memory for recent events while still having excellent long-term memory. Extreme memory loss, such as that seen in people with dementia, is not a normal age-related change.

Putting it all together!

- The nervous system receives, processes, and responds to information, helping the body to maintain a state of homeostasis.
- The nervous system is divided into the central nervous system and the peripheral nervous system. The central nervous system is made up of the brain and spinal cord. The peripheral nervous system is made up of the nerves.
- As we age, our reaction times become slower and we may experience slight memory loss.

The Sensory System

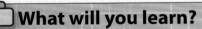

What will you learn?

When you are finished with this section, you will be able to:

1. Discuss the main functions of the sensory system.
2. Describe how we sense touch, position, and pain.
3. Describe how we experience taste and smell.
4. Describe how we experience sight.
5. Describe how we experience sound.
6. Describe the normal changes related to aging that occur in the sensory system.
7. Define the words **sensory receptors, cerumen, presbyopia,** and **presbycusis.**

Structure and Function of the Sensory System

The sensory system is the part of the nervous system that protects us from harm and lets us experience the world that we live in. The sensory system consists of sensory receptors. The **sensory receptor** picks up information, called a *stimulus*, and

Sensory receptors specialized cells or groups of cells associated with a sensory nerve

translates it into a nerve impulse, which is then sent to the brain for interpretation via the sensory nerve. Some sensory receptors are found in the *sense organs*—the eyes, the ears, the nose, and the taste buds. Other sensory receptors are found throughout the skin, and even in the tissues of internal organs.

General Sense

General sense is responsible for our sense of touch, position, and pain. The sensory receptors that are responsible for general sense are found throughout the body.

TOUCH. Our sense of touch allows us to feel textures and the shapes of objects. Sensory receptors are stimulated when something comes in contact with the surface of the body and presses on them, causing them to change shape. Some areas of the body, such as the fingers and lips, have more sensory receptors than others, and are therefore more sensitive to touch.

Some of the sensory receptors in the skin allow us to sense pressure, also known as *deep touch*. The discomfort caused by prolonged pressure is what makes us shift our position when we have been sitting in one position for a long time. A person who is unable to sense pressure (for example, a person who is paralyzed) does not become uncomfortable from being in one position for a long time.

POSITION. Sensory receptors found in the muscles, tendons, and joints keep the brain informed about the position of various body parts in relation to each other. For example, you can tell if your leg is bent or straight without actually looking down to check its position. These same receptors also relay information to the brain about the degree of muscle contraction, especially when the muscle is contracting against resistance (for example, when you are lifting weights). Position sense provides us with muscle tone and the ability to move our muscles in a smooth, coordinated way.

PAIN. Pain tells us that we have been injured, that we have overworked a muscle group, that an organ is not working properly, or that we are ill. Free nerve endings (dendrites) in the skin and the tissues of our internal organs allow us to detect pain.

Taste and Smell

Sensory receptors on the tongue and in the nose allow us to taste and smell. These sensory receptors detect chemicals in the food we eat, the beverages we drink, and the air we breathe. The chemical signal is changed to an electrical one and carried by sensory neurons to the brain, which tells us what we are tasting or smelling.

Sight

Our eyes contain sensory receptors for vision. The eyes are protected by the bones of the skull and by the eyelashes, eyebrows, and tears. Skeletal muscles located around the eyeball allow us to move our eyes. The eyeball is made up of three layers of tissue (Fig. 7-16):

- The *sclera* is the tough outer layer. The sclera is made of connective tissue. Although most of the sclera is white, the front of the sclera, which is called the *cornea*, is clear. Light passes through the cornea to the inside of the eye.
- The *choroid* is the middle layer. This layer contains the blood vessels that supply the retina and other parts of the eye. At the front of the eye, the choroid also forms the ciliary body and the iris. The *ciliary body* is a muscular structure that

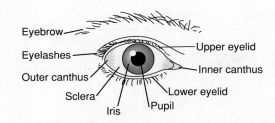

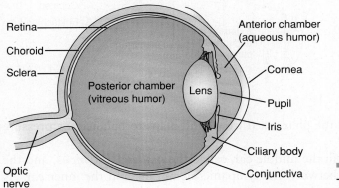

■ **FIGURE 7-16**

The eye.

attaches to the *lens*, a flexible, transparent, curved structure that adjusts to focus light rays onto the retina. The ciliary body changes the shape of the lens, allowing the eye to focus. The *iris* is the colored part of the eye. The iris is actually a round muscle with an opening in the center (the *pupil*). The iris controls the amount of light that enters the eye through the pupil.

■ The *retina* is the innermost layer. The retina contains sensory receptors, called rods and cones, which turn light into nerve impulses. The nerve impulses travel through the *optic nerve* to the brain for interpretation.

The eyeball also has two fluid-filled chambers (see Fig. 7-16):

■ The *anterior chamber* is located between the cornea and the lens. Special cells in the ciliary body secrete *aqueous humor*, a watery fluid that fills the anterior chamber. The aqueous humor passes through the anterior chamber and is reabsorbed back into the bloodstream.

■ The *posterior chamber* is located between the lens and the retina. The posterior chamber is filled with *vitreous humor*, a jelly-like substance that gives the eyeball its shape.

Hearing and Balance

The sense organ of hearing and balance is the ear (Fig. 7-17).

OUTER EAR. The outer ear consists of the part of the ear that you can see (called the *pinna* or the *auricle*) plus a short canal called the *external auditory canal*. The external auditory canal is lined with small hairs and special glands that secrete **cerumen**. The shape of the pinna allows it to collect sound waves and direct them down the external auditory canal toward the *tympanic membrane (eardrum)*.

MIDDLE EAR. The middle ear consists of an air space containing three small bones (called *ossicles*) and the opening of the *eustachian tube*. The eustachian tube

Cerumen a waxy substance that helps to protect the external auditory canal by trapping dirt and other particles; commonly referred to as "earwax"

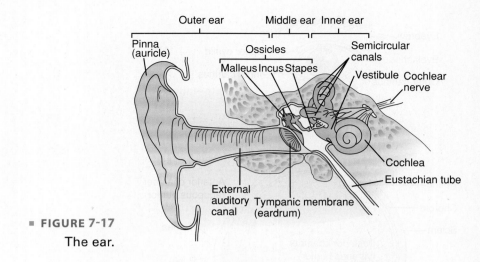

■ **FIGURE 7-17**

The ear.

connects the middle ear to the pharynx (throat) and helps to balance the pressure in the middle ear.

The three small bones in the middle ear, called the *malleus*, the *incus*, and the *stapes*, form a tiny bridge between the tympanic membrane and the inner ear. As the sound waves travel down the external auditory canal, they cause the tympanic membrane to vibrate. The tympanic membrane vibrations are then passed to the malleus, which sends the vibrations to the incus and then to the stapes.

INNER EAR. The inner ear contains the sensory receptors that make hearing and balance possible. Sensory receptors for hearing are found within the *cochlea*. The cochlea looks like a snail's shell and is filled with fluid. The stapes rests against a membrane at the opening of the cochlea called the *oval window*. When the stapes vibrates, it causes the oval window to vibrate, sending the vibrations through the fluid inside the cochlea. The moving fluid stimulates the sensory receptors inside the cochlea, which then send nerve impulses via the cochlear nerve to the brain. The brain interprets these nerve impulses as sound.

The other part of the inner ear consists of two sac-like structures called the *vestibule* and three *semicircular canals*. The vestibule and the semicircular canals, which are referred to together as the *vestibular apparatus*, help us to keep our balance. Like the cochlea, the semicircular canals are filled with fluid. When your body position changes, sensory receptors in the vestibular apparatus are stimulated. These sensory receptors then send nerve impulses via the vestibular nerve to the brain. These nerve impulses tell the brain what the body's position is relative to the ground.

The Effects of Aging on the Sensory System

Age-related changes that affect the sensory system can put an older person at risk for harm. They may also make it more difficult for the person to communicate with others.

■ **General sense.** The sense of touch becomes diminished because of the loss of sensory receptors in the skin. This can put the person at risk for accidental burns.

■ **Taste and smell.** The senses of taste and smell become weaker due to a decreased number of chemoreceptors on the tongue and on the roof of the nasal cavity. This can lead to a decrease in appetite. It can also put the older person at risk for injury. For example, an older person may not be able to tell that food has spoiled and so may become ill from eating it. Similarly, he or she may not be able to detect the smell of smoke or a gas leak.

- **Sight.** Changes in the eye as a result of aging can lead to **presbyopia** and dry eyes. In addition, older people need more time to adjust when moving from a brightly lit area to a dim one or vice versa.

- **Hearing.** Many older people gradually develop **presbycusis**. A person with presbycusis has trouble telling the difference between similar-sounding high-pitched sounds like *th* and *s*, which can lead to frequent misunderstandings. Many older people with presbycusis are mistakenly labeled "confused" or "disoriented" by family members, friends, or health care workers, but in fact, they just cannot hear well. A person with presbycusis may have trouble following conversations, especially when many people are talking at once or there is a lot of background noise. As a result, the person may start to avoid social situations because he or she cannot hear well and is embarrassed to have to keep asking others to repeat themselves. Avoiding social gatherings can lead to a feeling of isolation and a decreased quality of life for the older person. When speaking with a person with presbycusis, speak slowly and use a lower tone of voice. This may make it easier for the person to understand what you are saying.

Presbyopia age-related loss of the eye's ability to focus on objects that are close

Presbycusis age-related hearing loss

Putting it all together!

- Our sensory system protects us from harm and lets us experience the world that we live in.

- Sensory receptors are found throughout the body and allow us to sense touch, position, and pain.

- Sensory receptors are also located in the specific sense organs: the eyes, ears, nose, and tongue.

- Age-related changes that affect the sensory system can put the older person at risk for injury and may make it harder for the person to communicate with others. Normal age-related changes include a decreased sense of taste and smell, presbyopia (an inability to focus on objects that are close), and presbycusis (age-related hearing loss).

The Endocrine System

What will you learn?

When you are finished with this section, you will be able to:

1. Discuss the main function of the endocrine system.
2. List and describe the glands that make up the endocrine system.
3. List the hormones produced by the different glands of the endocrine system.
4. Describe the normal changes related to aging that occur in the endocrine system.
5. Define the word **hormones**.

Structure and Function of the Endocrine System

The endocrine system consists of glands throughout the body (Table 7-2). The endocrine system controls many of the body's processes, such as growth and development, reproduction, and metabolism. It does this by producing **hormones**, which are released into the bloodstream. The hormone travels in the blood until it reaches

Hormones chemicals that act on cells to produce a response

TABLE 7-2   The Endocrine System

Gland	Hormones	Effect on Body
Pineal gland	Melatonin	Regulates sleep–wake cycles
Pituitary gland	Adrenocorticotropic hormone (ACTH) Thyroid-stimulating hormone (TSH) Gonadotropins Prolactin Growth hormone Oxytocin Antidiuretic hormone (ADH)	Controls other glands in the endocrine system
Thyroid gland	Thyroxine	Sets the metabolism rate for the body's cells
	Calcitonin	Lowers the amount of calcium in the bloodstream by allowing calcium to be deposited in the bones and eliminated by the kidneys
Parathyroid glands (behind thyroid gland)	Parathyroid hormone (PTH)	Causes calcium to be released from the bones into the bloodstream
Thymus	Thymosin	Helps infection-fighting cells mature
Adrenal glands	Epinephrine Norepinephrine Glucocorticoids Mineralocorticoids Androgens	Help manage stress, metabolize fats and proteins, regulate the level of certain minerals in the body, and produce sex hormones
Pancreas	Insulin	Lowers blood glucose levels
	Glucagon	Raises blood glucose levels
Sex glands: Ovaries (female) Testes (male)	Sex hormones	Regulate reproduction

the specific cells that it acts on. Some hormones act on all of the body's cells, while other hormones act on only certain types of cells. Sometimes, the effects of the hormone occur over a long period of time. Other times, the effects of hormones occur more quickly. Hormones with short-term effects help the body to maintain homeostasis.

Pituitary Gland

The pituitary gland is connected by a stalk to the hypothalamus (part of the brain). The hypothalamus controls the pituitary gland. The pituitary gland releases hormones that affect other glands in the endocrine system. In this sense, the pituitary gland is like the "master gland." The pituitary gland has two parts, the posterior lobe and the anterior lobe (Fig. 7-18).

Thyroid Gland

The thyroid gland secretes thyroxine and calcitonin:

- *Thyroxine* sets the metabolism rate for the body's cells.
- *Calcitonin* (also called thyrocalcitonin) lowers the amount of calcium in the bloodstream by allowing the calcium to be stored in the bones and eliminated by the kidneys.

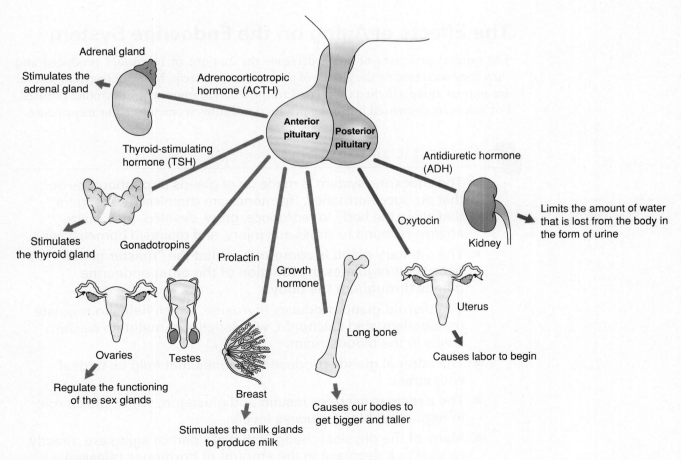

- **FIGURE 7-18**

The pituitary gland, or "master gland," releases hormones that affect other glands in the endocrine system.

Adrenal Glands

The adrenal glands are located on top of the kidneys. Each adrenal gland has two parts: the *medulla*, or inner portion, and the *cortex*, or outer portion. The medulla secretes *epinephrine* (adrenaline) and *norepinephrine*, two hormones that are responsible for the "fight-or-flight" response of the body in emergency situations. The cortex secretes:

- *Glucocorticoids*, which play a role in the metabolism of fats and proteins and help the body to maintain a reserve of glucose (sugar) that can be used in times of stress
- *Mineralocorticoids*, which help to regulate the level of certain minerals in the body, particularly sodium and potassium
- *Androgens*, which are changed by the body into the sex hormones *testosterone* (in men) and *estradiol* (in women)

Pancreas

The pancreas produces insulin and glucagon, which work together to keep the body's blood glucose levels stable:

- *Insulin* allows glucose to be transported from the bloodstream into the individual cells, where it is used for energy. In this way, insulin lowers the blood glucose level.
- *Glucagon* raises the blood glucose level by stimulating the liver to release stored glucose into the bloodstream.

The Effects of Aging on the Endocrine System

The normal processes of aging decrease the amount of hormones produced and slow their secretion by the glands of the endocrine system. Many of the changes that are part of aging are directly related to the smaller amounts of hormone released. For example, decreased hormone production causes women to enter menopause.

 Putting it all together!

- The endocrine system is made up of glands throughout the body that produce hormones. Hormones are chemical messengers that allow the body to reproduce, grow, develop, metabolize energy, respond to stress and injury, and maintain homeostasis.
- The pituitary gland is commonly called the "master gland" because it regulates the function of the other endocrine glands throughout the body.
- The thyroid gland produces thyroxine, which helps to regulate metabolism, and calcitonin, which helps to maintain calcium levels in the bloodstream.
- The adrenal glands produce hormones that help us to deal with stress.
- The pancreas secretes insulin and glucagon, which play a role in regulating blood glucose levels.
- Many of the physical changes that are part of aging are directly related to a decrease in the amount of hormones released throughout the body.

The Digestive System

What will you learn?

When you are finished with this section, you will be able to:

1. List and describe the main parts of the digestive system.
2. Discuss the main functions of the digestive system.
3. Describe the normal changes related to aging that occur in the digestive system.
4. Define the words **feces**, **peristalsis**, **digestion**, **enzymes**, **absorption**, and **constipation**.

Structure and Function of the Digestive System

The digestive system breaks down the food we eat into nutrients, which are then absorbed into the bloodstream for use by the body's cells. The digestive system also removes unusable digested food from the body, in the form of **feces**.

The digestive system is a long tube, or *tract*, consisting of the mouth, pharynx, esophagus, stomach, small intestine, and large intestine (Fig. 7-19). The walls of the "tube" are made up of four layers of tissue. The layers are basically the same throughout the digestive tract, although there is some variation from region to region. The inner layer, called the *mucosa*, secretes mucus and helps to protect us from germs and from the harsh chemicals found in stomach acid. The next layer, the *submucosa*, contains the blood vessels and nerves that supply the digestive tract. The *muscle* layer contains smooth muscle, which contracts and relaxes, allowing **peristalsis** to occur. The *serosa* is a tough outer layer of connective tissue.

In addition, several accessory organs—the teeth, salivary glands, liver, gallbladder, and pancreas—play a role in digestion but are not actually part of the digestive tract (see Fig. 7-19).

- The *teeth* are located in the mouth and assist with chewing food.
- The *salivary glands* produce and secrete saliva, a substance that helps with chewing and swallowing by moistening the food.
- The *liver* produces and secretes *bile*, a substance that helps us to digest fat.
- The *gallbladder*, a small pouch that is attached to the liver, stores bile produced by the liver that is not secreted directly into the small intestine.
- The *pancreas* produces substances that aid in digestion and secretes them into the small intestine. The pancreas also produces insulin and glucagon, hormones that are secreted directly into the bloodstream.

Mouth

Food is taken in through the mouth. **Digestion** begins in the mouth. First, we physically break the food into smaller pieces by chewing it. Next, **enzymes** in our saliva start to work on the smaller pieces of food, breaking them down even more.

Pharynx

From the mouth, the food moves into the pharynx (throat).

Feces the semi-solid waste product of digestion; stool

Peristalsis involuntary wave-like muscular movements, such as those that occur in the digestive system to move chyme (partially digested food) through the intestines

Digestion the process of breaking food down into simple elements (nutrients)

Enzymes substances that have the ability to break chemical bonds

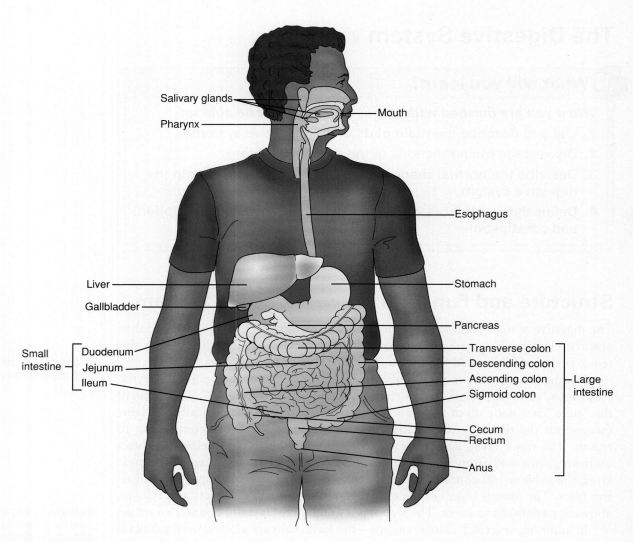

■ **FIGURE 7-19**

The digestive system.

Esophagus

From the pharynx, the food passes into the esophagus, a long, narrow tube that serves mainly as a passageway for food to get from the pharynx to the stomach. The esophagus passes through the chest cavity, behind the heart. After entering the abdominal cavity, the esophagus connects with the upper part of the stomach. The mucus secreted by the esophageal mucosa, as well as the action of the muscle layer, helps to move food downward and into the stomach. The *esophageal (cardiac) sphincter*, a circle of muscular tissue, surrounds the place where the esophagus enters the stomach and keeps food from going back up the esophagus after it has entered the stomach.

Stomach

The stomach is a hollow, muscular holding pouch for food. The food we eat stays in the stomach for 3 to 4 hours, where digestion continues to take place. Special glands in the stomach lining produce stomach acid and enzymes. The stomach acid and enzymes act on the pieces of food to break them down even further. The muscular action of the stomach helps to mix the food with the acid and enzymes, creating a liquid substance called *chyme*.

Small Intestine

The chyme leaves the stomach through the *pyloric sphincter*, a circle of muscular tissue that surrounds the place where the stomach empties into the small intestine and helps to prevent food from returning to the stomach once it enters the small intestine. The small intestine has three regions, called the *duodenum*, the *jejunum*, and the *ileum* (see Fig. 7-19). In the duodenum, the chyme mixes with bile (secreted by the liver) and digestive enzymes secreted by the pancreas. These substances cause further breakdown of the food.

When the chyme reaches the jejunum, **absorption** of nutrients begins. To reach the bloodstream, the nutrients pass through the mucosa and into the blood vessels in the submucosa. The mucosa of the small intestine has millions of tiny, finger-like structures called *villi* (Fig. 7-20). The villi increase the small intestine's ability to absorb nutrients by increasing the surface area of the mucosa.

Absorption transfer of nutrients from the digestive tract into the bloodstream

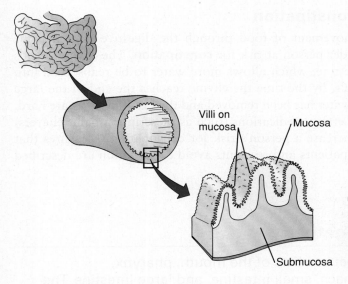

Villi on mucosa

Mucosa

Submucosa

■ **FIGURE 7-20**

Villi are finger-like projections that increase the small intestine's ability to absorb nutrients.

Large Intestine

After leaving the ileum of the small intestine, the chyme passes into the large intestine (*colon*). The large intestine also has several distinct regions (see Fig. 7-19):

- The *cecum* is like a "waiting room" for food that is leaving the small intestine and entering the large intestine. The *appendix* is a tiny, closed pouch that dangles from the cecum. Inflammation or infection of the appendix causes *appendicitis*.
- The *ascending colon* travels upward from the cecum.
- The *transverse colon* travels across.
- The *descending colon* travels down.
- The *sigmoid colon* is an S-shaped curve at the end of the descending colon.
- The *rectum* is the last segment of the colon. The place where the rectum opens to the outside of the body is the *anus*.

Although most of the absorption of nutrients takes place in the small intestine, the large intestine also plays a role in absorption. Bacteria that live in the large intestine act on the chyme to produce vitamin K and some B vitamins, which are absorbed by the body. The action of these bacteria on the chyme can also produce gas as a by-product.

As the chyme passes slowly through the large intestine, water is absorbed into the bloodstream. By the time the chyme reaches the rectum, all nutrients and most of the water have been removed, and the chyme has taken on the consistency of normal feces. The walls of the rectum gradually expand as the feces build up. At a certain point, the brain senses that the rectum is "full" and the urge to have a bowel movement occurs.

The Effects of Aging on the Digestive System

Difficulty Chewing and Swallowing

In older people, saliva production decreases, which may make chewing and swallowing more difficult. In addition, many older people have dental problems, such as missing or painful teeth. An older person may choke as a result of trying to swallow food that has not been chewed properly. Remember this when you are helping an older person to eat. Create a relaxed, social environment for eating and help the person to cut food up into small, easy-to-chew pieces.

Increased Risk for Constipation

Constipation a condition that occurs when the feces remain in the intestines for too long, resulting in hard, dry feces that are difficult to pass

In an older person, the movement of food through the digestive tract may be slower. This can put the older person at risk for **constipation**. The chyme spends more time in the large intestine, which allows more water to be reabsorbed into the bloodstream. As a result, by the time the chyme reaches the end of the large intestine, almost all of the water has been removed and the resulting feces are hard, dry, and difficult to pass. Certain medications (such as prescription pain relievers) and immobility can also increase a person's risk for constipation. Measures that you can take to help your patients and residents avoid constipation are described in Chapter 26.

Putting it all together!

- The digestive tract consists of the mouth, pharynx, esophagus, stomach, small intestine, and large intestine. The walls of the digestive tract are lined with a mucous membrane (mucosa) and contain smooth muscle, which contracts to move food through the digestive tract.

- The accessory organs of the digestive system play a role in digestion but are not actually part of the digestive tract. Accessory organs include the teeth, salivary glands, liver, gallbladder, and pancreas.

- The digestive system breaks down the food we eat into nutrients that can be used by the cells of the body. The digestive system also removes waste from the body in the form of feces. Most digestion takes place in the mouth and stomach. Most absorption takes place in the small and large intestines. Feces are what are left after all of the nutrients and most of the water have been removed from the chyme during its passage through the small and large intestines.

- As a person gets older, he or she may have more trouble chewing and swallowing food. In addition, the older person may be at higher risk for becoming constipated.

The Urinary System

What will you learn?

When you are finished with this section, you will be able to:

1. List and describe the main parts of the urinary system.
2. Describe the main functions of the urinary system.
3. Describe the normal changes related to aging that occur in the urinary system.
4. Define the words **filtrate** and **urine**.

Structure and Function of the Urinary System

The urinary system consists of the kidneys, the ureters, the bladder, and the urethra (Fig. 7-21). The main function of the urinary system is to remove waste products and excess fluid from the body. The urinary system also helps to regulate the acidity of the blood and the levels of minerals, such as sodium, calcium,

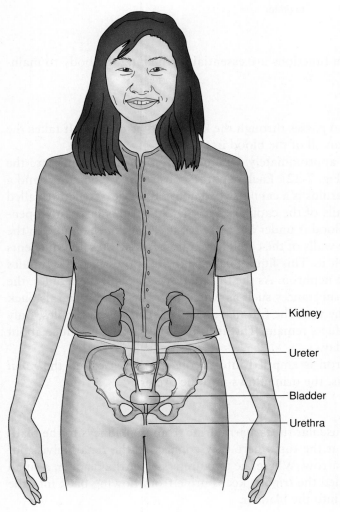

Kidney

Ureter

Bladder

Urethra

■ **FIGURE 7-21**

The urinary system.

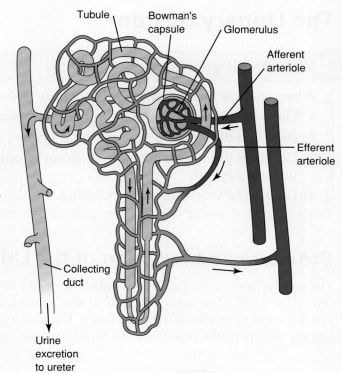

Tubule   Bowman's capsule   Glomerulus

Afferent arteriole

Efferent arteriole

Collecting duct

Urine excretion to ureter

■ **FIGURE 7-22**

Each nephron consists of a glomerulus and a series of tubules. Blood (*red*) enters the glomerulus through the *afferent* arteriole (*afferent* means "enter"). The glomerulus filters the blood, producing filtrate, the basis of urine (*yellow*). Filtered blood (*purple*) leaves the glomerulus through the efferent arteriole (*efferent* means "exit") and is returned to the circulation.

and potassium. All of these functions are essential for helping the body to maintain homeostasis.

Kidneys

We have two kidneys. Blood passes through the kidneys to be cleaned. It takes the kidneys half an hour to clean all of the blood in the body.

Inside each kidney are approximately 1 million tiny *nephrons*, which are the units that clean the blood (Fig. 7-22). Each nephron consists of a *glomerulus* and a series of *tubules*. The glomerulus is a capillary bed, located inside a structure called *Bowman's capsule*. The walls of the capillaries in the glomerulus have tiny openings in them. Because the blood is under a lot of pressure, a lot of the liquid in the blood squeezes through the walls of the capillaries, taking the wastes and nutrients that are dissolved in it with it. This liquid, called **filtrate**, flows into the tubules that make up the rest of the nephron. As the filtrate flows through the tubules, the capillaries reabsorb useful substances such as water, nutrients, and minerals back into the bloodstream. By the time the filtrate reaches the end of the tubules, only excess fluid and waste products remain. This is **urine**. The kidneys produce about 1 to 1.5 liters of urine per day.

Urine from each nephron is emptied into a collecting area called the *renal pelvis*. From the renal pelvis, the urine flows into the ureters.

Ureters

The ureters, two slender, muscular tubes, carry urine from the kidneys to the bladder. The ureters are wider at the top where they connect to the renal pelvis, but they quickly become very narrow. Where the two ureters enter the bladder, a small triangular fold of tissue called the *trigone* keeps urine from flowing back into the ureters after it has emptied into the bladder.

Filtrate the liquid that forms the basis for urine

Urine formed by the kidneys; consists of waste products that have been filtered from the bloodstream, along with excess fluid

The ureters are lined with a mucous membrane, which helps to protect against infection. Smooth muscle in the walls of the ureters contracts rhythmically, moving urine away from the kidney and toward the bladder.

Bladder

The bladder is a hollow sac that is a holding place for urine. Like the ureters, the inside of the bladder is lined with a mucous membrane. The walls of the bladder contain three layers of smooth muscle. When the walls of the bladder contract, urination occurs. The *internal sphincter*, a ring of involuntary muscle located where the bladder and the urethra join, keeps the bladder closed while it fills. The *external urethral sphincter*, a ring of voluntary muscle, relaxes to allow urine to pass during urination.

A moderately full bladder usually contains about 1 pint (470 mL) of urine. When about 200 to 300 mL of urine collects in the bladder, the internal sphincter opens and allows urine to flood the upper part of the urethra. At this point, the urge to urinate occurs. The person voluntarily relaxes the external urethral sphincter, and the muscles of the bladder contract, allowing urine to pass out of the body through the urethra. Although it is possible to delay urination for some time, eventually the bladder will empty itself automatically.

Urethra

The urethra is the tube that carries urine from the bladder to the outside of the body. The urethra begins just below the internal sphincter and ends at the *urinary meatus*. Male and female urethras are different in size and function (Fig. 7-23). In

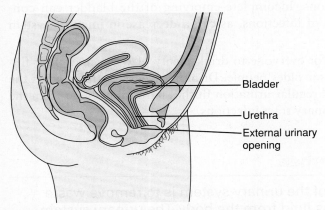

— Bladder

— Urethra

— External urinary opening

Female urethra: 1½ to 2½ inches and straight

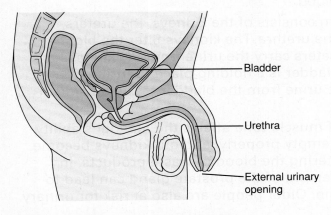

— Bladder

— Urethra

— External urinary opening

Male urethra: 6 to 8 inches and "S"-shaped

■ **FIGURE 7-23**

Female and male urethras.

women, the urethra is used only to pass urine. In men, the urethra serves as a passageway for both urine and semen.

The Effects of Aging on the Urinary System

The normal processes of aging affect the urinary system in many different ways:

- **Less efficient removal of waste from the blood.** After a person reaches 40 years of age or so, the number of functioning nephrons in the kidneys starts to decrease, decreasing the kidneys' ability to filter waste products from the bloodstream.

- **Decreased muscle tone.** Loss of muscle tone as a result of aging can reduce the amount of urine the bladder can hold and may contribute to stress incontinence. This type of urinary incontinence, which is most common in older women who have had children or are obese, can often be corrected with exercises or surgery.

- **Enlargement of the prostate gland (in men).** In older men, enlargement of the prostate gland is common. As the prostate gland enlarges, it pushes against the urethra, causing it to narrow. Total emptying of the bladder of urine becomes difficult. Because the bladder does not empty completely when the man urinates, it refills with urine quickly, and the urine simply overflows. As a result, the man may "dribble" urine in between visits to the bathroom.

- **Increased risk for urinary tract infections.** Older people are also more likely to get urinary tract infections. Incomplete emptying of the bladder can contribute to the development of infections, as can a decrease in immune system functioning.

Although it is important for everyone to drink plenty of water and other fluids, it is especially important for older people. Drinking plenty of fluids helps the kidneys to work properly, and regular urination flushes harmful bacteria from the bladder, helping to prevent urinary tract infections.

 Putting it all together!

- The main function of the urinary system is to remove waste products and excess fluid from the body. The urinary system also plays a role in homeostasis by regulating minerals and the acidity of the blood.

- The urinary system consists of the kidneys, the ureters, the bladder, and the urethra. The kidneys filter the blood to form urine. The ureters carry the urine from the kidneys to the bladder. The bladder is a holding place for urine. The urethra carries the urine from the bladder to the outside of the body.

- As we age, loss of muscle tone affects the bladder's ability to hold urine and empty properly, and our kidneys become less efficient at filtering the blood of waste products. In older men, enlargement of the prostate gland can lead to "dribbling" of urine. Older people are also at risk for urinary tract infections.

The Reproductive System

What will you learn?

When you are finished with this section, you will be able to:

1. List and describe the main parts of the female reproductive system.
2. Discuss the main functions of the female reproductive system.
3. List and describe the main parts of the male reproductive system.
4. Discuss the main functions of the male reproductive system.
5. Describe the normal changes related to aging that occur in the reproductive system.
6. Define the words **reproduction, sex cells, conception (fertilization), puberty, menopause, menstrual period, ovulation, lactation,** and **ejaculation.**

Structure and Function of the Reproductive System

Without a means of **reproduction**, human life would cease to exist. One of the main functions of the reproductive system in both men and women is to produce and transport **sex cells (gametes)**. Each species has a set number of genes, or chromosomes. For example, human beings have 46 chromosomes. This means that to keep the number of chromosomes the same from generation to generation, the father's sex cell (the *sperm*) contains 23 chromosomes and the mother's sex cell (the *egg* or *ovum*) contains 23 chromosomes. When the sperm joins the egg, **conception (fertilization)** occurs. During the 9 months leading up to the birth of a baby, the single original cell that formed at conception copies itself over and over again, forming all of the baby's tissues and organs.

The Female Reproductive System

The female reproductive system is designed to produce eggs, receive sperm cells, contain and nourish a developing baby, give birth, and provide nourishment after the baby's birth by producing breast milk. Each month during a woman's reproductive years (from **puberty** to **menopause**), her body prepares itself to become pregnant. If pregnancy does not occur, the woman has a **menstrual period**, and the cycle begins again.

INTERNAL ORGANS. The internal organs of the female reproductive system are the ovaries, fallopian tubes, uterus, and vagina (Fig. 7-24).

- **Ovaries.** When a girl baby is born, her ovaries contain all of the eggs she will ever have. The stored eggs are kept in a "holding pattern" until they are needed. Once a girl reaches puberty, **ovulation** occurs each month.
- **Fallopian tubes.** The fallopian tubes are slender tubes about 4 to 5 inches long that transport the egg from the ovary to the uterus. Fertilization, if it occurs, occurs in the fallopian tubes.

Reproduction the process by which a living thing makes more living things like itself

Sex cells (gametes) special cells contributed by each parent that contain half of the normal number of chromosomes

Conception (fertilization) occurs when the male and female sex cells join, forming a cell that contains the complete number of chromosomes

Puberty the period during which the secondary sex characteristics appear and the reproductive organs begin to function

Menopause the cessation of menstruation and fertility that women typically experience in their early 50s

Menstrual period the monthly loss of blood through the vagina that occurs in the absence of pregnancy

Ovulation the release of a ripe, mature egg from the female ovaries each month

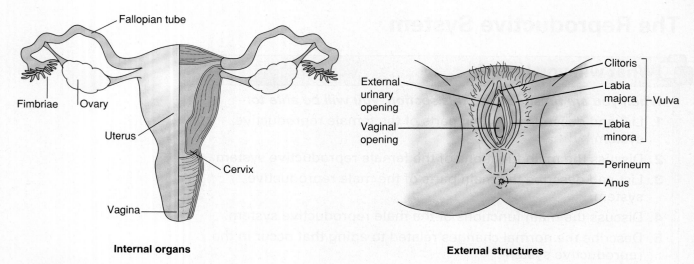

Internal organs

External structures

■ **FIGURE 7-24**

The female reproductive system.

■ **Uterus.** The uterus ("womb") is a hollow, muscular organ. If fertilization has occurred, the fertilized egg will attach to the lining of the uterus, called the *endometrium*, and continue to grow. (If fertilization has not occurred, the egg dissolves and is shed with the lining of the uterus during the menstrual period.) The muscular walls of the uterus expand to make room for the growing baby and then contract during labor to push the baby out. The *cervix* is the lower, narrow portion of the uterus. A very small opening allows sperm to enter and menstrual blood to leave. The cervix dilates during labor to allow a baby to be born.

■ **Vagina.** The vagina is a muscular tube about 3 inches long that connects the uterus to the outside of the body. The vagina is the receiving organ for sperm. It also serves as the birth canal through which a baby passes during birth.

EXTERNAL STRUCTURES. The external structures of the female reproductive system, sometimes collectively referred to as the *vulva*, are the vaginal opening, the labia, and the clitoris (see Fig. 7-24).

■ The **vaginal opening** is where the vagina opens to the outside of the body. The vaginal opening is located between the external urinary opening and the anus.

■ The **labia,** or "lips," are folds of tissue that surround the vaginal opening.

■ The **clitoris** is located at the top of the labia. This tissue, which is very sensitive to touch, helps a woman to become sexually aroused.

ACCESSORY ORGANS. The breasts (mammary glands) nourish the newborn baby. Although the female breasts develop during puberty, they do not produce milk until the end of pregnancy. The breasts are made up of lobes, or sections, that contain glandular tissue and fat (Fig. 7-25). When the breast tissue is stimulated by the hormone prolactin, **lactation** occurs. In response to the baby's suckling, the glandular tissue contracts, sending the milk through the ducts to the nipple.

Lactation the process by which the glandular tissue of the female breast produces milk

The Male Reproductive System

The male reproductive system is designed to produce sperm and deposit it inside the female's body. The organs and structures of the male reproductive system include the testicles (testes), the epididymis, the vas deferens, and the penis (Fig. 7-26). Accessory organs include the seminal vesicles and prostate gland.

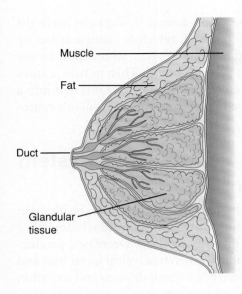

Muscle

Fat

Duct

Glandular
tissue

■ **FIGURE 7-25**

The breasts consist of glandular tissue
and fat.

■ **Testicles (testes).** The testicles are located in the *scrotum*, a loose, bag-like sac of skin that is suspended outside of the body between the thighs. The testicles secrete testosterone, the hormone that is responsible for the development of male secondary sex characteristics and for the proper functioning of the male reproductive system. The testicles also produce sperm cells. The testicles are located outside of a man's body because the temperature necessary for the proper development of sperm is lower than the temperature inside the body.

■ **Epididymis.** After the sperm cells leave the testes, they move into the epididymis, a series of coiled tubes where the sperm cells mature and develop the whip-like "tail" that gives them the ability to "swim" through the female reproductive tract in search of an egg to fertilize.

■ **Vas deferens.** From the epididymis, the sperm cells move into the vas deferens, a passageway that transports the sperm cells to the urethra. While in the vas deferens, the sperm cells are mixed with the secretions from the seminal vesicles and the prostate gland. These secretions, which nourish and protect the sperm cells, form *semen*, the fluid that carries the sperm cells out of the body. In the prostate gland, the vas deferens joins with the urethra, which is the final passageway through which the sperm cells leave the man's body.

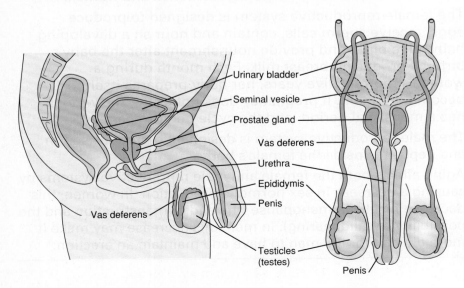

Urinary bladder

Seminal vesicle

Prostate gland

Vas deferens

Urethra

Epididymis

Penis

Vas deferens

Testicles
(testes)

Penis

■ **FIGURE 7-26**

The male reproductive system.

■ **Penis.** The male urethra is contained in the penis. Semen (and urine) leave the man's body by way of the external urinary opening, which is located at the tip of the penis. The urethra is surrounded by "spongy" tissue. Stimulation by the nervous system causes this spongy tissue to fill with blood. This, in turn, causes the penis to become hard and erect. When erect, the penis can be inserted into a woman's vagina, allowing sperm cells to be deposited into the woman's reproductive tract via **ejaculation**.

Ejaculation the forceful release of semen from the body; method by which sperm cells leave the man's body through the penis

The Effects of Aging on the Reproductive System

The Female Reproductive System

As a woman ages, her body produces lower amounts of sex hormones, resulting in menopause. Menopause can cause many uncomfortable symptoms, including "hot flashes," irritability, a loss of energy, and an inability to sleep. Decreased production of female sex hormones may also cause some women to develop facial hair and a coarse ("scratchy") voice. Some women experience vaginal dryness and irritation and may need to use a lubricant during sexual intercourse.

The Male Reproductive System

As they get older, many men find that the frequency and duration of their erections decrease. This is a result of decreased sex hormone production. A man's ability to have and maintain an erection may also be affected by the effects of aging on the cardiovascular system, which can result in decreased blood flow to the penis. Medications taken for hypertension and other common disorders can also affect a man's sexual abilities.

As a man ages, the prostate gland tends to enlarge. Because the prostate gland surrounds the urethra, this enlargement can make urination difficult. Prostate problems associated with aging are discussed earlier in this chapter.

Putting it all together!

■ Reproduction is the process by which a living thing makes more living things like itself. Although in both men and women the reproductive system produces cells and hormones that are necessary to create a new life, the organs that make up the reproductive system are very different in men and women.

■ The female reproductive system is designed to produce eggs, receive sperm cells, contain and nourish a developing baby, give birth, and provide nourishment after the baby's birth by producing breast milk. Each month during a woman's reproductive years, her body prepares itself to become pregnant. If pregnancy does not occur, the woman has a menstrual period, and the cycle begins again.

■ The male reproductive system is designed to produce sperm and deposit it inside the female's body.

■ Aging affects both the female and male reproductive systems by causing a decrease in sex hormone production. In women, this decrease results in menopause (the end of menstruation and the possibility of childbearing). In men, this decrease may make it more difficult for the man to have and maintain an erection.

WHAT DID YOU LEARN?

Multiple Choice

Select the single best answer for each of the following questions.

1. What is the purpose of epithelial tissue?
   a. To provide a frame for, and give shape to, the body
   b. To connect other types of tissue together
   c. To cover the body and line its cavities
   d. To conduct nerve impulses

2. The substance found in the epidermis that gives our skin, hair, and eyes color is called:
   a. Keratin
   b. Melanin
   c. Sebum
   d. Collagen

3. Which of the following is a normal age-related change affecting the integumentary system?
   a. The nails become thick and tough
   b. The body produces less sweat
   c. The skin becomes dry and fragile
   d. All of the above

4. Which of the following is a function of the skeletal system?
   a. It acts as a storage site for vitamin C
   b. It produces heat
   c. It produces blood cells
   d. All of the above

5. When a muscle atrophies, it becomes:
   a. Larger and stronger
   b. Thinner and weaker
   c. Stiff
   d. More flexible

6. Where does gas exchange take place in the respiratory system?
   a. In the alveoli
   b. In the bronchioles
   c. In the pharynx
   d. In the nasal cavity

7. What part of the respiratory tract is also known as the "windpipe"?
   a. Pharynx
   b. Epiglottis
   c. Larynx
   d. Trachea

8. The upper chambers of the heart are called the:
   a. Ventricles
   b. Atria
   c. Mitral valves
   d. Arterioles

9. Blood cells that contain hemoglobin and carry oxygen are called:
   a. Leukocytes
   b. Phagocytes
   c. Thrombocytes
   d. Erythrocytes

10. Varicose veins are commonly caused by:
    a. Loss of elasticity in the veins
    b. Forceful heart contractions
    c. Loss of elasticity in the arteries
    d. A decreased number of red blood cells

11. How does aging affect the nervous system?
    a. Older people usually become "senile" and forgetful
    b. Older people lose the ability to form or understand words
    c. Older people may take slightly longer to react to things
    d. Aging does not affect the nervous system because old neurons are constantly replaced

12. What is the fatty white substance covering a nerve fiber that helps speed the conduction of nerve impulses?
    a. Meninges
    b. Synapse
    c. Myelin
    d. Dendrite

13. What is the largest part of the brain?
    a. Cerebrum
    b. Cerebellum
    c. Brain stem
    d. Diencephalon

14. As a normal part of aging, many older people gradually lose the ability to hear high-pitched sounds. What is this called?
    a. Presbyopia
    b. Presbycusis
    c. Vestibular apparatus
    d. Cerumen

15. Hormones are chemical messengers that allow the body to:
    a. Metabolize energy
    b. Grow
    c. Reproduce
    d. All of the above

16. What hormone is secreted by the pancreas to help the body manage blood sugar levels?
    a. Insulin
    b. Thyroxine
    c. Glucocorticoids
    d. Antidiuretic hormone (ADH)

17. What is another term for the large intestine?
    a. Stomach
    b. Duodenum
    c. Cecum
    d. Colon

18. Bile helps to break down fats. Where is bile produced?
    a. Pancreas
    b. Liver
    c. Stomach
    d. Salivary glands

19. Normal changes in the digestive system related to aging include:
    a. More difficulty chewing and swallowing
    b. Sharper sense of taste and increased appetite
    c. Decreased risk for constipation
    d. All of the above

20. The tube that connects the kidneys to the bladder is called the:
    a. Ureter
    b. Urethra
    c. Trigone
    d. Sphincter

21. How much urine does an average adult pass each day?
    a. 200 mL of urine
    b. 500 mL of urine
    c. 1 to 1.5 liters of urine
    d. 160 to 180 liters of urine

22. How does aging affect the urinary system?
    a. The kidneys' ability to filter waste from the blood decreases
    b. The bladder is able to hold more urine
    c. The person's risk for constipation is increased
    d. The person's urine becomes darker

23. The complete ending of a woman's menstrual cycle that commonly occurs as part of the aging process is called:
    a. Puberty
    b. Pregnancy
    c. Menstrual period
    d. Menopause

24. What occurs when a male sex cell joins the female sex cell, forming a cell that contains the complete number of chromosomes?
    a. Ovulation
    b. Menstruation
    c. Menopause
    d. Conception

25. Where does conception usually occur?
    a. In the uterus
    b. In the vagina
    c. In the fallopian tube
    d. In the vas deferens

Matching

Match each organ system with its description.

_____ 1. Musculoskeletal system

_____ 2. Reproductive system

_____ 3. Endocrine system

_____ 4. Integumentary system

_____ 5. Digestive system

_____ 6. Respiratory system

_____ 7. Nervous system

_____ 8. Urinary system

_____ 9. Sensory system

_____ 10. Cardiovascular system

a. Provides a covering to protect the body

b. Allows the body to move

c. Provides oxygen and removes carbon dioxide

d. Transports oxygen and nutrients to the cells of the body

e. Receives, processes, and stores information

f. Protects us from harm and lets us experience the world we live in through the senses of touch, taste, sight, smell, and hearing

g. Controls body functions by secretion of hormones

h. Processes food and rids the body of waste

i. Filters the blood to remove excess fluid and waste

j. Provides the ability to produce children

 ## Stop *and* Think!

One of your residents, Mr. Conrad, has been suffering from a lung disorder for many years. He has difficulty breathing and seems to be prone to catch pneumonia. After learning about the function of the respiratory system, explain what effect a breathing disorder has on Mr. Conrad's body. What other body systems could this affect?

Common Disorders

Illnesses and injuries that result in disability are the main reasons a person will need the type of care that nursing assistants provide. You have learned about how the body functions when it is healthy. Now you will learn more about what happens to the body's organ systems as a result of illness or injury.

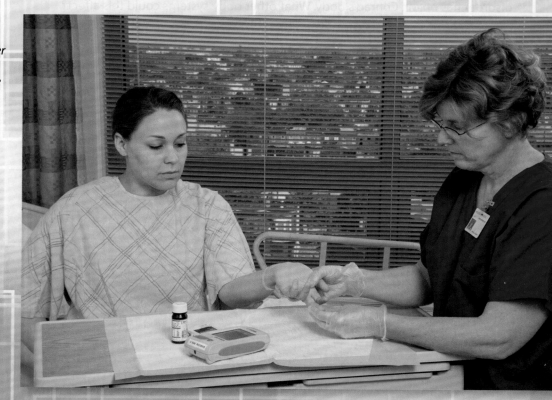

Photo: The nursing assistant checks the blood glucose level of a patient with diabetes, a disorder that occurs when the body is not able to produce or respond to the hormone insulin.

Introduction to Disorders

What will you learn?

When you are finished with this section, you will be able to:

1. Discuss the difference between acute and chronic disorders.
2. Describe the general categories used to describe the causes of disorders.
3. List factors that may put a person for risk for developing a certain disorder.
4. Define the words **disease**, **acute**, and **chronic**.

A disorder is something that affects the body's ability to maintain homeostasis. A disorder may also be called a "**disease**" or an "illness." A disorder can be **acute** or **chronic**. Disorders can be grouped into several broad categories based on their causes (Table 8-1).

Many factors can put a person at risk for developing a disorder or negatively affect his ability to recover from a disorder (Box 8-1). Awareness of the factors that can put your patients or residents at risk for a disorder will help you to better meet their individual needs.

Disease a condition that occurs when the structure or function of an organ or organ system is abnormal

Acute a word used to describe a disorder with a rapid onset and a relatively short recovery time; usually unexpected

Chronic a word used to describe a disorder that is ongoing and often needs to be controlled through continuous medication or treatment

TABLE 8-1 Types of Disorders

Type of Disorder	Cause	Examples
Infectious	Germs invade the body	Pneumonia, urinary tract infections, AIDS
Degenerative	The tissues of the body wear out or break down	Arthritis, osteoporosis, Alzheimer's disease
Nutritional	The person's diet is out of balance	Obesity, malnutrition
Metabolic (endocrine)	The body is unable to metabolize or absorb certain nutrients; often the result of producing too much of one type of hormone or not enough	Diabetes
Immunologic	The immune system does not work properly; the immune system may not be able to fight off infection, or the immune system starts to attack the body's own tissues	AIDS, rheumatoid arthritis, multiple sclerosis
Neoplastic	A tumor invades otherwise healthy tissues and prevents the tissues from functioning properly	Cancer
Psychiatric (mental)	The person is unable to maintain emotional balance	Depression, schizophrenia
Traumatic	The body's ability to function is changed by an outside force	Accidents, gunshot wounds, stabbing

BOX 8-1   Risk Factors for Disorders

- **Age.** Some disorders are more likely to occur in certain age groups. Age can also influence how a person reacts to disease. For example, an older person is much more likely to experience complications from the flu than a younger person is.

- **Gender.** Some disorders are more common in men than in women, and vice versa. For example, women are more likely to develop breast cancer than men are.

- **Heredity.** The genes that we get from our parents may put us at risk for developing certain diseases. For example, scientists now know that some types of cancer, diabetes, and heart disease are inherited.

- **Lifestyle.** A person's living conditions and health habits play a major role in the person's overall health status. For example, a person who smokes is more likely to develop cancer, lung disease, or heart disease than a person who does not.

- **Occupation.** Many jobs put a person at risk for certain diseases. For example, health care workers who do not take care to protect themselves are at risk for certain infections, such as HIV or hepatitis.

- **Chronic disease.** A person who has a chronic disease, such as diabetes or high blood pressure, is at increased risk for developing another disease. In addition, a person who has a chronic disease may be more likely to experience more severe problems from something that would not really affect a healthy person.

- **Emotional stress.** A person's emotional health can directly affect his or her physical health. Emotional stress can create physical problems such as headaches and digestive disorders, and it puts the body at higher risk for infection.

Putting it all together!

- When the body's ability to maintain homeostasis is altered, a disorder can result. A disorder can be acute (temporary) or chronic (long term).

- A disorder can be described as infectious, degenerative, nutritional, metabolic, immunologic, neoplastic, psychiatric, or traumatic in origin.

- Being aware of the factors that put a person at risk for disease will help you to provide better care for your patients or residents because you will have a better understanding of each individual's needs.

Integumentary Disorders

What will you learn?

When you are finished with this section, you will be able to:

1. Describe how an integumentary system disorder can place a person at risk for infection.
2. Describe what a burn is, and list the different types of burns.

3. Describe what a lesion is, and list the different types of lesions.
4. Discuss actions a nursing assistant can take to help promote comfort and skin healing in a person with a skin lesion.
5. Define the words **lesion** and **rash**.

Many people in your care will have a disorder of the integumentary system. Sometimes, this disorder is the reason the person is in the health care facility. For example, this might be the case for a person who has suffered severe burns or trauma. Other times, the disorder develops after the person is already in the health care facility. For example, a person might develop a pressure ulcer or have surgery that results in a surgical wound that must heal. Any break in the skin can allow germs to invade the body and cause an infection. If one of your patients or residents develops any type of skin disorder, you will need to report this to the nurse quickly so that measures can be taken to help the skin to heal and to prevent infection.

Pressure Ulcers

Pressure ulcers may form if a person is not able to move freely on his or her own. Pressure ulcers are discussed in detail in Chapter 22.

Burns

Burns are injuries to the skin and underlying tissues caused by contact with extreme heat, chemicals, or electricity. Burns are classified according to the depth of the damage:

■ **Superficial (First-degree) burns** cause injury to the outermost layer of the skin, the epidermis.

■ **Partial-thickness (Second-degree) burns** extend into the dermis. The loss of the epidermis increases the risk of infection.

■ **Full-thickness (Third-degree) burns** involve the epidermis and dermis, the subcutaneous layer, and often the underlying muscles and bones as well. Serious complications of third-degree burns include infection, scarring, and contractures (loss of motion in a joint resulting from shortening of the tendons).

People with second- and third-degree burns need very special care. Because of the risk of infection, caregivers must often wear sterile gloves and gowns when providing care, and bed linens may need to be sterilized before the bed is made.

Lesions

A **lesion** is a break in the skin (Table 8-2). Lesions often occur in groups, forming a **rash**. Rashes can be *localized* (limited to one area) or *systemic* (occurring all over the body). Rashes are often caused by an infection, such as chickenpox or the measles. In this case, the skin itself is not infected, but it is showing signs of an infection inside of the body. Shingles (herpes zoster) is a skin rash most commonly seen in people older than 65. It is caused by the same virus that causes chickenpox. A person with shingles should only be cared for by someone who has already been exposed to the chickenpox virus or has been immunized against chicken pox. It is possible to get chickenpox from a person with shingles if you have not been exposed to the virus before.

Lesion a general term used to describe any break in the skin

Rash a group of skin lesions

TABLE 8-2	Types of Skin Lesions
Lesion	**Description**
Macule	Small, flat, red lesions
Papule	Small, raised, firm bumps
Vesicle	Small, fluid-filled, blister-like lesions
Pustule	Small, pus-filled, blister-like lesions
Excoriation	Excoriation or abrasion (wearing away of the surface of the skin)
Fissure	A crack in the skin
Ulcer	A crater-like open sore

GUIDELINES BOX 8-1 Guidelines for Caring for a Person With a Skin Lesion

What you do	Why you do it
Check with the nurse or consult the nursing care plan to ensure that you are aware of any changes to the normal bathing and skin care routine that may be necessary.	*A special soap or lotion may have been ordered by the doctor as part of the person's treatment for the lesion. Or a product that is used as part of the normal bathing and skin care routine may be contributing to the skin problem and should no longer be used on the person.*
Help the person to choose clothing that does not rub or irritate the skin lesion.	*Protecting the lesion from additional irritation, such as that caused by clothing rubbing against it, is important to help it heal.*
Discourage the person from scratching itchy or irritated skin.	*Although scratching may bring temporary relief, it causes additional skin injury and puts the person at risk for infection.*
Observe the lesions for changes in color or for bleeding or drainage. Also note whether the lesions seem to be getting larger or spreading to other parts of the body. Report any changes to the nurse immediately.	*Your prompt reporting of any changes that you notice will help to ensure that the person receives the proper treatment.*
Make sure to follow your facility's infection control procedures when giving care to people who have skin lesions caused by an infection such as shingles or a localized infection.	*Following the proper infection control procedures will help to prevent the spread of the infection to other patients and residents and also to the people providing care to the person.*

Rashes may also be caused by contact with an irritant, such as poison ivy, bath soap, or laundry detergent. Itching, burning, or redness of the skin accompanies many skin lesions. When you are caring for a person with skin lesions, there are several things that you can do to increase the person's comfort and promote healing of the skin (Guidelines Box 8-1).

 ### Putting it all together!

- A break in the skin, such as that caused by wounds, burns, or lesions, puts the person at risk for infection.
- Burns are injuries caused by heat, chemicals, or electricity. Burns can be classified as first-degree (superficial), second-degree (partial-thickness), or third-degree (full-thickness) burns. People with second- and third-degree burn wounds require special care because of the very high risk of infection.
- Skin lesions can be caused by infections inside the body, infections of the skin itself, or irritation of the skin.
- As a nursing assistant, you will play a very important role in preventing the development of skin disorders, observing signs and symptoms of skin disorders, and helping people with skin disorders to heal.

Musculoskeletal Disorders

What will you learn?

When you are finished with this section, you will be able to:

1. Describe what osteoporosis is, and how to care for a person who has osteoporosis.
2. Describe three common types of arthritis.
3. Describe how to care for a person who has had hip-joint replacement surgery.
4. Describe how muscular dystrophy can cause disability.
5. Describe two ways that fractures are repaired, and discuss how to care for a person who has a cast.
6. Describe situations that can lead to amputation.
7. Define the terms **osteoporosis, arthritis, fracture, traction, amputation**, and **phantom pain**.

Osteoporosis

Osteoporosis a disorder characterized by the excessive loss of bone tissue

Although everyone experiences some loss of bone tissue as a normal part of aging, people with **osteoporosis** lose excessive amounts of bone tissue, causing the bones to become crumbly and very fragile. The bones most commonly affected by osteoporosis are the bones of the spine (Fig. 8-1), the pelvis, and the long bones in the arms and legs.

Osteoporosis is most common in older women. Other risk factors for the development of osteoporosis include:

- White race
- "Small bones"
- Smoking
- Inactivity or immobility
- Diseases of the thyroid and adrenal glands
- A diet lacking in calcium, vitamin D (necessary for the absorption of calcium), and protein
- Certain drugs, such as steroids

Osteoporosis causes bones to break more easily, and physical activity becomes very difficult. Guidelines for caring for a person with osteoporosis are given in Guidelines Box 8-2.

Arthritis

Arthritis inflammation of the joints, usually associated with pain and stiffness

There are many different types of **arthritis**. Three of the most common types are osteoarthritis, rheumatoid arthritis, and gout.

Osteoarthritis

Osteoarthritis is the leading cause of physical disability among elderly people. In osteoarthritis, the cartilage that covers the ends of the bones wears away, making

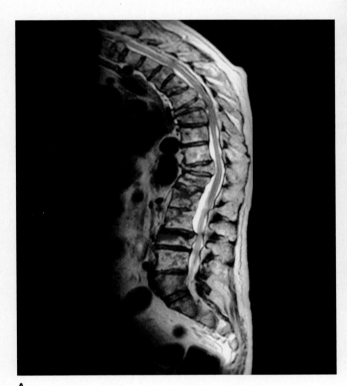

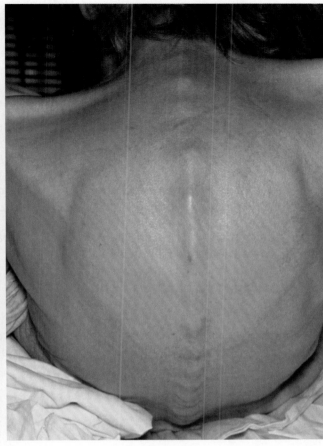

A   B

■ **FIGURE 8-1**

Osteoporosis. **(A)** A magnetic resonance imaging (MRI) scan of the spine of a 60-year-old patient with osteoporosis. This is a side view (the patient is standing, facing the left). The vertebrae (*brown*) enclose the spinal cord (*pink*). Some of the vertebrae (*orange*) have collapsed as a result of osteoporosis, causing the spine to curve. **(B)** This woman has a "dowager's hump" as a result of osteoporosis of the spine. The deformity occurs when the fragile bones of the spine crumble.

A, ©Zephyr/Science Photo Library; B, ©John Radcliffe Hospital/Science Photo Library.

movement of the joint difficult and painful. Osteoarthritis appears to be the result of normal wear and tear on the joint, which is why it is seen most often in elderly people. However, obesity, previous joint injury, or a family history of the disease may increase a person's risk of developing osteoarthritis earlier in life and more severely. Osteoarthritis usually affects weight-bearing joints, such as the knees, hips, and joints of the spine.

A person with osteoarthritis may take medications to decrease both the pain and swelling. Heat and cold applications, discussed in Chapter 27, can also increase a person's level of comfort. Mild exercise that places the affected joints through their range of motion helps to decrease stiffness and maintain joint function.

People who have very severe osteoarthritis may need joint replacement surgery, which involves removing the ends of the bones in the affected joint and replacing them with parts made from metal and plastic (Fig. 8-2). Hip and knee replacements are most common. Guidelines for caring for a person who has had hip replacement surgery are given in Guidelines Box 8-3.

GUIDELINES BOX 8-2   Guidelines for Caring for a Person With Osteoporosis

What you do	Why you do it
Remember to be gentle when helping the person to move.	*Sometimes bones are so brittle that a person can break them just by bumping into a piece of furniture. Bones that break are difficult to repair and heal slowly.*
Encourage exercise by having the person take frequent walks with you.	*Exercise helps to strengthen the bones and prevent complications of immobility.*
Carefully observe and document the types of foods and liquids the person eats and drinks, and encourage snacks that are high in calcium, such as milk, yogurt, ice cream, and cheese.	*Additional calcium can help slow bone loss.*
Be especially observant of loss of function, swelling, or complaints of pain.	*These signs and symptoms may indicate that a fragile bone has broken.*

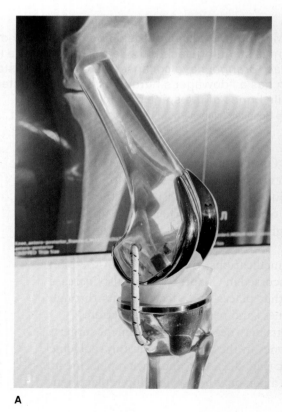

■ **FIGURE 8-2**
In joint replacement surgery, a damaged joint is replaced with an artificial (prosthetic) joint. **(A)** An artificial knee joint. **(B)** X-ray of an artificial knee joint in place. **A**

B

GUIDELINES BOX 8-3   Guidelines for Caring for a Person Who Has Had Hip Replacement Surgery

What you do	Why you do it
Assist the person with getting in and out of bed as necessary. Do not allow the person to bear weight on the affected joint without the doctor's approval.	*People who have had a joint replaced are not allowed to bear weight on the affected joint for a period of time after the surgery. The ligaments are weak, and placing weight on the joint can cause the joint to "give out."*
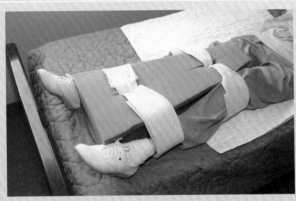 Use an abduction pillow to keep the person's legs abducted (spread apart) when the person is lying on his or her back or side.	*After the surgery, the muscles and ligaments that normally hold the hip joint in place are weak, making it very easy for the head of the femur (the thigh bone) to dislocate or pop out of joint. Keeping the legs abducted when the person is lying on his or her back or side helps to prevent this.*
Provide the person with a straight-backed chair to sit in.	*To prevent dislocation of the joint, the person's hips must be flexed no more than 90 degrees and the person's feet must rest flat on the floor. A straight-backed chair helps to ensure the proper sitting position.*
When assisting the person with elimination, use a special device to raise the height of the toilet seat, if necessary.	*Raising the height of the toilet seat helps to prevent flexion of the hip joint in excess of 90 degrees when the person is using the toilet.*
Ask to be present while the physical therapist is working with the person.	*This will enable you to learn the proper way to assist your patient or resident with getting in and out of bed and walking.*
Provide emotional support and encouragement.	*Recovering from surgery can be a long, difficult, and painful process. Your reassurance and encouragement are necessary to help keep the patient or resident focused on recovery.*

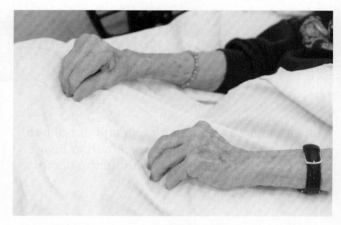

■ **FIGURE 8-3**

This woman has rheumatoid arthritis in the joints of her hands.

Rheumatoid Arthritis

Rheumatoid arthritis can cause severe joint deformities (Fig. 8-3). Researchers believe that rheumatoid arthritis is an autoimmune disorder. In autoimmune disorders, the body's immune system begins to attack the body's own tissues. So, for example, in rheumatoid arthritis, the immune system attacks and destroys the cartilage that covers the ends of the bones. Scar tissue develops within the joints, causing them to become stiff and useless. For many months, a person's rheumatoid arthritis may seem to be under control, but then the person will experience an acute flare-up of the disease. During the acute phases of the disease, the person may experience pain, swelling, redness, and heat in the joints, as well as fever and general weakness. Bed rest may be necessary, and splints can help decrease joint deformity. The gentle use of range-of-motion exercises (discussed in Chapter 18) helps to maintain joint mobility.

Gout

Gout is a type of arthritis caused by a disturbance in the body's metabolism. Uric acid, a waste product that is usually eliminated by the kidneys, builds up in the body. The uric acid forms crystals in the joints and causes inflammation and pain. While gout can affect any joint, the big toe is most commonly affected. Men past middle age are more commonly affected than women.

Muscular Dystrophy

Muscular dystrophy is a general term for a group of disorders that cause the skeletal muscles to become progressively weaker over time. These disorders are inherited. Some people with muscular dystrophy experience only moderate disability, while others may die from the disease. *Duchenne's muscular dystrophy* is the most common form of muscular dystrophy. It develops during childhood and usually causes death by the age of 20 years.

Myotonic muscular dystrophy is the most common type that affects adults. Myotonic muscular dystrophy causes a person to have difficulty relaxing the muscles after contracting them, and the muscles may spasm. Muscular dystrophy is a common reason why a younger person may become a resident of a long-term care facility.

Fractures

Fracture a broken bone

A **fracture** is usually caused by trauma. Older people are especially at risk for fractures because the bones become more fragile with age. Older people are also more

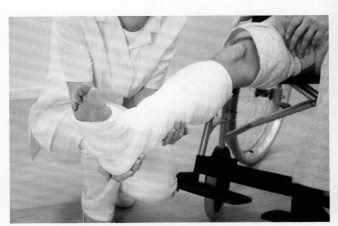

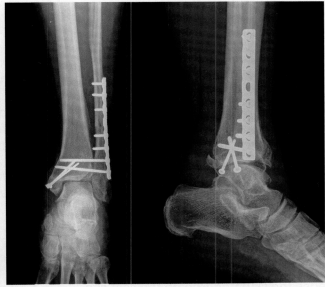

A

B

■ **FIGURE 8-4**

With any fracture, the broken ends of the bone need to be brought back together and then held in place so that healing can occur. The bone ends can be held together externally, using a cast **(A)**, or internally, using devices such as plates, screws, pins, or wires **(B)**.

likely to have diseases that weaken the bones and put them at risk for fractures, such as osteoporosis or bone cancer.

For a fractured bone to heal properly, the broken ends of the bone must be brought together (aligned) and then held in that position until the fracture heals. There are two ways to accomplish this:

■ If the fracture is not complicated, the doctor can move the broken ends into alignment and then apply a cast to keep the bone in the proper alignment until it heals (Fig. 8-4A). General guidelines for caring for a person with a cast are given in Guidelines Box 8-4.

■ If the fracture is complicated, surgery may be necessary, and metal plates, screws, rods, pins, or wires may be used to hold the broken ends of the bone in alignment (Fig. 8-4B).

Some fractured bones cannot be repaired surgically for a period of time, especially if the person's overall medical condition is unstable. In these cases, **traction** is used to keep the broken ends of the bone in alignment until the fracture can be permanently repaired by surgery or casting. When you are caring for a person who is in traction, be careful not to disturb the weights attached to the traction unit. When you lower the person's bed height, check to make sure the weights are not resting on the floor. They must hang freely to apply the correct amount of tension.

Traction a treatment for fracture in which the ends of the broken bone are placed in the proper alignment, and then weight is applied to exert a constant pull and keep the bone in alignment

Hip Fractures

Nursing assistants who work in a long-term care facility are very likely to care for people recovering from hip fractures. A *hip fracture* is a fracture that occurs at the top of the femur (thigh bone) (Fig. 8-5). Hip fractures are common in elderly people because they have an increased risk of falling and having fragile bones.

Most hip fractures are surgically reduced and stabilized with the use of plates, screws, or pins. Some people may also require joint replacement with an artificial

GUIDELINES BOX 8-4 Guidelines for Caring for a Person With a Cast

What you do	Why you do it
Do not cover the cast or place it on a plastic-covered pillow until it has dried completely.	The casting material produces heat as it dries. Covering the cast can cause the person's skin underneath the cast to burn.
Do not touch the cast with your fingertips until it is totally dry. If you must handle the cast, use the palms of your hands.	Touching the cast can cause it to dent, creating pressure spots against the person's skin.
Keep the casted body part elevated on a pillow for several days.	Elevating the casted body part helps prevent and reduce swelling around the fracture site.
Because the skin underneath the cast can start to itch, the person may try to slide an object between the cast and the skin in order to scratch the itchy area. Advise the person that placing objects inside of the cast should be avoided.	Sliding an object between the cast and the skin may injure the skin, which puts the person at risk for infection.
Make sure the person's toes (or fingers, if the cast is on the arm) are pink, warm, and moving. Report any complaints of increased pain, numbness, or tingling. Report any observations of cyanosis, increased swelling, cold toes or fingers, increased drainage on the cast, or a foul odor immediately.	Cyanosis; increased swelling; increased pain, numbness, or tingling; or cold fingers or toes may indicate that swelling inside the cast is interfering with blood flow. If the tissues do not receive enough oxygen and nutrients, tissue death and skin breakdown may occur. Increased drainage or a foul odor may indicate infection.
Keep the cast clean and dry.	Plaster cast material becomes soft again when it becomes wet.
Do not allow the person to place pressure or weight on the cast unless he or she has been specifically instructed to do so.	Placing too much pressure or weight on the cast can cause the cast to break.
Regularly inspect the condition of the cast and the skin around the edges of the cast.	A crack in the cast can cause the cast to become loose or break, which could delay healing of the bone. Rough edges on the cast can irritate or break the skin, putting the person at risk for infection and other problems.

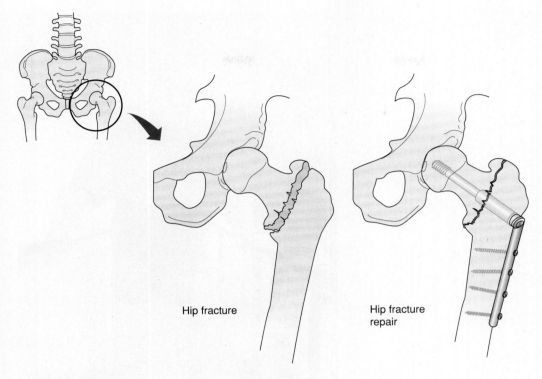

■ FIGURE 8-5

A hip fracture is a fracture that occurs at the top of the femur (the thigh bone). The fracture is often repaired using plates, pins, and screws.

Hip fracture

Hip fracture repair

(prosthetic) joint. During the recovery period, the person will need extensive rehabilitation to help regain strength and mobility.

Amputations

Amputation may be necessary as a result of trauma or disease. Diabetes-related foot problems are very common and account for many amputations in the United States. The loss of a body part, especially an arm or leg, is very emotionally traumatic for a person. The person's mobility, appearance, and sometimes even ability to earn a living or enjoy a hobby he or she used to love can be affected by an amputation. For some people who have had a body part either partially or completely amputated, a prosthetic (false) part may allow the person to regain mobility, function, and a more normal appearance (Fig. 8-6).

Many people experience **phantom pain** after an amputation. Aching, itching, and other sensations are all types of phantom pain. The sensations are caused by the healing of the nerves that were cut when the body part was removed. Phantom pain usually goes away a short while after surgery, but some people report having these episodes for years afterward.

Amputation the surgical removal of all or part of an extremity

Phantom pain the feeling that a body part is still present, after it has been surgically removed (amputated)

 Putting it all together!

- Disorders of the musculoskeletal system can make mobility difficult.
- Osteoporosis is the excessive loss of bone tissue, resulting in bones that break very easily.

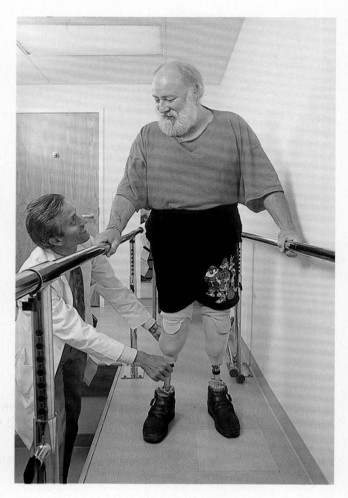

■ **FIGURE 8-6**

A prosthetic body part can help a person who has had an amputation regain function and mobility.

- Arthritis is inflammation of the joints. Osteoarthritis typically affects older adults and causes the cartilage covering the ends of the bones to become worn. People with osteoarthritis may eventually require joint replacement surgery. Rheumatoid arthritis typically affects younger people and can cause severe joint deformities.

- Gout is the build-up of uric acid that causes crystals to form in the joints. This causes inflammation and pain.

- Muscular dystrophy causes the skeletal muscles to become progressively weaker over time. Muscular dystrophy is a common reason why a younger person may become a resident of a long-term care facility.

- Older people are especially at risk for fractures, and fractures may take longer to heal in an older person. Fractures may be treated by casting or by surgical placement of plates, screws, pins, or wires.

- Amputation may become necessary because of trauma or because of complications related to a medical condition, such as diabetes.

Respiratory Disorders

What will you learn?

When you are finished with this section, you will be able to:

1. Describe three respiratory tract infections.
2. Describe how to collect a sputum specimen.
3. Describe the two types of chronic obstructive pulmonary disease (COPD).
4. List some general care measures that a nursing assistant may use to assist a person with a respiratory disorder.
5. Define the words **pneumonia**, **sputum**, **bronchitis**, **influenza**, **asthma**, **chronic obstructive pulmonary disease (COPD)**, **emphysema**, and **chronic bronchitis**.

Infections

Pneumonia

Pneumonia causes the alveoli to fill with fluid and pus, which prevents air from entering the alveoli. As a result, gas exchange (the transfer of oxygen into the blood and carbon dioxide out of it) cannot occur. Signs and symptoms of pneumonia include fever, pain when breathing, cyanosis (bluish skin as a result of decreased oxygen levels in the blood), and a productive cough. A productive cough is one in which a person coughs up **sputum**. You may be asked to assist in the diagnosis of pneumonia by collecting a sputum specimen for analysis (Guidelines Box 8-5).

There are many things you can do to help a person with respiratory problems, such as pneumonia, feel more comfortable:

- Raising the head of the bed so that the person can sit up in bed is often helpful. Some people are more comfortable when they assume a forward-leaning position using pillows on the over-bed table (Fig. 8-7).
- If the doctor has not placed any restrictions on the person's fluid intake, encourage the person to drink plenty of fluids. Fluids help to thin respiratory secretions so that they are easier to cough up.
- Providing frequent oral care will also help keep the person comfortable and will reduce the number of germs that are present in the mouth.

Bronchitis

Bronchitis may cause a dry, nonproductive cough that sounds like a "bark." Bronchitis can turn into pneumonia if the bronchial infection is not treated promptly.

Influenza

Influenza is very contagious. Most people who get influenza will recover in about a week. However, elderly people, very young children, and people with chronic illnesses who get influenza are at risk for developing serious complications, such as an extremely severe form of pneumonia. Residents of long-term care facilities are especially at risk for experiencing complications from influenza. An annual

Pneumonia inflammation of the lung tissue, caused by infection with a virus or bacterium, and resulting in impaired gas exchange

Sputum mucus and other respiratory secretions that are coughed up from the lungs, bronchi, and trachea; also known as *phlegm*

Bronchitis inflammation of the bronchi

Influenza an acute respiratory infection caused by the influenza virus; characterized by a sore throat, dry cough, stuffy nose, headache, body aches, weakness, and fever; commonly known as "the flu"

GUIDELINES BOX 8-5 Guidelines for Collecting a Sputum Specimen

What you do	Why you do it
Explain to the person that the sputum for the specimen should be coughed up from deep down in the respiratory tract.	*The sputum for analysis must come from the lungs because that is where most of the infection-causing germs are located. Explaining this to the person helps to ensure that she produces a specimen that will result in an accurate diagnosis. If you do not explain this to the person she may just cough up saliva, which will not result in an accurate diagnosis.*
Provide privacy.	*Having to spit mucus into a cup can be embarrassing and unpleasant for some people.*
Have the person rinse her mouth with water before coughing up the specimen.	*Rinsing with plain water helps to remove germs that are normally present in the mouth, resulting in a "cleaner" specimen.*
Do not have the person rinse with mouthwash before coughing up the specimen.	*The antiseptic effects of the mouthwash might kill the germs in the sputum specimen that are responsible for the infection, which will result in inaccurate test results.*
Have the person spit the specimen directly into a sterile specimen container and close the lid.	*Having the person spit directly into the sterile specimen container reduces the risk of contaminating the specimen and results in more accurate test results.*
Make sure that the specimen container is labeled properly and that the information is correct.	*Labeling errors can result in misdiagnosis or the need to repeat the test.*
Take the specimen container to the laboratory immediately after collecting the specimen or ask the nurse how to store it.	*Allowing a specimen to sit around or storing it the incorrect way can result in the need to repeat the test.*

"flu shot" for both staff members and residents can help to prevent outbreaks of influenza in long-term care facilities (Fig. 8-8).

Asthma

Asthma a condition that affects the bronchi and bronchioles of the lungs; triggers (such as cold weather, allergies, respiratory infections, stress, smoke, and exercise) cause the bronchi and bronchioles to become narrower, making breathing difficult

Asthma is a chronic disorder. When a person with asthma has an asthma attack, it can be very frightening for the person because breathing becomes almost impossible. A person with asthma may need to take medications on a regular basis to prevent attacks from occurring. These medications may be given by mouth, or they may be inhaled. If an attack does occur, it is usually treated with inhaled medications (Fig. 8-9).

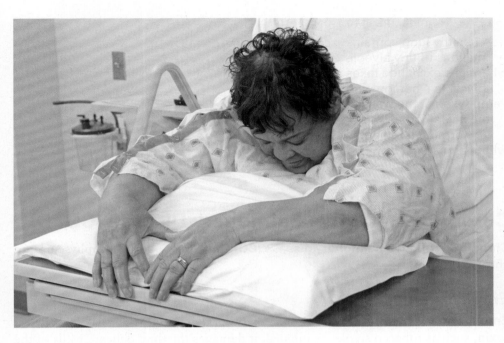

■ **FIGURE 8-7**

Certain positions make breathing easier for people with respiratory disorders. Many people find that leaning forward helps to make breathing easier.

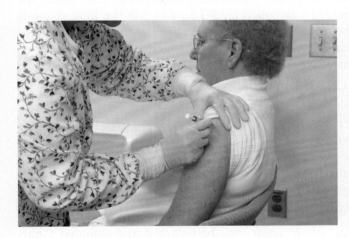

■ **FIGURE 8-8**

Flu shots are usually given to residents in the fall, before the start of flu season (November through April). Flu shots help to prevent infection with the influenza virus, which is very contagious and can cause serious complications in elderly people, very young children, and people with chronic illnesses.

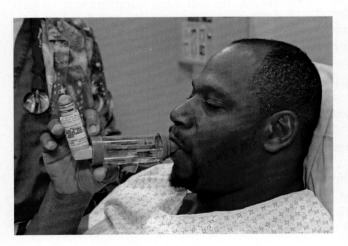

■ **FIGURE 8-9**

Asthma medications are often delivered through inhalers.

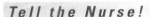

Tell the Nurse!

Signs and symptoms of respiratory disorders

■ Sudden onset of chest pain or difficulty breathing

■ Noisy breathing (for example, wheezing, "barking," or "crowing")

■ Fluid-like, gurgling sounds (this is especially important to report if the person is very weak or comatose)

■ Skin with a blue or gray tinge, either at rest or while exercising

■ Sputum that is discolored (green, frothy, brown, or red-streaked)

■ Shortness of breath during a physical activity that the person has performed without effort in the past

■ Respirations that are very slow and shallow or that stop

■ **FIGURE 8-10**

A healthy lung contains millions of tiny alveoli, where gas exchange takes place. In a person with emphysema, the walls of the alveoli break down, forming large areas where air can get trapped.

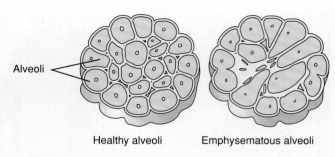

Alveoli

Healthy alveoli   Emphysematous alveoli

Chronic Obstructive Pulmonary Disease (COPD)

Chronic obstructive pulmonary disease (COPD) takes two forms: emphysema and chronic bronchitis.

Emphysema

Emphysema is a form of COPD that involves damage to the alveoli. When a toxin, such as tobacco smoke, is inhaled, it damages the thin, delicate walls of the alveoli. Over time, the damage causes the walls of the alveoli to break. Eventually, instead of having millions of tiny alveoli where gas exchange can take place, the person has fewer, large "merged" alveoli (Fig. 8-10). Because the lung tissue is damaged, it is no longer "springy," and the air gets trapped in the large, damaged alveoli. The trapped air cannot be exhaled and exchanged for new oxygen-rich air, which limits the amount of oxygen the lungs are able to supply to the body.

In addition, excess fluid can collect in the damaged alveoli, putting the person at risk for infection.

A person with emphysema has trouble getting a "proper breath." The person's breathing is shallow and rapid, and the person may have to stop to catch his breath quite frequently when talking or engaging in any type of physical activity. The person's chest may be enlarged and rounded ("barrel chest"). As the person's emphysema gets worse, he will need supplemental oxygen just to carry out even the simplest activities of daily living (ADLs).

Chronic Bronchitis

In **chronic bronchitis** ongoing irritation of the bronchi leads to the production of thick mucus, which blocks the flow of air through the airways. In addition, germs can collect in the mucus, leading to infection.

A person with chronic bronchitis has a nagging, productive cough. The person may complain of "tightness" in her chest or difficulty breathing. She is likely to have frequent respiratory tract infections. Like a person with emphysema, a person with chronic bronchitis will eventually need oxygen therapy.

Chronic obstructive pulmonary disease (COPD) a general term used to describe two related lung disorders, emphysema and chronic bronchitis; the leading cause of COPD is smoking

Emphysema a disorder caused by long-term exposure of the alveoli to toxins, such as tobacco smoke; one of two forms of chronic obstructive pulmonary disease (COPD)

Chronic bronchitis a disorder caused by long-term irritation of the bronchi and bronchioles, such as that caused by inhaling tobacco smoke; one of two forms of chronic obstructive pulmonary disease (COPD)

People who have chronic conditions of the respiratory system, such as asthma or COPD, may call you to the room frequently to ask for seemingly trivial things. Although this can be annoying, think about how you would feel if you had trouble breathing. Instead of giving in to the desire to avoid a "needy" patient or resident, understand the underlying fears the person may have. Spend more time with the person, and get into the habit of stopping by to check on him even when he has not called you. By addressing the person's underlying need for safety and security, you will be providing truly humanistic care.

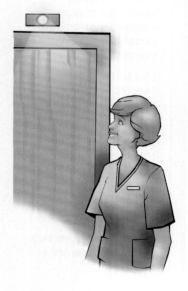

Cancer

In the United States, cancers involving the lungs and airway are the most common cause of cancer-related death in both men and women. Cancers that affect the respiratory system include tumors of the mouth, tongue, larynx, pharynx, bronchi, and lungs. People who smoke cigarettes are 10 times more likely to develop lung cancer than nonsmokers are. In addition, some cancers that begin in other body parts, such as the breast or intestines, commonly spread to the lungs.

Putting it all together!

- Pneumonia, bronchitis, and influenza are common infections of the respiratory system. If untreated, these infections can be life threatening for an elderly person.
- There are two forms of chronic obstructive pulmonary disease (COPD), emphysema and chronic bronchitis. The most common cause of COPD is smoking.
- Disorders of the respiratory system can make breathing very difficult. Not being able to breathe easily can be frightening for the patient or resident. Nursing assistants provide humanistic care by helping the person to feel safe and secure.
- When caring for a person with a respiratory disorder, nursing assistants may be asked to obtain a sputum specimen for analysis. Other responsibilities of the nursing assistant when caring for a person with a respiratory disorder include observing the person for signs that he is having trouble breathing and promoting comfort.

Cardiovascular Disorders

What will you learn?

When you are finished with this section, you will be able to:

1. Describe two types of disorders that can affect the blood vessels.
2. Describe risk factors for developing heart disease.
3. Describe how coronary artery disease can lead to angina pectoris, myocardial infarction, or both.
4. List the signs and symptoms of a myocardial infarction ("heart attack").
5. Describe how a pacemaker is used to help a person with heart block.
6. Define the words **atherosclerosis, plaque, embolus, arteriosclerosis, angina pectoris, myocardial infarction,** and **heart failure.**

Atherosclerosis blocking of the arteries, caused by the build-up of fatty deposits called plaque on the inside of the vessel wall

Plaque fatty deposits that build up on the inside of the artery wall, blocking blood flow to the tissues and making the artery wall brittle and prone to breaking

Embolus a blood clot in a vessel that breaks off and moves from one place to another

Arteriosclerosis "hardening of the arteries"; occurs when atherosclerotic plaque interferes with the elasticity of the arterial walls, making them brittle and prone to breaking

Tell the Nurse!

Signs and symptoms of cardiovascular disorders

- Chest pain or pressure
- Labored or difficult breathing
- A rapid or erratic pulse
- A slow, weak pulse
- A blood pressure reading that is either much higher or much lower than the person's usual reading
- Cyanosis of the face, lips, or fingers
- Decreased tolerance for usual exertion
- Red, painful, or swollen areas in the calves of the legs
- Unusual swelling of the legs, especially if it is accompanied by red, shiny skin
- "Dusky" (blue or grayish) coloring of the legs, especially if it is accompanied by a diminished pulse and coldness of the skin

■ **FIGURE 8-11**

In atherosclerosis, fatty plaque builds up on the inside of the arteries, blocking the free flow of blood. This is particularly dangerous when the artery supplies a vital organ such as the heart, brain, or kidneys.

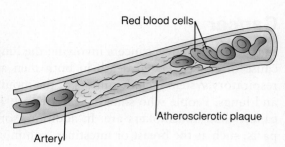

Red blood cells

Atherosclerotic plaque

Artery

Blood Vessel Disorders

Atherosclerosis

In **atherosclerosis, plaque** builds up on the inside of the vessel wall, blocking the flow of blood through the artery (Fig. 8-11). As a result, less oxygen and nutrients are delivered to the tissues. In addition, the plaque makes the normally smooth inner lining of the artery rough, which can cause blood clots to form. Sometimes a clot breaks off and becomes an **embolus**, which may be life threatening. The plaque also interferes with the elasticity of the arterial walls, leading to **arteriosclerosis**.

Venous Disorders

Loss of elasticity in the walls of the veins causes blood to "pool" in the legs, which can put the person at risk for several disorders:

- **Varicose veins.** In this condition, pooling of blood in the superficial veins (that is, the veins just underneath the skin) causes the veins to become swollen and "knotty" in appearance.
- **Phlebitis.** In this condition, pooling of blood in the vein causes the lining of the vein to become inflamed. The skin over the affected vein is reddened; the area feels hard and hot to the touch, and is very painful.
- **Venous thrombosis.** In this disorder, blood clots (thrombi) form in the veins where the blood pools, because the blood is moving so slowly. When the blood clots cause inflammation of the lining of the vein, you may hear this condition referred to as *thrombophlebitis*. When blood clots form in the deep veins, the condition is called *deep venous thrombosis* (DVT). People with DVT are at a high risk for pulmonary embolism that occurs when one of the blood clots breaks loose and travels to the lungs, becoming trapped in the pulmonary artery.
- **Venous (stasis) ulcers.** These ulcers are seen on the lower legs, usually in the ankle area. The pressure of the pooled blood in the veins forces plasma out of the blood vessels and into the surrounding tissues. Swelling occurs, and the skin becomes fragile and inflamed. Eventually the skin breaks down, forming an open sore.

Generally, people with venous disorders experience pain and difficulty with mobility. The doctor may order the use of leg exercises, antiembolism stockings, or both.

Heart Disorders

Perhaps more than any other organ system, the cardiovascular system is affected by the choices we make in life. Conditions that are known to increase a person's risk for developing a heart disorder are given in Box 8-2.

BOX 8-2 Risk Factors for Heart Disease

Conditions that are known to increase a person's risk of developing heart disease are called *cardiac risk factors*. We can control some of our risk factors for heart disease. Others are out of our control.

Risk factors for heart disease that we cannot change include the following:

- **Age.** The risk of developing heart disease increases with age.

- **Gender.** Men are at greater risk of developing heart disease at an earlier age than women are. However, after a woman goes through menopause, her risk of developing heart disease is the same as a man's.

- **Heredity.** People who have parents or siblings with heart disease are more likely to develop heart disease themselves.

- **Body build.** Some people tend to put on weight in the abdomen or chest ("apples"), while others tend to carry it in the buttocks or thighs ("pears"). "Apple"-shaped people are more likely to develop heart disease than "pear"-shaped people.

The following risk factors for heart disease can be controlled by making lifestyle changes:

- **Smoking**

- **Being physically inactive**

- **Being overweight or obese**

- **Consuming a diet high in saturated fat, cholesterol, and sodium**

- **Having poorly controlled hypertension**

- **Having poorly controlled diabetes**

Many national organizations, such as the American Heart Association, provide information and education about "healthy heart living." By following the advice of these organizations, many people are able to maintain good cardiovascular function well into old age. The keys to cardiovascular health are exercise; a diet that emphasizes fruits, vegetables, whole grains, and healthy fats (and low in unhealthy saturated fats); and avoidance of smoking.

- **Exercise** helps to keep the heart muscle strong and working efficiently. Exercise also helps us to maintain a healthy body weight and is an important measure for preventing or controlling conditions that can contribute to heart disease, such as diabetes and hypertension.

- **Eating a heart-healthy** diet helps to keep the heart muscle and blood vessels healthy. Like exercise, a heart-healthy diet also helps to prevent or control conditions that can contribute to heart disease, such as excess weight, diabetes, and hypertension.

- **Avoiding smoking** is important because chemicals in tobacco smoke cause the blood vessels to constrict, depriving the heart of the oxygen and nutrients it needs to function properly.

Coronary Artery Disease

The coronary arteries supply the heart muscle with blood containing oxygen and nutrients. Coronary artery disease occurs when the coronary arteries narrow as a result of atherosclerosis. At first, the heart muscle may receive enough oxygen to work properly when the body is at rest, but it may be unable to meet the increased needs brought on by activity. Eventually, one or more of the coronary arteries may become so narrow that no blood gets through, causing areas of the heart muscle to die. Coronary artery disease can be treated with medication, balloon angioplasty, the placement of a stent, or bypass surgery.

ANGINA PECTORIS. A person with coronary artery disease may have **angina pectoris**. Anginal pain varies among individuals. Some people describe it as a pain in the center of the chest. Others experience pain that starts in the chest and extends to the arm or neck. A person who is experiencing angina may feel as though he is suffocating and may become very anxious.

Angina pectoris the classic chest pain that is felt as a result of the heart muscle being deprived of oxygen

Many people experience angina quite frequently and know what it is. These people often keep nitroglycerin pills on hand to relieve the pain when it occurs. If you have been trained to help a person with his nitroglycerin, avoid handling the pills with your bare hands. The drug can be absorbed through the skin, causing a decrease in your blood pressure and a severe headache.

MYOCARDIAL INFARCTION. A **myocardial infarction** occurs when one or more of the coronary arteries become completely blocked. The lack of blood and oxygen causes the heart tissue to die. The dead tissue is called an *infarct*.

A myocardial infarction can be fatal. The severity of the myocardial infarction depends on how much tissue was damaged and which part of the heart was affected. Early recognition of the signs and symptoms of a myocardial infarction and prompt medical treatment can greatly increase a person's chances of surviving. If you suspect that one of your patients or residents is having a myocardial infarction, have the person lie down and raise the head of the bed to make breathing easier. Then report your observations to the nurse immediately.

Heart Failure

Heart failure has many causes. For example, disorders that cause the heart muscle to lose muscle tone and become large and flabby can cause heart failure. Heart failure can also occur as a result of a myocardial infarction that leaves the heart unable to function properly.

For people with heart failure, medications may be used to help increase the heart's ability to pump more effectively and to pull excess fluid from the tissues. Many people with severe heart failure have their fluids restricted and their intake and output very carefully monitored.

Heart Block

In heart block, the pathway that the heart uses to send the electrical impulses that cause contraction is blocked. Heart block causes the heart to slow down significantly, leading to dizziness or fainting episodes. Heart block is usually treated with a pacemaker, an electrical device that is surgically placed in the person's chest. When the person's heart rate drops below a programmed rate, the pacemaker sends an electrical impulse that stimulates the heart muscle to contract.

 Putting it all together!

- Disorders of the blood vessels include atherosclerosis and venous disorders. Atherosclerosis is especially dangerous when it affects arteries that supply vital organs, such as the heart, brain, or kidneys. Both atherosclerosis and venous disorders put the person at risk for developing an embolus, a potentially fatal condition.

- Several factors put us at risk for developing heart disease. Some we can control and some we cannot. Factors we can control include those related to diet, exercise, and smoking.

- The narrowing of the arteries that supply the heart muscle with oxygen and nutrients can lead to angina pectoris, myocardial infarction ("heart attack"), or both. Prompt medical treatment may prevent a person from dying from a heart attack.

Myocardial infarction a "heart attack"; occurs when one or more of the coronary arteries become completely blocked, preventing blood from reaching the parts of the heart that are fed by the affected arteries

Heart failure a condition that occurs when the heart is unable to pump enough blood to meet the body's needs

Tell the Nurse!

Signs and symptoms of a heart attack

- Pain or tightness in the chest that may extend to the neck or arm
- Excessive sweating
- Trouble breathing
- Pale, gray, or bluish color to the skin
- Anxiety
- Complaint of indigestion or heartburn pain
- Nausea and/or vomiting

- Heart failure results from the heart's inability to pump blood in sufficient amounts to supply the body.
- A person with heart block may have a pacemaker to ensure that the heart beats regularly.

Nervous System Disorders

What will you learn?

When you are finished with this section, you will be able to:

1. Discuss the difference between a transient ischemic attack (TIA) and a stroke.
2. List the signs and symptoms of a stroke ("brain attack").
3. Describe risk factors for having a stroke.
4. Describe the effects of a stroke.
5. Describe the effects of Parkinson's disease.
6. Describe the effects of multiple sclerosis (MS) and amyotrophic lateral sclerosis (ALS, Lou Gehrig's disease).
7. Describe the effects of spinal cord injuries and head injuries.
8. Define the terms **transient ischemic attack (TIA), stroke, hemiplegia, aphasia, Parkinson's disease, multiple sclerosis (MS), quadriplegia, paraplegia, coma,** and **persistent vegetative state.**

Transient Ischemic Attacks (TIAs)

A **transient ischemic attack (TIA)** occurs when blood flow to the brain is temporarily blocked. Small blood clots can form in the heart or the arteries that supply the brain. These clots can break off and travel into the narrow arterioles of the brain, where they temporarily block the blood flow. Low blood pressure, certain medications, cigarette smoking, or standing up suddenly after lying down can also lead to a TIA.

Symptoms of a TIA vary according to the part of the brain affected by the decreased blood supply. Common symptoms may include dizziness, nausea, blurring or loss of vision, double vision, paralysis on one side of the body or face (with or without loss of sensation), or the inability to speak or swallow. The symptoms of a TIA may only last a few minutes, or they may last for several hours. The person usually recovers completely within 24 hours.

If you suspect that one of your patients or residents is having or has just had a TIA, you should report this to the nurse immediately. TIAs are usually a warning that the person could have a stroke in the near future. A TIA may also be a sign of an underlying medical condition that needs to be addressed.

Transient ischemic attack (TIA) a temporary (transient) episode of dysfunction caused by decreased blood flow to the brain

Stroke

Unlike a TIA, a **stroke** causes permanent effects because the blocked blood flow lasts long enough for the brain tissue to die or become damaged. A stroke can

Stroke a disorder that occurs when blood flow to a part of the brain is completely blocked, causing the tissue to die; also known as a "brain attack" or cerebrovascular accident (CVA)

Hemiplegia paralysis on one side of the body

Aphasia a general term for a group of disorders that affect a person's ability to communicate with others; may be expressive (an inability to form words) or receptive (an inability to understand words); often occurs following a stroke

Parkinson's disease a progressive neurologic disorder that is characterized by tremor and weakness in the muscles and a shuffling gait

occur suddenly in a person who was previously healthy. Signs and symptoms vary, depending on the area of the brain that is affected. If you notice a change in a patient's or resident's usual behavior, appearance, or medical condition, keep the person lying down and report your observations to a nurse immediately.

Causes of Stroke

The most common cause of a stroke is a blood clot that blocks the flow of blood to a part of the brain. Therefore, people who smoke, have atherosclerosis, or have poorly controlled hypertension or diabetes are at high risk for having a stroke. Another, less common, cause of a stroke is cerebral hemorrhage. A cerebral hemorrhage occurs when a small artery in the brain bursts. The bleeding into the surrounding brain tissue puts pressure on the delicate tissue, damaging it. A cerebral hemorrhage is more likely in people with chronic hypertension, arteriosclerosis ("hardening of the arteries"), or certain deformities of the blood vessels in the brain.

Effects of Stroke

The effects of a stroke depend on the area of the brain that is affected and the amount of tissue that is damaged. The person may die or be left with disabilities. The most common disabilities resulting from a stroke are **hemiplegia** and **aphasia**.

HEMIPLEGIA. Depending on the amount of tissue damage, the hemiplegia may be mild or severe. A person with mild hemiplegia may have slight muscle weakness or shaking on the affected side, while a person with severe hemiplegia may not be able to move or feel any type of sensation at all on that side of the body. A person with severe hemiplegia who has lost sensation on one side of the body will need frequent repositioning to prevent pressure ulcers from forming. Care must also be taken to prevent other injuries, such as burns, because the person will not be able to feel extreme heat, cold, or pain on the affected side.

APHASIA. Aphasia affects the person's ability to communicate with others.

- **Expressive aphasia.** A person with expressive aphasia has trouble forming words. The person may also have trouble swallowing, increasing the risk of choking.
- **Receptive aphasia.** A person with receptive aphasia can speak clearly but no longer knows the meaning of the words. For example, a person with receptive aphasia may say "no" when she means "yes."

See Chapter 4 for tips on communicating with a person with aphasia.

Parkinson's Disease

In **Parkinson's disease** the body does not produce enough dopamine (a chemical that is necessary for proper functioning of the motor neurons). In a person with Parkinson's disease, the brain's instructions regarding muscle movement never reach the muscle because of the lack of dopamine. Without enough dopamine, the impulse cannot be passed on to the next neuron in line. Because of this nervous system "short circuit," the brain loses its ability to properly control body movement.

Parkinson's disease is a progressive disorder, which means that it gets worse with time. The average age for the onset of Parkinson's disease is 55 years. Men are affected more often than women.

Effects of Parkinson's Disease

The effects of Parkinson's disease can be easily remembered by thinking of the word "TRAP":

T stands for *tremor*. Parkinson's disease usually starts with a faint tremor that gets worse over a long period of time. The tremor is most apparent when the person is resting and decreases when the person attempts purposeful movement.

R stands for *rigidity*. The muscles become increasingly stiff. When rigidity is combined with the tremor, there is a cogwheeling effect. Cogwheeling is the term used to describe the jerky, ratcheting feel to the movement.

A stands for *akinesia* (lack of movement). *Bradykinesia*, or slowed movement, is also noted in Parkinson's disease.

P stands for *postural instability*. The person's ability to maintain his balance becomes increasingly worse, increasing the person's risk for falls.

As a result of these changes, the person has an abnormal gait. The person's steps are "shuffling," which means that they are short, there is a slight hesitation as the person tries to move the foot forward, and the foot barely comes off the floor. The person's posture is stooped forward, and he loses the natural arm swing that helps us to maintain balance (Fig. 8-12). The person has difficulty initiating movement, but once the person gets going, the short, shuffling steps and forward posture make

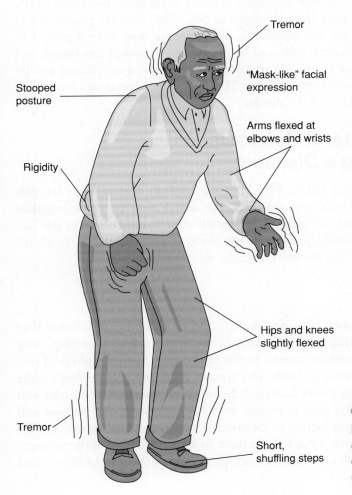

Tremor

"Mask-like" facial expression

Stooped posture

Arms flexed at elbows and wrists

Rigidity

Hips and knees slightly flexed

Tremor

Short, shuffling steps

■ **FIGURE 8-12**

People with Parkinson's disease often develop a characteristic shuffling gait with a forward lean.

it difficult for him to control his speed and maintain balance. In addition, the person has difficulty turning. Instead of twisting the body and pivoting on the toes, a person with Parkinson's disease turns his whole body as one unit, taking many small steps to complete the turn. Because of these abnormal movements, the person with Parkinson's disease is at very high risk for falling and significant injuries.

The person loses the ability to move the small muscles of the face that are responsible for facial expression, giving the face a "mask-like" appearance. Because the muscles used for swallowing are also affected, the person has trouble eating and is at high risk for choking and aspiration. Drooling is common.

The muscles used for speech are also affected. Picture boards and asking simple questions that can be answered with a nod or shake of the head can help improve the person's ability to express himself.

Other problems that are common with Parkinson's disease include skin disorders, sleep disturbances, constipation, and, as the disease progresses, incontinence. In the later stages of the disease, the person may develop dementia. In the end stage of Parkinson's disease, the person becomes totally dependent on others for care, and will be at risk for all of the complications of immobility.

Multiple Sclerosis (MS)

Multiple sclerosis (MS)
a disorder of the nervous system in which the myelin sheaths that cover the nerves are damaged, resulting in faulty transmission of nerve impulses

It is thought that **multiple sclerosis (MS)** is an autoimmune disorder. MS usually affects the nerves in the hands, feet, and eyes first and then moves inward toward the central nervous system. Muscle weakness, tingling sensations, twitching of the eyes, and vision problems may be early signs of MS. The disorder progresses at different rates, depending on the individual. Some people may have a period of remission (mild or no symptoms) followed by a relapse (the symptoms return and are much worse). In the late stages of the disease, the person may become totally paralyzed. At this time, there is no cure for MS, although some drugs have been shown to slow the progression of the disease.

Amyotrophic Lateral Sclerosis (ALS, Lou Gehrig's Disease)

Amyotrophic lateral sclerosis (ALS), like MS, is a nervous system disorder that causes progressive muscle weakness. In ALS, the nerves that transmit impulses between the spinal cord and the muscles are totally destroyed. People in the late stages of the disease are totally paralyzed, yet their minds remain sharp. Death occurs when a person loses the ability to breathe and swallow.

Head Injuries

Brain damage can result from falls, accidents, gunshot wounds, and events that cause a person to stop breathing for a period of time, such as near drowning, drug overdose, or choking. Traumatic injuries to the brain often result in physical disability, loss of mental function, or both. The type of disability will depend on the area and extent of the brain tissue damaged. Some people with head injuries will have paralysis similar to that seen in people who have had a stroke. Others will develop seizures, memory problems, or behavioral problems. Still others will be comatose. Some may need machines to help them to breathe. Many of the younger people who are in long-term care facilities are there because of a head injury that resulted in severe disability.

Spinal Cord Injuries

Injuries to the spinal cord are usually caused by trauma, but they can also be caused by birth defects or tumors of the spine. The effects of a spinal cord injury depend on the level of the spine where the injury occurred:

- An injury to the spinal cord in the neck area can result in **quadriplegia** (tetraplegia).
- An injury further down the spinal cord may result in **paraplegia**.

The paralysis may be partial or complete, depending on the severity of the injury.

For some people, the emotional effects of a spinal cord injury may be harder to overcome than the physical disabilities. Loss of control over one's body and the accompanying loss of independence can be devastating. Some people may not be able to return to their jobs, which can cause financial problems. Others may never be able to enjoy a favorite hobby again. When you care for a person with a spinal cord injury, it is very important to encourage the person to do as much as possible for herself. Doing so helps the person to maintain a sense of independence.

Quadriplegia paralysis from the neck down

Paraplegia paralysis from the waist down

Coma and Persistent Vegetative State

Coma can be caused by a head injury, a tumor, a lack of oxygen, exposure to toxins, or illness. A person who is comatose is unaware of his or her environment and cannot deliberately respond to people or things in it. The person cannot move on his or her own, and the person cannot talk or respond to commands. A coma generally lasts only 2 to 4 weeks.

Some people will come out of the coma and recover. Others will come out of the coma, but remain in a **persistent vegetative state**. A person in a persistent vegetative state has sleep–wake cycles, and is able to breathe on his or her own. In addition, it may seem like the person in a persistent vegetative state is responding to his or her environment. A person can live in a persistent vegetative state for years.

Coma a deep state of unconsciousness from which a person cannot be aroused

Persistent vegetative state a state of altered consciousness in which the person appears to be awake, but cannot respond in a deliberate or meaningful way to the environment

Putting it all together!

- Disorders of the nervous system can affect the brain, spinal cord, or nerves.
- Transient ischemic attacks (TIAs) are caused by a temporary decrease in blood flow to a part of the brain. Although the effects of a TIA are not lasting, a person who has had or is having a TIA needs medical attention because TIAs are often warnings that the person could have a stroke in the near future.
- A stroke occurs when blood flow to the brain is blocked, causing the brain tissue to die. The effects of stroke are permanent and can be mild or severe.
- Parkinson's disease affects the brain's ability to conduct motor impulses to the muscles. The person develops tremors and a shuffling gait. The person may have trouble expressing himself.
- Multiple sclerosis (MS) and amyotrophic lateral sclerosis (ALS) are disorders that cause muscle weakness that gets worse over time.
- Head injuries and spinal cord injuries result in varying degrees of disability, depending on the location and the severity of the injury.

Sensory Disorders

What will you learn?

When you are finished with this section, you will be able to:

1. Describe how conditions such as cataracts and glaucoma can lead to blindness.
2. Describe how to care for a person who is blind.
3. Describe special measures that can be taken to help a person who is deaf.
4. Define the words **cataract**, **glaucoma**, and **Braille**.

Cataracts

Cataract the gradual yellowing and hardening of the lens of the eye

Cataracts are common in older people, but they can occur in younger people as well. The person's vision becomes more and more cloudy as the cataract worsens (Fig. 8-13). Eventually, the person may become totally blind. Many people with cataracts have surgery to remove the cloudy lens and replace it with an artificial one.

Glaucoma

Glaucoma a disorder of the eye that occurs when the pressure within the eye is increased to dangerous levels

Glaucoma occurs when the aqueous humor in the anterior chamber of the eye is not reabsorbed into the bloodstream. As more and more aqueous humor is formed, it creates pressure, which builds up in the eye. The pressure squeezes the nerves and the blood vessels in the retina. Treatment is with medicated eye drops or surgery. If the glaucoma is not treated, eventually the nerves are destroyed and vision is lost.

Blindness

Braille a system that uses letters made from combinations of raised dots that allows a blind person to read

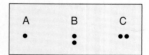

Blindness has many different causes and takes many different forms. Some people see nothing but darkness, but many others can see light, movement, shapes, and even colors, just not clearly enough to tell them apart.

A person who has recently lost his sight will be taught skills that will help him to regain his independence. He will be taught how to move around safely. He may learn how to read using **Braille** or how to work with a guide dog. At first, the person is likely to be frightened, especially of moving around on his own. However, with

■ **FIGURE 8-13**

Cataracts occur when the lens of the eye becomes yellow and hard over time, resulting in cloudy vision. This is what the world looks like to **(A)** a person with normal vision and **(B)** a person with cataracts.
Courtesy of the National Eye Institute, National Institutes of Health.

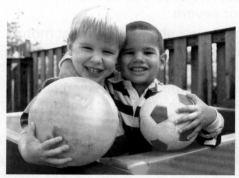

A. Normal vision

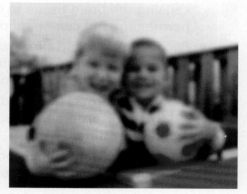

B. Cataract

time, most people who are blind adapt very well and are very independent. When caring for a person who is blind, treating the person with respect and allowing him to be as independent as possible are the best things you can do. Guidelines for caring for a person who is blind are given in Guidelines Box 8-6.

Deafness

Like blindness, deafness has many different causes and takes many different forms. Deafness can be partial or complete. A person with hearing loss may work with a speech therapist to learn how to speak more clearly. In addition, many adaptive devices are available to help a person with hearing loss maintain her independence. For example, telephone devices for the deaf (TDD) systems can be used in combination with a standard phone to allow a person with hearing impairment to communicate using the telephone. Television shows are available with "closed captioning," a system that prints the words that are being spoken at the bottom of the screen so that the person can read them. The person's doorbell, alarm clock, telephone, and smoke alarms may flash instead of ring. Tips for communicating with a person with hearing loss are given in Chapter 4.

 Putting it all together!

- Some eye disorders, such as cataracts and glaucoma, can lead to permanent vision loss if they are not treated.
- There are many different degrees of blindness. Most people who are blind manage quite well on their own. When you are caring for a person who is blind, it is important for you to announce yourself when you enter or exit the room and to describe what you are doing as you are doing it.
- There are many different degrees of hearing loss. When talking to a person with hearing loss, make sure that the person can see your face, take care to speak clearly, and clarify information as necessary.

Endocrine Disorders

 What will you learn?

When you are finished with this section, you will be able to:

1. Describe the difference between hyperthyroidism and hypothyroidism.
2. Describe the difference between type 1 diabetes mellitus and type 2 diabetes mellitus.
3. List and describe the three factors that must be balanced in order to keep blood glucose levels within the range of normal.
4. List signs and symptoms that a person's blood glucose level may be too high or too low.
5. Explain why it is important for people with diabetes mellitus to eat regular, nutritious meals and snacks.
6. Define the words **diabetes mellitus**, **hypoglycemia**, and **hyperglycemia**.

GUIDELINES BOX 8-6   Guidelines for Caring for a Person Who Is Blind

What you do	Why you do it
Speak in a normal tone of voice.	*Unless the person is hearing impaired as well as blind, there is no need to raise your voice.*
Describe the things you see around you. For example, tell the person that the sky is a beautiful shade of blue or that there are lovely yellow flowers blooming right outside the window.	*Most people who are blind appreciate your ability to share what you see with them through your descriptions.*
Ask the person about the extent of her blindness, and do not hesitate to ask the person what type of help she needs from you.	*Asking the person about her blindness will help you to better plan the person's care. You might be surprised at what the person is able to do for herself, with little or no assistance from you!*
When you enter the person's room, knock and tell the person who you are and why you are there. Similarly, when you leave, tell the person that you are leaving.	*If you do not announce yourself when you enter the room, you could startle the person. Similarly, if you do not tell the person that you are leaving, he may not be aware that you have left.*
Make sure that you explain procedures completely and descriptively. Throughout the procedure, tell the person what type of equipment you are using, what you are doing, and what you are going to do next.	*With all patients and residents, you should take care to explain procedures thoroughly. However, with a blind person, you may have to modify your approach a bit. For example, instead of just showing the person a piece of equipment, you will need to describe it to him or let him touch it. Also, you should tell the person what is happening as it happens so that the person is not left wondering where you are in the procedure, or what is coming next.*
Do not rearrange the furniture in the person's room, unless the person asks you to.	*The person is used to moving around the room on her own. If you move the furniture, the person could injure herself by running into something that has been moved and is now in an unfamiliar location.*
Leave the door either completely open or completely closed.	*If the door is partially open, the person may feel for the door, think that it is all the way open, and walk into the edge of the door.*
When helping a blind person to walk, do not propel the person in front of you. Instead, let the person walk beside you and slightly behind you as she rests a hand on your elbow. Walk at a normal pace. Let the person know when you are about to turn a corner, or when a curb or step is approaching (and whether or not you will be stepping up or down).	*In this way, you guide the person and reduce the risk of stumbles over unforeseen obstacles.*

Disorders of the endocrine system occur when the body produces too much or too little of a certain hormone. Thyroid gland disorders and diabetes are among the most common endocrine disorders.

Thyroid Gland Disorders

Hyperthyroidism

Hyperthyroidism is caused by the secretion of too much thyroid hormone (*hyper* = "above"). In a person with hyperthyroidism, the metabolic rate of the body's cells is increased. Signs and symptoms of hyperthyroidism include increased hunger, weight loss, an irregular heart beat, an inability to sleep, irritability, confusion, sweating, and intolerance to heat. Hyperthyroidism may be treated with surgery or radiation.

Hypothyroidism

Hypothyroidism results when thyroid hormone secretion is too low (*hypo* = "below"). In a person with hypothyroidism, the metabolic rate of the body's cells is decreased. Signs and symptoms of hypothyroidism include fatigue, weakness, depression, anorexia, weight gain, constipation, and intolerance to cold. Hypothyroidism may be treated with medication.

Diabetes

There are two types of **diabetes mellitus**, type 1 and type 2.

Diabetes mellitus an endocrine disorder that results when the pancreas is unable to produce enough insulin

Type 1 Diabetes

Type 1 diabetes occurs when the cells in the pancreas that produce insulin are destroyed. Most people who have type 1 diabetes are diagnosed while they are children or young adults.

Type 2 Diabetes

Type 2 diabetes (also called "glucose intolerance") is the most common type of diabetes. In people with type 2 diabetes, the pancreas still produces some insulin, but the cells of the body are unable to respond to the insulin. This results in higher blood glucose levels because the body is unable to move the glucose out of the blood and into the cells.

Type 2 diabetes is most often diagnosed later in life, although we are seeing an increase in the number of children with type 2 diabetes. People who are overweight or obese are at high risk for developing type 2 diabetes.

Management of Diabetes Mellitus

To keep blood glucose levels within the range or normal, three factors must be balanced: diet, exercise, and medication (Fig. 8-14). A change in any one of these factors can affect blood sugar control resulting in **hypoglycemia** or **hyperglycemia**. Box 8-3 reviews some of the causes and effects of hypoglycemia and hyperglycemia.

Hypoglycemia a dangerous drop in blood glucose levels

Hyperglycemia a state of having too much glucose in the bloodstream

DIET. A person with diabetes needs to eat a well-balanced, nutritious diet, with limited sweets and fats. Following a proper diet helps to keep blood glucose levels within the normal range. Meals and snacks should be eaten at regular times

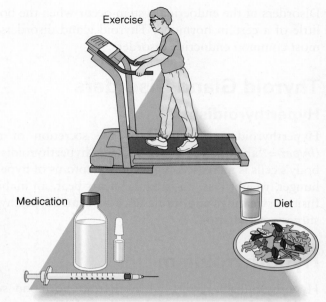

■ **FIGURE 8-14**

Exercise

Medication

Diet

Diabetes mellitus is managed with diet, exercise, and medication. A change in any one of these three factors can affect the blood glucose level.

throughout the day to help keep blood glucose levels steady (Fig. 8-15). You will need to pay attention to how much the person eats and what the person eats. Specific amounts of carbohydrates, sugars, fats, and proteins are needed to react with the medication the person takes for his or her diabetes. If the person does not eat at the recommended time after receiving insulin, the person's blood glucose level can drop too low.

Many people with diabetes understand how a balanced, nutritious diet can help them manage their blood glucose levels and prevent complications from developing. However, some people may not follow their diet as closely as they should. For a person with diabetes, eating too many sweets can result in hyperglycemia and lead to complications. Some of your patients or residents, especially the older ones, may keep stashes of candy. If you notice that a patient or resident is hoarding sweets, you should report this to the nurse.

EXERCISE. When we exercise, our muscles use glucose for energy. This helps to lower blood glucose levels. An older person's ability to exercise may be limited

■ **FIGURE 8-15**

It is very important for a person with diabetes to eat regular, nutritionally sound meals and snacks. If one of your patients or residents with diabetes refuses to eat or only eats part of a meal or snack, report this to a nurse immediately.

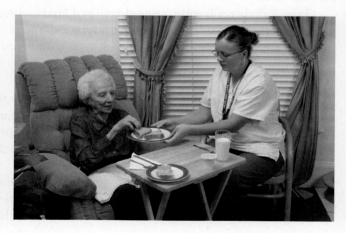

BOX 8-3 **Hypoglycemia and Hyperglycemia**

Hypoglycemia or hyperglycemia can result when diet, exercise, and medication are not in balance. A person's medication dose is planned to balance the person's usual food intake and amount of activity. A change in food intake or level of activity can lead to hypoglycemia or hyperglycemia if the person's medication dose is not adjusted accordingly. Both hypoglycemia and hyperglycemia can have serious consequences, including death, if they are not treated.

Hypoglycemia (low blood glucose levels)

Causes

- Missing a meal or a snack
- A delayed meal or snack
- Eating too little food
- Vomiting
- NPO status
- Increased level of activity
- Too much medication

Effects

- Cool, clammy skin
- Sweating
- Feeling "shaky"
- Confusion or difficulty concentrating
- Rapid heart rate and rapid breathing
- Headache
- Blurry or "double" vision
- Restlessness and irritability
- Trembling
- A tingling sensation in the mouth or tongue
- Hunger
- Loss of consciousness (insulin shock)

Hyperglycemia (high blood glucose levels)

Causes

- Eating too much food
- Decreased level of activity
- Too little medication
- Physical stress (illness or injury)
- Emotional stress
- Undiagnosed diabetes

Effects

- Excessive urination
- Excessive thirst
- Extreme hunger
- Unplanned weight loss
- Fatigue
- Blurry or "double" vision
- Headache
- Irritability
- Dry, flushed skin
- Sweet-smelling breath
- Dehydration
- Seizures
- Loss of consciousness (diabetic coma)

by a chronic health condition or disability. You should encourage the person to participate in whatever level of exercise the person can tolerate.

When you are caring for a person with diabetes, be aware that changes in the person's normal activity level could result in hypoglycemia or hyperglycemia. For example, a patient or resident with diabetes who is beginning a new physical therapy program should be watched closely for signs and symptoms of hypoglycemia (see Box 8-3), because the patient's or resident's activity level will be increased. Similarly, a decrease in the person's normal activity level could lead to hyperglycemia.

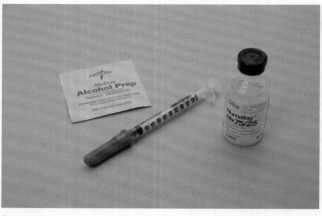

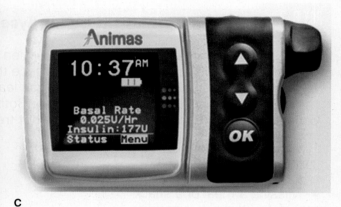

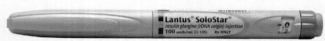

■ **FIGURE 8-16**

(A) A syringe or **(B)** and insulin pen can be used to administer insulin at regular intervals throughout the day. **(C)** A portable insulin pump allows for the continuous infusion of insulin.
B, Courtesy of Animas.

MEDICATION. Medications used to treat diabetes include insulin and oral medications:

■ Insulin. All people with type 1 diabetes mellitus, and some people with type 2 diabetes mellitus, require insulin. Insulin can be administered using a needle and syringe, a special insulin "pen," or a pump (Fig. 8-16). Several types of insulin are available. The types of insulin differ in the speed at which they start working and how long they last in the body. Most of your patients or residents who take insulin for the treatment of diabetes will receive multiple insulin injections each day.

■ Oral medications. Many people with type 2 diabetes mellitus take oral medications to help control their blood glucose levels. The different types of oral medications used to treat diabetes work in slightly different ways. Some stimulate the pancreas to produce more insulin, some act on the cells in the body to help them use the insulin that the body produces, and some decrease the amount of glucose that enters the bloodstream after eating.

Monitoring Blood Glucose Levels

As you have learned, diabetes control involves balancing diet, exercise, and medication. A person with diabetes needs to monitor his or her blood glucose levels regularly to make sure that the prescribed treatment is keeping the blood glucose level within the desired range. You will find the procedure for assisting a patient or resident with monitoring blood glucose levels in Chapter 24.

Complications of Diabetes

If not well controlled, diabetes can cause many serious complications:

■ Low insulin levels increase the release of lipids (fats) into the bloodstream. The lipids build up in the linings of the arteries, damaging them. Atherosclerosis, high blood pressure, heart disease, kidney disease, and blindness can result from the damaged blood vessels.

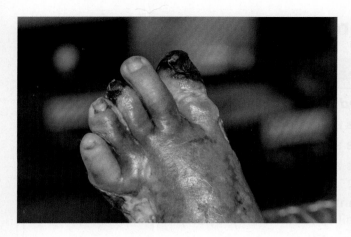

In a person with diabetes, a minor injury to the foot can cause major complications. Due to decreased blood flow to the tissues, the injury may not heal. If left untreated, gangrene (death of the tissue) can develop. In this case, the only treatment option may be amputation.

■ Nerve damage results from reduced blood flow to the neurons, causing decreased sensation in the arms and legs. This makes it harder for the person to detect injuries. Decreased blood flow in the feet and lower legs increases the risk of infection and poor tissue healing in the event of injury. Amputation of a foot or leg may be necessary if the person develops gangrene (death of the tissues due to lack of blood flow; Fig. 8-17).

Early detection of diabetes is essential for preventing complications. Once diabetes is diagnosed, there are many measures that can be taken to keep the disease under control and minimize the person's risk of developing complications. People who are overweight should try to lose the excess weight. In addition, exercising regularly, following the recommended diet closely, and taking prescribed medications correctly are also very important.

Putting it all together!

- Disorders of the endocrine system result from either too much hormone or too little hormone.

- Hyperthyroidism and hypothyroidism are disorders that occur when the thyroid gland produces too much thyroid hormone or not enough, respectively. These disorders affect the person's metabolic rate.

- People with type 1 diabetes require daily insulin injections because their bodies cannot produce insulin. The bodies of people with type 2 diabetes produce insulin, but the cells of the body do not respond to the insulin.

- To keep blood glucose levels within the range of normal, three factors must be balanced: diet, exercise, and medication.

- A person with diabetes needs to eat regular, nutritionally balanced meals and snacks. Nursing assistants play an important role in the care of people with diabetes when they serve meals and snacks at the scheduled time.

- People with diabetes are prone to hyperglycemia and hypoglycemia and must monitor their blood glucose levels carefully. Both hyperglycemia and hypoglycemia can have serious consequences if the person does not receive prompt treatment.

Digestive Disorders

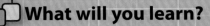

What will you learn?

When you are finished with this chapter, you will be able to:

1. Discuss symptoms a person with an ulcer may have.
2. Discuss symptoms a person with gallbladder disease may have.
3. Discuss symptoms a person with cancer involving the digestive system may have.
4. Discuss the different causes of hepatitis and how hepatitis can affect the liver's ability to function properly.
5. Define the word **hepatitis**.

Ulcers

Ulcers (sores caused by wearing away of the protective lining of the digestive tract) occur when the stomach produces too much stomach acid. Factors such as smoking, frequent use of over-the-counter pain medications, and infection with a bacterium called *Helicobacter pylori* can increase a person's chances of developing ulcers. A person with an ulcer may feel uncomfortably full or nauseated after eating. Stomach pain is common, especially within 3 hours of eating (or when the person does not eat). Most ulcers are chronic. The person will have periods of feeling well, interrupted by flare-ups of symptoms. Most ulcers can be treated with medication. People with severe ulcers may need surgery.

Gallbladder Disorders

Gallstones can form and block the flow of bile from the gallbladder into the duodenum. This can lead to inflammation and infection of the gallbladder. A person with a gallbladder disorder has episodes of severe pain. The pain may stay in the upper abdominal region, or it may spread to the back and shoulder on the person's right side. The person may also have indigestion, especially after eating foods that are high in fat. Medication or laser treatment may be used to dissolve the gallstones. In some cases, surgery to remove the gallbladder is needed.

Cancer

Any of the organs in the digestive system can be affected by cancer. A person with cancer involving the digestive system may experience loss of appetite, indigestion, pain, vomiting, constipation, changes in bowel movements, or blood in the stool. Depending on the location and type of cancer, treatment may involve surgery, radiation, chemotherapy, or a combination of these.

Hepatitis

Hepatitis inflammation of the liver

Hepatitis is most commonly caused by a viral infection, but it may also be caused by chemicals, drugs, or drinking alcohol. Some infections with a hepatitis virus are mild, producing no lasting effects on the liver. Others are chronic and affect the liver's ability to function over time. If the liver failure is severe, the person will die unless he receives a liver transplant.

 Putting it all together!

- Ulcers are caused by a wearing away of the protective lining in the digestive tract.
- Gallstones can block the flow of bile from the gallbladder into the duodenum, causing severe pain.
- Cancer can form in any of the organs in the digestive system.
- Hepatitis is inflammation of the liver, the organ that removes toxic substances from the bloodstream. Depending on the cause of the hepatitis, the person may recover fully from the illness, experience disabling symptoms for the rest of his or her life, or die.

Urinary Disorders

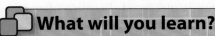 **What will you learn?**

When you are finished with this section, you will be able to:
1. Discuss common disorders of the urinary system.
2. List signs and symptoms that could indicate that a person has a urinary system disorder.
3. Describe how to care for a person who has kidney (renal) failure.
4. Define the word **dialysis**.

Urinary Tract Infections

Infections can affect any part of the urinary system. In younger people, symptoms of urinary tract infections include a frequent urge to urinate, burning, and cramping. However, many older people do not have these symptoms. You may be the first to notice a change in the appearance or odor of a patient's or resident's urine or a change in the person's urination habits (Fig. 8-18). These changes could mean that the person has a urinary tract infection and should be reported to the nurse immediately.

Neurogenic Bladder

Neurogenic bladder is a condition caused by problems with the nerves that control the bladder. Neurogenic bladder can be caused by a spinal cord injury, a stroke, a tumor, or complications from diabetes. The bladder is either overactive or underactive:

Tell the Nurse!

Signs and symptoms of urinary disorders

- Sharp, sudden pain in the abdomen, side, or back
- Cloudy urine
- Urine with an unusual odor or color
- Blood in the urine
- Difficulty passing urine
- Pain or a burning sensation when urinating
- A change in normal urination habits (the person has to go more often or less often than usual, or the person becomes unable to control her urination)
- A change in the amount of urine passed
- Increased confusion, decreased alertness, or unusual behavior

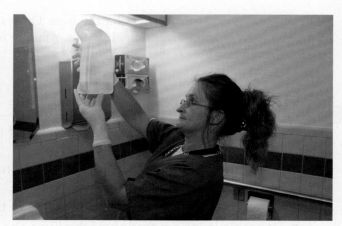

■ **FIGURE 8-18**
Urine that is cloudy, is an abnormal color, or has an abnormal odor may be a sign of a urinary tract infection. Always look at the urine before discarding it. If you notice anything unusual, get the nurse before discarding the urine.

■ An overactive bladder is spastic or highly sensitive to stimulation. The person experiences bladder spasms (involuntary contractions of the smooth muscle in the walls of the bladder) that result in the frequent, uncontrolled release of small amounts of urine from the bladder (urge incontinence). In this condition, the amount of urine the bladder is able to hold (that is, the bladder's capacity) is reduced.

■ An underactive bladder is flaccid or unable to contract forcefully. The smooth muscle that forms the walls of the bladder loses its tone, causing the bladder to "stretch out." As a result, the bladder's capacity is increased. Because of nerve damage, the person may not be able to sense that the bladder is full, resulting in reflex incontinence (the bladder empties itself automatically when it becomes too full). Or, the muscular walls of the bladder may not be able to contract strongly enough to empty the bladder of all urine, leading to urinary retention and overflow incontinence that leads to dribbling of urine as the bladder overfills.

Kidney Stones

Kidney stones are clumps of minerals that form in the kidneys and bladder. Factors that may increase an older person's risk of developing kidney stones include immobility, not drinking enough fluids, and infections of the urinary system. Kidney stones cause severe pain. Blood may also be seen in the urine.

A person with a kidney stone usually needs to drink plenty of fluids to help flush the stone through the urinary tract. Medication may be necessary to help control the pain. You may be asked to collect all of the person's urine after each voiding and strain it to retrieve the stone (Fig. 8-19). In some cases, the stone must be removed surgically.

Kidney (Renal) Failure

Kidney (renal) failure occurs when the kidneys are not able to filter the blood. As a result of kidney failure, waste products and fluid build up in the body, straining the heart and other organs. The person becomes very ill and can die if treatment is delayed.

People with kidney failure often need to have **dialysis**. Dialysis takes several hours and must be performed several times a week to keep the blood cleaned of waste products. You may be asked to monitor vital signs quite frequently after your patient or resident has had a dialysis treatment. Guidelines for caring for a person with kidney failure are given in Guidelines Box 8-7.

Dialysis a procedure that is done to remove waste products and fluids from the body when a person's kidneys fail and can no longer perform this task

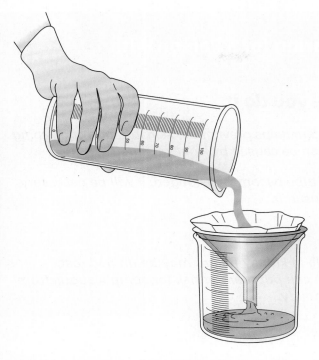

■ FIGURE 8-19

You may be asked to strain a person's urine to retrieve kidney stones. To strain urine, put a piece of filter paper or a 4″ × 4″ gauze pad in a graduate and then pour the urine into the graduate. The urine will pass through the paper or gauze pad, leaving any stones behind. The stones are then put in a specimen container and sent to the laboratory for analysis.

GUIDELINES BOX 8-7 Guidelines for Caring for a Person With Kidney Failure

What you do	Why you do it
Carefully measure the person's urine output and document the amounts accurately.	*The doctor will use this information to monitor how well the person's kidneys are functioning.*
Assist with obtaining urine samples as requested.	*Testing the urine for waste products is another way of monitoring how well the person's kidneys are functioning.*
Follow the person's care plan carefully with regard to food and fluid intake.	*To reduce the amount of work the kidneys have to do, the person's fluid intake may be restricted and a special diet that is low in salt and protein may be ordered.*
Monitor vital signs according to the person's care plan, and report any changes to the nurse immediately.	*Changes in fluid balance, especially after dialysis, can significantly raise or lower a person's blood pressure.*
If daily weights are ordered, make sure that you weigh the person at the same time each day and with the same amount of clothing on.	*Changes in a person's weight can indicate excess fluid that is being retained in the body.*
When measuring the blood pressure of a person who receives hemodialysis treatments, avoid measuring the blood pressure in the arm in which the person's fistula, graft, or shunt is located.	*Pressure can decrease blood flow through the fistula, graft, or shunt, which can lead to clots. Clots can make the fistula, graft, or shunt unusable for dialysis.*

(*box continues on page 198*)

GUIDELINES BOX 8-7 Guidelines for Caring for a Person With Kidney Failure (continued)

What you do	Why you do it
Provide frequent skin care.	*Skin care helps prevent the skin irritation and itching that can be caused by kidney failure.*
When assisting a person who receives peritoneal dialysis treatments with bathing or dressing, take care not to accidentally dislodge the tube used for peritoneal dialysis.	*If the tube becomes dislodged, it will be necessary to reinsert it.*
Provide care measures, such as frequent repositioning and range-of-motion exercises, to help prevent the complications of immobility.	*People in kidney failure may be on bed rest, which can put them at risk for complications from immobility.*

Putting it all together!

- Common disorders of the urinary system include infections, kidney stones, and kidney failure.
- The nursing assistant may be the first to notice signs and symptoms of a urinary problem that a patient or resident is having.

Reproductive System Disorders

What will you learn?

When you are finished with this section, you will be able to:

1. Discuss sexually transmitted infections (STIs) that may affect the male or female reproductive system.
2. Discuss cancers that may affect the male or female reproductive system.
3. Define the words **sexually transmitted infection (STI)** and **postmenopausal bleeding**.

Infections

Sexually transmitted infection (STI) an infection that is most commonly transmitted by sexual contact; also known as venereal disease

Sexually transmitted infections (STIs) are spread from one person to the next through contact with semen or vaginal secretions. Infection of the organs of the reproductive system is most common, although the mucous membranes of the eyes, mouth, or anus may also become infected following contact with infected semen

TABLE 8-3 **Sexually Transmitted Infections**

Disease	Description	Possible Complications	Treatment
Genital herpes	Painful blisters form around the vaginal opening and perineum (in women) or the external urinary opening (in men)	May cause blindness, brain damage, or both to child during birth	None
Gonorrhea	Men may notice a greenish discharge from the urethra and have a burning sensation during urination; women may not have any symptoms	Pelvic inflammatory disease, a condition that often results in severe pain and scarring that can lead to infertility (in women)	Antibiotics
Chlamydia	Often there are no signs or symptoms in men or in women	Infertility in both men and women	Antibiotics
Human papillomavirus (HPV)	Often there are no signs or symptoms in men or in women; small, wart-like growths may form around the vaginal opening, inside the vagina, or on the cervix (in women) or inside the urethra (in men)	Cervical cancer (in women). Tonsil and throat cancer (in men)	Removal of the growths with a laser. Vaccine is available and recommended for young men and women that can help prevent infection from some types of HPV
Syphilis	**Stage 1:** a painless lesion is seen on the genitals **Stage 2 (2 to 4 weeks later):** skin rash, fever **Stage 3 (20+ years later):** cardiovascular and neurologic problems	Dementia, paralysis	Antibiotics

or vaginal secretions. Some STIs, such as AIDS, involve the entire body. AIDS is discussed in detail in Chapter 31. Other common STIs are described in Table 8-3.

Cancer

Female Reproductive System

- **Cervical cancer** is cancer of the cervix, the lower region of the uterus.
- **Endometrial cancer** is cancer of the lining of the uterus. **Postmenopausal bleeding** may be the first sign of this type of cancer. Postmenopausal bleeding can also result from hormone imbalances.
- **Ovarian cancer** is a leading cause of cancer death for women.
- **Breast cancer** is the most commonly occurring cancer in women. Many breast lumps are not cancer, but the only way to be sure is to have them checked. Early detection and new treatment methods for breast cancer allow many women to be completely cured of this disease.

Postmenopausal bleeding
uterine bleeding after menopause

Male Reproductive System

- **Testicular cancer** can easily spread to other parts of the body before it is detected. Testicular cancer is most commonly found in young men.
- **Prostate cancer** typically grows slowly and has a good cure rate with early detection.
- **Penile cancer.** Occasionally, lesions that appear on the penis may be cancerous.

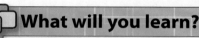

Putting it all together!

- Sexually transmitted infections (STIs) are spread through contact with semen and vaginal secretions. Common STIs include genital herpes, gonorrhea, chlamydia, human papillomavirus (HPV), syphilis, and AIDS. If not treated, STIs can lead to serious complications. Some STIs have no cure.
- Cancer can affect any organ in the male or female reproductive system.
- When you are assisting your patients or residents with bathing or elimination, you may notice signs of a problem involving the person's reproductive organs. Patients or residents may also tell you about problems they are experiencing.

Mental Health Disorders

What will you learn?

When you are finished with this section, you will be able to:

1. Describe what a mental health disorder is, and list some common mental health disorders.
2. Describe some of the emotional challenges an elderly person may face and how these challenges can affect an elderly person's mental health.
3. Define the words **coping mechanisms, defense mechanisms, depression, suicide, anxiety, delusions, hallucinations, addiction,** and **withdrawal**.

Mental health disorders affect a person's mind, causing the person to act in unusual ways, experience emotional difficulties, or both. (*Mental* means "mind.") There are many different types of mental health disorders and many different causes. Some types of mental health disorders run in families (that is, they are inherited). Others result from chemical imbalances in the brain. Finally, some mental health disorders may be caused by a person's environment.

Mental Health

A person who is mentally healthy is able to manage stress effectively. Sources of stress include:

TABLE 8-4 Defense Mechanisms

Defense Mechanism	Description	Example
Compensation	Substituting one thing for another	A person who feels lonely eats too much (the person is substituting food for affection)
Conversion	Changing one thing into another	A person who is depressed (an emotional problem) develops a stomachache (a physical problem) and then uses the physical problem as a reason to avoid participating in an activity
Denial	Refusing to believe something that is true	A person who is diagnosed with cancer believes that the doctor has made the wrong diagnosis and that he does not have cancer
Displacement	Shifting an emotion from one person to another	A resident who is angry with her daughter for moving her to a long-term care facility takes her anger out on a nursing assistant instead
Projection	Blaming someone else for your own uncomfortable or unacceptable feelings	A resident accuses a nursing assistant of breaking a vase when in fact the resident actually broke the vase himself
Rationalization	Making excuses for poor behaviors or actions	A student who does not study for a test and then fails it tells herself that she failed because the teacher is "too hard"
Regression	Turning back to an earlier state	An 8-year-old child who is hospitalized begins to suck his thumb, a behavior he outgrew when he was 4
Repression (suppression)	Refusing to remember or think about a frightening or painful memory	A person who was in a bad car accident cannot remember the accident

- Changes that affect us physically, such as illness or disability
- Life events, such as getting married, getting divorced, starting a new job, having a baby, moving, or losing a loved one
- Day-to-day activities, such as working, caring for a family, and world events

Too much stress can cause a person to feel sad and overwhelmed. However, most people with good mental health are able to use **coping mechanisms** and **defense mechanisms** (Table 8-4) to manage their stress and regain their balance (Fig. 8-20).

People who are mentally ill cannot cope effectively with stress. Treatment may include therapy, medication, or a combination of both. Some of the more common mental illnesses include anxiety disorders, mood disorders, schizophrenia, substance abuse disorders, and eating disorders.

Coping mechanisms conscious and deliberate ways of dealing with stress, such as exercising, praying, or enjoying a hobby

Defense mechanisms unconscious ways of dealing with stress

Anxiety Disorders

Although we all have experienced periods of increased **anxiety**, some people have periods of anxiety that continue to build until they can no longer function. Common anxiety disorders include:

Anxiety feeling of uneasiness, dread, apprehension, or worry

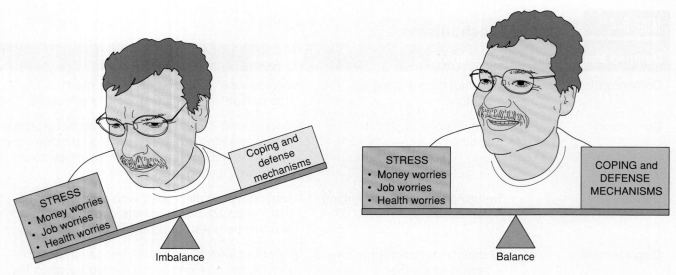

■ **FIGURE 8-20**

Stress can drag us down, causing the scale to tip out of balance, but a person who is mentally healthy is able to adjust to the stress and return to a state of emotional balance.

Depression an alteration in a person's mood that causes him or her to lose pleasure or interest in all usually pleasurable activities, such as eating, working, or socializing; a feeling of hopelessness

Suicide the act of taking one's own life intentionally and voluntarily

■ **Panic disorder.** The person has "panic attacks," during which he experiences sudden increases in anxiety, feelings of intense fear, and physical signs and symptoms, such as chest or abdominal pain, a rapid heart beat, shortness of breath, and dizziness.

■ **Obsessive-compulsive disorder.** The person has recurrent unwanted thoughts (*obsessions*) that are associated with rituals that the person cannot control (*compulsions*).

■ **Phobias.** The person has an excessive, abnormal fear of an object or situation.

■ **Post-traumatic stress disorder (PTSD).** Occurs after a person experiences an overwhelming traumatic event such as combat, natural disaster, serious injury, criminal assault, rape, or death of another person. PTSD can cause a person to have flashbacks (vivid memories of the event), panic attacks, nightmares, depression, and increased anxiety.

Mood Disorders

Mood disorders affect how a person feels emotionally.

Depression

People who are mentally ill may suffer from **depression**. When depression is severe and persistent, it is called *clinical depression*. A person who is clinically depressed loses interest in activities that she used to enjoy, such as eating and socializing. The person may cry frequently. She may sleep too much or not enough. The person may have feelings of guilt and worthlessness and struggle with thoughts of **suicide**. Physical complaints (*for example*, of pain or a stomach disorder) are also common. Prompt treatment is needed to help a clinically depressed person return to an enjoyable, productive life.

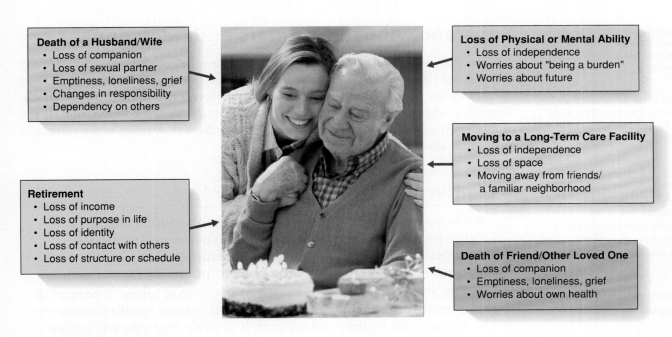

Death of a Husband/Wife
- Loss of companion
- Loss of sexual partner
- Emptiness, loneliness, grief
- Changes in responsibility
- Dependency on others

Loss of Physical or Mental Ability
- Loss of independence
- Worries about "being a burden"
- Worries about future

Moving to a Long-Term Care Facility
- Loss of independence
- Loss of space
- Moving away from friends/ a familiar neighborhood

Retirement
- Loss of income
- Loss of purpose in life
- Loss of identity
- Loss of contact with others
- Loss of structure or schedule

Death of Friend/Other Loved One
- Loss of companion
- Emptiness, loneliness, grief
- Worries about own health

■ **FIGURE 8-21**
As we age, we face very challenging life events. These additional stresses can put an elderly person at risk for clinical depression and other mental illnesses.

Clinical depression affects more than 19 million Americans each year. Clinical depression is also the most frequently treated mental health disorder among elderly people. As we age, we face many challenging life events (Fig. 8-21). Many elderly people are able to adjust to these changes, but others may struggle. Many older people who are depressed feel that their depression is just part of getting older and must be accepted. However, this is not the case. When you are caring for older patients or residents, pay attention to changes in their behaviors or moods that may be signs of clinical depression. By reporting these observations to the nurse, you play an important role in helping to ensure that the person receives treatment that will help him or her feel better.

Bipolar Disorder

The person has mood swings. Periods of excessive happiness and excitement that may cause the person to engage in impulsive or reckless behavior (*mania*) are followed by periods of excessive sadness and hopelessness (*depression*). Experts believe that bipolar disorder is caused by chemical imbalances in the brain that affect a person's moods. Bipolar disorder can be difficult to recognize and properly diagnose.

Schizophrenia

A person with schizophrenia has trouble determining what is real and what is imaginary. She may suffer from **delusions, hallucinations,** or both. The person's thinking and speech become disordered. Her behavior is often frightening and confusing to others. A person with severe schizophrenia that is untreated may be a danger to herself or to others.

Delusions false ideas or beliefs, especially about oneself

Hallucinations episodes when a person sees, feels, hears, or tastes something that does not really exist

Addiction a physical need for a substance that results in withdrawal signs and symptoms if the substance is withheld

Withdrawal an emotional and physical reaction that occurs when use of the addictive substance is discontinued

Substance Abuse Disorders and Addiction

Substance abuse disorders are disorders that involve the excessive or inappropriate use of drugs (legal or illegal), alcohol, or inhalants. Some people abuse more than one substance. A person with a substance abuse disorder can develop an **addiction**. When this occurs, the person must have the substance in order to function. If she cannot get the substance, she can experience **withdrawal**. Alcohol is the substance most often abused by older people.

Tell the Nurse!

Withdrawal is a medical emergency. Any of the following signs and symptoms should be reported to the nurse immediately:

- Body tremors
- Mental status and mood changes
- Delirium
- Hallucinations (such as a feeling that something is crawling all over the skin)
- Restlessness
- Anxiety and fear
- Insomnia
- Nausea and vomiting
- Sweating
- Heart palpitations and rapid pulse
- Seizures

Putting it all together!

- Mental health disorders affect a person's mind, causing the person to act in unusual ways, experience emotional difficulties, or both. Mental health disorders vary in their type, cause, and severity. They may be temporary or permanent.

- The additional stress of illness or injury that brings a person to a health care facility can cause a mild mental health disorder to worsen. As a nursing assistant, it is likely that you will notice changes in a patient's or resident's behavior that could be signs of a mental health disorder. Reporting your observations to the nurse immediately will help the patient or resident to get the help he needs.

WHAT DID YOU LEARN?

Multiple Choice

Select the single best answer to each of the following questions.

1. Which of the following is a factor that might put a person at risk for disease?
   a. Age
   b. Heredity
   c. Gender
   d. All of the above

2. Arthritis is an example of what category of disease?
   a. Infectious disease
   b. Metabolic disease
   c. Degenerative disease
   d. Neoplastic disease

3. An abrasion or wearing away of the top layer of the skin that is often caused by trauma is called a/an:
   a. Excoriation
   b. Fissure
   c. Macule
   d. Papule

4. Excessive loss of bone tissue is known as:
   a. Osteoarthritis
   b. Osteoporosis
   c. A normal effect of aging
   d. Fracture

5. Mr. Owen recently had hip replacement surgery for severe osteoarthritis. What are some specific care measures that you need to remember?
   a. Mr. Owen's legs must always be kept together (adducted).
   b. When assisting Mr. Owen with range-of-motion exercises, make sure to flex his hips beyond 90 degrees to maintain flexibility in the joint.
   c. Mr. Owen should use an abduction pillow to keep his legs spread apart when he is in a supine position.
   d. Mr. Owen can still safely sit on his soft couch.

6. A chronic lung condition that causes the alveoli to become enlarged and traps air that cannot be exhaled is called:
   a. Pneumonia
   b. Asthma
   c. Pleurisy
   d. Emphysema

7. The formation of artery-clogging plaque on the inside of arteries is called:
   a. Atherosclerosis
   b. Chronic obstructive pulmonary disease (COPD)
   c. Anemia
   d. Hypertension

8. Which of the following is a risk factor for cardiovascular disease?
   a. Poorly controlled hypertension
   b. A diet high in cholesterol and saturated fats
   c. Lack of physical activity
   d. All of the above

9. Another term that refers to a heart attack is:
   a. Chronic obstructive pulmonary disease (COPD)
   b. Stroke
   c. Myocardial infarction
   d. Transient ischemic attack (TIA)

10. Which of the following could be a sign of a heart attack?
    a. Slurred speech
    b. Excessive sweating
    c. Lower abdominal pain
    d. Headache

11. Mrs. Romanelli has had a stroke and has a lot of trouble forming words. What term is used to describe Mrs. Romanelli's difficulty with language?
    a. Aphasia
    b. Dysphasia
    c. Paraplegia
    d. Hemiplegia

12. Any condition that temporarily decreases blood flow to the brain can cause what to occur?
    a. A "senior moment"
    b. A transient ischemic attack (TIA)
    c. A heart attack
    d. A cerebral hemorrhage

13. Which nervous system disorder is characterized by a lack of the chemical dopamine?
    a. Multiple sclerosis (MS)
    b. Stroke
    c. Parkinson's disease
    d. Amyotrophic lateral sclerosis (ALS)

14. A gradual yellowing and hardening of the lens of the eye that causes a person's vision to gradually become more and more cloudy is known as:
   a. Glaucoma
   b. Cataracts
   c. Conjunctivitis
   d. Tinnitus

15. Diabetes mellitus is caused by a lack of the hormone:
   a. Insulin
   b. Glucagon
   c. Thyroxine
   d. Estrogen

16. Which endocrine disorder causes an increased metabolic rate, increased hunger, weight loss, an irregular heart beat, an inability to sleep, irritability, and intolerance to heat?
   a. Hyperthyroidism
   b. Diabetes
   c. Acromegaly
   d. Hypothyroidism

17. A mental illness that is characterized by recurrent unwanted thoughts and rituals that the person cannot control is known as:
   a. Schizophrenia
   b. Bulimia
   c. Depression
   d. Obsessive-compulsive disorder

Matching

Match each disorder with the organ system it affects.

_____ 1. Chronic obstructive pulmonary disease (COPD)

_____ 2. Gallbladder disease

_____ 3. Glaucoma

_____ 4. Urinary tract infection

_____ 5. Diabetes mellitus

_____ 6. Multiple sclerosis (MS)

_____ 7. Rheumatoid arthritis

_____ 8. Angina pectoris

_____ 9. Rashes

_____ 10. Endometrial cancer

a. Integumentary system
b. Musculoskeletal system
c. Respiratory system
d. Cardiovascular system
e. Nervous system
f. Sensory system
g. Endocrine system
h. Digestive system
i. Urinary system
j. Reproductive system

 Stop *and* **Think!**

Mrs. Detwiller has type 1 diabetes. She takes an insulin injection first thing every morning. Today, as you clear her breakfast tray, you notice that she ate very little of her breakfast. Why is this concerning, and what should you do?

 Stop *and* **Think!**

Mr. Cummings has just returned to the long-term care facility after having hip replacement surgery on his left hip. His favorite chair is an old, overstuffed couch by the window. He tells you that he wants to sit there now, barely 4 days after his operation. What should you do?

Rehabilitation and Restorative Care

Many of the disorders you have learned about can affect a person's ability to function independently. As a nursing assistant, you will help your patients or residents to return to their best level of functioning after an injury or an illness.

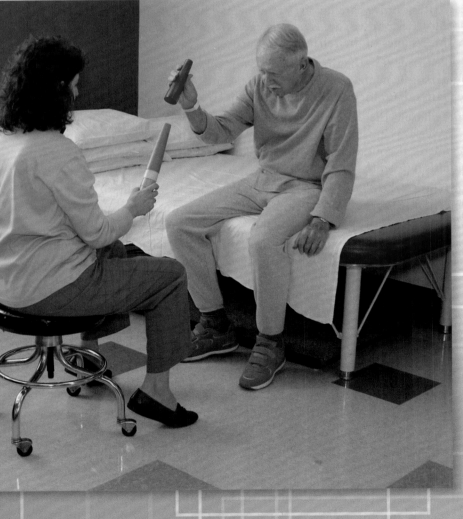

Photo: *This man has had a stroke. The exercise he is doing—stacking cones—will help him regain some use of his right arm.*

Introduction to Rehabilitation and Restorative Care

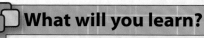

What will you learn?

When you are finished with this section, you will be able to:

1. Explain the goal of rehabilitation.
2. List and describe the three phases of the rehabilitation process.
3. List some of the members of the rehabilitation team.
4. State the Omnibus Budget Reconciliation Act (OBRA) requirements concerning rehabilitative services.
5. Define the words **disability**, **rehabilitation**, and **restorative care**.

Disability impaired physical or emotional function

Rehabilitation the process of helping a person with a disability to return to his highest level of physical, emotional, or economic function

Restorative care measures that health care workers take to help a person regain health, strength, and function; the means by which rehabilitation is achieved

Not all disorders and injuries result in death, but many of them leave the person with a **disability**. Disabilities can be temporary or permanent. They can be mild or severe.

The process of helping a person learn to manage his disabilities and live as independently as possible is called **rehabilitation**. Rehabilitation is started as soon as possible after the person's medical condition stabilizes. Rehabilitation is achieved through **restorative care**. Restorative care involves treatment, education, and the prevention of further disability. Restorative care is usually carried out by the nursing staff.

There are three stages of the rehabilitation process:

- **The acute phase** occurs in the first 24 hours after surgery, an injury, or a serious illness. The person is acutely ill and needs constant observation and care. The health care team's main focus during this phase is to keep the person alive.

- **The subacute phase** is the second phase of the rehabilitation process and usually lasts about 1 week. The health care team's focus during this phase is to stabilize the person's medical condition and prevent complications so that the person's best rehabilitation potential is maintained.

- **The chronic phase** is the phase in which the intense work of rehabilitation begins. The rehabilitation team develops a rehabilitation and restorative care program that is designed to meet the person's special needs.

Rehabilitation services can be provided in a hospital, in a subacute care facility, in a long-term care facility, in a facility that specializes in caring for people in need of a specific type of rehabilitation, in the person's home, or on an outpatient basis. Many people will receive rehabilitation in more than one of these settings during the course of their recovery.

Rehabilitation focuses on the individual needs and abilities of the patient or resident. Rehabilitation is a team effort. Members of the team include the patient or resident and his family members, the nurse, the nursing assistant, a doctor, and other specialists, depending on the type of rehabilitation and the goals of the effort.

Just as with any health care team, the patient or the resident is always the focus of

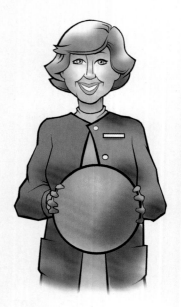

A person who has become disabled may feel frustrated, depressed, or guilty about her inability to do the things she used to be able to do. The person may become angry with caregivers, family, or herself because of these feelings. A holistic approach—considering the person's emotional needs, as well as her physical ones—is essential for the rehabilitative effort to be effective.

TABLE 9-1   Health Care Workers Who Specialize in Rehabilitation

Job Title	Responsibilities
Rehabilitation physician (physiatrist)	■ Works with the person's doctor to manage and direct the person's rehabilitation program
Rehabilitation nurse	■ Develops a nursing care plan to maximize the person's functioning and quality of life ■ Provides patient/resident and family education ■ Helps the person practice skills learned in therapy ■ Takes measures to prevent complications and monitors for complications
Occupational therapist	■ Helps the patient or the resident regain or maintain the ability to perform ADLs (for example, for eating, grooming, walking) ■ Teaches the person how to use assistive devices to carry out ADLs
Physical therapist	■ Helps the person regain or maintain strength, endurance, coordination, posture, and flexibility
Speech-language pathologist (speech therapist)	■ Helps the person regain or maintain the ability to communicate with others, chew, and swallow
Rehabilitation aide	■ Assists the occupational therapist, physical therapist, and speech therapist with carrying out the rehabilitation program
Orthotist	■ Fits the patient or the resident with supportive devices (such as braces or supports) to correct deformity, aid movement, and relieve discomfort
Prosthetist	■ Fits the patient or the resident with prosthetic devices (such as an artificial arm or leg)
Neuropsychologist	■ Helps the person regain or maintain cognitive skills

the rehabilitation team's efforts and the goal of the rehabilitation team is to provide holistic care. Many jobs within the health care field have rehabilitation as their specific focus (Table 9-1).

 The Omnibus Budget Reconciliation Act (OBRA) requires long-term care facilities to provide rehabilitative services that meet the specific needs of the residents who live in the facility.

Putting it all together!

- Rehabilitation is the process of helping a person regain independence and return to his or her highest level of function. Rehabilitation involves a team of people working together to address the needs of the patient or resident.
- There are three different phases of the rehabilitation process: the acute phase, the subacute phase, and the chronic phase.
- Rehabilitation takes place in many different types of health care settings.
- Restorative care is how rehabilitation is achieved. As a nursing assistant, you will play an important role in providing restorative care.

Types of Rehabilitation

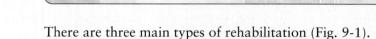

What will you learn?

When you are finished with this section, you will be able to:

1. Describe the different types of rehabilitation that a person may need.
2. Define the words **supportive devices**, **assistive devices**, **prosthetic devices**, and **contractures**.

There are three main types of rehabilitation (Fig. 9-1).

Physical Rehabilitation

Physical rehabilitation focuses on helping a person regain the physical ability to do certain tasks. There are three types of physical rehabilitation frequently used in the health care setting.

Physical rehabilitation: helps a person regain the ability to do certain tasks independently

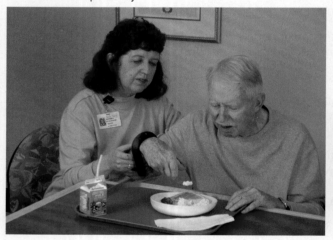

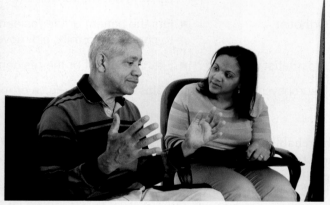

Emotional rehabilitation: helps the person come to terms with the disability and cope with loss

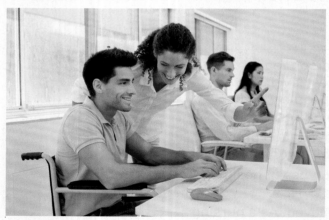

Vocational rehabilitation: helps the person learn or relearn skills he will need to return to work

■ **FIGURE 9-1**

The three main types of rehabilitation.

Physical Therapy

Physical therapy is used to help the person regain or maintain strength, endurance, coordination, balance, posture, and flexibility. The primary goals of physical therapy are to improve or maintain a person's ability to move and to prevent complications. As part of physical therapy, the person may learn how to use **supportive devices**, **assistive devices**, and/or **prosthetic devices** (Fig. 9-2).

Another major focus of physical therapy is to prevent complications that can result from the loss of function. When a person does not use a part of the body for a long time, she loses muscle mass in that part. As the muscle mass is lost, so is the person's strength. Exercise is used to help strengthen the muscles and prevent complications of immobility, such as muscle atrophy, **contractures**, and pressure ulcers. These complications can lead to failure of the rehabilitation effort and permanent disability.

Occupational Therapy

Occupational therapy is a rehabilitation specialty that focuses on helping a person regain or maintain the skills needed for everyday life, including those related to activities of daily living (ADLs). While physical therapy focuses on maintaining or improving the skills that involve bigger muscles and bigger movements, occupational therapy focuses more on maintaining or improving the skills that involve smaller muscles and smaller movements.

Speech-Language Pathology

Speech-language pathology is a rehabilitation specialty that focuses on helping the person regain or maintain the ability to communicate with others, chew, and swallow. Difficulty forming words, speaking, chewing, and swallowing can occur as a result of many different conditions. A licensed speech-language pathologist (sometimes called a speech therapist) works with the person to improve the person's ability to speak, chew, or swallow.

Emotional Rehabilitation

Adjusting to living with a disability can be very difficult emotionally. The person may struggle with depression, anger, or other feelings as he adjusts to the changes the disability has caused. Some people who have experienced a devastating illness or injury may even talk of suicide. Emotional rehabilitation helps the person learn to cope with the losses caused by the disability (see Fig. 9-1).

Vocational Rehabilitation

A *vocation* is a job. Vocational rehabilitation (see Fig. 9-1) helps the person to learn skills that she will need to work. In some cases, the person may need vocational rehabilitation to relearn the skills that she had before. In other cases, the person will need to learn a completely new set of skills that will allow her to get another type of job. Vocational rehabilitation may also help the person to find a new job, a new place to live, or a new mode of transportation that will allow her to become independent again.

Supportive devices devices that help to stabilize a weak joint or limb

Assistive devices devices that make certain tasks (such as walking, eating, or dressing) easier for a person with a disability

Prosthetic devices artificial replacements for legs, feet, arms, or other body parts

Contractures a condition that occurs when a joint is held in the same position for too long a time; the tendons shorten and become stiff, possibly causing permanent loss of motion in the joint

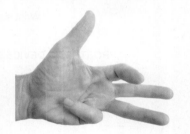

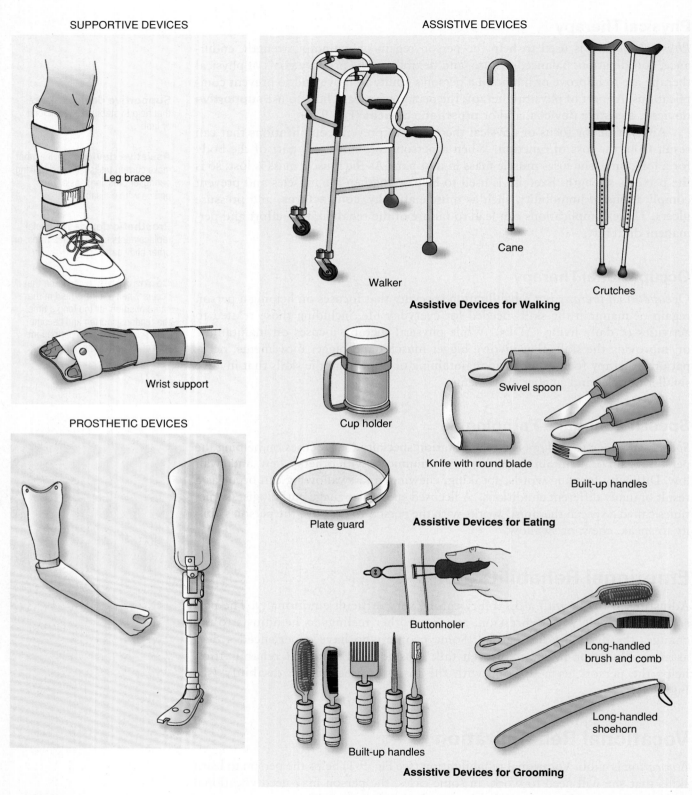

SUPPORTIVE DEVICES

Leg brace

Wrist support

PROSTHETIC DEVICES

ASSISTIVE DEVICES

Walker

Cane

Crutches

Assistive Devices for Walking

Cup holder

Swivel spoon

Knife with round blade

Built-up handles

Plate guard

Assistive Devices for Eating

Buttonholer

Long-handled brush and comb

Long-handled shoehorn

Built-up handles

Assistive Devices for Grooming

■ **FIGURE 9-2**

Supportive devices, assistive devices, prosthetic devices, or all three can help a person to do certain tasks independently.

Putting it all together!

- A person's specific disability and individual needs determine which type of rehabilitation is needed. Many patients and residents will need all three types of rehabilitation.

- Physical rehabilitation helps the person to regain the ability to do certain physical tasks independently. Physical rehabilitation may involve the use of physical therapy, occupational therapy, or speech-language pathology. During physical rehabilitation, the person may learn how to use special equipment, such as assistive devices, prosthetic devices, and supportive devices. In addition, exercise is used to help strengthen the muscles and prevent complications.

- Emotional rehabilitation helps a person to learn to cope emotionally with the disability.

- Vocational rehabilitation is used when a person's disability causes her to lose the skills that she needs to do the job that she had prior to becoming disabled.

The Role of the Nursing Assistant

What will you learn?

When you are finished with this section, you will be able to:

1. Understand the nursing assistant's responsibilities related to providing restorative care.
2. List observations a nursing assistant may make when providing restorative care that should be reported to the nurse.

Many of a nursing assistant's responsibilities are related to helping patients and residents to maintain their independence and return to their best level of functioning after an illness or injury. For example, nursing assistants are responsible for:

- Helping to prevent complications of immobility by assisting with repositioning (see Chapter 17) and exercise (see Chapter 18)

- Carrying out a bowel- or bladder-training plan by taking the person to the bathroom on schedule (see Chapters 25 and 26)

- Reinforcing the rehabilitation efforts and techniques that are being used with the patient or resident (Fig. 9-3)

    Guidelines for assisting with restorative care are given in Guidelines Box 9-1.

Concerns for Long-Term Care

Frailty is a special concern when caring for older adults. Age-related changes to skeletal muscles, combined with immobility or lack of exercise and poor nutrition, increase an older person's chances of being frail. A frail person has usually had unplanned weight loss, walks slowly, is easily

Tell the Nurse!

Providing restorative care

- The person's abilities have changed (for better or for worse)

- The person seems depressed, angry, or frustrated

- A new rehabilitation measure does not seem to be working for the person

- A supportive device is broken or not working properly

- The person has a change in vital signs during or after the rehabilitation activity

- The person has pain, swelling, or redness around supportive or prosthetic devices

- The person has skin breakdown or other signs of complications of immobility

fatigued, and generally has a low level of activity. Older people who are frail are more likely to be at high risk for falls, disability, hospitalization, nursing home admission, and death. Rehabilitation and restorative care can help a frail person to regain some strength and endurance and lower the risk of falling and other disability.

The Omnibus Budget Reconciliation Act (OBRA) requires nursing homes to provide each resident with the services the resident needs to reach and maintain her highest possible level of well-being and function. There are many specific OBRA requirements related to helping residents maintain or achieve their highest level of function. To be in compliance with OBRA, staff members must take steps to improve or maintain existing function and to prevent the loss of function.

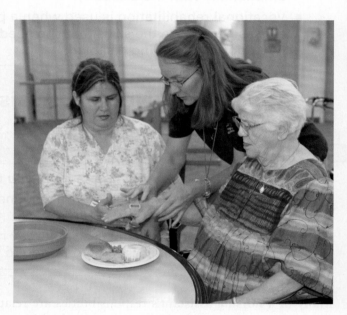

■ **FIGURE 9-3**

Ask the nurse or physical therapist to show you the special techniques and devices that are being used with your patient or resident. This will allow you to help your patient or resident more effectively. Here, a physical therapist is showing a nursing assistant how the resident can use a wrist supporter with a spoon attached to eat.

Putting it all together!

- The nursing assistant plays a key role in the successful rehabilitation of a patient or resident by providing physical and emotional care and by reporting observations about the person's progress and abilities.

- Rehabilitation focuses on the whole person, not just on the person's disabilities.

GUIDELINES BOX 9-1   Assisting With Rehabilitation and Restorative Care

What you do	Why you do it
Ask questions about new rehabilitation measures that have been planned for a resident or patient. Have the nurse or therapist explain to you how to use new equipment and show you how to help your patient or resident to use it.	*Knowing about the special techniques that are being used with the person will allow you to help the person to practice these techniques. Knowing how to use any special equipment will allow you to help the person to use the equipment properly.*
Monitor the person's emotional status.	*Working to regain or maintain function, or learning to adjust to a loss of function, can be a long, difficult, and painful process. It is very easy for patients or residents to become frustrated and discouraged. Reporting your observations about the person's emotional status to the nurse will enable the rehabilitation team to help the person work through these feelings so that the person can again focus on recovery.*
Focus on the person's abilities, and celebrate all successes, no matter how small.	*Achieving small goals gives the person an emotional boost and encourages him to keep working.*
Encourage and reassure the person, but be realistic in your encouragement and be careful not to compare the person with someone else.	*Each person will have individual responses to rehabilitation. Not all goals will be reached.*
Give the person the time she needs to complete a task independently. Offer assistance only as needed and only if the person seems overly frustrated.	*Although it may be faster or easier to just complete the task for the person, it is important for the person's self-esteem to let the person do as much for herself as possible.*
Be empathetic, but do not pity the person.	*When you pity someone, it means that you recognize his or her loss. When you empathize with someone, it means that you can imagine how the person feels about the loss. Empathy will help you deal more effectively with the person's anger and frustration.*
If you find yourself feeling frustrated with a patient or resident who is struggling with rehabilitation, you should talk to the nurse.	*If you let the person's frustration and anger affect you, you may not be able to provide the person with the best care possible. You may need a break or a short reassignment from that person to continue to provide the best care possible.*

WHAT DID YOU LEARN?

Multiple Choice

Select the single best answer to each of the following questions.

1. The process that helps a person with a disability to return to his highest level of physical, emotional, or economic function is called:
   a. Homeostasis
   b. Metabolism
   c. Prosthetics
   d. Rehabilitation

2. Which one of the following would you be responsible for when providing a patient or resident with restorative care?
   a. Assisting the person with range-of-motion exercises
   b. Taking the person to the bathroom at scheduled times as part of a bladder-training program
   c. Observing the person for changes in ability, positive or negative
   d. All of the above

3. What is it called when a joint is held in one position for too long, and the tendons shorten?
   a. A pressure ulcer
   b. A bed sore
   c. A contracture
   d. A shearing injury

4. The phase of rehabilitation in which the team focuses on stabilizing the person and preventing complications is known as the _____ phase.
   a. Acute
   b. Subacute
   c. Middle
   d. Chronic

Matching

Match each type of rehabilitation with its description.

_____ 1. Vocational rehabilitation

_____ 2. Physical rehabilitation

_____ 3. Emotional rehabilitation

a. Used to help a person manage the feelings caused by a disability

b. Used when a person's disability causes her to lose the skills that she needs to do the job that she had prior to becoming disabled

c. Used to restore strength and function to limbs that have been affected by illness or injury

STOP Stop *and* Think!

Amanda is assigned to care for Mrs. Webb, who recently had a stroke. When the stroke occurred, Mrs. Webb had been preparing dinner at the stove. As a result, when she fell, she also suffered severe burns on her arms. Now Mrs. Webb is receiving rehabilitation therapy for her left-sided weakness in addition to recovering from the skin grafts used to treat the burns on her arms. Mrs. Webb is a widow and her children live out of state. She cries frequently because she says there is "no one to help me and I will probably end up staying in the nursing home for the rest of my life." Every time Amanda tries to get Mrs. Webb to participate in bathing and feeding herself, Mrs. Webb shakes her head and says she "just doesn't feel up to the effort today." Mrs. Webb's grafts are healing well and she is doing great in therapy. Is there anything Amanda can do to help Mrs. Webb not feel so helpless? What can she say to her to encourage her to do more for herself and be less dependent?

STOP Stop *and* Think!

Jacob is working in the rehabilitation unit of his nursing facility. He has been assigned to care for Mr. Huff, who has recently had his right leg amputated (removed) above the knee. Jacob is to assist Mr. Huff in his transfers until he is able to do them himself. Mr. Huff is to do all of his own activities of daily living (ADLs), such as bathing, feeding, and dressing himself, with minimal help from Jacob. This morning when Jacob enters the room, he finds Mr. Huff on the floor between the bed and the wheelchair. Mr. Huff is struggling to climb into his wheelchair. When Jacob approaches him to help, Mr. Huff says angrily, "Leave me alone; I can do this. I'm OK, just leave me alone." Aside from helping Mr. Huff into his wheelchair, what could Jacob do to help Mr. Huff? What do you think about Mr. Huff's attempt to move from the bed to the wheelchair by himself?

Long-Term Care

The majority of nursing assistants are employed by long-term care facilities. The population of elderly people continues to increase dramatically due to advances and improvements in health care. The focus of this unit is on long-term care; the types of long-term care facilities, the people who reside in long-term care facilities, and people who have dementia.

Photo: *A nursing assistant pauses to visit with a resident.*

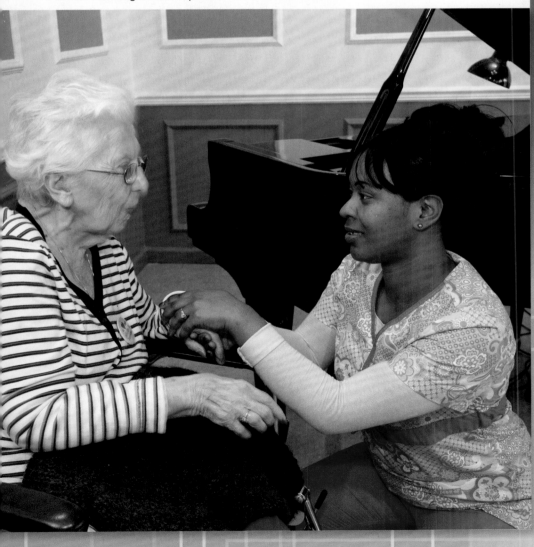

Overview of Long-Term Care

There are many different types of long-term care settings in the United States today. As the number of elderly people who need some type of assisted care continues to grow, the need for nursing assistants and other health care workers to work in these settings will continue to increase.

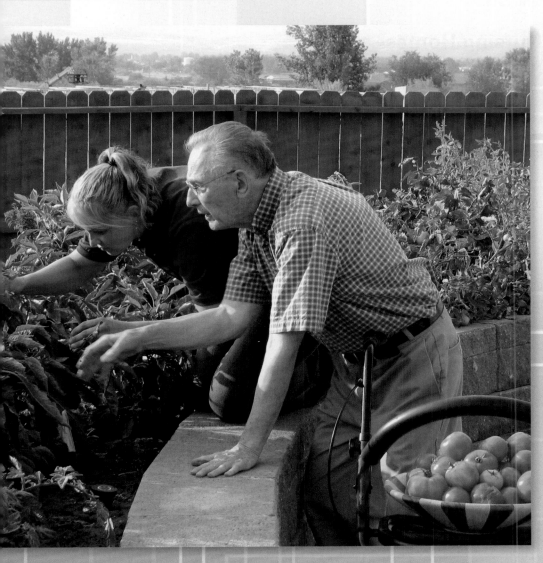

Photo: A resident of a Green House home enjoys gardening. The Green House project is an example of how long-term care is changing. (Photo courtesy of THE GREEN HOUSE Project.)

Types of Long-Term Care Settings

What will you learn?

When you are finished with this section, you will be able to:

1. Identify the various types of long-term care settings and discuss how they are different from one another.
2. Define the words **continuing care retirement community (CCRC)** and **continuum of care**.

A long-term care setting is a place where health care is provided for people who require ongoing nursing care, personal assistance, or both as the result of illness or disability. The three major types of long-term care settings are nursing homes, assisted-living facilities, and continuing care retirement communities (CCRCs). Some people also consider adult day care and home health services part of long-term care.

Nursing Homes

Nursing homes provide residents with around-the-clock nursing care and supervision. Typically, residents live in private or semi-private rooms grouped along a common hallway. Usually, there are also common areas where residents gather to socialize (such as dining rooms and activity rooms), a small chapel where religious services can be held, and patios and gardens that allow the residents access to outdoor activities (Fig. 10-1).

Nursing homes, also called *nursing facilities,* require that a registered nurse (RN) or licensed practical nurse (LPN) be on-site at all times. In addition to providing basic medical care and nursing services, nursing homes must also provide rehabilitation therapies, podiatry, dental, and medical specialty consultation services (for example, a cardiologist consult for a resident with a heart condition).

Levels of Nursing Home Care

Care in a nursing home is usually categorized as *intermediate care* (usually long-term) or *skilled* (usually short-term).

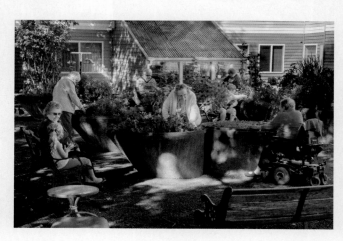

■ **FIGURE 10-1**

Residents of a nursing home enjoy time outside in the garden.

- Intermediate care is provided for people who are chronically ill or disabled and need assistance with the daily activities of living (ADLs). In addition, an increased focus on rehabilitation or restorative care (discussed in Chapter 9) helps residents to maintain or even improve their level of function and independence so that their abilities do not decline.

- Skilled care (sometimes referred to as skilled rehabilitation care) is provided for people who have recently required some type of acute care for an illness or injury. Typical reasons that a resident may be admitted for skilled care include stroke, fractured hip, and rehabilitation after an acute illness such as pneumonia or a heart attack. Many nursing homes provide skilled nursing care for people who will be returning to their own private homes after they have rehabilitated.

Another growing trend for long-term care facilities is the establishment of special care units (SCUs). These units are separate areas in the facility designed to meet the needs of residents with specific types of disorders. Rehabilitation, and dementia care units, or Alzheimer's units are examples of SCUs.

Assisted-Living Facilities

Assisted-living facilities provide residents with limited assistance with tasks such as personal care, medication administration, transportation, meals, and housekeeping. Residents of assisted-living facilities often live in small apartments that have a kitchen or kitchenette, a bathroom, a living area, and a bedroom. Most assisted-living facilities also have community dining rooms and common areas where residents can go to socialize.

Continuing Care Retirement Communities (CCRCs)

Continuing care retirement communities (CCRCs) provide many different levels of care and multiple services on the same campus. The CCRC campus provides a **continuum of care** by including facilities for independent living, assisted living, and nursing home care (Fig. 10-2). As age, health problems, or both cause a resident of a CCRC to become less independent, he is able to stay within the CCRC to obtain the care he needs. In addition, the CCRC campus may include restaurants or dining facilities, recreational and social facilities, facilities for worship, a small market where food and other items can be purchased, and a health center where residents can go for medical care.

Continuing care retirement communities (CCRCs) a type of long-term care setting that provides many different levels of care (for example, independent living, assisted living, and nursing home care) and multiple services on the same campus

Continuum of care the delivery of health care over time as a person moves from being independent to needing assistance with personal care, medical care, or both

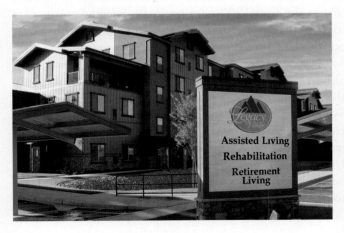

- **FIGURE 10-2**

A continuing care retirement community (CCRC) has facilities for independent living, assisted-living, and nursing home care, all on the same campus. As residents' needs change, they can obtain the care they need without moving away from the campus. Other buildings on campus might include restaurants, recreational facilities, facilities for worship, stores, and a health center where residents can go for medical care.
(Photo courtesy of Legacy Village, Layton, UT—A Continuing Care Senior Living Community.)

Putting it all together!

- The three major types of long-term care settings are nursing homes, assisted-living facilities, and continuing care retirement communities (CCRCs).
- Nursing homes provide residents with around-the-clock nursing care and supervision.
- Assisted-living facilities provide residents with limited assistance with certain tasks, such as meals and housekeeping.
- CCRCs provide residents with multiple levels of services, ranging from independent living to nursing home care, all on the same campus.

Long-Term Care: Past, Present, and Future

What will you learn?

When you are finished with this section, you will be able to:

1. Discuss the past, present, and future of long-term care.
2. Define the words **Social Security Act** and **pension**.

In past years, public opinion of long-term care, most specifically nursing homes, was very low. Many changes have occurred in the past that have helped improve the quality and reputation of long-term care.

The Journey From the Past to the Present

As long as there have been older, chronically ill, and disabled people, society has been challenged to care for them. Throughout history, family members or friends of those in need often took on the responsibility of caring for them. Those without family or friends (or the money to hire help) became the responsibility of the community. The community responded to this need by establishing *poorhouses* (community-supported facilities that provided shelter for those without the means of supporting themselves). From the mid-1800s, up until the Social Security Act was passed in 1935, many older, chronically ill, or disabled people lived in poorhouses. Conditions in the poorhouses varied quite a bit, but overcrowding, filth, and disease were common.

In 1935, President Franklin D. Roosevelt signed the **Social Security Act** into law. As a result of the Social Security Act, older people who were retired or unemployed were entitled to receive a **pension** from the government. Many elderly people could now afford to move to "boarding homes," places that provided housing, meals, and possibly other services for a fee. Rather than lose paying tenants as they became older and more frail, some boarding homes started to hire nurses to care for their tenants. This was the beginning of the "nursing home" that we know today.

The need for nursing homes and other types of long-term care continued to grow. Advances in the medical field and improvements in people's general health

Social Security Act an act that established a program designed to provide regular cash payments for retired people aged 65 years and older

Pension regular cash payments paid to a person, usually after retirement

allowed people to live longer. However, the quality of care provided in many nursing homes was poor. The "aides" who provided care were not required to receive any formal health care training. Neglect and abuse of residents were common. Many of the facilities were run by people who were more interested in making money than in caring for the older people and persons with disabilities.

In the 1980s, the Institute of Medicine (IOM) was given the task of studying nursing home care. The result of its report was the Omnibus Budget Reconciliation Act (OBRA) of 1987, which was put into effect in 1990. The strict OBRA legislation improved the quality of life for residents of nursing homes, by making sure that they received a certain standard of care. This care was required to take into account the residents' physical, emotional, spiritual, and social needs. In addition, OBRA set standards for the physical environment in the nursing home, as well as for the training and evaluation of the nursing assistants who worked in nursing homes.

The Future

In 1997, a small group of professionals working in long-term care met to share ideas and create a new vision for the future of long-term care. This group of long-term care professionals, which officially became known as the *Pioneer Network* in 2000, developed several models for long-term care.

The Green House® project is one representative of these changes in long-term care. The purpose was to create a place of warmth and growth for residents and staff. The design of a Green House home is much like that of a private home. Only 7 to 12 residents live in each Green House home. Each resident has a private bedroom and bathroom. Because only 7 to 12 residents live in each Green House home, there are no long hallways, so many residents are able to get around without using wheelchairs. Other features of the house include a large common living area, a laundry area, and an open patio and outdoor garden (Fig. 10-3).

The Green House® has been very successful. Some of the problems that residents frequently experience in more traditional long-term care settings, such as urinary incontinence (an inability to control urination), unexplained weight loss, depression, and a decline in abilities, are seen less frequently among residents of The Green House® homes. The Green House® model has other benefits as well. Nursing assistants receive additional education that enables them to make decisions and plan care. Staff turnover rates have been maintained well below the national average, and there have been fewer work-related injuries. Today, there are hundreds of Green House® homes open or under development in the majority of states across the United States.

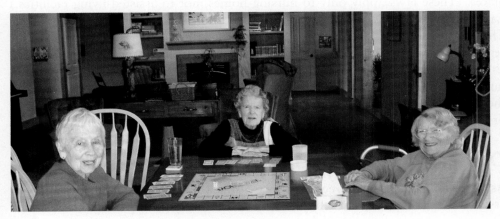

■ **FIGURE 10-3**

Residents of a Green House® home enjoy a board game together in the large common living area called "The Hearth."

(Photo courtesy of THE GREEN HOUSE® Project.)

Putting it all together!

- Only by understanding the past can we understand the present and future of long-term care.
- In the past, long-term care in the United States had many problems.
- Legislation, such as the Omnibus Budget Reconciliation Act (OBRA) of 1987, has greatly improved the quality of care provided in nursing homes.
- Today, leaders in long-term care continue to seek ways to improve the long-term care environment and the way care is delivered.

Oversight of Long-Term Care

What will you learn?

When you are finished with this section, you will be able to:

1. Describe some of the government and private agencies that provide oversight of long-term care.

Many different agencies—including the federal, state, and local government, as well as independent nonprofit organizations—are responsible for making that the care provided in long-term care facilities in the United States is safe and of high quality.

Oversight by the Federal Government

All types of long-term care facilities must follow the requirements of agencies, such as the Occupational Safety and Health Administration (OSHA), the Food and Drug Administration (FDA), and the Centers for Disease Control and Prevention (CDC). The functions of these agencies were reviewed in Chapter 1.

In addition, federal (OBRA) laws apply to every nursing home in the United States. (These laws apply only to nursing homes, not to assisted-living facilities.) Each nursing home is subject to routine inspection (surveys) by the government. The purpose of the survey is to make sure that the facility is following OBRA regulations and meeting the government's standards. The *Centers for Medicare & Medicaid Services (CMS)* is the government agency responsible for monitoring nursing homes to make sure that they are following OBRA regulations and meeting the government's standards. Government payment for services depends on whether or not the facility is meeting the required standards.

Oversight by State Governments

Assisted-living facilities are regulated by the state. Because no federal laws apply to assisted-living facilities, assisted-living services can vary greatly from state to state.

Nursing homes must comply with state laws, in addition to federal laws. Many state laws that apply to nursing homes follow OBRA, but some states have additional requirements that OBRA does not include.

Oversight by Local Governments

Local agencies (such as city or county health departments) are responsible for ensuring that the facility is in compliance with any regulations that the local government has established for long-term care facilities. Local officials may also have a role in checking to make sure that the facility is providing care according to state or federal standards.

Independent Nonprofit Organizations

In Chapter 1, you learned about The Joint Commission, an organization that sets national standards for all types of health care organizations and officially accredits organizations that meet these standards. Many long-term care facilities seek accreditation from The Joint Commission.

A similar organization, the *Continuing Care Accreditation Commission (CCAC)*, grants accreditation to CCRCs, as well as to some other types of organizations that provide long-term care services (such as adult day care centers). The CCAC is the only accrediting organization specifically for CCRCs.

 Putting it all together!

- Government agencies, as well as independent nonprofit organizations, provide oversight of the long-term care industry.
- Nursing homes in the Unites States must follow federal, state, and local regulations. Currently, there are no federal laws that govern assisted-living facilities.
- Independent nonprofit organizations, such as The Joint Commission and the CCAC, set standards for health care organizations and grant accreditation to organizations that meet the standards.

Paying for Long-Term Care

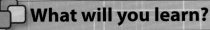 **What will you learn?**

When you are finished with this section, you will be able to:

1. Discuss how long-term care is paid for.
2. Define the word **benefit period**.

Long-term care is very expensive and not easily paid for by individuals or the government.

Paying for Nursing Home Care

In the United States, the average cost for nursing home care is more than $6,000 per month. Many people do not have the savings to pay for nursing home care if it is needed.

Medicare

Many people assume that Medicare will pay for nursing home care. In reality, what Medicare pays for is extremely limited. For Medicare to pay, several requirements must be met:

- The person must meet strict criteria for skilled health care services. Skilled health care services are those provided by nurses or other licensed health care professionals.
- Care must follow a hospital stay.
- Care must be provided in a nursing facility licensed to provide skilled care.

A **benefit period** begins when the person is hospitalized and ends when the person has not received any skilled health care services. A person can have up to 100 days of skilled care in one benefit period. A new benefit period cannot begin until 60 days without skilled services has passed.

Benefit period a unit of time used by the Medicare program to track how many days of skilled health care services a person uses, and how many are still available; begins with hospitalization and ends when a person has not received any skilled health care services, either in the hospital or in the nursing home

Medicaid

Many people need nursing home care but are not eligible for Medicare coverage. Some are admitted to a nursing facility as "private pay," meaning that they pay for care using their own money. Because nursing home care is so expensive, many people exhaust all of their savings and then must rely on Medicaid to pay for their care. Approximately 70% of those currently living in nursing homes are relying on Medicaid to pay for their care. Although Medicaid eases the financial burden for the person receiving care, the financial burden is transferred to the nursing facility, and to the state that is distributing the Medicaid payments.

Long-Term Care Insurance

Long-term care insurance is a private insurance policy that can be purchased by an individual to help pay for long-term care in the future, should it be needed. The benefit of long-term care insurance is that it can help to pay for long-term care services, which help to protect the person's savings and assets. The disadvantages are that long-term care insurance is very expensive and somewhat risky.

Long-term care insurance, like Medicare, does not pay for all costs associated with nursing home care. Even if the insurance pays for the nursing home stay, it may not cover additional expenses related to medications, supplies, or other special services and therapies.

Paying for Assisted-Living Care

The average cost for assisted-living care is approximately half the cost of nursing home care. Even though assisted-living care is less expensive, it is primarily a private pay expense. Medicare does not cover any portion of assisted-living care, and in most cases, Medicaid does not either. Payment by long-term care insurance depends on the type of policy that was purchased. Generally, long-term care insurance only covers certain expenses related to assisted-living.

Putting it all together!

- Long-term care is very costly and is not easily paid for by either the individual or the government.
- At an average cost of more than $6,000 per month for nursing home care, a lifetime of savings may not last very long.
- Medicare coverage for nursing home care is minimal. Those qualifying must meet very strict criteria for skilled health care. Medicare provides no payment for assisted-living care.
- Medicaid pays for most nursing home care in this country. This is causing financial strain for both the facilities and the government. Medicaid usually does not pay for assisted-living care.
- Long-term care insurance is private insurance that can help pay for long-term care.

WHAT DID YOU LEARN?

Multiple Choice

Select the single best answer for each of the following questions.

1. Which one of the following is an insurance policy for long-term care that can be purchased by an individual?
   a. Long-term care insurance
   b. Medicaid
   c. Medicare
   d. Pension

2. How is most assisted-living care paid for?
   a. Medicaid
   b. Medicare
   c. Private pay
   d. Long-term care insurance

3. What did the members of the Pioneer Network do?
   a. They started a movement to get older people out of poorhouses in the late 1800s
   b. They met to share ideas and create a new vision for the future of long-term care
   c. They investigated nursing home care and wrote the Omnibus Budget Reconciliation Act (OBRA) in 1987
   d. They developed the Social Security program in the 1930s

4. What is a benefit period?
   a. The period of time when a person receives nursing home care after using up all private funds
   b. The period of time when long-term insurance benefits are paid out to a person who has purchased a policy
   c. The period of time when a person is eligible for Medicare benefits
   d. The period of time that Medicaid pays for a person's nursing home care

Matching

Match each numbered item with its appropriate lettered description.

_____ 1. Pension

_____ 2. Continuing care retirement community (CCRC)

_____ 3. Centers for Medicare and Medicaid Services (CMS)

_____ 4. Omnibus Budget Reconciliation Act (OBRA)

_____ 5. Continuum of care

a. A long-term care facility that provides multiple levels of care and multiple services on one campus

b. The delivery of health care over time as a person moves from being independent to needing assistance with personal care, medical care, or both

c. Tough regulations put into action to improve the quality of care and quality of life for residents of nursing homes

d. The government agency that provides oversight to ensure nursing home compliance with OBRA regulations

e. Monthly income provided to older Americans as a result of the Social Security Act of 1935

 Stop *and* **Think!**

How would your life change if you had to take in an elderly, dependent family member because there were no other options available to provide care? What difficulties would you encounter? What would be the benefits?

The Long-Term Care Resident

In Chapter 5, you learned about human growth and development and meeting human needs. In this chapter, you will build on this knowledge by learning more specifically about the residents and the families that you will care for in the long-term care setting. As you begin your nursing assistant career in long-term care, it is important that you have knowledge about the people in this setting as well as their circumstances.

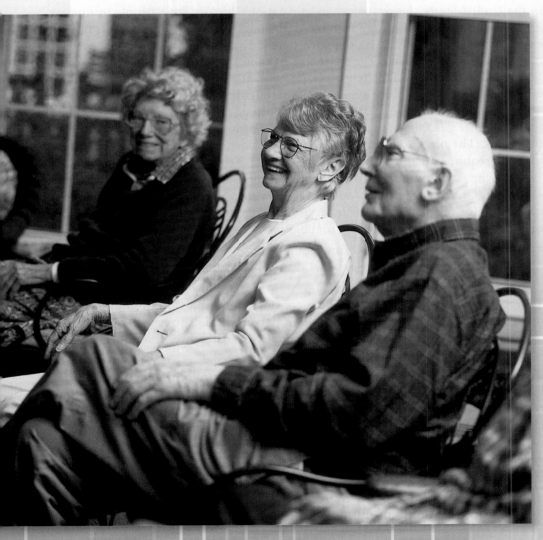

Photo: *Most residents of long-term care facilities are older with multiple care needs. Here, a group of residents enjoy an activity together. (Photo courtesy of Copper Ridge.)*

Our Aging Population

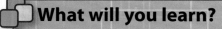

What will you learn?

When you are finished with this section, you will be able to:

1. Discuss why the number of people aged 65 years and older living in the United States is increasing every year.
2. Describe what effect the increasing number of older people could have on the long-term care industry.
3. Define the words **chronic condition** and **degenerative condition**.

Although people of all ages are cared for in nursing homes, most of the residents of nursing homes are 65 years and older, with the highest number of people being 85 years and older. Each year, the number of people living in the United States who are 65 years and older increases. As a society, we need to be prepared to care for this growing segment of the population.

In 2010, there were more than 40 million people aged 65 years and older living in the United States. Never before in our nation's history have people in this age group represented such a large segment of the population. In addition, this trend is expected to continue. By 2030, the government expects that there will be nearly 72 million people older than 65 years of age living in the United States.

In 2010, there was approximately 1.3 million people aged 65 years and older who were residents of some type of long-term care facility. Although only about 5% of the older adult population resides in a long-term care facility at any given time, a higher percentage will need some form of long-term care at some point in their lives. The oldest old, those 85 years and older, are the people who are most likely to require care in a long-term care facility.

So, why is the number of older people in the United States steadily increasing each year? One major reason is advances in health care. These advances have made it possible for people to recover from (or continue to live with) conditions that at one time would have caused them to die. For example:

Chronic condition a condition that is ongoing and often needs to be controlled through continuous medication or treatment (for example, diabetes, heart failure, or hypertension)

Degenerative condition a condition that gets progressively worse over time (for example, dementia)

- In the past, many people died from acute illnesses for which there were no treatments. Many illnesses, such as heart disease, cancer, and infectious diseases are now treatable or preventable.

- In the past, conditions that are now considered **chronic conditions** or **degenerative conditions** might have caused a person to die sooner. Today, we have medications and treatments that help people live with chronic and degenerative conditions, while in the past we did not.

These changes in cause of death are reflected in our current population. We have large numbers of people who are living longer and longer lives, but with chronic conditions. As more and more people live longer lives, many with one or more chronic conditions, the need for long-term care services will increase.

Putting it all together!

- People in the United States are living longer because of improvements in public health and advances in medical care and technology. Because of this, the number of people who are 65 years and older living in the United States is increasing each year.

■ One third to one half of all people aged 65 years and older will need some type of long-term care sometime before they die. People aged 85 years and older are the most likely to require long-term care.

Factors Leading to Long-Term Care Admissions

What will you learn?

When you are finished with this section, you will be able to:

1. Discuss why a person might need long-term care.
2. Discuss the expected length of stay for someone in long-term care.
3. Define the words **activities of daily living (ADLs)**, **instrumental activities of daily living (IADLs)**, **co-existent medical conditions**, and **cognitive impairment**.

There are several reasons why a person might be admitted to a nursing home:

■ A person may be admitted to a nursing home on a temporary basis to recover from the lingering effects of an acute illness (such as a stroke) or injury (such as a broken hip).

■ A person may be admitted to a nursing home because she needs continuous monitoring and treatment as a result of one or more chronic conditions.

■ A person may be admitted to a nursing home because he needs help meeting his physical needs as the result of a degenerative condition.

■ A person may be admitted to a nursing home because it is no longer safe for the person to live on her own, due to physical or mental impairment (or both).

Short-Stay Admissions

The use of nursing homes for short-stay admissions (3 months or less) has been steadily increasing. This increase in short stays is primarily due to changes to how health care is paid for. As a result of these changes, hospitals are discharging patients "quicker and sicker." Many of these patients are admitted to long-term care facilities to receive the care they need until they are well enough to return home. Providing this care in a nursing home instead of in a hospital saves the government insurance programs significant money, and this helps to control overall health care spending.

Extended-Stay Admissions

Although the use of nursing homes for short-stay admissions has been increasing, most people cared for in nursing homes are there for longer periods of time (for example, 1 year or more). What are the factors that make nursing home admission necessary?

People come to live in nursing homes because they have physical or mental disabilities that make it impossible for them to care for themselves properly. Many times, the level of care they require is beyond what family members are able to provide, or there simply are no family members to provide care.

Activities of daily living (ADLs) routine tasks of daily life, such as bathing, eating, and grooming

Instrumental activities of daily living (IADLs) more complex tasks that a person must be able to do in order to continue to live independently, such as using the telephone or handling money

Most residents of nursing homes need help with **activities of daily living (ADLs)**. At least 75% of nursing home residents need help with three or more of their ADLs. About 75% of nursing home residents also need help with at least some **instrumental activities of daily living (IADLs)**, and more than 50% need help with all of them. Several factors can cause a person to need help with his or her ADLs and IADLs:

- Medical conditions or the effects of aging can affect the person's strength, endurance, or coordination.
- Medical conditions that affect a person's ability to think and remember (such as dementia) can cause the person to forget how to do these routine tasks.
- Sensory deficits, such as impaired vision or hearing, can make it harder for the person to function independently.

Co-existent medical condition more than one medical condition at the same time in the same person

It is very common for a resident to have **co-existent medical conditions**. Nearly all residents of nursing homes have more than one medical condition at the time of admission. More than half of them have three or more.

The most common medical conditions among nursing home residents are cardiovascular disease, respiratory disease, stroke, dementia, depression, diabetes, and arthritis. These are all examples of chronic conditions that require continuous medical monitoring and care. These conditions may also significantly impact a resident's ability to perform ADLs and IADLs.

Cognitive impairment problems processing, learning, or remembering information

Cognitive impairment, especially when it is accompanied by physical problems, is the reason why many people come to live in nursing homes. Seventy percent of the residents in nursing homes have either short-term or long-term memory loss, or both. Almost half of the residents have some form of dementia (discussed in Chapter 12).

Nursing assistants are responsible for providing most hands-on care in the nursing home setting. In many instances, the nursing home resident requires special consideration when receiving that care, often due to advanced age. You will see sections titled "Concerns for Long-Term Care" throughout this textbook that will point out areas of special consideration related to the topic being discussed. Pay special attention to these concerns. Your role as a caregiver in this type of health care setting is very important, and you have the opportunity to improve the comfort and quality of life for each person you care for.

 Putting it all together!

- Medical need, triggered by acute, chronic, or degenerative illness, often makes long-term care necessary. Most residents have three or more co-existent medical conditions.
- Most people who live in nursing homes need help with activities of daily living (ADLs) and instrumental activities of daily living (IADLs) because of physical disability, mental disability, or both.

Making the Adjustment to Long-Term Care

What will you learn?

When you are finished with this section, you will be able to:

1. Describe and discuss the challenges a person may face when he or she comes to live in a long-term care facility.

2. Describe and discuss the challenges a family may face when one of it its members comes to live in a long-term care facility.

The move to a nursing home is often preceded by some crises, such as an unexpected accident or illness. Box 11-1 gives a couple of examples of the different types of crises that can cause a person to need to be placed in a nursing home.

Can you imagine what it would be like if you suffered an unexpected injury or medical crisis that made it impossible for you to return home to live? Perhaps someone else made the decision about where you would live, and you did not even

BOX 11-1   Situations That Can Initiate a Move to a Nursing Home

- An elderly widow living alone has had a stroke. Suddenly, she is taken from home to the hospital for intensive medical care. She needs extensive rehabilitation that the hospital cannot provide, so she is transferred to a nursing home for that care. Despite months of therapy, she is unable to regain enough self-care skills to live independently anymore. Living with her son or daughter is not an option because their homes are not set up for someone with a disability and besides no one is home during the day. Without much time for emotional preparation, the woman must adjust to the loss of her independence and the loss of her home. Her son and daughter must also adjust to the changes brought on by their mother's stroke.

- An elderly man is living with family members because he has dementia and diabetes. He is no longer able to take care of any of his own needs. As the dementia progresses, he becomes more and more difficult to care for. The family struggles to get him to take his medication. He is no longer able to find the bathroom and has begun to urinate in inappropriate places throughout the house. His odd behaviors are scaring the grandchildren.

He requires supervision 24 hours a day. He has wandered away from home several times, once in the middle of the night. The last time, the police had to be called to help find him. The family is exhausted and family relationships are suffering. The family can no longer continue to provide the care that the man needs, so the decision is made to admit him to a nursing home. Even though this situation is not as sudden as the situation described in the first example, there is still a crisis (in this case, calling the police for assistance) that spurs action toward nursing home placement.

Many of your residents are coping with multiple losses and life changes. For example, in the case of the elderly widow who suffered a stroke, she must not only cope with the loss of her home, but with the fact that her body no longer functions as it used to. She has to re-learn many tasks that she took for granted when her body worked normally. The man with dementia from the second example is thoroughly confused in his new environment. He is unable to understand the reason for the change, and he does not recognize anything or anybody. How upsetting and frightening this must be!

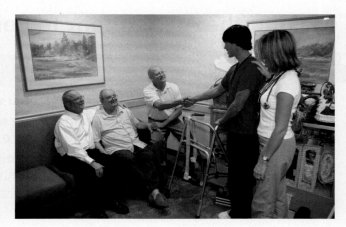

■ **FIGURE 11-1**
Being admitted to a nursing home is often stressful for the resident, as well as his or her family members. As a nursing assistant, it is important for you to take steps to make the transition easier for everyone. The first step is understanding what the resident and family may be feeling.

get a say in the matter. This happens frequently—most nursing home residents are "placed" in the long-term care facility, they do not choose to come live there.

Similarly, how would you feel if you were the one who had to make the decision to admit your mother, father, sibling, husband, wife, or child to a nursing home? When a person comes to live in a nursing home, it is often a difficult adjustment for both the person and his or her family members (Fig. 11-1). As a nursing assistant, there are many things that you can do to help ease the transition to long-term care for both the resident and the family (Box 11-2).

The Resident

Most people do not *plan* to come live in a nursing home, and to be honest, it is not something most people *want* to do. People do not choose illness or infirmity. All of us, given the choice, would prefer to remain healthy and in our own homes.

Residents of nursing homes often have many fears and anxieties. They may worry about how their medical problems will affect their health and independence in the future. Because long-term care is expensive, they may have concerns about their finances. They worry about how the move to the nursing home will affect their family members, and they may be sad to be separated from them.

The nursing home environment itself can be frightening and uncomfortable, full of strange noises and smells and unfamiliar people. The resident must learn to develop trusting relationships with many new people under very difficult

---

BOX 11-2   **Helping Residents and Family Members Adjust**

- Be knowledgeable about the resident's condition.
- Be knowledgeable about the circumstances that necessitated the move to the long-term care facility.
- Know your resident. Learn about his or her likes, dislikes, relationships, and interests.
- Allow the resident to make choices about his or her care.

- Be sensitive to both resident and family needs.
- Be flexible!
- Welcome family members and include them in the resident's care when appropriate.
- Be sensitive to the resident's environment. Accommodate needs for privacy.

circumstances. Moving to a nursing home means having to give up your home and move to a place where you may have to share a room with a stranger. Space is limited, and you may only be able to bring a few of your own possessions. Moving to a nursing home also means having to adjust to the loss of a certain amount of independence. It means not being able to do whatever you want to do, whenever you want to do it. You may have to adapt your usual routines to your new situation.

People who become residents of a nursing home often feel that they are at the mercy of the health care industry. While some are cheerful, compliant, and grateful, others may be depressed, angry, anxious, or unpleasant. When you must care for a resident who makes you wish you had never chosen to be a nursing assistant (and you can be certain you *will* encounter residents like this), stop and think for a moment about the reason that person may be out of sorts. When you look beyond the illness or condition, past the technical duties and procedures, and into that person's eyes, you will find your reason for choosing to be a nursing assistant . . . a *person* who needs you very much.

The Family

Admitting a family member to a nursing home is often a traumatic event for the family as well as for the person who is actually being admitted. Like the resident, the family may have a hard time adjusting to the fact that admission to a nursing home is necessary. In some instances, family members do not get along with each other, and that can lead to conflict within the family. Sometimes, family members take out their stress on the person being admitted to the nursing home, leading to abuse.

Adjusting to Changing Roles Within the Family

Within a family, each family member has familiar and expected roles. A decline in health or function for any one member of the family often disrupts expected roles and relationships for all of the family. Many adult children experience "role reversal" as their parents become more dependent. The child becomes the parent, and the parent becomes the child. We are used to our parents caring for *us*. It is physically and emotionally difficult to assume basic care for a parent. Caregiving responsibilities take a lot of time, and sometimes even financial resources away from other family members. This can also create tension, conflict, and stress within the family.

Family members may look to you for direction and support. (Unfortunately, some will also look to you as a target for their stress and frustration.) Admission of a family member to a nursing home affects the whole family. As a nursing assistant, it is your responsibility to care for the resident as well as the family.

Giving Up the Role of "Primary Caregiver"

You might think that admitting a loved one to a nursing home is a relief to family members because it relieves them of their caregiving responsibilities. In reality, it is not a relief, just a change. Family members must learn to trust other people—usually people they do not know—with providing care for their loved one.

Family members often feel guilty about not being able to provide care themselves. Family members who provided care to their loved one before the person was admitted to the nursing home usually have a great deal of knowledge about how to care for the person. Adjusting to a new role (that of "visitor" instead of "primary caregiver") may be particularly difficult for these family members. When

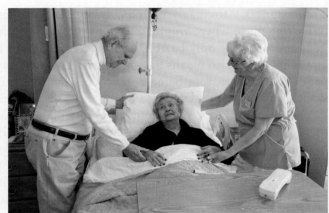

■ **FIGURE 11-2**

As a nursing assistant, you can help family members adjust by helping them to feel included and involved in the ongoing care of their loved one.

the family member tries to share knowledge about the resident's care with a staff member, the staff member may feel that the family member is interfering or lacks confidence in his or her abilities. This may create tension between the family and the staff.

Families want to see that staff members are interested in their loved one as a human being. They expect staff members to ask questions about their loved one's preferences and dislikes. They want to feel as if their input provides the staff with knowledge that is welcomed and valued. As a nursing assistant, you can help family members adjust by helping them to feel included and involved in the ongoing care of their loved one (Fig. 11-2).

Losing a Life Partner

For couples, admission of one partner to a long-term care facility can be particularly difficult both for the partner who is left behind and for the partner who is moving to the long-term care facility. No longer being able to live together can trigger a tremendous sense of loss for both partners. The need to share intimate moments with a life partner, whether sexual or not, is important throughout one's entire life. As a nursing assistant, you can help to make the transition easier by ensuring that couples have privacy during their visit.

 Putting it all together!

- Adjusting to admission to a nursing home is difficult both for the person being admitted and for his or her family members. It involves coping with many changes, accepting losses, and adapting to new roles and relationships.
- Family members must adjust to the changed health status of their loved one and adapt to the new surroundings.
- Family roles and relationships change when a loved one moves to a long-term care facility.
- Families need to be welcomed and included to the best extent possible.
- Provision of privacy for family visits is essential, especially for couples.

Living With a Chronic Condition

What will you learn?

When you are finished with this section, you will be able to:

1. Explain how chronic conditions can affect a person.

As you have just learned, most residents have one or more chronic conditions. A chronic condition affects our self-image (how we see or feel about ourselves). Many people with chronic conditions find it difficult to accept that their bodies no longer function as they should.

A chronic condition often affects how others act toward the person with the condition. Some people become overprotective of the person. Or the person with the chronic condition may let others do everything for him, when in reality he is capable of doing many things independently. This can cause problems with relationships, as those around the person with the chronic condition become frustrated and impatient.

Medications that are used to treat chronic conditions usually have to be taken for a long period of time. The person may have to learn to live with side effects that are unpleasant. Living with chronic conditions often causes the person to have to make lifestyle changes that are not always welcome. Changes in activity, diet, or other habits may be necessary. Making changes in the way we live can be difficult even when we want to make these changes. Imagine how it must feel to be told that you *must* make these changes or risk further health problems.

It is common for those with chronic conditions to experience problems with mental health. Some see the disease as taking over their lives and become angry, frustrated, or depressed. Some will just continue to deny that they have the disease. Some chronic conditions, such as arthritis, are painful. Living with pain can disrupt a person's life. Constant pain or discomfort reduces a person's physical abilities and limits the person's ability to interact socially with others.

For a person with a chronic condition, there will be good days when the person feels well and there will be bad days when symptoms make it hard to function. This can become very tiresome for the person. The person may have to be hospitalized repeatedly for acute flare-ups. As the condition progresses, it may cause the person to experience a decline in her level of health or function.

As a nursing assistant, it is important to understand the roller-coaster ride of living with a chronic condition. Most of your residents will have co-existent medical conditions, not just one condition. You cannot expect your residents to perform at the same level every day. You must adapt to their good days and bad days by being flexible with your approach and the amount of assistance that you provide. Learning about each resident's conditions will help you to understand each resident's struggles and limitations. Your encouragement and support can help your residents maintain their sense of independence and dignity.

Putting it all together!

- Most residents of nursing homes are living with one or more chronic health conditions. Chronic conditions become part of who we are and can significantly affect our day-to-day life.

■ When caring for people with chronic conditions, nursing assistants must adapt care approaches as necessary to accommodate the person's "good days" and "bad days."

The Young Resident

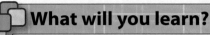

What will you learn?

When you are finished with this section, you will be able to:

1. List reasons why a younger person might become a resident of a long-term care facility.
2. Explain some of the special considerations that must be taken into account with younger residents.

Although most people living in nursing homes are 65 years of age or older, younger people receive care in nursing homes as well. You may care for residents who are in their 20s. Children and adolescents who are severely disabled may also require long-term care, but usually they are cared for in long-term care facilities that specialize in the care of children and adolescents, rather than in regular nursing homes. Traumatic injuries (such as severe brain and spinal cord injuries), degenerative neurological conditions (such as multiple sclerosis), and developmental disabilities (such as cerebral palsy or Down syndrome) are some reasons why a younger person might be cared for in a nursing home.

For many younger residents, the disease or injury that results in the need for nursing home care is an unexpected event. Understandably, many younger residents experience anger, frustration, and depression. It may take a younger person longer to adjust to placement in a long-term care facility. When caring for a younger resident, you will need to have empathy and patience. Be flexible, and give the person opportunities to exercise personal choice whenever possible. Having the opportunity to make decisions about everyday matters helps the resident maintain a sense of control and personal identity and is important for maintaining the resident's self-esteem.

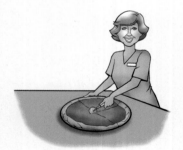

Young adults are usually busy completing their educations, starting or advancing in their careers, and possibly finding life partners and starting families. Can you imagine what it would be like to have your normal life shattered by disease or injury and to find yourself living in a facility where most of the other residents are significantly older than you are?

Because younger residents are living in an environment that is not reflective of their age group or interests, special accommodations will need to be made. The person's preferences in the types of food, music, leisure activities, and clothing choices will be different than the older residents and should be accommodated. Phone and computer access can help younger residents keep up with the outside world, and a pleasant area where younger residents can "hang out" with friends should be available (Fig. 11-3). Helping a younger resident find ways to enjoy and participate in life and interests outside of the facility greatly enhances the resident's quality of life and provides a sense of hope for the future.

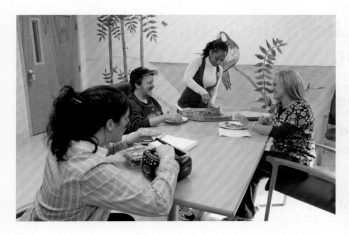

■ FIGURE 11-3

Providing opportunities for younger residents to enjoy the same things that others their age enjoy can greatly improve the younger resident's quality of life.

Being involved in life outside of the long-term care facility also includes being involved in family life. Being separated is hard on all members of the family. Family relationships can be strained by these changes. Finding ways to help the resident continue to participate in family life is very important. Providing for phone and e-mail access, ensuring that a private space is available for family visits, and encouraging the family to participate in events held at the facility are all measures you can take to help maintain connections among family members.

As you learned in Chapter 5, sexuality and intimacy are basic human needs for everyone, young and old. Younger residents face many of the same challenges older residents face in meeting these needs. For young residents who are married or in a committed relationship, admission to a nursing home disrupts the normal intimate relationship between the two partners. Other young residents may not be in such a relationship, but will still have the need to establish and maintain intimate relationships with others. In a nursing home environment, it can be especially difficult for a younger resident to find someone to develop an intimate relationship with, and privacy can be an issue. As a nursing assistant, you will need to recognize the importance of sexual expression as part of the human experience and take measures to help your younger resident meet his needs related to sexuality and intimacy.

Caring for a younger resident can pose some unique challenges for a nursing assistant. You may find it difficult to maintain professional boundaries. Younger residents often interact more with staff members than with the other older residents or even with their friends outside of the nursing home. As a result, a younger resident may interpret your professional interest and caring as a sign of personal friendship, and become interested in developing a personal, or even a sexual, relationship with you. Although it is important for you to have a friendly and warm attitude toward all of your residents, you must make sure that you keep your relationships with your residents professional at all times.

 ## Putting it all together!

- Although people aged 65 years and older make up most of the population in nursing homes, younger people may also live in long-term care facilities.
- Special accommodations need to be made to give the younger resident the opportunity to socialize with peers, engage in age-appropriate activities, and connect with the world outside of the nursing home.

Quality of Life in the Long-Term Care Setting

What will you learn?

When you are finished with this section, you will be able to:

1. Discuss the importance of promoting quality of life in the long-term care setting.
2. Explain how assisting with activities can help improve your residents' quality of life.

Quality of life has to do with getting satisfaction and comfort from the way we are living. As you recall, the Omnibus Budget Reconciliation Act (OBRA) was put in place to protect residents' quality of life. As you have learned, the changes a person experiences when faced with being admitted to a long-term care facility take away many of the things that he or she felt gave life quality. Many factors contribute to quality of life, including:

- The ability to be free from physical and emotional discomfort.
- The ability to make decisions for oneself, based on one's own personal values and sense of what is best for oneself.
- The ability to engage in activities that one finds enjoyable.

When you take a humanistic approach to health care, you help to ensure that your residents enjoy a good quality of life. Respecting residents' rights, as outlined in the *Residents' Rights* portion of OBRA, also helps to protect your residents' quality of life.

Activities

In order to enjoy a good quality of life, we must get pleasure from life. One of the ways that we get pleasure from life is by engaging in hobbies or activities that interest us. Participating in activities that we enjoy provides an outlet for our creativity, prevents boredom, reduces stress, improves sleep, and allows us to feel a sense of purpose and accomplishment. Many activities also give us the opportunity to interact with people who share similar interests, so they help us to meet our need to socialize with others.

Participating in activities benefits us physically as well as mentally. Because participation in activities has so many benefits, and is so important for maintaining quality of life, OBRA specifies that nursing homes must provide for meaningful activity for residents (Fig. 11-4). The activity program must include a variety of activities that allow residents to socialize with others and pursue personal interests.

The activity program is developed and managed by the Activities (or Therapeutic Recreation) Department. However, all staff members play an important role in making sure that each resident has the opportunity to participate in activities that provide pleasure and increase the resident's satisfaction with the quality of his or her life. As a nursing assistant, you will support the facility's activity staff by ensuring that residents are ready on time for scheduled activities and by helping to transport residents to the area where the activity is taking place.

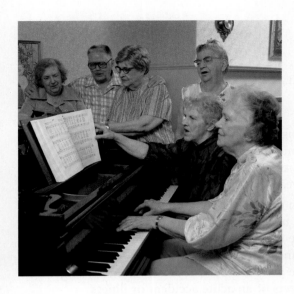

■ **FIGURE 11-4**

Activities provide entertainment and an opportunity to socialize with others.

Many residents will express the need to feel useful, rather than just sitting around watching other people work. While it is not acceptable to require a resident to perform work in a facility, it is acceptable to allow a resident to help wipe tables, water plants, and perform other simple chores on the unit, if that is what the resident wants to do. Positive activities like this often do a great deal to help boost a resident's self-esteem and sense of worth. The resident's desire to assist with chores on the unit should be documented appropriately in the resident's care plan, so that it is clear that the resident's participation in these sorts of activities is voluntary.

Putting it all together!

- We are responsible for helping our residents to maintain a good quality of life.
- Participating in enjoyable activities benefits residents physically, emotionally, and socially, and contributes to their overall quality of life.

WHAT DID YOU LEARN?

Multiple Choice

Select the best answer for each of the following questions.

1. As more people live into old age, you would expect:
   a. All of them to need long-term care
   b. An increase in long-term care use
   c. A decrease in long-term care use
   d. No change in long-term care use

2. Most residents of nursing homes fall into what age group?
   a. Younger than 65 years
   b. 65 to 74 years
   c. 75 to 84 years
   d. 85 years and older

3. Mrs. Merkle has been a resident at the Golden Harvest Nursing Center for almost 2 years. You know that this length of stay is:
   a. Typical for most nursing home residents
   b. Unusual (most people stay for 3 months or less)

   c. Longer than most stays (the average stay is 6 months to 1 year)
   d. Shorter than most stays (the average stay is 3 years or more)

4. Which of the following are reasons that someone might need long-term care?
   a. The family can no longer provide for care at home
   b. The person needs to recover from the lingering effects of an acute accident or illness
   c. The person is no longer able to care for himself
   d. All of the above

5. A younger resident may need care in a nursing home because of:
   a. A spinal cord injury from a diving accident
   b. A developmental disability
   c. Progressive multiple sclerosis
   d. All of the above

Matching

Match each numbered item with its appropriate lettered description.

_____ 1. Acute illness

_____ 2. Chronic condition

_____ 3. Degenerative condition

_____ 4. Activities of daily living (ADLs)

_____ 5. Instrumental activities of daily living (IADLs)

_____ 6. Co-existent medical conditions

_____ 7. Cognitive impairment

a. Problems processing, learning, or remembering information

b. A condition that gets progressively worse over time

c. Examples include dressing, eating, bathing, toileting, and moving

d. More than one illness at the same time in the same person

e. A condition that is ongoing

f. Examples include using the telephone and balancing a checkbook

g. An unexpected illness with a rapid onset and a relatively short recovery time

(STOP) Stop *and* Think!

■ You are working the day shift on a very busy day. One of your co-workers went home sick, so everyone had to pick up the care for additional residents. You are behind in your work, and the charge nurse has just told you that Mrs. Wilkins, a new resident, is arriving any minute and you have been assigned to Mrs. Wilkins' care. You wish the charge nurse would have told you this earlier. There is only an hour left on your shift, and you have to leave on time because you have a doctor's appointment after work. You still need to answer Mr. Jones' call light, and now you see Mrs. Wilkins arriving in a wheelchair. How are you feeling about this new admission? What mood will you be in when you enter Mrs. Wilkins' room to greet her? If you are not careful, what impression could you give Mrs. Wilkins and her family members? What impression do you want to give Mrs. Wilkins and her family members?

Caring for People With Dementia

Dementia is a terminal illness that affects a person's ability to remember and think. More than half of the residents in long-term care facilities are there because they have dementia and are no longer able to care for themselves. People who have dementia also need care in other types of health care settings. In this chapter, you will learn about some of the types of dementia and about the special care needs of people with dementia.

Photo: *Dementia robs a person of her identity and sense of self. (Courtesy of Stanley Healthcare Solutions.)*

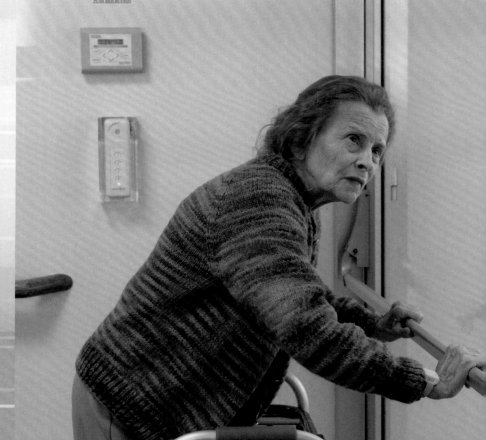

Introduction to Dementia

What will you learn?

When you are finished with this section, you will be able to:

1. Describe problems related to thinking and remembering that a person with dementia experiences.
2. Explain the difference between dementia and delirium.
3. Describe changes in a normally alert person that could signal delirium and should be reported to the nurse.
4. Define the words **dementia** and **delirium**.

A person with **dementia** experiences:

- Problems with memory, especially short-term memory
- Difficulty communicating
- Problems with judgment (the person is not able to make good decisions)
- Confusion (the person is not oriented to person, place, or time)
- An inability to manage activities of daily living (ADLs)

In the early stages of dementia, the person is usually aware that he is having trouble remembering things. He may try to cover up the memory loss. As the disease progresses, the person may have problems remembering words. He may act "out of character." The person loses the ability to recognize others and, eventually, the ability to remember his own identity. In the final stage of the disease, the person dies.

If a patient or resident who is normally alert and oriented begins to act confused, report your observations to the nurse immediately. The person may be experiencing **delirium**. Unlike dementia, delirium is temporary. Delirium is a sign of an underlying problem, such as an infection. Once the cause of the delirium is discovered and treated, the delirium goes away.

> **Dementia** the permanent and progressive loss of the ability to think and remember

> **Delirium** a temporary state of confusion

Putting it all together!

- Dementia is the permanent and progressive loss of the ability to think and remember, caused by damage to the brain tissue. There is no cure for dementia.
- Dementia should not be confused with delirium. Delirium is confusion in a person who is normally alert and oriented. Delirium goes away when the underlying cause is treated.

Tell the Nurse!

Delirium

The person is normally alert and oriented, but is now:

- Hallucinating
- Unable to recognize someone familiar
- Restless, especially at night
- Confused
- Unable to remember recent events
- Lost or wandering aimlessly

Types of Dementia

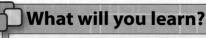

What will you learn?

When you are finished with this section, you will be able to:
1. List and describe the three stages of dementia.
2. Describe the two most common types of dementia.

There are many different types of dementia. People with all types of dementia show similar behaviors and have similar disabilities in the late stages of the disease. Two of the most common types of dementia are Alzheimer's disease and vascular dementia.

Dementia has a very gradual onset, with symptoms appearing over a period of several months or a few years. On average, a person with dementia will live 8 to 10 years after the first symptoms appear. During this time, the person will pass through three major stages (Box 12-1). Although medications are available that may help to slow the progression of the dementia, there is currently no cure for dementia.

Alzheimer's Disease

Alzheimer's disease is the most common type of dementia. Alzheimer's disease is most often seen in people older than 65 years; however, people as young as 40 years may also get the disease. Because the risk of developing Alzheimer's disease increases with age, people 85 years and older are at the highest risk for developing Alzheimer's disease.

BOX 12-1 Stages of Dementia

Early Stage

- The person begins to experience memory loss. Because the person is aware of these memory changes, she may become fearful, anxious, or depressed. The person may become angry at other people.

Middle Stage

- The person begins to have difficulty communicating. She may have difficulty using words, understanding words, or both.

- The person begins to have difficulty recognizing familiar people and things.

- The person begins to have difficulty remembering the steps that are necessary to complete familiar tasks, such as getting dressed.

- The person's personality may change, and she may begin to behave differently, often in challenging ways.

- The person begins to experience incontinence.

Late Stage

- The person loses the ability to walk and sit independently and eventually becomes bedridden.

- The person is no longer able to speak, swallow, or smile.

- The person becomes totally incontinent of urine and feces.

- The person dies.

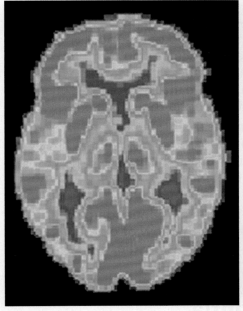

A. Healthy

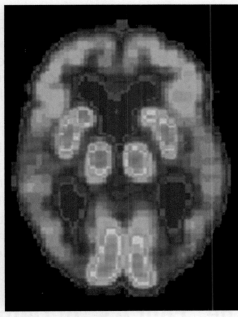

B. Alzheimer's disease

■ **FIGURE 12-1**

(A) Brain scan of a healthy person. **(B)** Brain scan of a person with Alzheimer's disease, the most common type of dementia. The blue areas indicate areas where brain activity is lost.
(Alzheimer's Disease Education Referral Center, a service of the National Institute on Aging.)

Physical changes occur in the brains of people with Alzheimer's disease. Abnormal deposits of protein, called *plaques* and *tangles,* develop in the brain. These protein deposits interfere with the way that the nerves inside the brain communicate with each other. Brain scans done on people with Alzheimer's disease show large areas in the brain where there is no activity (Fig. 12-1).

Vascular (Multi-Infarct) Dementia

Damage to the blood vessels that supply the brain can decrease the amount of oxygen and nutrients that are delivered to the brain tissue. In people with vascular (multi-infarct) dementia, mental functions are lost because multiple areas of the brain tissue die due to a lack of oxygen and nutrients.

Vascular dementia most often affects people between the ages of 55 and 75 years. It is more common in men than in women. Conditions that put a person at risk for developing vascular dementia include:

- Myocardial infarction (heart attack)
- Hypertension (high blood pressure)
- Diabetes mellitus
- Peripheral vascular disease
- Transient ischemic attacks (TIAs)
- Obesity
- Smoking
- High blood cholesterol levels

Symptoms may appear suddenly, and they may vary from person to person, depending on which areas of the brain are affected. Like Alzheimer's disease, vascular dementia is irreversible and incurable.

Putting it all together!

- There are several types of dementia. Two of the most common types are Alzheimer's disease and vascular (multi-infarct) dementia. All people with dementia show similar behaviors and have similar disabilities in the late stages of the disease, no matter what specific type of dementia they have.

- In people with Alzheimer's disease, the brain tissue is damaged by abnormal protein deposits called plaques and tangles. Alzheimer's disease progresses through a number of stages, with each progression causing the person to become more and more dependent on others for care.

- In people with vascular (multi-infarct) dementia, damage to the blood vessels in the brain blocks the flow of oxygen and nutrients, causing parts of the brain tissue to die.

The "Four A's" of Dementia

What will you learn?

When you are finished with this section, you will be able to:
1. Describe the "four A's" of dementia.
2. Define the words **amnesia**, **aphasia**, **agnosia**, and **apraxia**.

Amnesia difficulty remembering

Aphasia difficulty using language

Agnosia difficulty recognizing information obtained using the five senses

Apraxia difficulty coordinating the steps needed to complete a task

No matter what the underlying cause of dementia is, all people with dementia experience changes in the brain that lead to the "four A's" of dementia: **amnesia**, **aphasia**, **agnosia**, and **apraxia**. Understanding these "four A's" will allow you to provide better care for your residents with dementia because you will be better able to understand what they are experiencing, thinking, and feeling.

Amnesia

Amnesia is memory loss. During the early stage of dementia, memory loss generally only affects short-term (recent) memory, and long-term memory remains intact. As dementia progresses, the person's long-term memory will begin to be affected as well. The person can lose years of memory, causing her to forget about entire periods of her life. Because this person is literally living in the past, she will not be able to understand references to her current situation.

Because of amnesia, people with dementia have a limited ability to think through the changes in their routine and to remember what they are supposed to be doing. As a result, a change in the normal routine causes a person with dementia a great deal of stress.

Aphasia

Aphasia is difficulty in communicating. During the middle stage of dementia, the person begins to experience aphasia. The person may have:

- *Expressive aphasia* (difficulty using words): a person with expressive aphasia may have difficulty finding the right word and use the wrong word for objects or people. The person may also group words together that do not make sense.
- *Receptive aphasia* (difficulty understanding words): a person with receptive aphasia may not respond appropriately to your questions or directions.

Some people with dementia experience both expressive and receptive aphasia. The inability to make oneself understood or to understand others can be a great source of stress and frustration for the person.

Agnosia

Agnosia is difficulty in recognizing information received through the eyes, ears, nose, taste buds, or sense of touch. The person may have difficulty recognizing objects or difficulty recognizing people she knows. In addition to not recognizing others, a person who has agnosia may not even recognize herself in a mirror.

Apraxia

Apraxia is difficulty coordinating the steps needed to complete a task. Simple, everyday activities become very difficult for a person with dementia. The person may have difficulty getting dressed because he might put clothes on in the wrong order. Or, he cannot remember how to use the knife and fork at mealtime. The frustration the person experiences because of the inability to perform these tasks can cause a behavioral outburst.

Putting it all together!

- All people with dementia experience changes in the brain that lead to the "four A's" of dementia: amnesia (difficulty remembering), aphasia (difficulty using language), agnosia (difficulty recognizing information obtained using the five senses), and apraxia (difficulty coordinating the steps needed to complete a task).

Behaviors Associated With Dementia

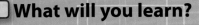

What will you learn?

When you are finished with this section, you will be able to:

1. Describe behaviors that are common in people with dementia.
2. Describe strategies for managing difficult behaviors in people with dementia.
3. Define the word **validation therapy**.

People with dementia often show a wide range of behaviors, especially as the dementia progresses. Some of these behaviors can be dangerous for the person, such as the tendency to wander. Others are not dangerous, but they can be very annoying to caregivers or other residents. Many of these behaviors occur because

BOX 12-2 **Situations That Can Cause Dementia-Related Behaviors**

- The person is in a room that is too large or too small.
- The person is in a room that is overstimulating (cluttered, noisy, or decorated with fabrics and wallpapers with "busy" patterns).
- The person is in a place that is new or unfamiliar (for example, the person is hospitalized for treatment of an acute problem).
- The person is being asked to do something that is too complicated, has too many steps, or is unfamiliar.
- The person is trying to express a physical or emotional need.

of changes in the brain caused by the disease. People with dementia lose their ability to communicate effectively as the dementia progresses. The only way they can express themselves is through their behavior. A change in a person's "normal" behavior is a cause for concern and should be reported to the nurse. The person may have a medical problem or be in pain.

To understand why a behavior is happening, use your observation skills to answer the following questions:

- **What** is the behavior? Describe the behavior in as much detail as possible.
- **Who** is the behavior associated with? For example, does the person act this way only in the presence of certain people?
- **When** does the behavior occur?
- **Where** does the behavior occur?

Box 12-2 lists common situations that can trigger dementia-related behaviors. Simple solutions such as offering the person a snack, taking the person to the bathroom, or finding a quieter place for a person to sit may be enough to stop the behavior. Table 12-1 lists common types of behaviors that a person with dementia may have and also gives suggestions of actions you can take to help manage them.

TABLE 12-1 **Behaviors Associated With Dementia**

Behavior	Common Causes	Ways to Manage the Behavior
Wandering: The person moves about without a specific destination in mind.	■ Inability to recognize surroundings	■ Provide distracting activities (for example, ask the person to sit down and look at a photo album with you). ■ Allow the person to wander in a safe area (such as an enclosed outside courtyard or a secure area inside the facility). ■ If a wanderer monitoring system or pressure-sensitive alarm system (see Chapter 15) is being used with the person, ensure that the sensor is in place on the person's bed, wheelchair, or body.
Pacing: The person moves back and forth within a confined area.	■ Unmet physical needs ■ A noisy, stimulating environment ■ Feeling scared or lost	■ Make sure the person's physical needs are met (for example, offer food or a trip to the bathroom). ■ Make sure that the person's emotional needs are met (for example, take the person to a quieter area). ■ If the pacing cannot be stopped, allow the person to pace in a safe area.

Behavior	Common Causes	Ways to Manage the Behavior
Repetition (perseveration): The person does the same thing over and over again (for example, repeats a word or phrase; folds and unfolds a napkin).	■ Boredom ■ Decreased ability to communicate	■ Provide distracting activities.
Rummaging: The person goes through drawers, closets, or boxes looking for an item he is never able to find.	■ Short-term memory loss	■ Ask the person what he is looking for and offer to help find it. ■ Provide distracting activities. ■ Give the person a special drawer or box filled with small personal items that he can rummage through.
Delusions: The person may think she is someone else, such as the Queen of England.	■ Changes in the brain as a result of the disease	■ Use validation therapy. ■ Provide distracting activities.
Hallucinations: The person sees, hears, tastes, or smells something that is not really there, such as a cat in the room or bugs on the bed.	■ Changes in the brain as a result of the disease	■ Use validation therapy (for example, ask the cat to leave; sweep the bugs off the bed). ■ Provide distracting activities.
Agitation: The person becomes very upset and excited and may shout or strike out at caregivers or other residents.	■ Pain or infection ■ Unmet physical needs ■ Feeling threatened or overwhelmed	■ Make sure that the person's physical needs are met (for example, offer food or a trip to the bathroom). ■ Provide a quiet, calm environment.
Catastrophic reactions: The person over-reacts to something that would cause a healthy person minimal or no stress; the person becomes very agitated and may begin to scream.	■ Feeling threatened or overwhelmed ■ Fatigue	■ Provide simple explanations of what you are doing or what you would like the person to do. ■ Provide a quiet, calm environment. ■ Calm the person by using gentle touch, playing soothing music, or singing to the person.
Sundowning: The person's behaviors worsen in the late afternoon and evening.	■ Fatigue ■ Decreased vision	■ Provide periods of rest and quiet during the day to reduce fatigue. ■ Turn on the lights earlier in the evening. ■ If the person wears vision aids, make sure that they are in place.
Inappropriate sexual behavior: The person attempts sexual relations with staff or other residents or masturbates or undresses in public.	■ Inability to recognize other people ■ Changes in the brain as a result of the disease	■ Provide distracting activities. ■ Protect people who are unable to give consent to, or protect themselves from, unwelcome sexual advances.

TABLE 12-2 Validation Therapy

Example	Response That Reflects the Nursing Assistant's Reality	Response That Reflects the Patient's or Resident's Reality (Validation Therapy)
Mrs. Rivera is trying to leave the facility. She is very agitated. She keeps repeating that she needs to go home to take care of her mother.	Nursing assistant: "Don't you remember? Your mother died 20 years ago. You are staying here with us." ↓ *Mrs. Rivera's agitation increases. She may continue to insist on going home, or begin to grieve her mother's death.*	Nursing assistant: "You want to go home to see your mother. Aren't mothers wonderful? Here, sit down and tell me about your mother." ↓ *Mrs. Rivera is diverted from wanting to go home. She happily sits down with the nursing assistant to discuss mothers.*
Dr. Carroll, a retired family doctor, believes that he needs to leave the facility and go to the hospital to deliver babies and make rounds on his patients.	Nursing assistant: "I'm sorry. Don't you remember that you are retired? You live here in the nursing home with us now. We can't let you leave because you might get lost or hurt." ↓ *Dr. Carroll becomes agitated because what the nursing assistant is saying does not match his current reality.*	Nursing assistant (leading Dr. Carroll to the nurse's station): "I bet we can find you a nurse who would love to have you make rounds with her and see the patients here." ↓ *Dr. Carroll is diverted while still thinking that he has some value as a doctor.*

Validation therapy a technique used for interacting with people who have dementia, in which the caregiver acknowledges the person's reality; rather than correcting the person, the caregiver attempts to distract the person and redirect the conversation whenever possible

Validation therapy is a technique you can use to respond to some behaviors. To "validate" something means to confirm it. This technique is especially useful when the person has long-term memory loss. When you use validation therapy, you acknowledge the person's reality instead of trying to get the person to accept your reality. Instead of correcting the person, you respond to what the person is telling you while gently redirecting the conversation (Table 12-2).

Putting it all together!

- A person with dementia often shows a wide range of behaviors, especially as the dementia progresses. These behaviors occur as a result of changes in the brain resulting from the disease.

- As the dementia progresses, the person loses the ability to communicate through normal channels. A change in behavior or an increase in a certain type of behavior could mean that the person is trying to communicate with you about an unmet physical or emotional need. Report a change in the person's "normal" behavior to the nurse immediately.

- Validation therapy is a way of responding to the person with dementia. When you use validation therapy, you try to understand what is "real" for the person with dementia and respond accordingly. You do not try to correct the person or make the person understand your reality.

Caring for a Person With Dementia

What will you learn?

When you are finished with this section, you will be able to:

1. Describe special considerations you should keep in mind while helping a person with dementia with activities of daily living (ADLs).
2. Describe special care measures that are taken to help maintain quality of life for a person with dementia.
3. Define the word **reminiscence therapy**.

General guidelines for caring for a person with dementia are given in Guidelines Box 12-1.

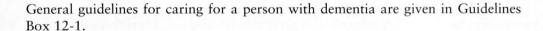

GUIDELINES BOX 12-1   Guidelines for Caring for a Person With Dementia

What you do	Why you do it
Maintain a calm, structured environment.	*A person with dementia can become overwhelmed very easily. When the person becomes overwhelmed, difficult behaviors are likely to increase.*
Approach the person with dementia slowly, announcing yourself before touching her.	*Many people with dementia also have hearing problems, vision problems, or both. If you approach quickly without warning, you may startle the person, triggering a catastrophic reaction.*
Avoid arguing or disagreeing with the person.	*A person with dementia exists in a different reality from the rest of the world. Trying to force the person with dementia to understand or acknowledge anything other than her own reality will increase the person's agitation.*
When asking a person with dementia to do something, use short words and short sentences. Avoid negatively worded instructions (such as, "Don't put that there!"). Avoid instructions that require the person to remember more than one action at a time.	*Because a person with dementia has problems with short-term memory, he will not be able to remember or understand long words and sentences. A positively worded command ("Please put that here") is easier to understand than a negative one. Failing at a task increases the person's frustration. When you give the person instructions in a way that he can understand, you increase the person's chances of successfully completing the task.*

(*box continues on page 256*)

GUIDELINES BOX 12-1   Guidelines for Caring for a Person With Dementia (continued)

What you do	Why you do it
Give a person with dementia enough time to respond to questions and directions.	*It may take the person a while to think of the word or words she needs to answer your question or the actions she must take to follow your directions. Feeling rushed can cause the person to become agitated.*
"Listen" to the person by paying attention to body language. Make good use of your observation skills.	*As a person's dementia gets worse, he loses the ability to communicate effectively. Often, body language and behaviors become the person's main way of expressing himself.*
When managing difficult behaviors, be aware that solutions that work today may not work tomorrow. Be creative, and do not give up.	*Dementia is a progressive disease. Therefore, the person's abilities, disabilities, and needs change over time, and your approaches to managing difficult behaviors may also need to change.*
Help the person with dementia to feel secure and loved by showing affection (kind words, a gentle touch) and smiling.	*Like all people, people with dementia have emotional needs that must be met.*
Allow the person with dementia to do as much as he can for himself for as long as possible.	*This is important for maintaining the person's dignity and self-esteem. No one likes to feel helpless or useless.*
Use visual cues to orient the person to place and time. For example, place a large-faced clock in the person's room, decorate for the holidays, and post names and other reminder signs in prominent places. (For example, if a person keeps trying to walk out the front door, apply a big red and white "stop" sign to the inside of the door.)	*Using visual cues can help the person to maintain independence longer, which is important for the person's self-esteem.*
Help the person to exercise her mind by getting the person involved in activities that relate to the person's former interests and experiences.	*Participating in activities helps to prevent boredom and increases the person's sense of purpose and accomplishment.*
Protect the person from physical injury.	*People with dementia often become clumsy as a result of their disease, which increases their risk of falling. In addition, they lose the ability to make good decisions related to their well-being. For example, a person with dementia might walk in front of an oncoming car, leave the house without a coat in the middle of a snowstorm, or drink the contents of a bottle found under the sink.*

What you do (continued)	**Why you do it** (continued)
Maintain the person's hygiene and good grooming habits.	*This is important for the person's health as well as for self-esteem.*
Be as tolerant as possible of the person.	*The person's behaviors are a result of her dementia, and are beyond the person's control. The person is not purposely trying to frustrate or annoy you.*
When you become tired and frustrated, take time out, be good to yourself, and share your feelings with the nurse. Know that these emotions and thoughts are normal.	*Caring for a person with dementia is emotionally draining and physically difficult. If you do not take measures to protect your own mental health, you run the risk of "burn-out." In addition, you place the resident at risk for abuse should you lose your temper.*

Meeting the Physical Needs of a Person With Dementia

For a person with dementia, everyday activities such as bathing, dressing, eating, and using the bathroom can be challenging. The person cannot remember how to do these things and, as a result, may become very frustrated. Sometimes the person will resist doing what you need him to do.

When you are helping a person with dementia with his ADLs, there are several general things you can do to make the task go more smoothly:

- **Speak clearly, in a calm tone of voice.**
- **Gently rest one of your hands on the person's arm or hand.** Many people with dementia respond positively to touch.
- **Remind the person at each step what she needs to do next.** The person may be able to complete tasks independently if you provide the appropriate guidance. Allowing a person to complete tasks independently for as long as possible is important for the person's self-esteem.
- **Use hand gestures in addition to spoken instructions.** For example, if you are trying to get the person to sit down at the table and eat, pat the seat of the chair as you ask the person to come sit down.
- **Plan for the procedure in advance.** Many routine procedures are very stressful for a person with dementia. Being prepared and having everything you need before you begin a procedure will allow you to accomplish the task as quickly as possible, which can help to reduce the amount of stress the person feels.
- **Keep to a regular schedule.** A person with dementia responds best to a very structured environment. To a person with dementia, the world is very confusing. Structuring the person's world as much as possible by following an established routine can reduce the person's confusion and fear.

Assisting With Bathing

Bath time can be a frightening time for a person with dementia. The person may not remember what a bath or shower is or why he needs to take one. The sound

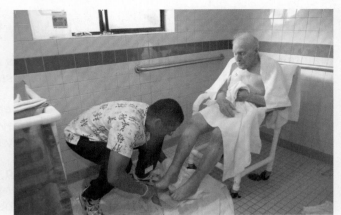

■ FIGURE 12-2

Bath time can be very frightening for a person with dementia. Making every effort to maintain the person's modesty is important.

of running water, the bright lights, and the shiny surfaces in the tub room can be upsetting. Being naked makes the person feel exposed and vulnerable. The person may be afraid of falling.

As a result, the person may become agitated when you tell him that it is "time to take a bath." If this is the case, try to avoid the word "bath." Instead, say "Let's go freshen up" or "It's time for an activity you will enjoy." If the person seems very agitated, try singing to the person or playing soothing music. Singing and music can have a calming effect on people with dementia.

Make sure that the tub room is warm, and fill the tub ahead of time so that the person does not become frightened by the sound of the running water. Put a folded towel on the shower chair for comfort. Allow the person to wear his robe as long as possible and consider draping a bath blanket or towel over the person's shoulders while he is bathing (Fig. 12-2). The bath blanket or towel will make the person feel less exposed, and it will provide some warmth. Hand the person a washcloth and let the person assist as much as possible.

Assisting With Dressing

Many people with dementia have trouble choosing an outfit to wear. They often want to wear the same clothes every day. Limiting the number of outfits the person has to choose from and asking family members to purchase several identical outfits for the person can help to solve these problems.

For a person with dementia, putting on and fastening clothing can also be difficult. To help make dressing less frustrating for the person, choose articles of clothing that are simple rather than complex. For example, a shirt that pulls over the head is easier to manage than a shirt that buttons up the front. Pants with elastic waistbands are easier to manage than pants with zippers and buttons.

Assisting With Eating

It may be difficult to get a person with dementia to focus on eating at meal times. The person may forget why she is at the table or become distracted by others at the table. A quiet setting and limited food choices can help.

The person may not recognize eating utensils or may forget how to use them. You may have to remind the person how to eat by placing your hand over the person's hand. Together, you bring the fork or spoon with the bite of food to the person's mouth (Fig. 12-3). Some people with dementia find "finger foods," such

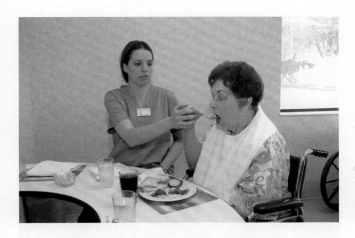

■ **FIGURE 12-3**

You may have to remind a person with dementia how to eat.

as sandwiches, cut-up vegetables or fruit, or a stuffed baked potato, easier to manage.

Make sure that the person is swallowing the food after chewing it. A person with dementia has the tendency to chew the food and then pack it into her cheek instead of swallowing it. This increases the person's risk for choking.

People in the advanced stages of dementia lose the ability to eat independently. You may be trained in special feeding techniques to use with these patients or residents. As always, be especially observant for signs of choking.

Assisting With Fluid Intake

People with dementia lose the ability to relate the sensation of being thirsty to the action of getting a drink. As a result, they are at risk for becoming dehydrated. Offer the person water and other favorite beverages frequently (unless the person has a medical condition that requires fluid restriction). A plastic cup with a lid and a straw or a spout may be easier for the person to manage.

Assisting With Elimination

A person with dementia may forget where the bathroom is or fail to recognize the toilet. Sometimes, the person will have an accident because she is unable to move her clothing out of the way fast enough. Taking the person to the bathroom on a regular schedule (for example, every 2 hours) can help. So can helping the person to select clothing with fasteners that are easy to manage. If a person suddenly seems to be having a lot of accidents, report this to the nurse. The person may have a medical problem, such as a urinary tract infection, that needs to be addressed.

Eventually, the person will become totally incontinent of urine and feces. As with all incontinent patients or residents, it is important to provide good skin care to prevent skin breakdown.

Meeting the Emotional Needs of a Person With Dementia

Helping a person with dementia to meet his emotional needs is just as important as helping the person to meet his physical needs. Just like everyone else, a person with dementia needs to feel loved and needed.

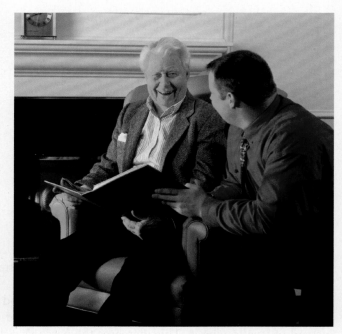

■ **FIGURE 12-4**

Reminiscence therapy increases a person's self-esteem and happiness by encouraging him to remember the past.
(Courtesy of Copper Ridge.)

Reminiscence Therapy

Reminiscence therapy
a technique used for interacting with people who have dementia, in which the person with dementia is encouraged to remember and share experiences from his or her past with others

Reminiscence therapy encourages the person to talk about the past. Talking about the past diverts the person's attention and increases his self-esteem. Reminiscence therapy can be used in a "one-on-one" setting or in a group setting (Fig. 12-4).

Activity Therapy

Participating in activities helps a person with dementia to feel useful and gives her a sense of purpose and accomplishment. Activities may be planned for a group of residents or just for one resident (Fig. 12-5). There are many different types of activities that a person with dementia can enjoy:

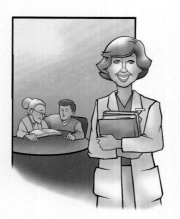

For family members, having a loved one with dementia can be particularly hard. Because dementia lasts for many years, dementia is sometimes referred to as "the long good-bye." Throughout the course of the person's illness, family members will constantly have to deal with loss, as the person they knew and loved slowly slips away. Imagine how hard it would be if someone you loved no longer remembered or recognized you.

- Creative activities (flower arranging, painting, baking)
- Intellectual activities (looking at a book of photographs, reading the newspaper aloud together, attending a play)
- Social activities (hosting a tea party, going on a picnic)
- Physical activities (taking a walk, participating in a group exercise class)

When planning an activity, take care to choose one that relates to the former interests and abilities of the person or people who will be participating in it.

Other Therapies

Music therapy and pet therapy are other therapies that are commonly used to help meet the emotional needs of people with dementia.

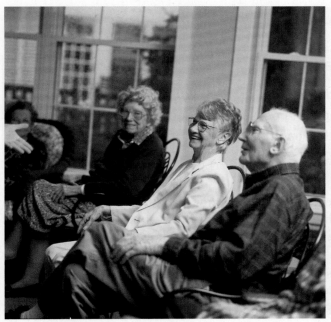

Activity therapy

■ **FIGURE 12-5**

Activities can be planned for an individual or for a group of residents.
(Courtesy of Copper Ridge.)

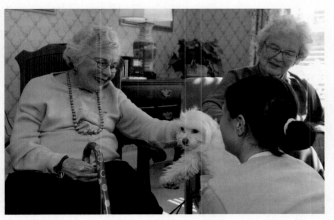

Pet therapy

■ **FIGURE 12-6**

Pet therapy can improve the quality of life for many residents with dementia.

- **Music therapy.** Music can have a calming effect on people with dementia. Often, activities are planned that involve music.
- **Pet therapy.** Spending time with animals can have many benefits for people with dementia (Fig. 12-6). Volunteers may bring animals to the facility to visit. Or, the facility may have a pet cat, dog, or bird that lives on the unit. A person with dementia may get pleasure simply by watching the animal or by holding the animal and stroking its fur. Pet therapy can also prompt the person to remember and talk about a pet he had in the past.

 Putting it all together!

- People with dementia need help to accomplish their ADLs. Preparing for procedures in advance, providing clear step-by-step instructions in a calm voice, using hand gestures and gentle touch as necessary, and keeping to a regular schedule are actions you can take to help ensure that procedures go smoothly.
- Reminiscence therapy, activity therapy, music therapy, and pet therapy are used to help meet the emotional needs of the person with dementia. These therapies promote self-esteem and help to prevent boredom.

Effects on the Caregiver

What will you learn?

When you are finished with this section, you will be able to:

1. Describe how caring for a person with dementia can affect you.
2. Discuss strategies that can help you to cope.

Caring for people with dementia is very important work. The difference you make in the life of the person with dementia, as well as those of her family members, is significant. However, caring for a person with dementia can take its toll on you, physically and emotionally.

- A person with dementia is prone to outbursts of anger and can become agitated very easily. You may be cursed at, spit on, slapped, hit, scratched, or pinched.
- Many of the behaviors of people with dementia can be very annoying because they are repetitious.
- Caring for a person is hard physical work. Exhaustion and fatigue can put you on edge, making it difficult for you to keep your emotions in check.

Try to remember that a person with dementia cannot be held responsible for her actions. If you still feel angry, make sure that the person is safe and walk away. Ask a co-worker or the nurse for help with the person. Sometimes you may need to ask to be assigned to another resident for a while. If your frustration or anger moves you to the point of actually causing a resident physical harm, you could lose your job.

Putting it all together!

- Caring for a person with dementia can be difficult both physically and emotionally.
- To provide the best care to your patients or residents, you need to care for yourself.

WHAT DID YOU LEARN?

Multiple Choice

Select the single best answer for each of the following questions.

1. Which one of the following is experienced by a person with dementia?
   a. Problems with memory, especially short-term memory
   b. Confusion and disorientation
   c. An inability to manage activities of daily living (ADLs)
   d. All of the above

2. When caring for a person with dementia, it is helpful to:
   a. Be understanding and see the person's behaviors as part of the disease
   b. Take the same approach with every resident
   c. Correct the person to bring him back to the "here and now"
   d. Avoid acknowledging your own feelings

3. When communicating with a person with dementia, what is the best approach to take?
   a. Speak loudly and quickly to get the person's attention
   b. Speak clearly, in a calm tone of voice
   c. Avoid touching the person or using hand gestures
   d. Avoid talking about the past

4. Which statement about validation therapy is true?
   a. Validation therapy stresses the importance of bringing the person with dementia back to the "here and now."
   b. Validation therapy is based on the belief that people with dementia are able to return to the present if given enough information to do so.
   c. Validation therapy stresses the importance of acknowledging the person's reality.
   d. Validation therapy encourages the caregiver to correct the person to help the person to stay on track.

5. A person with dementia may show which one of the following behaviors?
   a. Pacing and wandering
   b. Hallucinations
   c. Agitation
   d. All of the above

6. What is sundowning?
   a. Increased confusion, restlessness, and insecurity that occur late in the day, as it becomes darker outside
   b. Aimless wandering after dark
   c. Worry and increased suspicion
   d. Crying inconsolably for a long time

7. When you come on duty at 3:00 PM, Mr. Antonio asks you what time dinner will be served. You tell him that dinner is served at 5:30 PM and show him where "5:30" is on the clock. When you return to his room at 3:30 PM, he asks you again what time dinner will be served. You give him the same response as you did before. He leaves the room, and heads toward the dining room. You hear him ask another staff member what time dinner will be served. You understand this behavior is most likely a symptom of:
   a. Aphasia
   b. Amnesia
   c. Apraxia
   d. Agnosia

8. What is a catastrophic reaction?
   a. A response to a situation that is more extreme than would normally be expected
   b. An abnormal protein deposit that is found in the brains of people with Alzheimer's disease
   c. The belief that you are someone you are not (for example, the President of the United States)
   d. The reaction family members have on learning that a loved one has Alzheimer's disease

9. When helping a person with dementia with her activities of daily living (ADLs), such as bathing, eating, and dressing, what should you remember?
   a. Keep to an established routine as much as possible
   b. Prepare for the procedure ahead of time
   c. Many ADLs are very frightening or frustrating for the person with dementia
   d. All of the above

🛑 Stop *and* Think!

You work in the dementia unit of a long-term care facility. Mrs. Darden, one of the residents you are responsible for, needs a great deal of help with all of her activities of daily living (ADLs). Lately, Mrs. Darden has started having a catastrophic reaction every time you help her bathe. What are some things you could do to make bathing easier and less frightening for Mrs. Darden?

🛑 Stop *and* Think!

You work in a long-term care facility. One day, you go to the room of one of your residents, Mrs. Craven, to answer her call light. When you enter the room, Mrs. Craven cries out to you in a frightened voice, "Get them out of here! Get them out of here now!" You don't know what she is talking about—you don't see anybody or anything in the room. You ask Mrs. Craven to explain what she means, and she tells you that there are spiders crawling all over the walls. Normally, Mrs. Craven is alert and oriented, but today, she definitely seems "out of it." What do you think is wrong with Mrs. Craven? What should you do?

🛑 Stop *and* Think!

Mrs. Rowan has Alzheimer's disease. You have cared for Mrs. Rowan for a long time and know pretty much what to expect from her in terms of behavior. Although she does tend to pace and to rummage quite frequently, she is usually calm and pleasant. Today in the dining room, however, when you are trying to help Mrs. Rowan eat lunch, she becomes angry and strikes out at you. What might be the explanation for this behavior?

Safety

As a nursing assistant, one of your most important responsibilities is to keep your patients or residents safe. Keeping yourself safe while you are at work is important too. Maintaining safety is the focus of Unit 4.

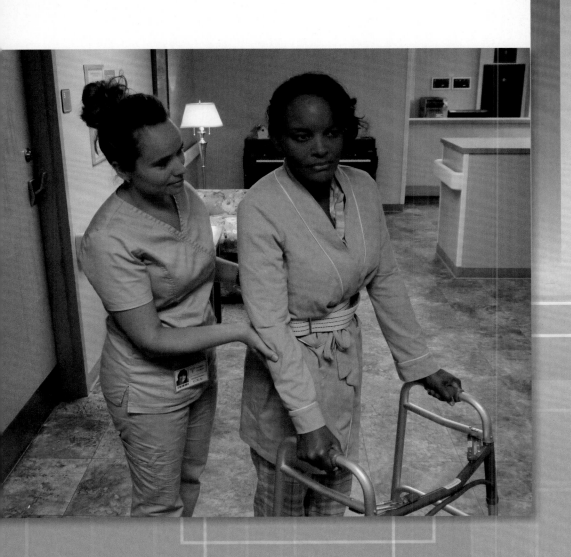

Infection Control

An infection is an illness caused by germs. Many (but not all) infections are *communicable*, which means that they can be spread from one person to another. There are many factors that come together in the health care setting to make it easy for infections to spread. In this chapter, you will learn how to minimize these factors so that you can protect your patients or residents, yourself, and your family members from getting a communicable infection.

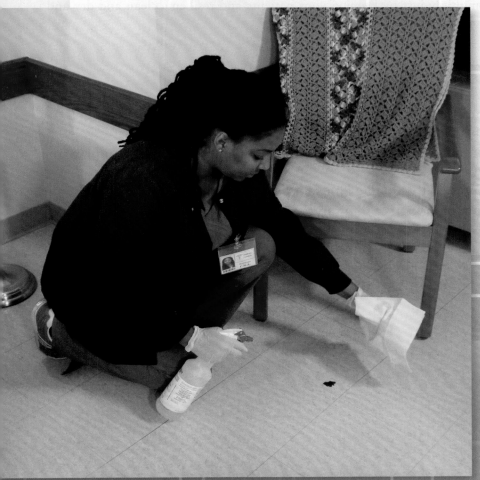

Photo: *A nursing assistant wears personal protective equipment (PPE) to protect herself from infection while cleaning up a spill.*

Causes of Infection

What will you learn?

When you are finished with this section, you will be able to:

1. Briefly describe the different types of germs that can cause disease.
2. Discuss the conditions that promote the growth of germs.
3. Define the words **microbe** and **pathogen**.

Microbe a living thing that cannot be seen with the naked eye; examples include bacteria and viruses

Pathogen a microbe that can cause illness

There are many different types of **microbes**. Microbes can be classified as bacteria, viruses, fungi, or parasites (Table 13-1). Some microbes are harmless or even helpful. But others can cause disease. A microbe that can cause disease is called a "germ" or a **pathogen**.

Pathogens, like any other type of living thing, require certain conditions to grow and multiply. Most pathogens prefer an environment that is warm, moist, and dark. Some pathogens need oxygen to live, while others do not. When you are caring for people in a health care setting, you can make it harder for pathogens to grow and multiply just by keeping your patients and residents clean and dry and their environment clean, dry, and well lighted.

Putting it all together!

- Communicable infections are infections that can be spread from one person to another.
- Microbes are generally classified as bacteria, viruses, fungi, or parasites.
- Microbes that cause illness are called pathogens.
- Most pathogens prefer an environment that is warm, moist, dark, and with proper amounts of oxygen.

TABLE 13-1 Types of Microbes

	Type	Examples of Commonly Caused Infections
	Bacteria	Strep throat, urinary tract infections, abscesses, tuberculosis (TB), bacterial meningitis, Lyme disease, Rocky Mountain spotted fever, syphilis
	Viruses	HIV/AIDS, hepatitis, fever blisters, common cold
	Fungi	Ringworm, athlete's foot, vaginal yeast infections (candidiasis), oral yeast infections (thrush)
	Parasites Insects	Scabies, pediculosis (lice)
	Helminths (worms)	Pinworm infestation
	Protozoa	Malaria, amebic dysentery (traveler's diarrhea)

Defenses Against Infection

What will you learn?

When you are finished with this section, you will be able to:
1. Explain the defense mechanisms the body uses to fight infection.
2. Define the word **antibodies**.

The Immune System

Some of the body's defenses against pathogens are *nonspecific*, which means that they help to protect us from all infections. Other defenses are *specific*, which means that they help to protect us only from certain infections.

Nonspecific Defense Mechanisms

Our first line of defense against infection includes healthy skin and mucous membranes:

- Skin that is without cuts, scrapes, or wounds physically prevents pathogens from entering the body. Keeping the skin clean and dry helps to reduce the number of pathogens on the skin, also reducing the risk of infection.

- Mucous membranes line all of the organ systems that open to the outside of the body (the respiratory system, the digestive system, the urinary system, and the reproductive system). The sticky mucus they secrete traps and destroys pathogens. Practicing good oral hygiene and drinking plenty of fluids help to keep mucous membranes functioning properly.

If a pathogen manages to get past these first lines of defense and an infection results, the body activates a general immune response that helps to fight off the infection:

- Blood vessels around the site of the infection dilate (widen), allowing more blood flow to the area. The increased blood flow causes the area to become red, hot, swollen, and painful. But the increased blood flow also brings more oxygen and nutrients to the tissues, along with large numbers of white blood cells (leukocytes). White blood cells destroy pathogens that invade the body either by eating them (Fig. 13-1) or by secreting substances that cause them to die.

- The person may also develop a fever (high body temperature). The fever causes the pathogen's environment to become too hot, and the pathogen dies. Fever is a normal response in many infections.

As a nursing assistant, it is important for you to watch for signs of infection in your patients or residents. Some infections, if not treated at an early stage, can be very dangerous.

Specific Defense Mechanisms

Our bodies produce **antibodies** following exposure to certain pathogens. This exposure may come from a previous infection with the pathogen or through a vaccination (shot). For example, the antibodies that build up in the body following an episode of chickenpox are the reason most of us only get this "childhood disease" once. Similarly, when you get your annual "flu shot," what you are getting

---

Tell the Nurse!

Signs of infection

- Fever (elderly people may only have a slight increase in body temperature, or even no increase at all)
- A rapid pulse, a rapid respiratory rate, or changes in blood pressure
- Pain or difficulty breathing
- Redness, swelling, or pain
- Foul-smelling or cloudy urine
- Pain or difficulty urinating
- Diarrhea or foul-smelling feces
- Nausea or vomiting
- Lack of appetite
- Skin rashes
- Fatigue
- Increased confusion or disorientation
- Any unusual discharge or drainage from the body

Antibodies specialized proteins produced by the immune system that help our bodies to fight off specific pathogens, preventing infection

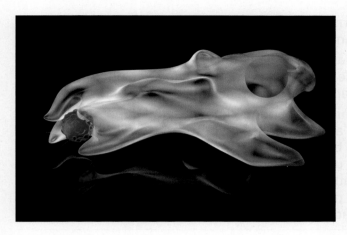

■ **FIGURE 13-1**

In this photograph, a white blood cell (*white*) is killing a pathogen (*red*) by eating it. This is a process called phagocytosis (*phago-* means "eat" and *cyt-* means "cell").

is a dose of the virus strains that cause the flu. The viruses have been killed, so that you do not actually get sick, but the exposure is enough to cause your immune system to begin producing antibodies against those particular strains of the virus. That way, if you are exposed later, you will not get sick.

Medications

Many medications are available to help us fight infections:

- *Antibiotics* are used to treat bacterial infections.
- *Antimicrobial agents* are used to treat fungal and parasitic infections.
- *Antiviral agents* are used to treat viral infections.

Although these medications help us to treat many infections, not all infections can be treated with medications. In some cases, no medication has been found that is effective against the pathogen. In other cases, a medication that used to work against the pathogen no longer works. These bacteria, known as "multidrug-resistant organisms (MDROs)," are resistant to one or more types of antibiotics that could have been effectively used against them in the past. Two particular MDROs, methicillin-resistant *Staphylococcus aureus* (MRSA) and vancomycin-resistant enterococcus (VRE), are easily spread from person to person in a health care setting, usually via the hands of health care workers. Bacteria that have become resistant to antibiotics can cause serious problems for people in health care settings.

Sometimes, the powerful antibiotics that are used to treat infections destroy other bacteria that help keep us healthy. When this happens, other bacteria that are not destroyed will grow rapidly. One such bacterium, *Clostridium difficile* (commonly called *C. diff*) is a major cause of health care-associated diarrhea. *C. diff* is easily spread from person to person in a health care setting and has been responsible for large outbreaks that can be fatal for patients or residents already weakened by illness or advanced age.

Putting it all together!

- The immune system's nonspecific defense mechanisms against pathogens include the physical barriers provided by the skin and mucous membranes and the general immune response. Many of the signs and symptoms of infection, such as a redness, warmth, pain, swelling, and fever, are the result of the general immune response.

- The immune system's specific defense mechanisms against pathogens include antibodies. A person can develop antibodies either by having an infection or receiving a vaccination.

- Antibiotics, antimicrobial agents, and antiviral agents are medications that are used to treat some kinds of infections. Not all infections can be treated with medications. In some cases, medications that used to work against certain pathogens no longer work because the pathogens have developed resistance. Some antibiotics destroy bacteria that help keep us healthy, allowing other bacteria to grow rapidly and make us sick.

Ways Infections Are Transmitted

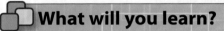

What will you learn?

When you are finished with this section, you will be able to:

1. Describe the airborne route of transmission.
2. Describe the direct route of transmission.
3. Describe the oral–fecal route of transmission.
4. Describe the bloodborne route of transmission.
5. Identify body fluids that are most likely to contain bloodborne pathogens.
6. Define the words **airborne pathogens**, **oral–fecal route**, **bloodborne pathogen**, and **body fluids**.

Airborne Transmission

Airborne pathogens pathogens that can be transmitted through the air

Some infections can be spread through the air. When the person coughs or sneezes, **airborne pathogens** leave the body through particles of saliva or sputum. As these particles spray through the air, they dry out and remain in the air for a long time. The dried-out droplets containing pathogens are in the air we breathe and on the surfaces we touch. Infection spreads when a person breathes the air containing the pathogens. Infections that are transmitted in this way include tuberculosis (TB), measles, and chickenpox.

Direct Transmission

Many infections are spread directly from one person to another when an uninfected person touches an infected person. Infection can also spread when an uninfected person touches objects that the infected person has touched, such as drinking glasses, bedpans, or bed linens. Infections that are transmitted in this way include herpes and conjunctivitis ("pink eye").

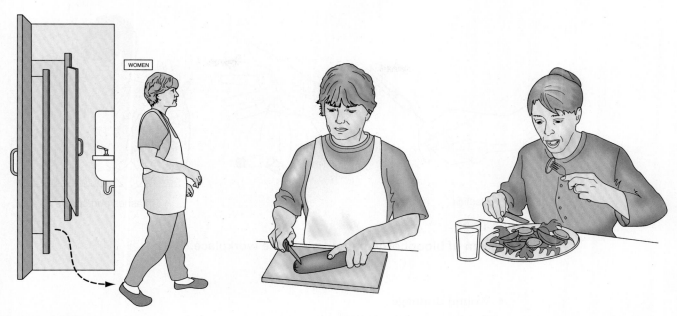

■ **FIGURE 13-2**

The oral–fecal route of transmission. The virus lives in an infected person's digestive tract and leaves the body through the feces. If the person's hands become contaminated with feces and then the person handles food, the infection could be passed on to the person who eats the contaminated food.

Oral–Fecal Transmission

Some pathogens are transmitted through the **oral–fecal route**. The pathogen lives in an infected person's digestive tract and leaves the body in the feces. The feces can contaminate food or water. Then, when another person eats or drinks the contaminated food or water, he becomes infected. Proper hand hygiene and sanitation help to prevent infections that are spread through the oral–fecal route (Fig. 13-2). Infections that are transmitted in this way include hepatitis A, hepatitis E, vancomycin-resistant enterococcus, and some types of parasitic infections.

Oral–fecal route a method of transmitting an infection; occurs when feces containing a pathogen contaminate food or water, which is then consumed by another person

Bloodborne Transmission

For a **bloodborne pathogen** to be transmitted from one person to another, blood or **body fluids** from an infected person must enter the bloodstream of a person who is not infected. There are several ways this could occur in the workplace:

- Needlesticks (puncture wounds caused by used needles)
- Cuts from contaminated, broken glass (such as that from a broken blood tube)
- Direct contact between infected blood and broken skin, mucous membranes, or the eyes (Fig. 13-3)

    Body fluids that are most likely to contain bloodborne pathogens include:

- Blood
- Semen
- Vaginal secretions

Bloodborne pathogens pathogens that can be transmitted to another person through blood or other body fluids

Body fluids liquid or semiliquid substances produced by the body, such as blood, urine, feces, vomitus, saliva, drainage from wounds, sweat, semen, vaginal secretions, tears, cerebrospinal fluid, amniotic fluid, and breast milk

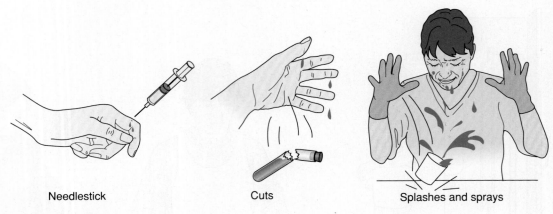

Needlestick   Cuts   Splashes and sprays

■ **FIGURE 13-3**

Transmission of bloodborne pathogens in the workplace.

- Wound drainage
- Cerebrospinal fluid (CSF)
- Amniotic fluid
- Breast milk

Infections that are transmitted this way include hepatitis B, hepatitis C, hepatitis D, and HIV infection/AIDS.

 Putting it all together!

- Some infections are transmitted through the air. The person becomes infected when he or she breathes contaminated air.
- Some infections are transmitted through contact with an infected person or objects that the infected person has used.
- Some infections are transmitted when feces containing a pathogen contaminate food or water that is then consumed by another person.
- Some infections are transmitted when blood or body fluids from an infected person enter the bloodstream of a noninfected person. Bloodborne pathogens are not found in sweat and tears. They are most likely to be found in blood, semen, vaginal secretions, wound drainage, cerebrospinal fluid (CSF), amniotic fluid, and breast milk.
- Needlesticks, cuts from contaminated glass, and splashes and sprays of contaminated body fluids can put a health care worker at risk for a bloodborne disease.

The Chain of Infection

What will you learn?

When you are finished with this section, you will be able to:

1. List and describe the six key conditions that must be met for an infection to be spread from one person to another.
2. Explain how the chain of infection can be broken.

For a person to get a communicable infection, six key conditions must be met. These six key elements are known as the chain of infection (Fig. 13-4). The chain

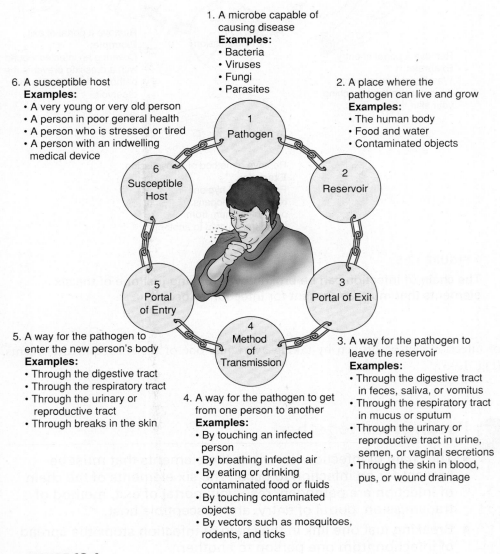

1. A microbe capable of causing disease
   Examples:
   • Bacteria
   • Viruses
   • Fungi
   • Parasites

2. A place where the pathogen can live and grow
   Examples:
   • The human body
   • Food and water
   • Contaminated objects

3. A way for the pathogen to leave the reservoir
   Examples:
   • Through the digestive tract in feces, saliva, or vomitus
   • Through the respiratory tract in mucus or sputum
   • Through the urinary or reproductive tract in urine, semen, or vaginal secretions
   • Through the skin in blood, pus, or wound drainage

4. A way for the pathogen to get from one person to another
   Examples:
   • By touching an infected person
   • By breathing infected air
   • By eating or drinking contaminated food or fluids
   • By touching contaminated objects
   • By vectors such as mosquitoes, rodents, and ticks

5. A way for the pathogen to enter the new person's body
   Examples:
   • Through the digestive tract
   • Through the respiratory tract
   • Through the urinary or reproductive tract
   • Through breaks in the skin

6. A susceptible host
   Examples:
   • A very young or very old person
   • A person in poor general health
   • A person who is stressed or tired
   • A person with an indwelling medical device

1 Pathogen
2 Reservoir
3 Portal of Exit
4 Method of Transmission
5 Portal of Entry
6 Susceptible Host

■ **FIGURE 13-4**

The chain of infection. For a person to get an infection, all six links in the chain must be present.

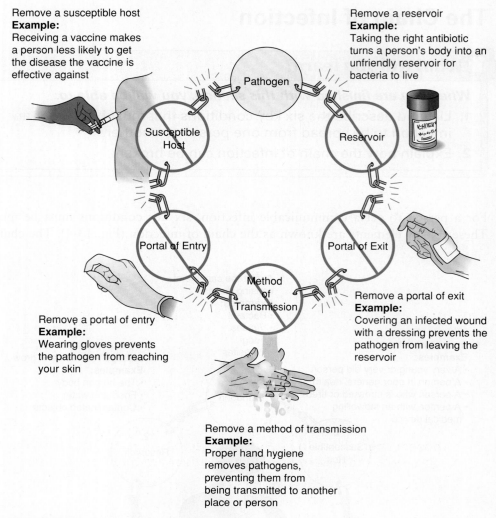

Remove a susceptible host
Example:
Receiving a vaccine makes a person less likely to get the disease the vaccine is effective against

Remove a reservoir
Example:
Taking the right antibiotic turns a person's body into an unfriendly reservoir for bacteria to live

Remove a portal of exit
Example:
Covering an infected wound with a dressing prevents the pathogen from leaving the reservoir

Remove a portal of entry
Example:
Wearing gloves prevents the pathogen from reaching your skin

Remove a method of transmission
Example:
Proper hand hygiene removes pathogens, preventing them from being transmitted to another place or person

■ **FIGURE 13-5**
The chain of infection can be broken by removing just one of the six elements that must be present for infection to occur.

of infection can be broken by taking away just one of the six required elements (Fig. 13-5).

Putting it all together!

- The chain of infection describes the elements that must be present for an infection to occur. The six elements of the chain of infection are pathogen, reservoir, portal of exit, method of transmission, portal of entry, and susceptible host.
- Breaking just one link in the chain of infection stops the spread of infection from one person to another.

Methods of Infection Control

What will you learn?

When you are finished with this section, you will be able to:

1. Discuss ways that a person could get an infection within the health care system.
2. List the four major methods of infection control.
3. Describe the four techniques that make up the practice of medical asepsis.
4. Explain why proper hand hygiene is the single most important method of preventing the spread of infection, and give examples of when you should wash your hands or use an alcohol-based hand rub.
5. State how personal protective equipment (PPE) is used in infection control.
6. Explain how isolation precautions are used to help prevent the spread of infection.
7. Explain when airborne precautions, droplet precautions, contact precautions, and standard precautions are used.
8. Describe tuberculosis (TB), an airborne infection that poses a special risk to health care workers.
9. Describe four diseases caused by bloodborne pathogens that pose a special risk to health care workers, and explain how the viruses that cause these diseases affect the body.
10. Demonstrate proper hand hygiene, gloving, masking, gowning, and double-bagging techniques.
11. Define the words **health care–associated infections (HAIs)**, **nosocomial infections**, **medical asepsis**, **transient flora**, **contaminated**, **personal protective equipment (PPE)**, **tuberculosis (TB)**, and **standard precautions**.

All health care facilities follow basic practices that are designed to decrease the chance that an infection will be spread from one person to another. These practices are called infection control. Practicing infection control in health care facilities is essential to reduce the number of **health care–associated infections (HAIs)**. Exposure to pathogens is increased in health care facilities. In addition, most of the people in health care facilities are there because they are not in good overall health. Therefore, their potential to get an infection is increased (Box 13-1). The chance of a patient or resident getting an infection while in a health care facility is so great that there is even a name for it: **nosocomial infections**. General guidelines for keeping the environment clean and reducing the spread of pathogens are given in Guidelines Box 13-1.

There are four major methods of infection control—medical asepsis, surgical asepsis, barrier methods, and isolation precautions.

Health care–associated infections (HAIs) infections that patients or residents get while receiving treatment in a hospital or other health care facility, or that health care workers get while performing their duties within a health care setting

Nosocomial infections infections that patients or residents get while receiving treatment in a hospital or other health care facility; a type of HAI

BOX 13-1 Risk Factors That Increase a Person's Risk for Infection

- **Very young or very old age.** The very young and the very old are more likely to get an infection. The young have not had time to develop an effective defense mechanism for fighting infections, and the elderly lose their defenses as they age.

- **Poor general health.** A person who is sick or debilitated ("worn down") is more at risk for infection because the body's defenses are already weakened by illness. Therefore, the person is not able to fight off the pathogen as easily. In addition, certain medical treatments, such as chemotherapy and radiation therapy, can affect the functioning of the body's immune system and put a person more at risk for infection.

- **Stress and fatigue.** Lack of rest and emotional stress can affect the body's ability to defend itself from pathogens.

- **Indwelling medical devices.** Medical devices, such as catheters, feeding tubes, and intravenous (IV) lines, increase a person's risk of infection by making it easier for pathogens to enter the body.

Medical Asepsis

Medical asepsis techniques that are used to physically remove or kill pathogens

Medical asepsis is achieved through processes involving soap and water, antiseptics, disinfectants, or heat. The goal of medical asepsis is to remove pathogens from surfaces, equipment, and the hands of health care workers. There are four techniques that make up the practice of medical asepsis (Table 13-2). More than one of these techniques may be used to remove pathogens from an object. For example, equipment must be properly cleaned with soap and water before it can be disinfected or sterilized.

Hand Hygiene

As a nursing assistant, the technique of medical asepsis that you will use most frequently is hand hygiene. Hand hygiene consists of both thoroughly washing your hands, using soap and water, and the use of alcohol-based hand rubs. According to the Centers for Disease Control and Prevention (CDC 2002), *handwashing is still the best method of decontaminating the hands and the consistent use of both methods of hand hygiene the most important method of preventing the spread of infection.* While you are taking care of your patients or residents, you will collect **transient flora** on your hands. These microbes could then be easily transferred to the next patient or resident you care for, yourself, or one of your family members. In fact, most HAIs are caused by transient flora—the hands of the health care worker serve as the method of transmission from one person to another. Transient flora are removed by proper hand hygiene.

Transient flora microbes that are picked up by touching contaminated objects or people who have an infectious disease

Procedure 13-1 describes the basic handwashing procedure. Although the specifics of how handwashing is performed vary from setting to setting, one aspect of handwashing always remains the same—it must be performed thoroughly, properly, and consistently. Box 13-2 describes when handwashing, instead of using an alcohol-based rub, is required.

While nothing can replace the effectiveness of good handwashing to remove visible dirt, blood, or other body fluids or substances, the Centers for Disease Control and Prevention (CDC) issued guidelines in October 2002, recommending the

GUIDELINES BOX 13-1   Guidelines for Maintaining a Clean Environment

What you do	Why you do it
Wash your hands, instead of using an alcohol-based hand rub, after contact with any body fluid, whether it is your own or another person's. Examples of body fluids include blood, saliva, vomitus, urine, feces, vaginal discharge, semen, wound drainage, pus, mucus, and respiratory secretions.	*Pathogens often leave the body through the gastrointestinal tract, reproductive or urinary tract, respiratory tract, or breaks in the skin. In addition, some pathogens are transmitted in blood and other body secretions, such as breast milk.*
Handwashing, instead of hand hygiene with an alcohol-based rub, should be used when caring for a person who may have certain infections, such as *C. diff.*	*Alcohol-based hand rubs may not be effective against certain microorganisms.*
Wash your hands frequently, especially after using the bathroom, and before handling food, drink, or eating utensils. Perform hand hygiene before and after any contact with a patient or resident.	*Frequent hand hygiene eliminates a method of transmission for pathogens.*
Cough or sneeze into a tissue or into your sleeve at the elbow, and teach your patients and residents to do the same. Dispose of tissues properly by placing them in a waste container.	*Some pathogens are transmitted in particles of saliva or sputum. Coughing or sneezing into your sleeve or a tissue contains these particles and helps to prevent the spread of infection.*
Provide each patient or resident with individual personal care items, such as toothbrushes, drinking glasses, towels, washcloths, and soap. Disposable items are preferred when possible.	*If not properly cleaned after use, these items can spread pathogens. Therefore, it is better to limit their use to one person.*
Keep contaminated or dirty items, such as soiled linens, away from your uniform.	*Pathogens can be transferred from the dirty item to your uniform, which can then act as a fomite.*
When cleaning, take care not to stir up dust. For example, wiping dusty surfaces with a damp cloth or mop helps to prevent the movement of dust and lint into the air. Do not shake linens when making beds.	*Dust can carry pathogens from one area to another.*
Dispose of trash properly. Follow established procedures for preparing dirty linens and clothing for the laundry.	*If not disposed of properly, trash can provide an ideal environment for pathogens to grow, especially if the trash contains food or other materials that can rot. Soiled items and clothing can spread pathogens and must be handled in a way that will lessen the chance of someone else coming in contact with the dirty item.*
Maintain good personal hygiene, and help your patients or residents to do the same. Bathing, washing hair, brushing teeth, and wearing clean clothing are all grooming practices that help to prevent the spread of infection.	*Personal grooming practices help to reduce the number of pathogens present on the skin.*

TABLE 13-2 Techniques of Medical Asepsis

Technique	Description
Sanitization 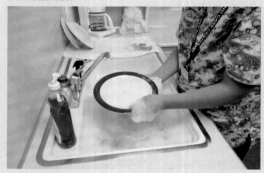	Practices associated with basic cleanliness, such as hand hygiene, cleansing of eating utensils and other surfaces with soap and water, and providing clean linens and clothing
Antisepsis 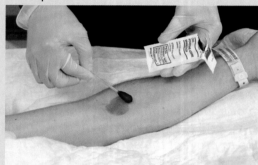	The use of mild chemicals (such as rubbing alcohol and iodine) to kill microbes or stop them from growing on skin
Disinfection 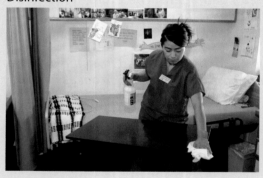	The use of strong chemicals (such as a bleach solution) to kill microbes on nonliving objects, such as bedpans, urinals, and over-bed tables
Sterilization 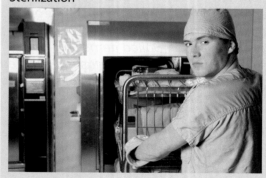	The use of pressurized steam heat or very strong chemicals to kill microbes on equipment that will be placed in a patient's or resident's body, such as surgical instruments

BOX 13-2   When Handwashing is Required

Handwashing, instead of using an alcohol-based rub, is required:

- When you first arrive at your facility
- When hands are visibly dirty
- When hands are visibly soiled with or in contact with blood or other body fluids
- When caring for patients or residents who may have certain infections, such as *C. diff*
- Before you go on break and before you leave your shift

- Before and after drinking, eating, or smoking
- Before and after inserting contact lenses
- After using the bathroom
- After coughing, sneezing, or blowing your nose
- After touching anything that may be contaminated with blood or other body fluids or substances
- After handling your hair or applying make-up or lip gloss

use of alcohol-based hand rubs for routine hand decontamination. Alcohol-based hand rubs have several advantages:

- Using an alcohol-based hand rub is quicker than washing your hands at the sink, which means that during duties that require frequent handwashing, using an alcohol-based hand rub can save time.
- Alcohol-based hand rubs are gentler on the skin than soap and water.
- Alcohol-based hand rubs are used without water, so they can be used anywhere. In many facilities, alcohol-based hand rubs can be dispensed at the patient's or resident's bedside, saving many trips back and forth to the sink. Many even come in containers small enough to be carried in your uniform pocket.

It is very simple to use an alcohol-based hand rub. The label on the product will tell you how much product to use. Procedure 13-2 describes how to use an alcohol-based hand rub. Box 13-3 describes when alcohol-based hands are appropriate to use.

Microbes can get trapped underneath long or false fingernails and jewelry worn on the hands and wrists, such as rings and bracelets. For the sake of efficiency and cleanliness, it is best to keep your fingernails short and unpolished and to leave your jewelry at home when performing your duties as a nursing assistant. Because

BOX 13-3   Using Alchohol-Based Rubs

Alcohol-based hand rubs are appropriate to use:

- When hands are not visibly soiled
- Before entering a patient's or resident's room
- Before and after patient or resident contact or contact with surfaces in the patient's or resident's room
- Before entering a "clean" supply room
- Before obtaining clean linen from a linen cart

- Before handling a person's meal tray
- After picking up an object from the floor
- After removing or changing disposable gloves, including those times when you are replacing a torn glove
- When moving from a dirty body site to a clean body site when providing care

frequent hand hygiene can cause the skin to become excessively dry, leading to cracking, applying a lotion or hand cream after washing is recommended. Remember, your own intact skin is important to help protect you from infection too.

Surgical Asepsis

Surgical asepsis is used for procedures that involve entering a person's body, such as surgical procedures, injections, insertion of intravenous (IV) catheters, and insertion of urinary catheters. Because these procedures involve putting a foreign object inside the person's body, all instruments and equipment used must be *sterile* (totally free from microbes). In most states, performing procedures that require surgical asepsis is not within a nursing assistant's scope of practice.

Personal protective equipment (PPE) barriers that are worn to physically prevent microbes from reaching a health care provider's skin or mucous membranes, such as gloves, gowns, masks, and protective eyewear

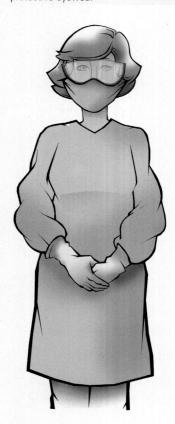

When caring for a person with a communicable disease, it is very important to remember the person's feelings. We work hard to follow all of the procedures that help to prevent the spread of infection, and this is a very important part of providing care. However, sometimes it is easy to forget about how the person with the infection might feel. How would you feel if a health care worker had to wear gloves or a mask every time he came near you? How would you feel if you had to stay in your room most of the time with the door shut? When you are caring for a patient or resident with a communicable disease, checking on the person frequently and taking the time to talk with the person when you are providing care can help to make the person feel better.

Barrier Methods

Barrier methods involve the use of **personal protective equipment (PPE)**. In many situations, you may need to wear more than one article of PPE. The best order for putting on PPE is as follows: gown, mask, protective eyewear, and gloves. The order for removal when it is time to take off the PPE is: gloves, protective eyewear, gown, and mask. After use, PPE is considered contaminated. Removing PPE in the correct sequence helps to protect you from infection. For instance, you would not want to remove your mask first because this would mean that you would have to touch your face with your contaminated gloves.

Gloves

Gloves are worn in the following situations:

- When there is a possibility that you will come in contact with body fluids
- When you are assisting with perineal care (cleaning of the area between the legs)
- When you are assisting with oral care (care of the gums and teeth)
- When you are shaving a patient or resident
- When you are caring for a patient or resident who has an open wound or other break in the skin
- When you have a cut on your hands

   Guidelines for using gloves are given in Guidelines Box 13-2. Procedure 13-3 describes the proper way to remove gloves.

Gowns

A gown should be worn when your uniform may become soiled with body fluids. Each gown is worn only once. A gown is considered contaminated if it becomes wet. Procedures 13-4 and 13-5 describe how to put on and take off a gown.

GUIDELINES BOX 13-2 Guidelines for Using Gloves

What you do	Why you do it
If the glove tears when you are putting it on, discard it.	*A glove that has a hole or tear will not protect your hands from contamination.*
Choose gloves that fit properly.	*Gloves that are too tight are uncomfortable and may tear. Gloves that are too loose will not stay on your hands.*
Use gloves made from another material if you or the person you are caring for is sensitive to latex.	*Depending on the severity of the allergy, exposure to latex can cause redness and cracking of the skin, a severe rash, or problems breathing.*
Remove contaminated gloves before touching any other surface. You may need to change gloves several times during one procedure.	*Replacing your gloves when they become contaminated prevents the transfer of pathogens from dirty areas to clean areas. If you touch a surface (such as the side rail, light switch, or doorknob) with your contaminated gloves, the pathogens will be transferred from your gloves to that surface. The next person who touches the surface could then pick up the pathogens you left there with your contaminated gloves.*
Perform hand hygiene after removing gloves.	*Gloves are easily torn or may have holes too small to see, causing your hands to become contaminated. Proper hand hygiene removes any microbes that may be on your hands.*

Masks

Masks cover your nose and mouth, and are worn when there is a chance that you will be exposed to pathogens that are transmitted through the air or in droplets of saliva. You could be exposed to these pathogens when a person talks, coughs, or sneezes. A mask is also worn if there is a possibility that blood or other body fluids may splash or spray toward your face.

Surgical masks are most commonly used, but if you are caring for a person with TB, you may be required to wear a special high-filtration mask (Fig. 13-6). Surgical masks are "one size fits all," but high-filtration masks are available in various sizes, and you must be fitted for them in advance. All masks are used only once. You must discard and replace your mask if it becomes wet or soiled. Procedure 13-6 explains how to put on and take off a mask. Procedure 13-7 explains how to remove more than one article of PPE.

Protective Eyewear

Goggles, face shields, and other types of protective eyewear are used to protect your eyes from body fluids that may splash (Fig. 13-7). Goggles fit close to your face and can be worn over prescription eyeglasses. Face shields may be attached to a mask or to an elastic band that fits around the head.

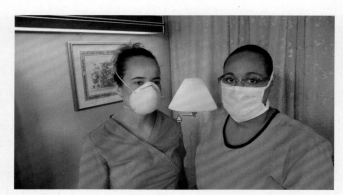

■ **FIGURE 13-6**

Masks cover your nose and mouth and protect you from inhaling pathogens transmitted in the air or in saliva. (*Left*) A high-filtration respirator mask, worn when caring for people with tuberculosis (TB). (*Right*) A surgical mask.

Isolation Precautions

Isolation precautions are guidelines that we follow to contain pathogens and limit others' exposure to them as much as possible.

Transmission-Based Precautions

Transmission-based precautions are used when a person is known or thought to have an infection that is transmitted a certain way.

AIRBORNE PRECAUTIONS. Airborne precautions (Box 13-4) are used when caring for people infected with airborne pathogens. Airborne pathogens enter the respiratory tract of people breathing the same air as the infected person. Therefore, airborne precautions involve placing the patient or resident in a private room with the door closed, wearing a mask when caring for the person, and minimizing the amount of time the person spends out of her private room. When the person must leave her room, she must wear a mask. Examples of diseases caused by airborne pathogens include measles, chickenpox, and **tuberculosis (TB)**. TB is described in more detail in Box 13-5.

Tuberculosis (TB) an airborne infection caused by a bacterium that usually infects the lungs

DROPLET PRECAUTIONS. Droplet precautions are used when caring for people with diseases caused by pathogens that are transmitted by direct exposure to droplets released from the mouth or nose (for example, when the person coughs, sneezes, or talks). Droplet precautions must also be taken when performing procedures that involve contact with an infected person's mouth or nose. Droplet

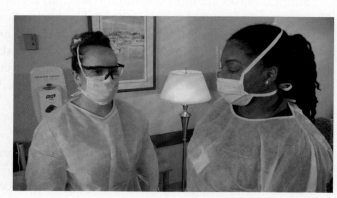

■ **FIGURE 13-7**

Face shields (*right*) and goggles (*left*) are used to protect your eyes from substances that may splash.

BOX 13-4   Airborne Precautions

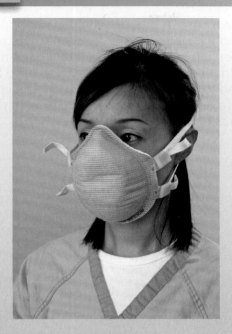

1. Patients or residents known or suspected to be infected with an airborne pathogen are to be placed in private rooms, called "airborne infection isolation rooms (AIIR)", that are equipped with special ventilation and filtration systems.

2. Health care workers should wear masks when caring for patients or residents with known or suspected tuberculosis (TB). If the health care worker has not been exposed to (or been vaccinated against) measles or chickenpox (and is therefore not immune), then he is at risk for these diseases, and a mask should be worn when caring for patients or residents with measles or chickenpox. If the health care worker is immune to measles or chickenpox, a mask is not necessary.

3. A mask should be placed over the patient's or resident's face if she must be transported from one location to another. Transport of the patient or resident should be kept to a minimum.

4. All precautions for preventing transmission of TB should be implemented if the patient or resident is known or suspected to have TB.

precautions are similar to airborne precautions, except that it is usually only necessary to wear a mask when you are within 3 ft of the infected person. Examples of diseases caused by pathogens that can be transmitted in droplets include influenza, whooping cough, strep throat, scarlet fever, rubella, meningitis, pneumonia, diphtheria, and epiglottitis.

CONTACT PRECAUTIONS. Contact precautions are used when caring for people with diseases caused by pathogens that are transmitted directly (by touching the person) or indirectly (by touching contaminated objects). Diseases that can be transmitted by contact include skin and wound infections, digestive tract infections, and some respiratory tract infections. Contact precautions involve using PPE whenever you must touch the infected person or items used by the person. Contaminated linen and waste materials must be contained and disposed of properly. Procedure 13-8 describes how to transfer contaminated items out of a person's room when contact precautions are being followed.

Standard Precautions

Because of the type of work you do, you will come in contact with body fluids that carry bloodborne pathogens. Bloodborne pathogens that pose the greatest risk to health care workers in the workplace are hepatitis B virus (HBV), hepatitis C virus (HCV), hepatitis D virus (HDV), and human immunodeficiency virus (HIV). The

BOX 13-5 Tuberculosis (TB)

Tuberculosis (TB) is an airborne infection that usually involves the lungs, but may also involve the kidneys or bones. The infection is spread when the person coughs, sneezes, speaks, or sings. People who have close, frequent contact with a person who has TB are most likely to get the disease. A person infected with TB may have the disease for years before she shows any symptoms. TB is usually diagnosed following a routine skin test (used to screen for the disease) or chest x-ray. Treatment is complicated and involves taking many different drugs for a long period of time. If not treated, tuberculosis can be fatal.

Because health care workers are at risk for getting TB from patients or residents, health care facilities regularly screen employees for TB using a simple skin test. A small amount of test material, called tuberculin, is placed under the skin on the arm using a needle or tines. In a few days, the area is checked. A person who has been exposed to the bacterium that causes TB will develop redness and swelling in the area,

as shown here. A person who has not been exposed will not have any reaction to the tuberculin. Testing positive on a skin test does not mean that you have TB, just that you have been exposed to it. Additional tests, such as a chest x-ray, are necessary to determine whether a person actually has TB.

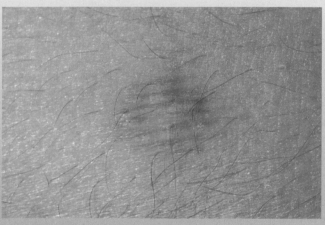

© Dr P. Marazzi/Science Photo Library.

diseases caused by these pathogens are potentially life threatening (Box 13-6). In many cases, you will not be able to easily identify patients or residents who are infected with bloodborne pathogens. This is why you must treat each patient or resident you have contact with as if he *may be* infected with a bloodborne pathogen. To protect yourself from exposure to bloodborne pathogens, you will take **standard precautions** with every patient or resident (Box 13-7). *For these methods to be effective, they must be used consistently!*

Three new elements have been added to the existing standard precautions guidelines that focus on helping to protect patients and residents:

- "Respiratory hygiene/cough etiquette" is used to help prevent the spread of any undiagnosed respiratory infection from patients, residents, and also any visitors in a health care facility to others.

- "Safe injection practices" are used to prevent the spread of infection by using a new, sterile syringe and needle each time a medication is drawn from a multidose vial for IV injection.

- "Infection control practices for special lumbar puncture procedures" require that health care workers wear a surgical mask when assisting with any type of lumbar puncture procedure.

Standard precautions
precautions that a health care worker takes with each patient or resident to prevent contact with bloodborne pathogens; include the use of barrier methods (such as gloves) as well as certain environmental control methods

BOX 13-6 — Hepatitis B, C, and D and HIV/AIDS

Methods of transmission

Bloodborne diseases that pose the most risk to health care workers include hepatitis B, hepatitis C, hepatitis D, and HIV/AIDS. The viruses that cause these diseases are found in blood, as well as in other body fluids, such as semen and vaginal secretions. This means that these viruses can be transmitted through transfusion of infected blood or blood products, across the placenta from mother to infant, through unprotected sexual intercourse, and by sharing needles used to inject drugs of abuse. These viruses can also be transmitted to health care workers through needlestick injuries, cuts with contaminated glass, or direct contact with blood.

Consequences of infection

Hepatitis B

Infection with hepatitis B virus (HBV) causes inflammation of the liver, the organ that removes toxic substances from the blood. Infection with HBV causes an acute illness in most people, but between 5% and 10% of HBV infections become chronic. People with chronic infections may never have symptoms but they can still pass the virus on to others. Or, they may have flare-ups of symptoms every so often, resulting in months of disability. Some people who are infected with HBV will eventually develop liver failure or liver cancer as a result of the infection. These conditions are potentially fatal.

A vaccine against HBV is available and is recommended for all health care workers.

Hepatitis C

Infection with hepatitis C virus (HCV) also causes inflammation of the liver. The illness that results from infection with HCV tends to be more chronic and serious than that resulting from infection with HBV. As many as 85% of people with hepatitis C develop chronic disease, and of these, 20% go on to develop liver failure or liver cancer. Many people with hepatitis C will eventually require a liver transplant to save their lives. Currently, no vaccine against HCV is available.

Hepatitis D

Hepatitis D virus (HDV) is found only in people who are already infected with HBV. Vaccination against HBV protects against HDV.

HIV/AIDS

Acquired immunodeficiency syndrome (AIDS) is caused by infection with human immunodeficiency virus (HIV). HIV invades the body's T cells, special white blood cells that help to protect the body from infection. Instead of killing the T cell immediately, HIV uses the T cell to make copies of itself and increase its numbers. Eventually, the virus kills the T cell, and then the virus and all of its copies move on to repeat the process in other T cells. Over time, the number of T cells in the body decreases. The body becomes unable to fight off infections and the person dies. To date, there is no cure for AIDS and no vaccine against HIV.

Risk to the health care worker

Of the bloodborne pathogens that you may be exposed to, HIV is the least likely one that you will catch. Your chances of becoming infected with HBV or HCV on the job are much higher (approximately 30%) than your chances of becoming infected with HIV (less than 0.1%). However, it is important for you to know that although your work as a nursing assistant does put you at risk for being exposed to bloodborne pathogens, your behavior outside of work could put you at much higher risk for getting a bloodborne disease. Having unprotected sexual intercourse is the most common way of getting hepatitis B and HIV.

BOX 13-7   Standard Precautions

1. Gloves must be worn if the *possibility* exists that the hands could come in contact with blood or other body fluids. Gloves must also be worn when touching any surface or linen that could be contaminated with infected materials. Remember that you cannot see a virus with the naked eye.

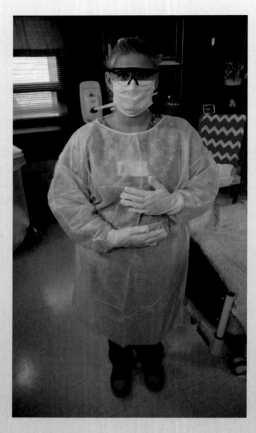

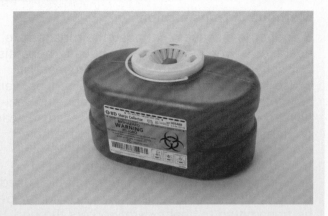

4. Sharps, such as used needles, razors, or broken glass, must be disposed of properly in labeled, OSHA-approved containers. Contaminated, broken glass items should not be handled, even with gloved hands. They should be swept or vacuumed up for disposal.

5. Spills of blood or other body fluids must be cleaned up promptly with an approved viricidal cleaning agent or a solution of 1 part household bleach to 10 parts water. Personal protective equipment (PPE), such as gloves and a gown, should be worn while cleaning up spills.

2. A waterproof (impervious) gown must be worn if the *possibility* exists that your clothes could become soiled with blood or other body fluids.

3. A mask, face shield, and eye goggles must be worn if the *possibility* exists that blood or other body fluids could splash or spray.

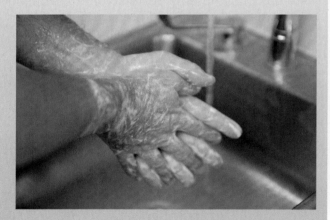

6. ***Proper hand hygiene is the most important method of preventing the spread of infection!*** Hands must be washed when you remove your gloves. If accidental exposure to blood or other body substances occurs, hands must be washed thoroughly and immediately.

Putting it all together!

- Infections can spread easily through a health care facility. Many of the people you will care for will have risk factors for infection. A major part of your responsibility in caring for other people involves protecting them from infection.

- Infection control is achieved through medical asepsis, surgical asepsis, barrier methods, and isolation precautions.

- Medical asepsis, or the process of physically removing pathogens from surfaces, is achieved through processes involving soap and water, antiseptics, disinfectants, or heat.

- Proper hand hygiene is the single most effective method of preventing the spread of infection. For hand hygiene to be effective in preventing the spread of infection, it must be performed thoroughly, properly, and consistently.

- Barrier methods prevent a pathogen from gaining access to a health care worker's body. Commonly used barrier methods include gloves, gowns, masks, and protective eyewear [personal protective equipment (PPE)].

- Isolation precautions are used to contain the spread of a pathogen. There are two main types of isolation precautions: transmission-based precautions and standard precautions. Transmission-based precautions are used when a person is known or thought to have an infection that is transmitted a certain way: airborne precautions (used when caring for people infected with pathogens that can be transmitted through the air), droplet precautions (used when caring for people infected with pathogens that are transmitted by direct exposure to droplets released from the mouth and nose), and contact precautions (used when caring for people infected with pathogens that are transmitted by direct contact with the infected person or objects that the infected person has touched). Standard precautions are taken with every patient or resident.

- Tuberculosis (TB) is an airborne infection that poses a risk to health care workers. A person can have TB and not know it. If not treated, TB can be fatal.

- Hepatitis B virus (HBV), hepatitis C virus (HCV), hepatitis D virus (HDV), and human immunodeficiency virus (HIV) are bloodborne pathogens that a health care worker may be exposed to. All of these viruses can cause serious—possibly even fatal—illnesses.

Occupational Safety and Health Administration (OSHA) Bloodborne Pathogens Standard

What will you learn?

When you are finished with this section, you will be able to:

1. Describe the standards set by the Occupational Safety and Health Administration (OSHA) to protect health care workers from exposure to bloodborne pathogens in the workplace.

2. Explain how the employer and the employee share responsibility for maintaining the employee's safety in the workplace.

Your employer is responsible for making sure that you have the equipment and training you need to maintain your safety in the workplace. To help employers to meet their responsibilities toward their employees, OSHA has created certain standards that all employers must follow (Box 13-8).

BOX 13-8 OSHA Bloodborne Pathogens Standard

- People working in an area where exposure to bloodborne pathogens is possible must receive training on the risks associated with bloodborne pathogens and on the methods they can use to safeguard themselves. Proof of initial training (at orientation) is to be on file in the employee's records, and training must be updated annually.

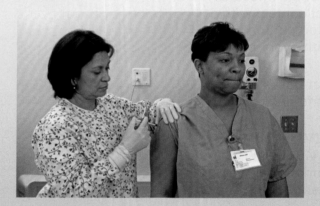

- Employers must make the hepatitis B vaccine available to workers who are at risk, free of charge. If an employee refuses the vaccination, a disclaimer signed by the employee must be kept on file. If the employee decides to accept the vaccine at a later date, the employer must provide it.

- The employer must provide adequate personal protective equipment (PPE), as required by the employee's duties. This includes gloves (non-latex, if the employee has allergies), face and eye protection, gowns and aprons, and scrub attire. It is the employee's responsibility to use the PPE consistently and conscientiously.

- Environmental control methods must be used to protect both the employees and the patients or residents. Environmental control methods include special ventilation systems to keep the air clean, procedures for the disposal of liquid waste, the availability of sharps disposal containers, and procedures for handling contaminated linen and trash. Housekeeping and cleaning methods must also meet OSHA's standards.

- Each health care facility must have an exposure-control plan in place in case an employee is exposed to blood or other body fluids from a patient or resident. This plan must be up to date, available in written form, and available to all employees. It is the employee's responsibility to report any exposure incidents so that the employer can arrange for appropriate medical tests and treatment.

Any health care facility that does not follow the OSHA Bloodborne Pathogens Standard risks heavy fines and serious penalties, such as closure of the facility. For health care workers who do not follow standard precautions, the penalty can be even greater—a deadly illness. Additionally, if you have an exposure accident and are not following the recommended precautions, you may not be covered by worker's compensation if you become sick as a result of the exposure. The consequences of not following proper procedures in the workplace are not worth the risk.

Putting it all together!

- You and your employer share the responsibility for protecting you from exposure to bloodborne pathogens in the workplace. You are responsible for taking standard precautions with each and every patient or resident. Your employer is responsible for following the standards outlined by the Occupational Safety and Health Administration (OSHA) to ensure that the work environment is safe (the OSHA Bloodborne Pathogens Standard).

PROCEDURE 13-1
Handwashing

Why you do it: According to the CDC, handwashing continues to be the best method of decontaminating the hands.

1. Gather needed supplies if not present at the handwashing area: *soap or the cleansing agent specified by your facility, hand lotion* (optional), *paper towels, an orangewood stick or disposable nail cleaner* (optional).
2. Stand away from the sink, so that your uniform does not touch the sink. Push your sleeves up your arms 4 to 5 in if you are wearing a watch, push it up too.
3. Turn on the water and adjust the force so that it does not splash on your uniform. Use warm, not hot water.
4. Wet your hands, keeping your fingers pointed down. This will cause the water to run off your fingertips and into the sink. Do not allow water to run up your forearms.
5. Press the hand pump or step on the foot pedal to dispense the cleaning agent into one cupped hand.
6. Lather well, keeping your fingers pointed down at all times. Make sure the lather extends at least 1 in past your wrists.
7. Rub your hands together in a circular motion, washing the palms and backs of your hands. Interlace your fingers to clean the spaces between your fingers. Continue for at least 15 seconds.

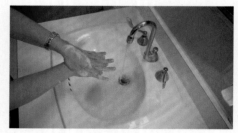

STEP 7 ■ Interlace your fingers.

8. Rub the fingernails of one hand against the palm of the opposite hand to force soap underneath the tips of the fingernails, or clean underneath the tips of the fingernails with the blunt edge of an orangewood stick or a disposable nail cleaner.

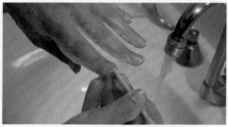

STEP 8 ■ Clean under your fingernails.

9. Rinse your hands, keeping your fingers pointed down at all times.

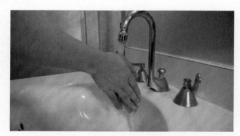

STEP 9 ■ Always point your fingertips down.

10. Dry your hands thoroughly with a clean paper towel, beginning with the fingers and moving upward to the wrists. Dispose of the paper towel in a facility-approved waste container, being careful not to touch the container.
11. With a new paper towel, turn off the faucet. Carefully dispose of the paper towel without touching it to the other clean hand.
12. As you leave the handwashing area, if there is a doorknob, open the door by covering the doorknob with a clean paper towel. If there is no doorknob, push the door open with your hip and shoulder to avoid contaminating your clean hands.
13. After leaving the handwashing area, apply a small amount of hand lotion to keep your skin supple and moist.

PROCEDURE 13-2
Using an Alcohol-Based Hand Rub

Why you do it: Proper hand hygiene is the most important method of preventing the spread of infection.

1. Gather needed supplies: *facility-approved alcohol-based hand rub, hand lotion* (optional).
2. Check the product label for the correct amount of product you should use.
3. Apply the correct amount of the hand rub to the palm of one hand.
4. Rub your hands together, covering your hands and fingers (front and back), and in between the fingers with the product. Make sure to clean the fingertips and rub the fingernails against your palms to force the product under the nails.
5. Continue rubbing your hands together until they are dry.
6. Apply hand lotion if desired.

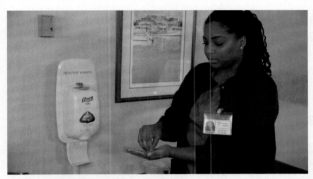

STEP 4 ■ Rub your fingernails against your palms to force the product under the nails.

PROCEDURE 13-3
Removing Gloves

Why you do it: Removing your gloves properly prevents you from contaminating your skin or uniform.

1. With one gloved hand, grasp the other glove at the palm and pull the glove off your hand. Keep the glove you have removed in your gloved hand. (Think, "glove to glove.")

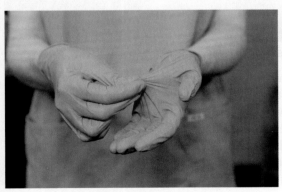

STEP 1 ■ "Glove to glove."

2. Slip two fingers from the ungloved hand underneath the cuff of the remaining glove, at the wrist. Remove that glove from your hand, turning it inside-out as you pull it off. (Think, "skin to skin.")

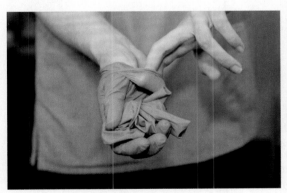

STEP 2 ■ "Skin to skin."

3. Dispose of the soiled gloves in a facility-approved waste container.
4. Perform hand hygiene.

PROCEDURE 13-4
Putting on a Gown

Why you do it: Putting on a gown properly prevents your uniform from becoming soiled with body fluids.

1. Gather needed supplies: a gown, gloves.
2. Remove your watch and place it on a clean paper towel or in your pocket. (If you are wearing jewelry, remove that as well.) Roll up the sleeves of your uniform so that they are about 4 to 5 in above your wrists.
3. Perform hand hygiene.

5. Secure the gown around your neck by tying the ties in a simple bow or by fastening the Velcro strips.

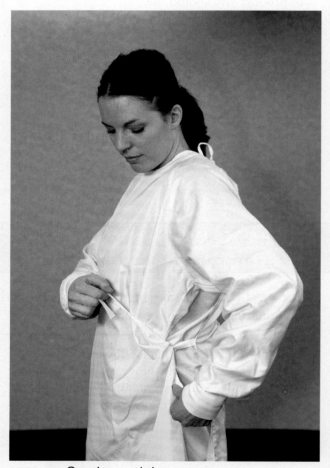

STEP 6 ▪ Overlap and tie.

6. Reach behind yourself and overlap the edges of the gown so that your uniform is completely covered. Secure the gown at your waist by tying the ties in a simple bow or by fastening the Velcro strips.
7. Put on the gloves. The cuffs of the gloves should extend over the cuffs of the gown.

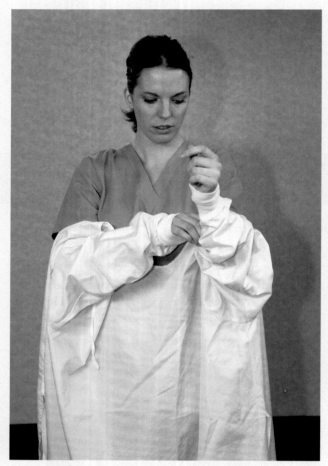

STEP 4 ▪ Slip your arms into the sleeves.

4. Put on the gown by slipping your arms into the sleeves.

PROCEDURE 13-5
Removing a Gown

Why you do it: Removing a gown properly prevents you from contaminating your skin or uniform.

1. Remove and dispose of your gloves as described in Procedure 13-3. (If your gown ties in the front, untie the waist strings before removing your gloves.)
2. Untie the waist ties (or undo the Velcro strips at the waist).
3. Untie the neck ties (or undo the Velcro strips at the neck). Be careful not to touch your neck or the outside of the gown.
4. Grasping the gown at the neck ties, loosen it at the neck and allow the gown to fall away from the shoulders.
5. Be careful to touch only the inside of the gown and pull it away from your body and off your arms.

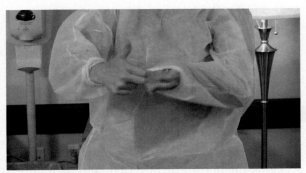

STEP 5 ■ Be careful not to touch the outside of the gown.

6. Holding the gown away from your body, roll it downward, turning it inside out as you go. Take care to touch only the noncontaminated side of the gown.

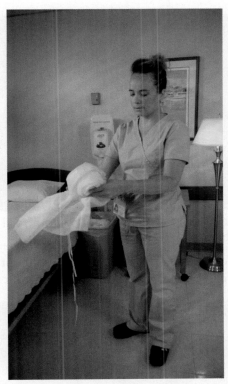

STEP 6 ■ Hold the gown away from your body and roll it downward, turning it inside out.

7. After the gown is rolled up, contaminated side inward, dispose of it in a facility-approved container.
8. Perform hand hygiene.

PROCEDURE 13-6
Putting on and Removing a Mask

Why you do it: Putting on a mask properly prevents pathogens that are transmitted through the air or in droplets from entering your nose and mouth. Removing a mask properly prevents you from contaminating your skin or uniform.

PUTTING ON A MASK

1. Gather needed supplies: *a mask*.
2. Perform hand hygiene.

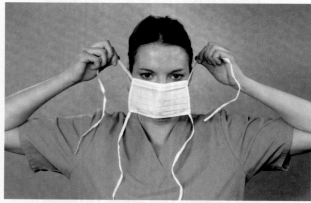

STEP 3 ▪ Be careful not to touch your face with your hands.

3. Place the mask over your nose and mouth, being careful not to touch your face with your hands.

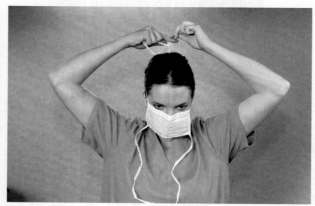

STEP 4 ▪ Tie the top strings securely.

4. Tie the top strings of the mask securely behind your head.

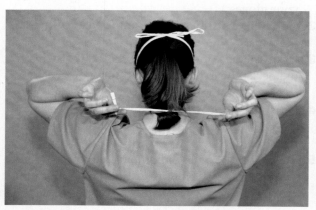

STEP 5 ▪ Tie the bottom strings securely.

5. Tie the bottom strings of the mask securely behind your neck. Make sure that the mask fits snugly around your face. You want to breathe through the mask, not around it.

REMOVING A MASK

1. Perform hand hygiene. (You do not want to touch your face with dirty hands.)
2. Untie the bottom strings first, and then untie the top strings.
3. Remove the mask by holding the top strings. Dispose of the mask, holding it by its ties only, in the facility-approved container located inside the patient's or resident's room.
4. Perform hand hygiene.

PROCEDURE 13-7
Removing More Than One Article of Personal Protective Equipment (PPE)

Why you do it: Remove PPE at the doorway before leaving the patient room.

1. Remove and dispose of your gloves as described in Procedure 13-3.
2. Remove your protective eyewear. Handle only by the "clean" headband or ear pieces.
3. Untie the gown's waist ties (or undo the Velcro strips at the waist). If the gown ties in the front, untie the waist tie before removing your gloves.

4. Untie the gown's neck ties (or undo the Velcro strips at the neck), and loosen the gown at the neck. Remove and dispose of the gown as described in Procedure 13-5.
5. Remove and dispose of the mask as described in Procedure 13-6.
6. Perform appropriate hand hygiene immediately after removing PPE.

PROCEDURE 13-8
Double-Bagging (Two Assistants)

Why you do it: Double-bagging helps to keep any pathogens that may be on the outside of the bag from spreading to other places.

1. The nursing assistant inside the person's room places the contaminated items into an isolation bag (usually a color-coded plastic bag) and secures the bag with a tie.
2. Another nursing assistant, referred to as the "clean" nursing assistant, stands outside of the person's room, holding a plastic bag cuffed over her hands. The cuff at the top of the bag protects the "clean" nursing assistant's hands.
3. The nursing assistant inside the isolation unit deposits the bag of contaminated items into the bag held by the "clean" nursing assistant.
4. The "clean" nursing assistant secures the top of the plastic bag tightly and disposes of the double-bagged items according to facility policy.

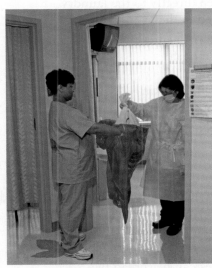

STEP 3 ▪ The assistant inside the room places the bag of contaminated items in the bag held by the nursing assistant outside of the room.

WHAT DID YOU LEARN?

Multiple Choice

Select the single best answer for each of the following questions.

1. When you wash your hands, you should:
   a. Use the hottest water possible
   b. Scrub with a brush for 3 minutes
   c. Rinse with your fingers pointed up
   d. Rinse with your fingers pointed down

2. When should you wash your hands instead of using an alcohol-based hand rub when performing hand hygiene?
   a. When hands are not visibly soiled
   b. When hands have come in contact with blood or other body substances
   c. After performing routine care, such as taking a person's blood pressure
   d. When changing gloves during a care procedure

3. You have been told to follow contact precautions with one of your residents. Therefore, this resident's soiled linen should be:
   a. Thrown away
   b. Bagged prior to removing it from the room
   c. Taken directly to the laundry
   d. Placed in the linen hamper

4. Bacteria may enter the body through:
   a. The mouth
   b. The nose
   c. Cuts in the skin
   d. All of the above

5. Which statement about the handwashing procedure is correct?
   a. As long as soap is used, the temperature of the water does not matter
   b. The faucet is clean and may be touched during handwashing
   c. Wash at least 1 inch above the wrist
   d. All of the above

6. Microbes can be spread by:
   a. Looking at a person with a communicable disease
   b. Coughing or sneezing
   c. Touching a person with a communicable disease
   d. Both "b" and "c"

7. Which one of the following statements about gowns is true?
   a. The outside is considered the "clean" side
   b. The gown opens in the front
   c. A gown may be used more than once
   d. A gown is considered contaminated when wet

8. Which one of the following must be present in order for infection to spread?
   a. A nursing assistant
   b. An indwelling medical device
   c. A susceptible host
   d. A patient or resident who looks ill

9. Hepatitis B virus (HBV), a bloodborne pathogen, can be found in all of the following body fluids except:
   a. Blood
   b. Semen
   c. Wound drainage
   d. Sweat

10. When are goggles a necessary part of personal protective equipment (PPE)?
    a. Whenever blood is present
    b. Whenever blood may splash or spray
    c. Whenever you are taking care of a person with tuberculosis (TB)
    d. Goggles are not really a necessary part of PPE

11. Human immunodeficiency virus (HIV) can be transmitted through all of the following means except:
    a. Blood splash to mucous membrane
    b. Sexual intercourse
    c. Sharing needles
    d. A mosquito bite

12. A vaccination against which one of the following bloodborne diseases is available?
    a. Lyme disease
    b. AIDS
    c. Hepatitis C
    d. Hepatitis B

13. Hepatitis B is a viral disease of the:
    a. Spleen
    b. Liver
    c. Blood
    d. Heart

14. For health care workers, which of the following is the most important method of preventing the spread of infection?
    a. Standard precautions
    b. Proper hand hygiene
    c. Wearing gloves
    d. Wearing gowns and goggles

15. Personal protective equipment (PPE) refers to:
    a. Sterilization and disinfection
    b. Security personnel
    c. Disposable gloves, face masks, and gowns
    d. Isolation precautions

Matching

Match each word with its definition.

_____ **1.** Communicable disease

_____ **2.** Pathogen

_____ **3.** Leukocyte

_____ **4.** Health care–associated infection (HAI)

_____ **5.** Antibodies

a. Special proteins that help fight specific pathogens

b. Can be transferred from one person to another

c. Microbe that can cause illness

d. White blood cell that helps to fight pathogens

e. Infection acquired in the health care setting

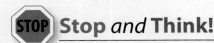 **Stop** *and* **Think!**

You are providing care to Mr. Torres, who has hepatitis B. This morning, while you are helping Mr. Torres to brush his teeth, he coughs, spraying your uniform and arms with bloody mucus. You are wearing gloves, but no gown or mask. Is it possible that you have been exposed to an infectious disease? What should you do?

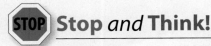 **Stop** *and* **Think!**

Today you have a new resident on your acute care unit who has just been transferred from another facility. He has a productive cough, and you were informed in report that the nurse is waiting for the results of his tuberculosis (TB) test. What precautions should you take when caring for him?

Workplace Safety

In Chapter 13, you learned about one threat to safety in the health care setting—infectious disease. In this chapter, we will explore other threats to the safety of people who work or live in a health care facility and the measures you can take to minimize these threats.

Photo: A nursing assistant uses good body mechanics to protect herself from injury while assisting a resident to stand.

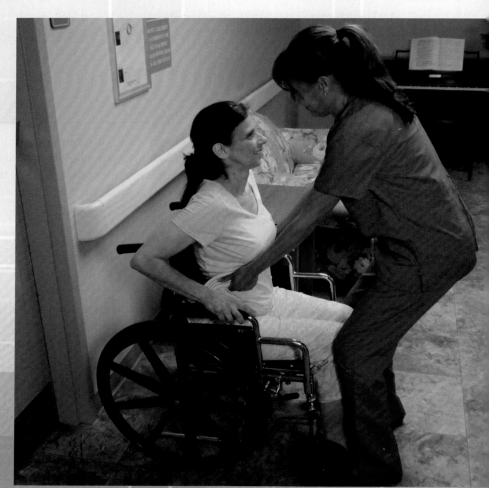

Protecting Your Body

What will you learn?

When you are finished with this section, you will be able to:

1. Discuss why people who work in a health care setting are at an increased risk for injury.

2. Describe and demonstrate the "ABCs" of proper body mechanics.

3. Explain how the proper use of body mechanics promotes safety and makes the body more effective when working.

4. Demonstrate proper lifting technique, and explain how using proper lifting technique can help to prevent back injuries.

5. Define the words **ergonomics, body mechanics, alignment, balance,** and **coordinated body movement**.

As a nursing assistant, you will place stress on your body as you lift, push, pull, stoop, and bend repeatedly on a daily basis. In addition, in many cases, you will need to move a person or piece of equipment that is larger and heavier than you are. By practicing good body mechanics and learning proper lifting techniques, you can minimize your risk for physical injury.

Ergonomics

The Occupational Safety and Health Administration (OSHA) recognizes that health care workers encounter many physical hazards when performing routine duties in the health care setting. The physically demanding nature of duties performed by nurses and nursing assistants, such as manual lifting and transferring and repositioning patients and residents, places these health care workers at an increased risk of injury, particularly back injuries. Nursing assistants who work in nursing homes have been identified as being more than twice as likely to be injured on the job.

To better protect workers in health care settings, OSHA guidelines recommend that workers should be provided with **ergonomics** training. The use of ergonomics basically entails adjusting the work environment and how workers perform work-related practices so that injuries are prevented. Work-related practices that nursing assistants face on a daily basis in the health care setting include:

Ergonomics the practice of designing equipment and work tasks to conform to the capability of the worker

- *Force*, which is the amount of physical effort that is required to perform a task, such as during heavy lifting or repositioning a patient or resident.

- *Repetition*, where the same motion or series of motions are performed continually or frequently.

- *Awkward postures*, where a person assumes positions that place stress on the body, such as reaching above shoulder height, kneeling, squatting, leaning over a bed, or twisting the torso while lifting.

OSHA also recommends that manual lifting of residents in long-term care facilities be minimized in all cases and eliminated whenever possible by using mechanical lifts.

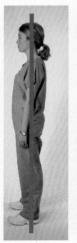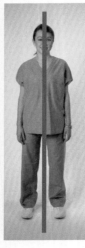

■ FIGURE 14-1

Proper body alignment. On the side view, you should be able to draw an imaginary line connecting the ear, shoulder, hip, knee, and ankle. From the front view, you should be able to draw an imaginary line connecting the nose, sternum (breastbone), and navel and continuing between the legs, dividing that space equally in half.

Body mechanics the efficient and safe use of the body

Alignment good posture

Balance stability produced by even distribution of weight

Coordinated body movement using the weight of the body to help with movement

Body Mechanics

The "ABCs" of good **body mechanics** are **alignment, balance,** and **coordinated body movement:**

■ **Alignment.** When the body is held in proper alignment, the back is in a "neutral" position, with the curve of the lower spine intact (Fig. 14-1). Holding the body in proper alignment prevents strain on the joints and muscles.

■ **Balance.** When you are standing, your *base of support* is your feet, and your *center of gravity* is your torso, the heaviest part of your body. Bringing your center of gravity closer to your base of support makes it easier for you to stay balanced (Fig. 14-2).

■ **Coordinated body movement** involves using the weight of your body to help with movement. For example, when moving a person up in bed, you stand facing the bed with your feet apart. As you step sideways to move the person's head and shoulders up, you transfer your weight from one foot to the other, and the momentum helps you to move the person.

Lifting and Back Safety

As a nursing assistant, you will be required to lift people and objects. If you fail to use proper technique when you are lifting, you may injure your back. Back injuries are the most common work-related injury in the nursing field. Back injuries can be serious enough to end your career and prevent you from participating in other activities that you enjoy. Proper lifting technique is summarized in Figure 14-3 and in Guidelines Box 14-1.

■ FIGURE 14-2

Maintaining balance. Spreading your feet apart and bending at the hips and knees improve your ability to stay balanced.

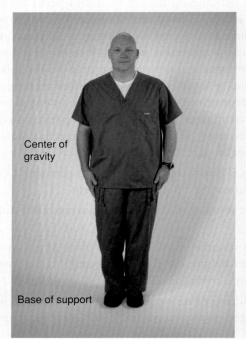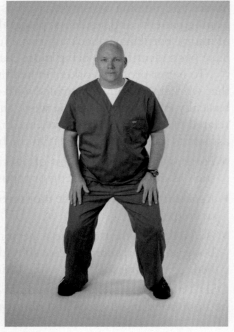

Center of gravity

Base of support

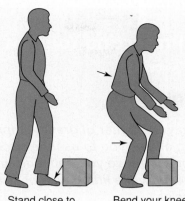

Plan your lift and ask for help if you need it.

Stand close to the object and widen your base of support.

Bend your knees and keep your back straight.

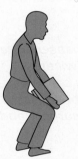

Tighten your stomach muscles.

Lift with your leg muscles.

■ **FIGURE 14-3**
Proper lifting technique.

GUIDELINES BOX 14-1 Guidelines for Protecting Yourself From Physical Injury

What you do	Why you do it
Make a habit of practicing good posture.	*Keeping the body in proper alignment, regardless of the activity, reduces stress and fatigue to the muscles and joints.*
Create a solid base of support by moving your feet apart, either by widening your stance or by placing one foot in front of the other.	*A solid base of support improves your balance, reducing the chance that you will injure yourself during the maneuver.*
Allow the weight of your body to assist in pulling or pushing heavy objects.	*Using coordinated body movement to move something minimizes the stress on your body while making the task you are trying to accomplish easier.*
When moving or lifting people or objects, place your body as close as possible to the object being moved.	*Bringing your body's center of gravity closer to the object improves your balance and allows the strong muscles of the shoulders and upper arms to assist in the move.*

(*box continues on page 304*)

GUIDELINES BOX 14-1 Guidelines for Protecting Yourself From Physical Injury (continued)

What you do	Why you do it
Squat—do not lean over—to lower your center of gravity when lifting.	*Lowering your center of gravity improves your balance. Squatting allows you to use the strong muscles of your lower body to move yourself, and the weight, upward. Leaning over while lifting weight strains the back joints and muscles.*
Use the large, strong muscles of the hips, buttocks, and thighs to do the lifting.	*Using the strong muscles of the legs to move yourself upward avoids placing strain on the muscles of the back, which are not meant to be used to lift substantial amounts of weight.*
Do not twist your spine when lifting.	*Vertebral discs are "cushions" of cartilage that separate the vertebrae of the spine from each other. Twisting your spine when lifting is the most common cause of a herniated disc (rupture of one of the vertebral discs). This is a painful condition that may require surgery and a long recovery period.*
Do not lift heavy objects from a position higher than your head. Use a step stool or a short safety ladder to raise your entire body closer to the desired level.	*Attempting to lift a heavy object from an awkward position (for example, with your arms raised above your head) interferes with your ability to balance and places you at risk for injury.*
If an object is very heavy, do not attempt to lift it. Instead, pull, push, or roll the object.	*Pushing, pulling, or rolling a heavy object places less strain on your body because you can use your body weight to help you accomplish the task.*
Use assistive devices whenever possible to make the job easier.	*Hand carts and dollies permit the easy movement of objects by placing them on wheels. Gait belts, draw sheets, and mechanical lifts (discussed in detail in Chapter 17) help make moving people easier.*
Ask for help when lifting or moving heavy people or objects. You should also get help when you need to move a person who cannot offer any assistance or is combative.	*Heavy or awkward loads increase your risk of injury (and, if you are attempting to lift a person, increase that person's risk of injury as well). A person who is "dead weight" or uncooperative is both heavy and awkward.*
Keep your body in good physical condition by exercising regularly, eating nutritious foods, and getting enough rest.	*Your body must be properly maintained in order to provide you with years of solid performance.*

Putting it all together!

- Ergonomics entails making adjustments in the work environment and how workers perform work-related duties to help prevent injuries.
- Practicing good body mechanics allows you to use your body effectively when lifting and moving people and equipment and helps to protect you from injury as you perform your daily duties. The "ABCs" of good body mechanics are alignment, balance, and coordinated body movement.
- Using proper lifting technique is critical for preventing back injuries.

Following Procedures

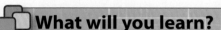 **What will you learn?**

When you are finished with this section, you will be able to:

1. Explain why nursing assistants follow procedures when providing patient or resident care.
2. List the steps that are taken before and after every patient or resident care procedure and explain why these steps are taken.
3. Define the word **procedure**.

To ensure that the care you provide is safe and correct, you will follow specific **procedures**. Following the recommended steps of a procedure helps to protect the person you are caring for, and it protects you.

The steps of the procedures you learn may differ somewhat depending on where you work and what state you receive your training in. The steps of the procedures in this book reflect general practice and may be a little different than what your instructor teaches. Always be sure to follow the policies of the facility or the state where you work so that the care you provide is safe and consistent.

Certain steps, called *pre-procedure actions*, are followed before performing any procedure on a patient or resident. In this book, we call these actions "Getting Ready" steps. "Getting Ready" always begins with checking the patient's or resident's care plan. The care plan will tell you the specifics about providing care for each individual person. Care plans change, sometimes frequently, so they correlate with changes in the patient's or resident's condition and abilities. That is why you will need to check the care plan frequently, especially if you work in an acute care type of setting.

A simple mnemonic has been created to help you remember the "Getting Ready" steps: "WEAVERS." Guidelines Box 14-2 lists and explains each of these actions.

Similarly, there is a group of actions that are routinely performed at the end of each procedure, called *post-procedure actions*. In this book, we call these actions "Finishing Up" steps (Guidelines Box 14-3). The mnemonic to help you remember the "Finishing Up" steps is: "ALSO Wash & Document." As you review the procedure boxes throughout this book, you will see references to these "Getting Ready" and "Finishing Up" steps in each of them. You must learn these steps and perform them before and after every procedure.

Procedure a series of steps followed in a particular order when providing care to a patient or resident that help to ensure that the care provided is safe and correct

GUIDELINES BOX 14-2 Guidelines for Getting Ready (Pre-procedure Actions) WEAVERS

What you do	Why you do it
To prepare for any type of care you provide, always check the person's care plan.	The person's care plan gives you specific information about the type of care you need to provide and will change as the person's condition and abilities change.
WASH Perform proper hand hygiene. Apply gloves and follow standard precautions if contact with blood or body fluids is possible.	Proper hand hygiene and using standard precautions prevent the spread of infection.
EQUIPMENT Gather all needed supplies.	Having everything you need before you start promotes efficiency.
ANNOUNCE Knock on the door and identify yourself by name and title to the person.	Knocking before you enter protects the person's right to privacy. Identifying yourself respects the person's right to know who is providing care.
VERIFY Identify the person, and greet him or her by name. Methods of identifying patients and residents will vary depending on where you work. Common methods of identifying people in health care facilities include wrist bands and photographs.	Identifying the person ensures that the procedure is being done on the correct patient or resident. Greeting the person by name is courteous.
EXPLAIN the procedure and encourage the person to participate as appropriate.	Explaining the procedure lets the person know what to expect and helps him to understand how he can help.
RESPECT THE PERSON'S PRIVACY by showing any visitors where they may wait, if necessary, until you have completed the procedure. Close the door and the curtain. Drape the person for modesty as appropriate.	Asking visitors to leave the room, closing the door and curtain, and draping the person for modesty protect the person's right to privacy.
SAFETY Take safety precautions by following standards of body mechanics, equipment use, and infection control. In procedures that involve getting a person out of bed, lower the bed to its lowest position. This decreases the distance between the bed and the floor, should the person fall. In procedures that involve providing care while the person remains in bed, raise the bed to a comfortable working height, usually around elbow-level of the caregiver. This protects your back. When using a bedside table to hold items used to provide personal care, keep the table close to the bed so that you do not have to turn or move away from the patient or resident.	Following standards of body mechanics, equipment use, and infection control keeps you and your patients or residents safe.

GUIDELINES BOX 14-3 Guidelines for Finishing Up (Post-procedure Actions) ALSO Wash & Document

What you do	Why you do it
ALIGNMENT Confirm that the person is comfortable and in good body alignment.	*Proper body alignment is most comfortable for the person. It relieves strain on the muscles and joints, promotes good heart and lung function, and helps prevent contractures and pressure ulcers.*
LIGHT Leave the call light control, telephone, and fresh water within easy reach of the person.	*Having necessary items nearby promotes independence and helps to prevent falls.*
SAFETY Return the bed to the lowest position, lock the wheels, and raise the side rails (if side rails are in use).	*Lowering the bed, locking the wheels, and raising the side rails (if side rails are in use) help to prevent falls.*
OPEN the curtain and door if desired by the patient or resident, and inform visitors that they may return to the room.	*Opening the curtain and door and letting visitors know that they can return help to prevent feelings of isolation.*
WASH Perform hand hygiene. If gloves were worn during the procedure, remove them, discard according to facility policy, and perform hand hygiene before touching clean items. Perform hand hygiene again before leaving the patient's or resident's room.	*Performing proper hand hygiene helps to prevent the spread of infection.*
DOCUMENT Report and record actions as required by your facility.	*Reporting lets the nurse know that you have completed the task and allows you to update the nurse about any changes in the patient's or resident's status. Recording formally documents the care that was provided and ensures that all members of the health care team have the same information about the patient's or resident's status and care.*

Putting it all together!

- Following procedures when providing patient or resident care helps to ensure that the care you provide is safe and correct.
- Pre-procedure actions ("Getting Ready" steps) are taken before every patient or resident care procedure. These actions promote efficiency, safety, and respect of the patient's or resident's rights.
- Post-procedure actions ("Finishing Up" steps) are taken after every patient or resident care procedure. These actions promote comfort, safety, and communication among members of the health care team.

Fire Safety

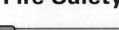

What will you learn?

When you have finished with this section, you will be able to:

1. List the elements necessary for a fire to start and continue to burn.
2. Describe precautions that are taken in the health care setting to prevent fires.
3. Describe the RACE fire response plan.
4. Demonstrate how to use a fire extinguisher.

In a health care facility, a fire that gets out of control can have tragic consequences. As a nursing assistant, you must know how to prevent fires in the workplace and what to do in the event when a fire does occur.

Preventing Fires

For a fire to occur, three elements must be present: fuel (something to burn), heat (something to light the fuel), and oxygen (Fig. 14-4). In a health care facility, many patients and residents receive oxygen therapy. Oxygen therapy increases the amount of oxygen in the air. Safety precautions that are used to prevent fires (Guidelines Box 14-4) are extremely important when oxygen therapy is in use.

Reacting to a Fire Emergency

The general actions that are taken in the event of a fire emergency are known as the RACE *fire response plan* (Fig. 14-5). Be familiar with your facility's fire safety policies and know the location of all exits in case an evacuation is necessary. In the event of an evacuation, knowing the shortest, safest route to an exit will allow you to move your patients or residents to safety faster.

(text continues on p. 312)

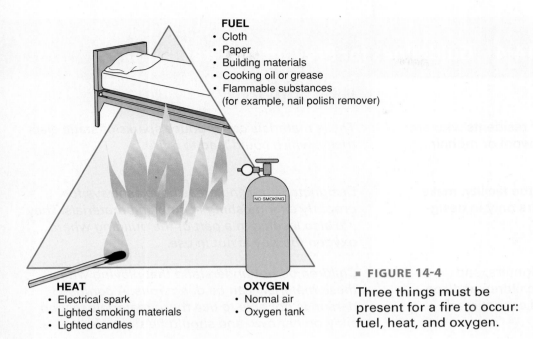

FUEL
- Cloth
- Paper
- Building materials
- Cooking oil or grease
- Flammable substances
  (for example, nail polish remover)

HEAT
- Electrical spark
- Lighted smoking materials
- Lighted candles

OXYGEN
- Normal air
- Oxygen tank

■ **FIGURE 14-4**

Three things must be present for a fire to occur: fuel, heat, and oxygen.

GUIDELINES BOX 14-4　Guidelines for Preventing Fires

What you do	Why you do it
Supervise patients or residents who are disoriented or who may fall asleep while smoking, any time when they smoke.	*A sleepy or disoriented person is not paying close attention to the lighted smoking material, which increases the chance that a fire will start.*
Do not allow any patient or resident to smoke in bed, especially if the person is receiving oxygen therapy.*	*A person who smokes in bed is bringing all three elements necessary for a fire together (fuel = bed linens; heat = lighted smoking material; oxygen = surrounding air). Smoking in bed is especially dangerous because the person is more likely to fall asleep and forget about the lighted smoking material. In addition, the use of oxygen therapy increases the oxygen content in the immediate area. If burning ashes from a cigarette should happen to drop on the bed, a fire would be more likely to start and would burn much faster as a result of the added oxygen.*

(*box continues on page 310*)

GUIDELINES BOX 14-4   Guidelines for Preventing Fires (continued)

What you do	Why you do it
Do not provide patients or residents who are receiving oxygen therapy wool or mohair blankets.	*These materials can produce sparks of static electricity, which could lead to a fire.*
If smoking is permitted in the facility, make sure that all smoking occurs only in designated smoking areas.	*Designated smoking areas have ashtrays for properly extinguishing lit smoking materials. They are also located in a part of the building where oxygen therapy is not in use.*
Keep smoking materials, lighters, and matches in a place where children and confused patients or residents cannot reach them.	*Children do not understand that playing with these materials can be dangerous. A confused person is not able to use these materials responsibly on her own and should be supervised.*
Keep all electrical equipment in good working order.	*A spark from a frayed wire, an improperly grounded plug, or an electrical "short" can start an electrical fire.*
Handle flammable substances safely and clean up any spills immediately. Do not use flammable substances near a heat source such as a hair dryer or heater or while smoking.	*Flammable substances ignite easily and burn quickly. Therefore, if they come in contact with a heat source, a fire is likely to start.*
Report any malfunctioning smoke detectors immediately.	*A smoke detector is the best early fire detection device available, but only if it is functioning properly.*
Promptly investigate smoke or smells of anything burning. Be aware of the location of fire alarms and fire extinguishers and know how to activate and use them.	*Early investigation and quick action can help to contain a fire before it gets out of control.*
Be familiar with your facility's fire safety policies and know the location of all exits.	*If a fire does occur, you may need to evacuate patients or residents. You will be much more effective in your duties if you are able to remain calm, and your calmness will also help to calm others.*

*Although health care facilities prohibit smoking in patient or resident rooms, some people may forget or disregard the rules.

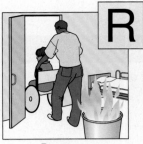

Remove any patients or residents who are in immediate danger to safety. Escort people who can walk. Use wheelchairs for unsteady people. People who cannot get out of bed should be moved in their beds, if possible. If the bed cannot be moved out of the room, or if stairs must be used, the patient or resident can be pulled to safety using the linens from the bed.

Remove

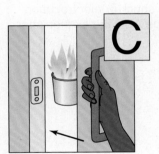

Activate the alarm according to your facility's policy. You may be required to pull the fire alarm, or use the intercom or telephone system.

Alarm

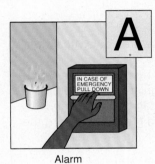

Contain the fire by closing doors and windows. This action helps to slow the spread of the fire.

Contain

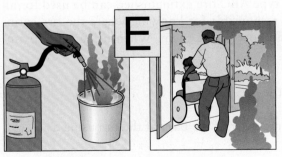

Extinguish the fire, OR, if the fire is large or spreading quickly, evacuate the building.

Extinguish   or   Evacuate

■ **FIGURE 14-5**

The RACE fire response plan.

TABLE 14-1   Types of Fires

Type	Description	Method of Extinguishing
A	Fueled by wood, paper, cloth, leaves, or grass	These fires can be put out using water, a type A, or a type ABC fire extinguisher.
B	Fueled by a petroleum product (for example, gasoline, automotive oil), cooking oil, or grease	Do not try to put these fires out with water! Instead, smother the fire by sprinkling baking soda on it or by using a type B or type ABC fire extinguisher. A stovetop fire that starts in a pan can be extinguished by covering the pan and removing it from the heat source.
C	An electrical fire	Attempting to put an electrical fire out with water can result in shock or electrocution. Use a type C or type ABC fire extinguisher instead.

Using a Fire Extinguisher

All health care facilities must have easily accessible fire extinguishers. The most common type of fire extinguisher, a type ABC fire extinguisher, can be used for all types of fires (Table 14-1). You are responsible for knowing where the fire extinguishers are kept in your facility and how to use them. When using a fire extinguisher, remember the word **PASS**:

Pull the safety pin out.
Aim the hose toward the base of the fire.
Squeeze the handle.
Spray the contents of the fire extinguisher at the base of the fire using a sweeping motion.

Putting it all together!

- Three elements are necessary to start a fire and keep it burning: fuel, heat, and oxygen.
- The RACE fire response plan describes the general actions that are to be taken in the event of a fire emergency: **R**emove people in the immediate area, activate the **A**larm, **C**ontain the fire, and **E**xtinguish or **E**vacuate as indicated by the situation.

■ Not all fires are alike. When using a fire extinguisher, make sure that it is effective against the type of fire you are trying to put out. Type ABC fire extinguishers are effective against all types of fires (A, B, and C).

Preventing Chemical and Electrical Injuries

What will you learn?

When you are finished with this section, you will be able to:

1. Describe OSHA requirements for employers with regard to chemicals in the workplace.
2. Explain how a nursing assistant can find out how to handle a chemical properly and what to do in the event of a chemical exposure.
3. Discuss safety precautions that are taken to lower the risk of electrical shock and electrical fires.
4. Define the word **Safety Data Sheets (SDSs)**.

Preventing Chemical Injuries

Health care workers use many chemicals on a daily basis. Many of these chemicals can be harmful if they are inhaled, swallowed, absorbed through the skin, or splashed in the eyes. Some chemicals can become dangerous if accidentally mixed with another product.

OSHA requires all employers to maintain a list of the chemicals that are used in the facility, from household cleaners to highly toxic solutions, and to inform and educate all workers about the chemicals that are in use in their workplace. One way of communicating information about chemicals to employees is through **Safety Data Sheets (SDSs)**, which the manufacturer of the chemical is required to supply. The SDSs for each chemical in use must be readily available to all employees of the health care facility. Container labels also provide information about the chemicals in the container, and all containers must be clearly labeled. As a nursing assistant, it is your responsibility to be familiar with the chemicals that you may come in contact with in your facility and to know the proper, safe way to handle each chemical in use.

Safety Data Sheets (SDSs) a document that summarizes key information about a chemical, its composition, which exposures may be dangerous, what to do if an exposure should occur, and how to clean up spills

Preventing Electrical Injuries

Many electrical appliances are used in the health care setting, including electric adjustable beds, call-light controls, lamps, hair dryers, curling irons, and electric razors. Improperly used or maintained electrical equipment can lead to electrical shocks (the passing of electrical current through the body) or fire. Guidelines for preventing electrical injuries are given in Guidelines Box 14-5.

GUIDELINES BOX 14-5 Guidelines for Preventing Electrical Injuries

What you do	Why you do it
Use grounded appliances (which have special three-pronged plugs) and outlets with ground-fault breakers whenever possible.	*Grounded appliances and outlets with ground-fault breakers return stray electrical current to the outlet so that the risk of electrical shock and fire is reduced.*
If more than two items must be plugged into an outlet, use a facility-approved power strip.	*Overloading the outlet or using an extension cord increases the risk of electrical shock and fire.*
Remove appliances with frayed cords or loose plugs from use immediately. Follow your facility's policy for tagging the item and sending it for repair.	*Frayed cords and loose plugs increase the risk of electrical shock or fire.*
Do not operate electrical appliances around sinks, showers, and bathtubs.	*Electricity and water do not mix! Using electrical appliances around water increases the risk of electrical shock or fire.*

 Putting it all together!

- Health care facilities use many chemicals in their daily operation. OSHA requires employers to inform and educate all workers about the chemicals used in their workplace. Information about how to respond to a chemical exposure is found on the SDSs and on the labeled container.
- Knowing how to safely operate and maintain electrical equipment in the workplace helps to create a safe working environment for you and a safe living environment for your patients or residents by minimizing the risk of electrical shock and fire.

Disaster Preparedness

 What will you learn?

When you are finished with this section, you will be able to:
1. List disaster situations that may affect a health care facility.
2. Define the word **disaster**.

A **disaster** can be caused by an act of nature (such as a tornado, earthquake, hurricane, flood, blizzard, or ice storm), or it may be the result of an explosion, accident, or act of war or terrorism. Every health care facility has a *disaster preparedness plan*, which directs the actions of the health care team in the event of a disaster. Know the particular duties that will be required of you in the event of a disaster and remain calm.

> **Disaster** a sudden, unexpected event that causes injury to many people, major damage to property, or both

Putting it all together!

- Your facility's disaster preparedness plan will detail your responsibilities in the event of a disaster. Be familiar with the plan so that you can act efficiently and calmly if a disaster does occur.

Workplace Violence

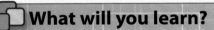

What will you learn?

When you are finished with this section, you will be able to:

1. Describe factors that may lead to workplace violence in the health care setting.
2. Define the word **workplace violence**.

Violent acts are increasing in areas where the victims are the most vulnerable, such as schools, churches, and health care facilities. As a result of this increased threat to people who work in health care settings and to those they care for, OSHA has issued recommendations and guidelines aimed at preventing **workplace violence**. These new guidelines are intended to advise employers on the risks of violent acts that may occur in their specific types of work environment and how to train their employees to recognize and respond to these risks.

Health care workers may be victims of violent acts from many sources. External parties such as robbers or muggers can attack a worker as he or she walks from the parking lot to the building going to and from work. Internal parties that may inflict violence include co-workers, patients and residents, and their family members or other visitors. Table 14-2 lists factors that OSHA has released that increase the health care worker's risk of work-related assaults.

> **Workplace violence** defined by the National Institute for Occupational Safety and Health (NIOSH) as "violent acts (including physical assaults and threats of assaults) directed toward persons at work or on duty."

Putting it all together!

- Workplace violence is increasing as a risk to the health care worker.

TABLE 14-2 **Factors That Increase the Risk of Workplace Violence in the Health Care Setting**

- The prevalence of handguns and other weapons among patients, their families, or friends
- The increasing use of hospitals by police and the criminal justice system for criminal holds and the care of acutely disturbed, violent individuals
- The increasing number of acute and chronic mentally ill patients being released from hospitals without follow-up care
- The availability of drugs or money at hospitals, clinics, and pharmacies, making them likely robbery targets
- Factors such as the unrestricted movement of the public in clinics and hospitals and long waits in emergency or clinic areas that lead to client frustration over an inability to obtain needed services promptly
- The increasing presence of gang members, drug or alcohol abusers, trauma patients, or distraught family members
- Low staffing levels during times of increased activity, such as mealtimes, visiting times, and when staff members are transporting patients
- Isolated work with clients during examinations or treatments
- Solo work, often in remote locations with no backup or way to get assistance, such as communication devices or alarm systems
- Lack of staff training in recognizing and managing escalating hostile assaultive behavior
- Poorly lit parking areas

WHAT DID YOU LEARN?

Multiple Choice

Select the single best answer for each of the following questions.

1. In the event of a fire in a resident's room, your first action should be to:
   a. Remove the resident to a safe place
   b. Get the fire extinguisher
   c. Sound the fire alarm
   d. Notify the nurse

2. When lifting, remember to use the large muscles of your:
   a. Chest
   b. Hips, buttocks, and thighs
   c. Back
   d. Shoulders

3. Using good body mechanics to lift an object off the floor means that you would:
   a. Use a mechanical lift
   b. Kneel down to get the broadest base of support and lift up
   c. Squat and lift with your legs
   d. Lean over at the waist, keeping your back flat

4. Unsafe conditions in a health care facility can be caused by:
   a. Health care workers who allow patients or residents to get out of bed
   b. Health care workers who stop doing an assigned task to clean up a spill
   c. Overloaded outlets and extension cords
   d. Patients and residents who smoke in "smoking only" areas

5. All of the following actions could cause a fire except:
   a. Using a grounded appliance
   b. Emptying an ashtray into a wastebasket
   c. Smoking in a room where a person is receiving oxygen therapy
   d. Placing a stack of linens on a heating unit to warm them

6. Where should you direct the foam when using a fire extinguisher to put out a fire?
   a. At the base of the fire
   b. In a circle around the fire, to prevent the fire from spreading
   c. At the top of the fire
   d. Anywhere in the general area of the fire

7. What are the "ABCs" of good body mechanics?
   a. Assess, Balance, Complete
   b. Assign, Begin, Complete
   c. Alignment, Balance, Coordinated movement
   d. Attempt, Brace, Change

8. You are a new nursing assistant and have been assigned to clean the room of a resident who has just been discharged. The nurse shows you the cleaning closet, which contains towels, rags, and containers holding liquids and powders of various colors and odors. How can you find out what cleaning products are appropriate for your assigned task?
   a. Read the nursing care plan
   b. Read the product label
   c. Use your senses—smell the contents of each container and use whichever has the most pleasant smell
   d. There is no need to find out which product is most appropriate—the cleaning closet contains only products used for cleaning

9. Following pre-procedure and post-procedure actions before and after each procedure is important to:
   a. Prevent the patient or resident from becoming confused
   b. Ensure that the care you give is safe and correct
   c. Make the nurse happy
   d. Pass the certification exam

10. Workplace violence can result from either internal or external parties. Which of the following is an example of an external party?
    a. Confused resident
    b. Mugger in the parking lot
    c. Angry co-worker
    d. Mentally ill patient

(STOP) Stop *and* Think!

You work on the second floor of a large long-term care facility. As you are on your way from the nurses' station to answer a resident's call light, you see smoke coming from another resident's room. You know that the occupant of that room, Miss Verna, smokes. Although Miss Verna knows she is not supposed to smoke, she often tries to "sneak" a cigarette. She has emphysema and is receiving oxygen therapy. When you enter the room, you see that Miss Verna has dozed off, dropping a lit cigarette onto her bed linens. The sheets have begun to smolder and catch on fire. What should you do first—sound the fire alarm? Turn off the flow of oxygen? Wake Miss Verna up and assist her to safety? Explain the logic behind your answer.

Patient and Resident Safety

Safety is a basic human need. If we feel safe, we can relax and rest and we feel secure and comfortable. One of your primary responsibilities as a nursing assistant is to help keep those in your care safe.

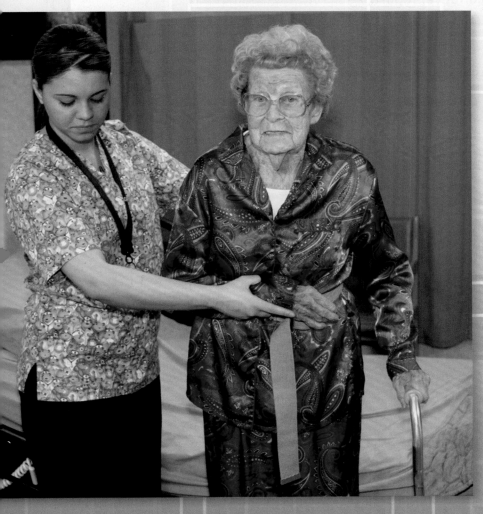

Photo: A nursing assistant helps a resident to get out of bed safely.

Accidents and Incidents in the Health Care Setting

What will you learn?

When you are finished with this section, you will be able to:

1. Discuss how accidents and incidents can threaten the safety of a person in a health care setting.
2. Identify risk factors that may put people in a health care setting at higher risk for accidents and injury.
3. List and describe special needs that residents in a long-term care setting may have related to safety.
4. Describe measures that a nursing assistant can take to prevent accidents in a health care setting.
5. Demonstrate how to assist a patient or resident who is falling.
6. Understand the importance of reporting an accident, if one occurs, and completing the necessary follow-up paperwork.
7. Define the words **accident, incident, entrapment,** and **incident (occurrence) report.**

Accidents and Incidents

Following safety guidelines to help keep the patients and residents we care for safe, as well as ourselves, is very important in the health care setting. Unfortunately, even with the best of care, an **accident** or an **incident** can still occur. Accidents and incidents can involve patients or residents, staff, or visitors to the facility.

Accident an unexpected, unintended event that has the potential to cause bodily injury

Incident an occurrence that is considered unusual, undesired, or out of the ordinary and disrupts the normal routine for the patient or the resident, the health care facility, or both

Risk Factors for Accidents

Recognizing the factors that can increase a person's chances of having an accident will help you to minimize the chance that an accident will occur.

Age

The young and the older people are at high risk for accidents:

- **Infants** can wriggle, roll, and twist themselves into dangerous situations very quickly.
- **Young children** lack knowledge about things that are dangerous, which puts them at risk for injuries, such as falls, burns, poisoning, and drowning.
- **Elderly people.** The physical and mental effects of the aging process (or of disease) can affect an elderly person's ability to be safe.

Medication

Medications, especially if they are not taken properly, can cause side effects, such as dizziness and confusion, that put a person at higher risk for accidents.

Poor Mobility

An inability to move easily can put a person at risk for falling. A person's mobility can be affected by:

- Pain and stiffness (for example, from arthritis)
- Paralysis (such as that resulting from a spinal cord injury or stroke)
- Conditions that cause a shuffling gait, such as Parkinson's disease or stroke
- Knee surgery or a broken leg

Sensory Impairment

We rely on our five senses to give us information about our environment and to keep us safe:

- **Vision.** Poor vision can increase a person's risk of falls, especially on stairs or over objects left on the floor. Poor vision can also increase a person's risk of accidental poisoning because the person cannot see medication labels clearly.
- **Hearing.** Poor hearing affects a person's ability to detect danger. For example, a person who does not hear well may not be able to hear the sounds of approaching traffic or warning alarms, such as the sound made by a smoke detector.
- **Touch.** People with an impaired sense of touch, such as that resulting from paralysis or complications of diabetes, may not be able to detect pain, heat, or cold. This puts the person at risk for burns, frostbite, and other injuries.
- **Taste and smell.** A decreased ability to taste and smell (such as often occurs as part of the normal aging process) can leave a person unable to detect spoiled food, a natural gas leak in the home, or smoke.

Confusion and Disorientation

Confusion and disorientation can cause a person to act in a way that puts him at risk for injury. For example, a person who is confused or disoriented may not be able to remember to call for help before getting out of bed. Or he might wander away from the facility and get lost. Confusion and disorientation can be caused by:

- Reactions to medication
- Infections and other acute medical conditions
- Head injuries
- Dementia
- Changes in the environment (such as moving from home to a long-term care facility)
- Sensory impairment

Loss of Consciousness

A person who is unconscious is totally unable to respond to her environment and will rely on you to remain safe.

Concerns for Long-Term Care

Residents in long-term care settings often have special needs regarding safety. In fact, the Omnibus Budget Reconciliation Act (OBRA) requires the facility to maintain an environment that lowers the risk of accidents and incidents to the greatest extent possible. In addition, OBRA requires that all residents receive the supervision and assistance needed to prevent accidents and incidents from occurring. To fulfill those requirements, all facility staff must be alert for any potentially unsafe conditions that exist in the environment for each resident.

■ Physical Changes of Aging

The majority of people who reside in a long-term care facility are elderly people. The normal physical changes that occur with aging can affect a resident's ability to be safe. For example:

- Neurological changes can cause an older person to take longer to regain balance, increasing the risk of falling.
- Sensory changes can cause an older person to have difficulty detecting and responding to dangerous situations.
- Musculoskeletal changes that result in the loss of muscle tissue can cause an older person to become easily fatigued and frail.
- Urinary changes can cause an older person to experience urinary frequency and make him or her rush to the bathroom.
- Respiratory changes can cause an older person to feel short of breath and weak during physical activity.
- Skin changes can cause an older person to have fragile skin and increase the risk of bruising and skin tears during routine care.

■ Effects of Medical Conditions or Treatments

Most of the residents in the long-term care setting will have chronic health conditions. The health condition, its treatment, or both can increase the resident's risk for accidents or incidents. Many of your residents will take one or more medications to treat their chronic health conditions. These medications can affect a person's ability to be safe. For example, some medications can cause an elderly person to become dizzy when he stands up or even cause confusion, especially if they are not taken properly.

■ Environmental Conditions

The risk for accidents and incidents is also increased simply by the nature of the long-term care environment itself. Consider the following points:

- Something as simple as moving into a long-term care facility can cause a new resident to become confused or disoriented, increasing the resident's risk for an accident or incident.
- In a long-term care facility, there are many residents living under the same roof, each with varying degrees of mental disability, physical disability, or both.
- Long-term care facilities are very busy places. The hustle and bustle of people and equipment creates an environment where accidents and incidents are likely to occur.
- Environmental hazards (such as clutter, slippery surfaces, poor lighting, and sun glare) can also affect resident safety.

As you see, there are many factors that can affect a person's safety in the health care setting. When several of these risk factors are combined, complex safety issues can result.

Preventing Accidents

Many accidents and incidents that occur in the health care setting could have been prevented. Most safety measures only require taking an extra step or two. Take that extra step to help ensure the safety of those you care for.

Preventing Falls

Falls are the leading cause of nonfatal and fatal injuries in the United States and of accidental death among elderly people. Falls are the most common cause of functional decline, hospital admission, emotional trauma, and eventual placement in some type of nursing facility for older people. Falls are also the most common type of accident that occurs in the health care setting. Guidelines for preventing falls are given in Guidelines Box 15-1.

GUIDELINES BOX 15-1   Guidelines for Preventing Falls

What you do	Why you do it
Check the person's clothing and shoes. Clothing should fit properly. Shoes should provide good foot support and have nonskid soles.	*Long or loose clothing or shoes that provide inadequate foot support or have slippery soles could lead to tripping.*
Encourage the person to use rails along hallways and stairways while walking.	*The additional support offered by rails may be all that is needed to allow a person to move about safely and independently.*
Observe the person for signs of unsteadiness and offer physical assistance as needed.	*Offering assistance as needed allows the person to remain as independent as possible while minimizing the risk of falls.*
Encourage and assist the person to ambulate and exercise according to his or her care plan and abilities.	*Gait and balance training, along with exercise and restorative care can help reduce falls in the elderly person by improving strength and mobility.*
Observe the person's ability to use walking aids, such as canes and walkers, and correct incorrect use.	*Using a piece of equipment improperly can be just as hazardous as not using it at all.*
Check equipment, such as walkers and wheelchairs, to ensure that it is in good condition. Nonskid tips should be intact on walkers. Wheelchair wheel locks should function properly.	*Malfunctioning or broken equipment increases a person's risk for falls.*
Make sure a patient or resident who needs glasses is wearing them when he is out of bed.	*A person who cannot see clearly is more at risk for falls.*
Remove any clutter or obstacles from walkways and provide adequate lighting. Use night lights along walkways at night.	*Removing objects a person could trip over is an easy way to minimize falls. Proper lighting enhances the ability to see.*

(box continues on page 324)

GUIDELINES BOX 15-1   Guidelines for Preventing Falls (continued)

What you do	Why you do it
Create clear pathways in the person's room leading to the door and the bathroom. Keep heavy or large pieces of furniture away from the bedside and walkways.	*Keeping walkways clear of obstacles reduces the risk of falling. It also prevents a person from hitting his head against a piece of large furniture in the event of a fall.*
Keep beds in the lowest position. Keep bed wheels locked. Use beds that lower closer to the floor for elderly people who are at an increased risk of falling out of bed.	*Keeping the bed in the lowest position minimizes the distance from the bed to the floor, should the person fall out of bed. Keeping the wheels on the bed locked prevents the bed from rolling. A rolling bed could result in injury to the patient or resident, the nursing assistant, or both.*
Keep side rails up or down, according to the care plan for that particular person.	*Side rails can prevent a person from falling out of bed. Because side rails are considered a form of restraint, they should always be lowered, unless the person's medical condition is such that she needs the protection that is offered by having the side rails raised. Some patients or residents will benefit from having the side rails raised on one side of the bed so that they can be used to assist with repositioning or getting out of bed.*
Use cushioned floor mats beside the bed for people who are likely to fall out of bed.	*Floor mats can help prevent or lessen an injury caused by falling out of a low bed. However, they should be used with caution because they can actually cause a person to fall when they stand up.*
Always make sure the call-light control is within easy reach of the person. Answer call lights promptly, and offer to help the person with toileting frequently.	*Many falls are the result of a person trying to get up without assistance.*
Wipe up any spills immediately.	*Wet floors may not be obvious (especially to people who cannot see well) and greatly increase the risk of slipping.*
Keep people who are at risk for falling and disoriented close to the nurses' station. Offer frequent assistance with walking.	*Keeping a person who is disoriented and at risk for falling close to the nurses' station allows staff to keep an eye on the person and also minimizes the chance that a person who feels lonely will attempt to get up to look for company. A person who is offered help with walking on a fairly regular basis is less likely to attempt to get up on his own, thereby minimizing the chance of a fall.*
Orient a newly admitted patient or resident to the unit and her room.	*Falls often occur when a person is unfamiliar with her surroundings.*

If you are assisting a person who begins to fall, follow the steps in Box 15-1 to minimize the risk of injury for you and for the patient or resident.

Preventing Burns

A burn can be life threatening to a patient or resident. Measures for preventing burns include the following:

- If you will be assisting a person with a tub bath or shower, always check the water temperature first using a bath thermometer. The water temperature should be between 105°F (40.5°C) and 110°F (43.3°C). If the person is elderly, the water temperature should be at the lower end of this range.
- If you will be giving a person a bed bath, measure the temperature of the water in the basin. The water in the basin can be a little warmer than the water in a bathtub or shower because it cools off quickly and the person will not be immersed in it. The temperature range for a bed bath is between 110°F (43.3°C) and 115°F (46°C).
- Teach patients or residents who will be bathing themselves to check the water temperature with a thermometer or a hand or wrist before getting into the bathtub or shower.
- Use extreme care with heat applications (discussed in detail in Chapter 27).
- Warn people that a food or beverage is hot before giving it to them. Some people may need a cup with a lid for their coffee or tea if weakness or unsteadiness puts them at risk for spilling.
- Follow the guidelines for using electrical appliances that are given in Chapter 14. Electrical burns can occur if an appliance malfunctions or is used near water.

Preventing Entrapment

Beds in health care settings usually have side rails, which can be raised to help prevent the person from falling out of bed. Some patients or residents may also use a side rail that is raised only on one side of the bed for assistance when they are repositioning themselves in bed or getting up. Any time the side rails are in use, there is a risk for **entrapment** (Fig. 15-1). Patients and residents who are confused and those with physical disabilities are at the highest risk for entrapment. Mattresses that do not fit the bed frame properly also increase the risk of entrapment because it results in extra space left in between the mattress and the side rail. To help prevent entrapment, you should:

Entrapment occurs when a person becomes trapped in the side rail, or between the side rail and the mattress

- Always use the side rails as ordered in the person's care plan
- Check on the person frequently, especially if he has risk factors for entrapment
- Use devices that are specially designed to reduce the risk for entrapment by covering the open spaces between the side rails or between the side rail and the mattress

Preventing Accidental Poisonings

Many people think that accidental poisonings only occur with children. However, elderly people are at risk for accidental poisoning too. Poor eyesight, confusion, or a decreased sense of taste or smell can cause an elderly person to eat or drink something that will cause her harm. To minimize the risk of accidental poisonings:

- Never store household cleaners or other chemicals in containers meant for food or beverages.
- Keep household cleaners and chemicals in a locked cabinet.

BOX 15-1   Minimizing the Risk of Injury as a Result of a Fall

1. If the person complains of dizziness or seems unsteady, help him to sit in a chair. If a chair is not close by, help the person to sit on the floor. Stay with the person and call for assistance. This action can prevent a fall completely.

2. If a fall cannot be avoided, place your body behind the person and place your arms around his torso, pulling him close to your body. Do not grab the person's arm in an attempt to prevent the fall because doing so may actually cause more extensive injuries in some people (such as elderly people, who may have brittle bones, and people with weaknesses on one side of the body).

3. With the person's body pulled close to yours, widen your base of support by placing one foot behind the other, and allow the person to slide down your body toward the floor.

4. As the person slides down, squat while still supporting his body and gently lower him to the floor. Lower yourself to the floor and assume a sitting position with the person's head in your lap.

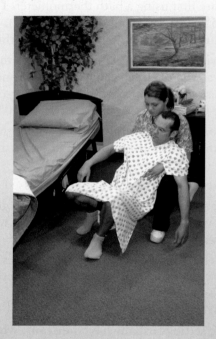

5. Stay with the person and call for assistance.

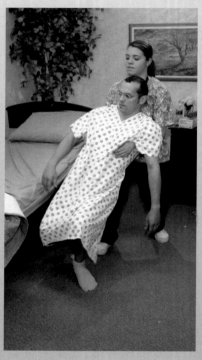

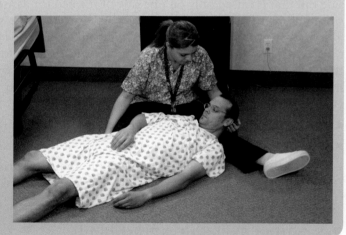

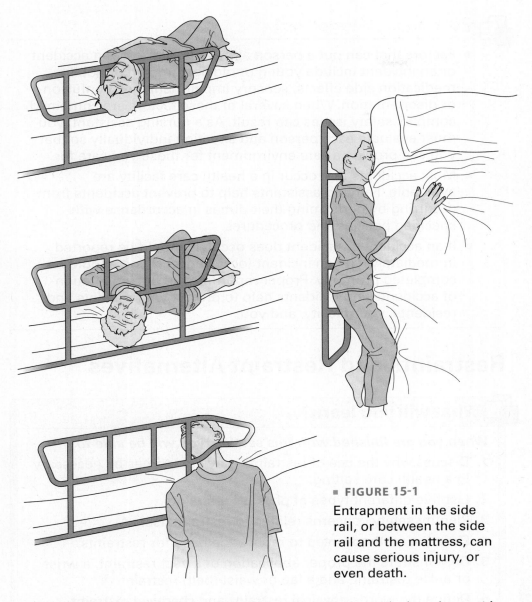

■ **FIGURE 15-1**

Entrapment in the side rail, or between the side rail and the mattress, can cause serious injury, or even death.

- Make sure that the contents of all containers are clearly marked on the outside.
- Provide help with reading labels as necessary.

Reporting Accidents and Incidents

Accidents and incidents can happen even when all safety measures have been followed carefully. Some accidents occur as a result of faulty equipment or from unfamiliarity with new equipment. Other accidents are the result of carelessness. When an accident does occur, you must know your facility's policy for reporting and documenting the incident. In all cases, information about the accident or incident should be provided in a straightforward and factual manner, without opinion or blame.

All accidents and incidents are to be reported immediately to the nurse. In addition, most facilities will require you to complete an **incident (occurrence) report**. The quality assurance department will look at the completed incident (occurrence) report and compare it to others to identify trends or patterns. In this way, they may be able to prevent similar accidents and incidents from happening again.

Incident (occurrence) report a preprinted document that is completed following an accident involving a patient or resident

Putting it all together!

- Factors that can put a person at increased risk for an accident or an incident include young or old age, impaired mobility, medication side effects, sensory impairment, and confusion or disorientation. When several of these factors are combined, complex safety issues can result. As a nursing assistant, you must evaluate each person and situation individually so that you can provide a safe environment for those you care for.

- Most accidents that occur in a health care facility are avoidable. Nursing assistants help to prevent accidents from occurring by performing their duties in accordance with specified policies and procedures.

- If an accident or incident does occur, it should be reported immediately, and an incident (occurrence) report should be completed promptly. Proper reporting and documentation of accidents and incidents help to protect your patients and residents, your facility, and you.

Restraints and Restraint Alternatives

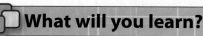

What will you learn?

When you are finished with this section, you will be able to:

1. Discuss why the use of restraints may sometimes be necessary in a health care setting.
2. List five different types of physical restraints.
3. Identify safety concerns related to restraint use.
4. Describe methods used to reduce the need for restraints.
5. Demonstrate the proper application of a vest restraint, a wrist or ankle restraint, and a lap or waist (belt) restraint.
6. Define the words **physical restraint** and **chemical restraint**.

Restraints ("reminder devices") are sometimes necessary to help keep a person safe. A *restraint* is something that limits a person's freedom of movement. Restraints may be physical or chemical.

A **physical restraint** is attached to or near a person's body and cannot be easily removed by the restrained person. A device is not considered a restraint if a person has the physical and mental ability to release the fastener. Examples of physical restraints include:

- Devices that are applied to parts of the body, such as the wrists, hands, elbows, ankles, chest, or waist (Table 15-1)

- "Lap buddies" and tray tables that are attached to a chair and which a person cannot remove independently (Fig. 15-2)

- Raised side rails

Physical restraint a device that is attached to or near a person's body to limit a person's freedom of movement or access to his or her body

TABLE 15-1 Physical Restraints

Type of Restraint	Use
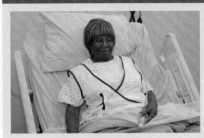 Vest restraint (no sleeves, flaps cross in the front)	Applied to the person's chest to prevent the person from falling out of bed or a chair
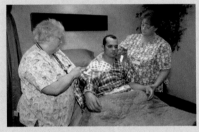 Jacket restraint (sleeves, closes in the back)	Applied to the person's chest to prevent the person from falling out of bed or a chair
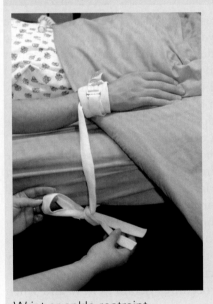 Wrist or ankle restraint	Applied to the person's wrists or ankles to prevent the person from moving his arms or legs; may be used to confine a person to bed, but more common use is to prevent a person from removing tubes or catheters
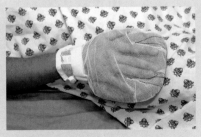 Mitt restraint	Applied to the person's hand to restrict finger movement; prevents the person from grasping tubes or catheters, but allows for more freedom of arm movement than a wrist restraint

(table continues on page 330)

TABLE 15-1   Physical Restraints (continued)

Type of Restraint	Use
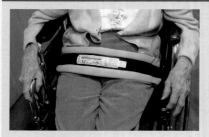 Lap restraint	Applied to the person's waist to prevent a person from sliding out of a chair

- Tightly tucked sheets
- Not permitting a person free access to other rooms or parts of the facility

Chemical restraint any medication that alters a person's mood or behavior, such as a sedative or tranquilizer

A **chemical restraint** is a medication used to assist in the control of anxiety, combative behavior, or agitation. These medications should help the person to feel less anxious. They should not make the person sleepy or unable to function in a normal fashion.

Use of Restraints

Many complications can result from the use of restraints (Box 15-2). Restraints are never used as punishment or for the staff's convenience. They are used to provide postural support, to protect the patient or resident from harm, and/or to protect the staff from harm (in the case of a combative or violent patient or resident) (Fig. 15-3). Restraints are to be used only if all other methods of ensuring safety have failed (Box 15-3). These measures, known as restraint alternatives, taken to avoid the use of restraints on a person must be documented before resorting to the use of restraints. Restraints are used only with a doctor's order.

The use of restraints is clearly defined in guidelines issued by OBRA, The Joint Commission, and the Food and Drug Administration (FDA). The *Resident Rights* portion of OBRA addresses a person's right to be free from physical and chemical restraints. According to OBRA, the improper use of restraints can be considered holding a person against her will (false imprisonment). Standards of care set forth by The Joint Commission and the Centers for Medicare and Medicaid Services (CMS) require that health care facilities minimize their use of restraints. Today, many health care facilities, especially long-term care facilities, are almost restraint-free.

Each health care facility has policies and procedures detailing how and when restraints are to be used. As a nursing assistant, you must understand your facility's

■ **FIGURE 15-2**
Lap buddies and tray tables are considered restraints if the person cannot remove the lap buddy or tray table independently.

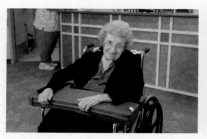
Lap buddy

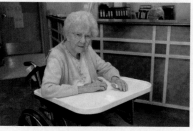
Chair with a tray table

BOX 15-2 Complications of Restraint Use

- Strangulation, which can lead to death, can occur if a vest restraint is improperly applied or if the restraint gets tangled in a piece of furniture.

- Bruises, nerve damage, and skin abrasions can result if a restrained person pulls at the restraint or if the restraint is applied too tightly.

- Permanent tissue damage as a result of decreased blood flow can occur if a restraint is placed incorrectly or too tightly.

- Broken bones and other serious injuries can occur if a restrained person tries to get out of the restraint.

- Complications of immobility, such as pneumonia, pressure ulcers, and blood clots, can occur if a person is left in a restraint for too long.

- Incontinence (an inability to control one's bowel, bladder, or both) can occur if a restrained person is not taken to the bathroom regularly.

- Loss of independence can occur when decreased mobility from restraint use leads to a decrease in bone and muscle strength.

- The mental effects associated with the use of restraints can be serious and include agitation, increased confusion, humiliation, and embarrassment.

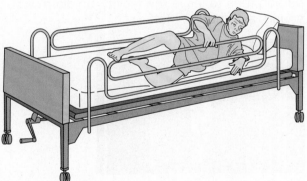

A person who is at risk for falling but will not stay in his bed or a chair and will not call for help may need to be restrained.

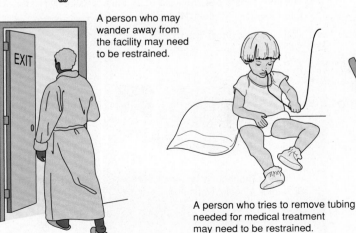

A person who may wander away from the facility may need to be restrained.

A person who tries to remove tubing needed for medical treatment may need to be restrained.

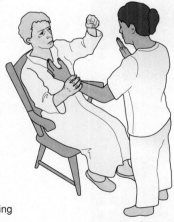

A person who is combative (physically aggressive) may need to be restrained.

■ **FIGURE 15-3**

The use of restraints is a last resort. However, in some situations, the use of a restraint may be appropriate. A restraint is never applied without a doctor's order.

BOX 15-3 Alternatives to Restraint Use

- Provide an environment in which the person feels safe and secure. Placing a confused person close to the nurses' station allows the staff to keep an eye on the person and keeps the person from feeling lonely. Taking time to speak to the person often or sitting beside her while you complete paperwork offers the person company and companionship. Soft music, television, or other methods of entertainment can be calming.

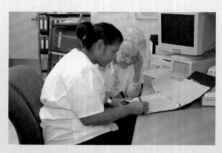

- Provide frequent attention to the person's physical needs. Take the person to the bathroom and offer a drink or snack regularly, per facility policy or more frequently if necessary. Assist the person with walking or change his position frequently to help maintain comfort. Answer call lights promptly, and make sure that the call-light control is within easy reach of the person.

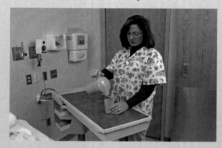

- Explain procedures and reassure the person. Being in a situation or having a condition that requires the use of restraints can be confusing and embarrassing.

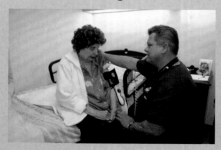

- Provide company and diversion. Don't be afraid to ask for help from family members, volunteers, and other residents of the facility.

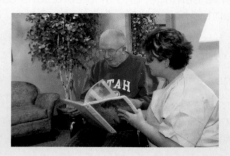

- Use restraint methods that are less restrictive. Pressure-sensitive alarm systems are placed on a person's mattress or wheelchair seat. If the person tries to get up without help, the alarm will sound, alerting the staff. Wanderer monitoring systems have a sensor that is attached to the person's wheelchair or placed around the person's wrist or ankle. If the person tries to leave the facility, an alarm will sound, alerting the staff.

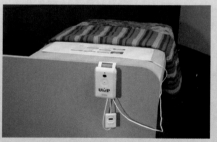

Pressure sensitive alarm system. Courtesy of Stanley Health Care Solutions, Lincoln, Nebraska

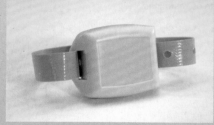

Wanderer monitoring system. Courtesy of Stanley Health Care Solutions, Lincoln, Nebraska

policies, and your responsibilities, regarding the use of restraints. Failure to follow these policies can result in a situation that is dangerous for your patient or resident, and it can put you and your facility at risk for lawsuits.

Applying Restraints

Restraints are dangerous even when used properly, but doubly so if they are not. A person who is restrained is eight times more likely to die than a person who is not restrained. Guidelines for the safe use and application of restraints are given in Guidelines Box 15-2.

GUIDELINES BOX 15-2 Guidelines for Using Restraints

What you do	Why you do it
Do not use a restraint without a written doctor's order that states the reason for the restraint.	OBRA and state laws protect patients and residents from being unnecessarily restrained.
Never use a restraint to "punish" a patient or resident or for your own convenience.	Physically and emotionally, the use of restraints has a very negative impact on the person's quality of life. Therefore, restraints are only used when absolutely necessary, after all other methods of ensuring the person's safety have failed.
Use the least restrictive restraint for the least amount of time.	Minimizing the use of restraints is important to preserve the person's quality of life.
Follow the manufacturer's instructions, nurse's direction, and facility policy for applying restraints.	Improper application of restraints can lead to serious medical complications, injury, or even death.
Use a restraint that is the correct size and in good condition.	If the restraint is too large, the person may be able to remove it, either completely or partially. This puts the person at risk for falling and strangulation. If the restraint is too small, complications such as restriction of blood supply to areas beyond the restraint can result. If the restraint is in poor condition, it may not properly restrain the person or the person may be injured when the restraint is applied.
Use commercial restraints. Do not use makeshift restraints, such as bed sheets or locks.	Using anything other than a commercial restraint to restrain a person is unprofessional and dangerous.
Restraints are always applied over clothing, pajamas, or a gown.	Clothing offers a layer of protection between the restraint and the person's skin.
Never put a vest restraint on backward (for example, with the back of the vest on the person's chest and the flaps crossed in the back).	Putting the vest restraint on backward can cause the person to strangle if she slides down in the chair or bed, because the back of the restraint is higher than the front.

(*box continues on page 334*)

GUIDELINES BOX 15-2   Guidelines for Using Restraints (continued)

What you do	Why you do it
Restraints are to be tied in simple, easy-to-release knots placed out of reach of the patient's or resident's hands. Some restraints are manufactured with quick-release buckles or airline-type buckles instead of ties.	*Easy-to-release knots or buckles must be used in case a person needs to be released from the restraint quickly due to an emergency (for example, choking).*
Ensure that you have enough help when applying a restraint.	*Attempting to apply a restraint to an uncooperative, combative person can lead to injury of the person, you, or both.*
Check on the restrained person every 15 minutes to make sure that feeling and blood flow are normal in any restrained extremity (arm or leg).	*A restraint that is applied too tightly can lead to poor blood flow, which in turn can lead to permanent tissue or nerve damage. In addition, checking on the person regularly helps to prevent him from feeling abandoned.*
Make sure that wheelchair wheels are locked and the front swivel wheels are facing forward when a person is restrained in a wheelchair.	*Locked wheels and forward-facing front wheels help make the wheelchair more stable and less likely to tip over.*
Completely remove the restraint every 2 hours, for a total of 10 minutes. Provide range-of-motion exercises and reposition the person.	*Releasing the restraint allows you to reposition the person and perform exercises to prevent loss of mobility and skin breakdown. All patients and residents should be repositioned at least every 2 hours, whether they are restrained or not.*
Attend to the person's needs for nutrition, hydration, toileting, and general comfort.	*A restrained patient or resident is unable to get a drink of water or go to the bathroom if they need to.*
Side rails should always be raised when a person is restrained in bed.	*Raising the side rails decreases the chances that a restrained person could slide out of bed and become tangled in the restraint.*
Record any care given to a restrained person promptly and according to your facility's policy.	*In a legal situation, any action not recorded is considered not done. You can provide the best care possible, but if you do not record it, your effort will not protect you or your facility if legal action is taken.*
Make sure that the call light control is within the restrained person's reach and respond to the call light promptly.	*The ability to call for help if needed and knowing that someone will respond quickly help to make the restrained person feel safe.*
Use restraints only if you have been properly trained in their use.	***Incorrect use of restraints can result in death!***

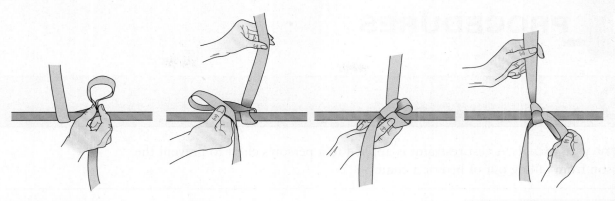

■ **FIGURE 15-4**

 To make a quick-release knot, make a regular overhand knot, but slip a loop (instead of the end of the strap) through the first loop.

The procedures for applying a vest restraint, a wrist or ankle restraint, and a lap or waist (belt) restraint are given in Procedures 15-1, 15-2, and 15-3, respectively. Any restraint that is tied should be tied with a "quick-release" knot (Fig. 15-4). A quick-release knot, or slip knot, will hold tightly if the restrained person pulls against it, but can be undone quickly by pulling on its "tails." The use of a quick-release knot will allow you to free a person from a restraint quickly in the event of an emergency.

Most facilities require either a registered nurse (RN) or a licensed practical nurse (LPN) to apply the restraint, but as a nursing assistant, you will be responsible for caring for the person while she is restrained. For example, you must check on the person every 15 minutes and help her with repositioning, range-of-motion exercises, and meeting food, fluid, and elimination needs. You will also be responsible for observing the person's response to the restraint and reporting any signs of trouble to the nurse immediately. Be sure to consider how frightening and humiliating it can be for a person to be restrained. Do not forget to provide the care necessary to meet the person's emotional as well as physical needs. Record all care that you give to a restrained person promptly.

Physically and emotionally, restraints have a very negative impact on a person's quality of life. As a nursing assistant, there are many things that you can do that may eliminate or reduce the need for restraints. These things require planning and effort, but the effort is considered part of the quality, individualized care that should be given to each person.

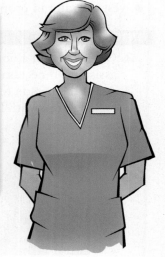

Putting it all together!

- Restraints are sometimes necessary to keep a person safe. Because the use of restraints can be associated with complications (and possibly even death), restraints are used only when all other measures to ensure a person's safety have failed.

- Restraints are never used to punish a person or for the convenience of the staff.

- Restraint alternatives can be effectively used in many situations.

- Physically and emotionally, restraints have a very negative impact on a person's quality of life. The use of restraints requires extra care on the part of the nursing assistant to protect the patient's or resident's safety and dignity.

Tell the Nurse!

Complications from a restraint

- Shortness of breath or difficulty breathing

- The hand or foot beyond the restraint is pale, blue, or cold

- Pain, numbness, or tingling at or below a restrained body part

- The skin beneath a restraint is red, blistered, broken, or bruised

- Increased confusion, sleepiness, disorientation, or agitation

---

PROCEDURE 15-1
Applying a Vest Restraint

Why you do it: A vest restraint is applied to a person's chest to prevent the person from falling out of bed or a chair.

GETTING READY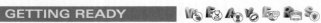

1. Complete the "Getting Ready" steps.

SUPPLIES

- vest restraint in proper size

PROCEDURE

2. Get help from a nurse or another nursing assistant, if necessary.
3. Assist the person to a sitting position by locking arms with her.

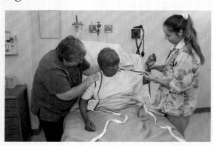

STEP 4 ▪ Support the person's back and shoulders while slipping her arms through the armholes of the vest.

4. Support the person's back and shoulders with one arm while slipping the person's arms through the armholes of the vest using your other hand. Apply the restraint according to the manufacturer's instructions. The vest should cross in the front, across the person's chest.
5. Make sure that there are no wrinkles across the front or back of the restraint.
6. Bring the ties through the slots.

7. Help the person to lie or sit down.
8. Make sure that the person is comfortable and in good body alignment.

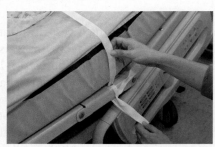

STEP 9 ▪ Attach the straps to the bed frame, never the side rails.

9. If the person is in a chair, thread the straps under the armrests and tie behind the chair (to keep the person seated), according to the manufacturer's directions. If the person is in bed, attach the straps to the bed frame out of the person's reach, never the side rails. Always use the quick-release knot approved by your facility.

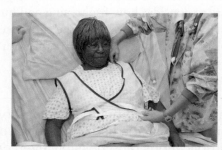

STEP 10 ▪ Check to make sure that the restraint is not too tight.

10. Make sure the restraint is not too tight. You should be able to slide a flat hand between the restraint and the person. Adjust the straps if necessary.

11.
   a. Raise the side rails if the person is in bed.
   b. Lock the wheels and make sure the front wheels are facing forward if the person is in a wheelchair.

FINISHING UP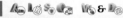

12. Complete the "Finishing Up" steps.
13. Check on the restrained person every 15 minutes.
14. Release the restraint every 2 hours and:
   a. Reposition the person.
   b. Meet the person's needs for food, fluids, and elimination.
   c. Give skin care and perform range-of-motion exercises.
15. Reapply the restraint.

WHAT YOU DOCUMENT

- Type of restraint used
- Time restraint was applied
- Person's response to the restraint
- Position of the patient or resident (when repositioned)
- Food or fluids taken by the person
- Elimination results
- Skin care given
- Range-of-motion exercises completed

PROCEDURE 15-2
Applying Wrist or Ankle Restraints

Why you do it: Wrist or ankle restraints are applied to keep a person from moving his arms, legs, or both.

GETTING READY

1. Complete the "Getting Ready" steps.

SUPPLIES

- appropriate number of wrist restraints, ankle restraints, or both

PROCEDURE

2. Get help from a nurse or another nursing assistant, if necessary.
3. Apply the wrist or ankle restraint following the manufacturer's instructions. Place the soft part of the restraint against the skin.

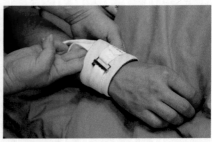

STEP 4 ▪ You should be able to slip two fingers between the person's wrist and the restraint.

4. Secure the restraint so that it is snug, but not tight. You should be able to slide two fingers under the restraint.
5. Attach the straps to the bed frame. Always use the quick-release knot approved by your facility.

6. If applying more than one restraint, repeat steps 3 through 5.
7. Raise the side rails if the person is in bed.

FINISHING UP
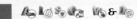

8. Complete the "Finishing Up" steps.
9. Check on the restrained person every 15 minutes.
10. Release the restraint every 2 hours and:
    a. Reposition the person.
    b. Meet the person's needs for food, fluids, and elimination.
    c. Give skin care and perform range-of-motion exercises.
11. Reapply the restraint.

WHAT YOU DOCUMENT

- Type of restraint used
- Time restraint was applied
- Person's response to the restraint
- Position of the patient or resident (when repositioned)
- Food or fluids taken by the person
- Elimination results
- Skin care given
- Range-of-motion exercises completed

PROCEDURE 15-3
Applying Lap or Waist (Belt) Restraints

Why you do it: Lap restraints are used to prevent a person from sliding out of a chair. Waist (belt) restraints can be used to secure a person in a chair or in a bed.

GETTING READY

1. Complete the "Getting Ready" steps.

SUPPLIES

■ lap or waist restraint in proper size

PROCEDURE

2. Get help from a nurse or another nursing assistant, if necessary.
3. If the person is in a chair, assist him to a proper sitting position, making sure that the person's hips are as far back against the back of the chair as possible. (If the person is in a wheelchair, make sure the brakes are locked first, the front wheels are facing forward, and position the footrests to support the person's feet.)
4. Wrap the restraint around the person's abdomen, crossing the straps behind the person's back.
5. Bring the ties through the loops at the sides of the restraint, according to the manufacturer's directions.
6. Make sure the person is comfortable and in good body alignment.
7. Thread the straps under the armrests and secure the straps out of the person's reach, at the back of the chair. If the person is in the bed, secure the straps to the bed frame, not the side rails, out of reach of the person. Always use the quick-release knot approved by your facility.
8. Secure the restraint, making sure it is not too tight. You should be able to slide a fist between the restraint and the person.
9. Raise side rails if the person is in bed.

FINISHING UP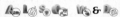

10. Complete the "Finishing Up" steps.
11. Check on the restrained person every 15 minutes.
12. Release the restraint every 2 hours and:
    a. Reposition the person.
    b. Meet the person's needs for food, fluids, and elimination.
    c. Give skin care and perform range-of-motion exercises.
13. Reapply the restraint.

WHAT YOU DOCUMENT

■ Type of restraint used
■ Time restraint was applied
■ Person's response to the restraint
■ Position of patient or resident (when repositioned)
■ Food or fluids taken by the person
■ Elimination results
■ Skin care given
■ Range-of-motion exercises completed

WHAT DID YOU LEARN?

Multiple Choice

Select the single best answer for each of the following questions.

1. After applying a restraint to a patient or resident:
   a. Try to ignore the person's complaints; he just wants attention
   b. Check the restraint every 6 hours
   c. Change the restraint once a day
   d. Remove the restraint at least every 2 hours

2. Vest restraints are applied so that the flaps:
   a. Cross in the back
   b. Cross in the front
   c. Are left open
   d. Are wrapped tightly around the person's chest

3. Which one of the following should not be done when applying a restraint to a patient or resident?
   a. Explain the procedure to the patient or resident
   b. Introduce yourself by name and title
   c. Make sure the patient or resident is asleep
   d. Make sure you have a written doctor's order for the restraint

4. While you are walking with Mrs. Davis in the hallway, she complains of chest pains and dizziness. Your first response should be to:
   a. Assist her to the floor and call for help
   b. Assist her to the floor and go get help
   c. Ask Mrs. Davis to breathe deeply and reassure her that everything will be fine
   d. Encourage Mrs. Davis to continue walking because she needs the exercise

5. What is the leading cause of accidental death among elderly people?
   a. Burns
   b. Falls
   c. Poisonings
   d. Drowning

6. Mary is helping Mr. Watkins to get out of bed when he becomes dizzy, loses his balance, and falls. How should Mary report this accident?
   a. She should tell the nurse about it
   b. She should fill out an incident (occurrence) report
   c. She should tell the nurse about it and fill out an incident (occurrence) report
   d. She should tell the doctor about it

7. Why is a restraint used?
   a. To make caregiving easier for the staff
   b. To punish residents or patients who refuse to follow the rules
   c. To protect a person from harming himself or others when all other methods of keeping the person safe have failed
   d. All of the above

8. You work in the pediatrics unit of a hospital. One of your small patients has a nasogastric feeding tube that is causing her discomfort, and she keeps trying to pull it out. What should you do to prevent the child from removing the feeding tube?
   a. Apply a mitt restraint
   b. Report your observations to the nurse
   c. Explain to the child that she has to leave the tube alone
   d. Use a sensor alarm

STOP Stop *and* Think!

Mr. Lovell, one of the residents with dementia at the long-term care facility where you work, has become very agitated. He is prone to falling, and should not get up without help. However, today he is refusing to stay in his bed or his wheelchair. You get him situated, and then as soon as you leave the room, he tries to get up again. This has happened twice, and you are only in the first hour of your shift. You are very concerned that Mr. Lovell will fall and hurt himself, but you cannot stay with him all day because you have other residents to attend to. Describe some things that you could do to help protect Mr. Lovell.

Basic First Aid and Emergency Care

Any condition that requires immediate medical attention to prevent a person from dying or having a permanent disability is an *emergency*. An emergency can occur as a result of an accident or a medical condition. Emergency situations can occur anywhere, even in a health care setting. As a nursing assistant, you must be prepared to provide care for a person in an emergency situation.

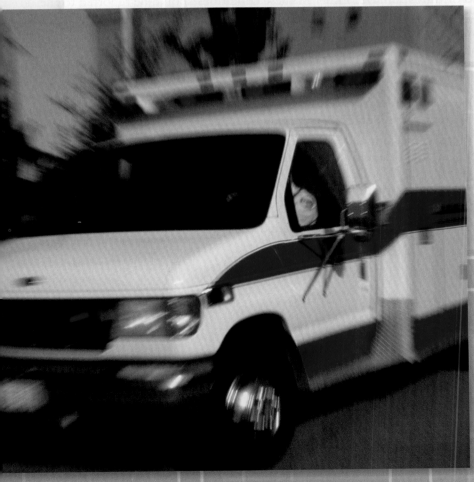

Photo: *An ambulance speeds through the city streets to aid a person in need.*

Responding to an Emergency

What will you learn?

When you are finished with this section, you will be able to:

1. Discuss your role in an emergency situation.
2. Define the words **disoriented**, **unresponsive**, and **basic life support**.

As a nursing assistant, you will spend more time with your patients and residents than any other member of the health care team. Because of this, you may be the first person to find a patient or resident who has fallen or had some other kind of an accident. You may also be the first person to notice that a patient or resident has signs or symptoms of a medical emergency (Fig. 16-1).

Many medical emergencies start out with only a slight change in a person's condition. For example, the first sign of a stroke is often just a slight slurring of speech or a small change in a person's personality. The people you care for will have varying levels of ability and awareness, and you will come to learn what is normal for each person. A person who is usually alert and oriented can suddenly become **disoriented** or **unresponsive**. Either of these conditions should be reported to the nurse immediately. By quickly reporting signs or symptoms that seem unusual or give you cause for alarm to the nurse, you may help to prevent an emergency situation from worsening.

In an emergency situation, your responsibilities as a nursing assistant are clear. You should:

1. **Recognize that an emergency exists.** Use your observation skills and familiarity with the patient or resident to detect changes in behavior or physical condition.
2. **Decide to act.** Stay calm and organize your thoughts. Check the scene to make sure that you are not entering a situation that is potentially dangerous for you or for other members of the health care team. Acting hastily can make the problem worse in many situations.
3. **Check for consciousness.** If it is safe to do so, gently shake the person and call to him. The person may have just fainted ("passed out"), in which case you

Disoriented the state of being unable to answer basic questions about person, place, or time; a state of confusion

Unresponsive a person who is unconscious and cannot be aroused, or conscious but not responsive when spoken to or touched

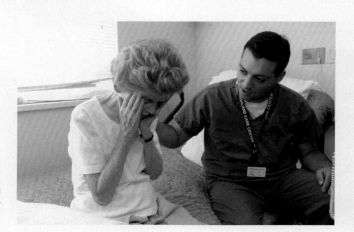

■ **FIGURE 16-1**

Being able to recognize an impending emergency is a life-saving skill.

will need to call the nurse for help. Keep the person lying down until the nurse arrives. The nurse will make sure that no other injuries are present and work to find out why the person fainted. If the person does not respond when you gently shake his arm and call to him, then you will need to . . .

4. **Activate your facility's emergency response system.** Every health care setting has a network of resources (including people, equipment, and facilities) that is organized to respond to an emergency. Hospitals typically have a code or procedure for calling for assistance from within the facility. Home health care agencies, assisted-living facilities, and long-term care facilities may require you to dial "911" or some other emergency telephone number. Know your facility's or agency's policy so that you can get help quickly. Early activation of the emergency response system allows the person to get advanced medical care as soon as possible. This greatly increases the person's chances of survival.

5. **Provide appropriate care until the emergency personnel arrive.** Start first aid or **basic life support (BLS)** measures according to the situation and your level of training. (As in any situation, you should perform only those procedures that you have been trained to do and that are within your scope of practice.) Speak gently and calmly to the person, and reassure him that more help is on the way.

Basic life support (BLS) basic emergency care techniques, such as rescue breathing and cardiopulmonary resuscitation (CPR)

Putting it all together!

- Any situation where a person needs immediate medical attention to prevent death or permanent disability is considered an emergency. Emergencies can result from medical conditions (such as a heart attack or stroke) or from an accident (such as a fall).

- Your knowledge of your patient's or resident's usual condition may allow you to recognize a potential emergency situation. By communicating what you have observed to the nurse, you may be able to prevent the emergency from getting worse.

- In an emergency situation, you will be responsible for (1) recognizing that an emergency exists, (2) deciding to act, (3) checking for consciousness, (4) activating the facility's emergency response system, and (5) providing appropriate care per your training and scope of practice until the emergency personnel arrive.

An emergency can be very frightening for the person experiencing it. Although you will be focused on the person's physical needs, try not to forget about the other needs that the person and his or her family members have. Reassure the person and family members that more help is on the way.

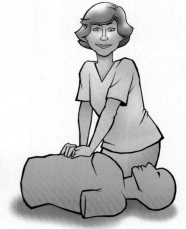

Basic Life Support (BLS) Measures

What will you learn?

When you are finished with this section, you will be able to:

1. List and discuss the measures included in BLS.
2. List some of the organizations that offer approved training in BLS measures.
3. Define the words **respiratory arrest** and **cardiac arrest**.

Respiratory arrest the condition where breathing has stopped

Cardiac arrest the condition where the heart has stopped

Any process that negatively affects our ability to take air into our lungs or to send oxygen-rich blood to the tissues of the body is an emergency. The goal of BLS is to prevent **respiratory arrest, cardiac arrest,** or both. If the person is already in respiratory or cardiac arrest, BLS is used to keep the person alive until advanced medical assistance arrives. BLS measures include rescue breathing, cardiopulmonary resuscitation, and the use of an automated external defibrillator (AED).

- In *rescue breathing*, the rescuer blows air into the person's mouth to perform the function of breathing for the person until the person begins breathing again on her own.

- In *cardiopulmonary resuscitation (CPR)*, the rescuer uses a combination of rescue breathing and chest compressions to sustain breathing and circulation for a person who has gone into respiratory or cardiac arrest. The emphasis is now on starting chest compressions initially and then adding breathing to the cycle after performing 100 chest compressions.

- An *automated external defibrillator (AED)* is a small, portable device that automatically detects a person's heart rhythm and delivers an electrical shock to the heart to stop fast, abnormal heartbeats and restore the heart's normal rhythm. If the facility where you work has an AED, you should know exactly where it is located.

Recent revisions made by the American Heart Association (AHA) have changed the sequence of BLS. You will find the 2010 AHA Guidelines for BLS in Box 16-1. If you find one of your patients or residents in a state of respiratory or cardiac arrest, be sure you know the person's wishes for resuscitation before beginning BLS.

You may receive training in BLS techniques, such as rescue breathing and CPR, as part of your nursing assistant training course. If this training is not included as part of your nursing assistant training course, you can learn these techniques in courses offered by organizations such as the American Red Cross (ARC), the National Safety Council (NSC), and the American Heart Association (AHA).

Putting it all together!

- In an emergency situation, BLS measures are used to keep a person alive until more advanced emergency help is available.

- BLS guidelines include chest compressions, airway, and breathing.

- Training in BLS measures, whether required by your employer or not, will prepare you for emergency situations that may arise in your workplace, home, or community.

Emergency Situations

What will you learn?

When you are finished with this section, you will be able to:

1. List the signs and symptoms of a "heart attack" and describe how you would assist a person who is having those symptoms.

2. List the signs and symptoms of a stroke.

3. Describe how you would assist a person who complains of feeling faint or who has fainted.

4. Describe how you would assist a person who is having a seizure.

5. Describe how you would assist a person who is bleeding uncontrollably (hemorrhaging).

6. Describe some of the types and causes of shock and how you would assist a person who is in shock.

7. List situations that can put a person at risk for choking.

8. Demonstrate how to perform abdominal thrusts or chest thrusts to clear an obstructed airway.

9. Define the words **syncope**, **epilepsy**, **hemorrhage**, **pulse points**, and **aspiration**.

BOX 16-1 | 2010 American Heart Association Guidelines for BLS*

"C" is for "compressions." Initially check for unresponsiveness. If the person is unresponsive, check the person's pulse. You can feel an adult's or child's pulse by placing your fingers on either side of the Adam's apple, over the carotid artery in the neck. An infant's pulse is felt over the brachial artery, in the upper arm. A person in an emergency situation may have a rapid, weak, erratic (irregular), or very slow pulse. As you are checking the pulse, also check by looking at the person's chest to see if she is breathing normally. A person with no pulse or normal breathing needs immediate chest compressions and defibrillation. Chest compressions should be started within 10 seconds.

minute), open the person's airway by tilting her head back and lifting her chin. This prevents the person's tongue from falling backward against the back of the throat, blocking the flow of air into the lungs.

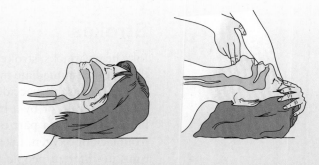

"B" is for "breathing." Give the person two breaths and continue on with chest compressions. If the person does have a definite pulse but is not breathing normally, you should proceed to open the airway and give one breath every 3 seconds. Recheck the pulse every 2 minutes.

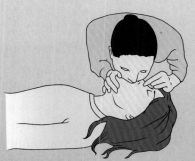

"A" is for "airway." After completing one cycle of chest compressions (100 compressions in a

*These recommendations by the AHA have changed the sequence of BLS from "ABC" to "CAB," have eliminated the "Look, Listen, and Feel" step, and should be used for all adult and pediatric patients with the exclusion of newborns.

Heart Attacks

A "heart attack," also called a *myocardial infarction or MI*, can occur suddenly with very little prior warning. A heart attack is a life-threatening situation that requires emergency care. During a heart attack, the blood vessels that supply the muscular layer of the heart (the myocardium) become blocked and are not able to deliver oxygen and nutrients to the tissue, causing them to die. As a result, the heart is unable to pump blood effectively throughout the body. If the damaged area of the heart is large enough, cardiac arrest can occur.

The signs and symptoms of a heart attack can vary greatly from one person to the next. Signs and symptoms of a heart attack may include:

- Pain or tightness in the chest, which may extend to the neck, back, or arm
- Pale, blue, or grayish skin color
- Excessive sweating
- Trouble breathing
- Nausea or heartburn-like pain

If you observe signs that a person may be having a heart attack, have the person lie down. Raise the person's head to help make breathing easier, and call the nurse or activate the EMS system immediately. Prompt medical treatment can help to minimize damage to the heart muscle. If the person goes into cardiac arrest, you will need to begin basic life support.

Strokes

Like heart attacks, strokes also can occur suddenly and are life-threatening situations that require immediate medical attention. Strokes are also known as "brain attacks" or cerebrovascular accidents (CVAs). They can be caused by a blocked blood vessel in the brain or by a blood vessel that suddenly ruptures. In either circumstance, blood supply to a part of the brain is cut off, causing that part of the brain to die from lack of oxygen. Like a heart attack, a stroke can cause different signs and symptoms in different people. A stroke's results on a person can vary widely—anywhere from only mild physical changes to severe enough to cause a loss of consciousness or a coma. Signs and symptoms of a stroke could include any of the following:

- The person is unconscious or difficult to arouse from sleep
- The person suddenly seems confused or disoriented
- The person slurs his or her speech or is unable to speak clearly
- The person is drooling
- One of the person's eyelids or the corner of the mouth is drooping
- The person complains of the sudden onset of a severe headache
- The person complains of weakness, paralysis, tingling, or numbness of an arm or leg or the side of the face
- There is a change in a the person's vital signs, especially the blood pressure or the pulse

If you think that a person is having or has had a stroke, report your observations to the nurse and activate the EMS system. Keep the person lying down and watch for signs of respiratory arrest until advanced care arrives. New advances in the treatment of stroke have resulted in improved outcomes for some patients, when treatment is started early.

Fainting

Fainting **(syncope)** occurs when the blood supply to the brain suddenly decreases, causing a loss of consciousness. Hunger, pain, extreme emotion, fatigue, certain medications, a stuffy room, excessive heat, or just standing for a long period of time are common causes of fainting. Fainting can also be an early sign of a serious medical condition, such as a heart attack or a stroke.

A person who is about to faint may complain of dizziness or a temporary loss of vision. The person's skin may be pale and clammy, and the pulse may be weak. Have the person lie down and elevate her feet and lower legs. Or you can have her sit down and place her head between her knees (Fig. 16-2). These actions will help to increase the flow of blood to the brain, which may prevent the person from losing consciousness and falling. Stay with the person and call the nurse for assistance. If the person does lose consciousness, keep her airway open and monitor her breathing.

Syncope fainting

Seizures

Seizures, also called *convulsions*, occur when electrical brain activity is interrupted. Seizures can result from head injuries (either recent or past), strokes, infections, high fevers, poisonings, brain tumors, and **epilepsy.**

The severity of a seizure can vary greatly from person to person. Some seizures are mild. The person may simply stop speaking in mid-sentence and stare into space. Other seizures cause violent jerking of the muscles all over the body followed by disorientation and possible loss of consciousness. The person may lose control of her bladder or bowels, and saliva may pool in the mouth. Seizures can last anywhere from just a few seconds to longer than 10 minutes. The person may have no memory of the episode afterward.

A person having a seizure is at risk for injury from falling. The person could also injure herself by striking nearby objects or by biting her tongue and lips.

Epilepsy a disorder characterized by chronic seizure activity

Tell the Nurse!

What to report when a person faints

- What time the person fainted

- Whether there was a change in the person's level of consciousness, and if so, how long this change lasted

- Whether the person vomited

- The person's appearance at the time of the incident (for example, overheated, pale, sweaty)

- Whether the person complained of anything before the incident (for example, loss of vision, dizziness, nausea)

- The actions you took to assist the person

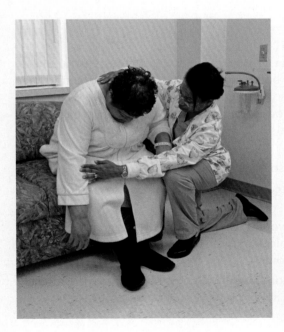

■ **FIGURE 16-2**

Having a person sit with her head between her knees increases blood flow to the brain and may prevent a fainting episode.

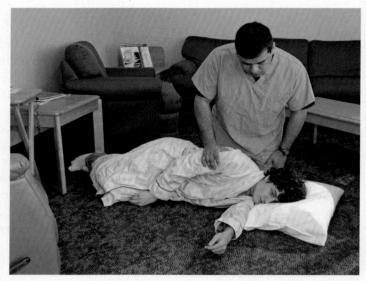

■ **FIGURE 16-3**

After the seizure has passed, place the person in the recovery position and allow secretions to drain from the mouth (this prevents choking).

Emergency care for a person having a seizure involves protecting the person from injury until the seizure is over and keeping the airway open during the period of reduced consciousness afterward:

■ If the person is sitting or standing, gently help the person to the floor and move furniture out of the way.

■ Protect the person's head by placing a pillow or folded towel underneath it and call for help while allowing the seizure to run its course.

■ Never attempt to place anything in the person's mouth or between the teeth. You may hurt the person or get bitten.

■ After the seizure is over, provide warmth and a quiet environment. Place the person in the recovery position and allow secretions to drain from the mouth (Fig. 16-3).

Hemorrhage

Hemorrhage can be caused by trauma or certain illnesses, such as gastric ulcers. Hemorrhage can occur outside of the body and be plainly visible. Or hemorrhage can occur within the body. In this case, the hemorrhage might not be seen unless the person vomits blood or passes blood through the rectum. If hemorrhage is not controlled quickly, the person will die.

If a person is hemorrhaging:

■ Call for help and make sure the person is lying down.

■ Take standard precautions to protect yourself from exposure to bloodborne pathogens.

■ Apply firm, steady pressure to the wound using a sterile dressing, a clean towel, or whatever else is clean and available. Continue to apply pressure to the wound until more advanced medical help comes.

■ If the direct pressure does not stop or slow the flow of blood, raise the affected body part (if it is an arm or leg) and apply pressure to a **pulse point** between the wound and the heart (Fig. 16-4).

Hemorrhage severe, uncontrolled bleeding

Pulse point the points where the large arteries run close enough to the surface of the skin to be felt as a pulse

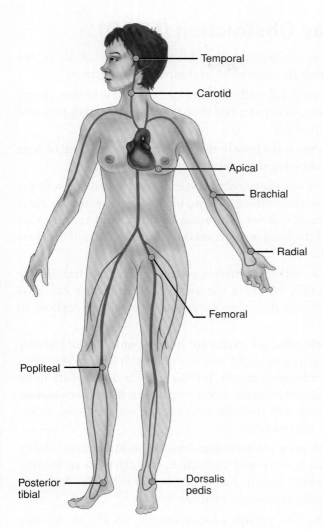

Temporal

Carotid

Apical

Brachial

Radial

Femoral

Popliteal

Posterior tibial

Dorsalis pedis

■ **FIGURE 16-4**

The pulse points.

Shock

Shock occurs when the tissues of the body do not receive enough oxygen-rich blood. There are many different causes and types of shock. For example:

- **Cardiogenic shock** can occur after a heart attack because the heart is too weak to pump enough blood throughout the body to meet the tissues' need for oxygen.

- **Hemorrhagic (hypovolemic) shock** results from massive blood loss. There is simply not enough blood to supply the tissues of the body.

- **Septic shock** is caused by a severe bacterial infection that involves the entire body.

- **Anaphylactic shock** is caused by a severe allergic reaction. These reactions can cause the airways in the lungs to close off, preventing the person from breathing.

A person entering into a state of shock will have low blood pressure that continues to decrease. Her pulse will be rapid and weak. Her skin will be cool, clammy, and pale. She may be disoriented and her breathing may be rapid. Keep the person warm and calm. Elevate the feet and lower legs, and make sure that advanced medical help is on the way.

Aspiration the accidental inhalation of foreign material (such as food, liquids, or vomitus) into the airway

Foreign-Body Airway Obstruction (FBAO)

Aspiration can lead to an airway obstruction that blocks the flow of air to the lungs. Some people are at high risk for aspiration and airway obstruction:

- Children often do not chew their food well; they may attempt to continue eating while running, playing, laughing, or crying; and they tend to place small toys and other foreign objects in their mouths.

- Older patients and residents often have poorly fitting dentures or missing or sore teeth that prevent them from chewing their food properly.

- People who are not conscious or who have weak coughing or swallowing reflexes as a result of paralysis or medication effects are unable to keep the airway clear by coughing. These people are at risk for aspirating vomitus, saliva, and other fluids that pool in the mouth if the head is not turned to the side to drain the fluid and help keep the airway clear.

An airway obstruction can be either partial or complete. In a partial airway obstruction, the object is not totally blocking the airway and some air can pass through. In a complete airway obstruction, the object totally blocks all airflow to the lungs.

- **Partial airway obstruction with good air exchange** (that is, an adequate ability to breathe). The person is coughing strongly and has good skin color. Stay with the person and allow her to continue to cough. If the person is not already in an upright position, assist her into one to make breathing easier. If the person does not quickly cough up the object, call for help because the object could move, resulting in a complete airway obstruction.

- **Partial airway obstruction with poor air exchange** (that is, an inadequate ability to breathe). The person's cough is weak and ineffective, and attempts to breathe result in a high-pitched, "crowing" sound. The person's skin is bluish. A person with this type of airway obstruction needs immediate help.

- **Complete airway obstruction.** The person cannot cough, speak, or breathe and will lose consciousness quickly if the object that is blocking airflow is not removed. The person will be frightened, and may run to the bathroom if the obstruction occurs in a public place, such as in the dining room. (If you suspect that someone who has left the table is choking, you should follow him.) The person may grab his throat in what is considered the universal choking sign (Fig. 16-5).

When a person is choking, call for advanced medical assistance as soon as possible. While you wait for help, perform abdominal thrusts repeatedly, until the airway is open again and the person starts breathing on his own. (In abdominal thrusts, pressure is applied to the abdominal cavity, forcing the air out of the lungs and dislodging the object that is blocking the airway. In the past, this procedure was called the *Heimlich maneuver* after the man who invented it.) If the person does not start breathing on his own, perform rescue breathing after the airway is cleared. You may need to start CPR if the person goes into cardiac arrest.

The procedures for relieving an obstructed airway in a person who is conscious and in a person who is unconscious are given in Procedures 16-1 and 16-2, respectively. The procedure for relieving an obstructed airway in a person who is obese or pregnant is given in Procedure 16-3.

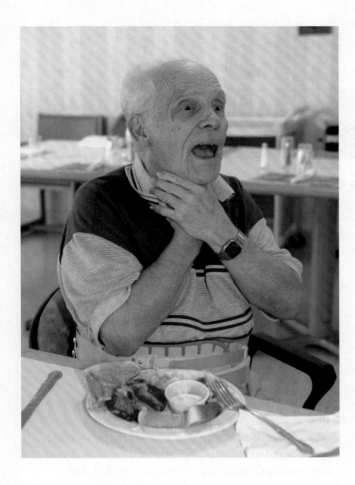

■ **FIGURE 16-5**

Grasping the throat is the universal sign for "I'm choking!"

Putting it all together!

- A heart attack can occur suddenly and is a life-threatening condition that requires immediate emergency treatment.

- The symptoms of a stroke can be very mild or result in unconsciousness or coma.

- Although fainting is not life threatening, it could put the person at risk for injury from falling. If a person complains of feeling faint, have the person lie down or place her head between her knees to increase blood flow to the brain.

- First aid for a person who is having a seizure involves protecting the person from injury during the seizure and keeping the airway open after the seizure.

- Hemorrhage is controlled by applying direct pressure to the wound or to a pulse point above the wound.

- Shock results when the organs and tissues of the body do not receive enough oxygen-rich blood. Keep a person who is in shock warm and calm until emergency personnel arrive.

- Airway obstructions block the flow of oxygen into the lungs and can quickly result in death if the obstruction is not cleared quickly.

PROCEDURE 16-1
Relieving Foreign-Body Airway Obstruction in Conscious Adults and Children Older Than 1 Year

Why you do it: If the object is not removed from the airway, allowing air to get to the lungs, the person will die.

1. Check the person's ability to breathe and speak by tapping her on the shoulder and saying, "Are you okay? Can you talk? I can help you." A person who cannot breathe or speak needs immediate help.

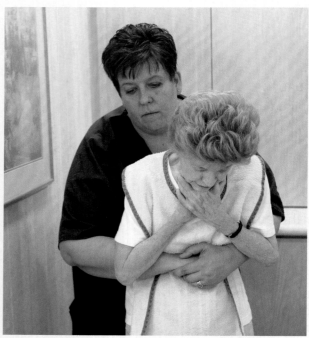

STEP 5 ■ Place your fist just above the person's navel and below the sternum.

2. If the person starts to cough, wait and see whether the coughing will dislodge the object. If the person's cough is weak and ineffective, or if the person is in obvious distress, continue with step 3.

3. Stay with the person and call for help. Have the person who is helping you activate the facility's emergency response system.

4. Stand behind the person with the obstructed airway and wrap your arms around her waist. The person may be sitting or standing.

5. Make a fist with one hand and place the thumb of the fist against the person's abdomen, just above the navel and below the sternum (breastbone). Grasp your fist with the other hand. (Do not tuck your thumb inside your fist.)

6. Being careful not to put pressure on the person's ribs or sternum with your forearms, press your fist inward and pull upward, using quick thrusting motions, until the object is expelled, the person begins to cough forcefully, or the person loses consciousness. Give each thrust with the intent of relieving the obstruction. (In a child, less force is applied to the abdomen to avoid injuring the child's ribs, sternum [breastbone], and internal organs.)

    a. If the object is expelled, stay with the person, and follow the nurse's directions.

    b. If the person begins to cough, wait and see whether the coughing results in expulsion of the object. If it does not, continue giving abdominal thrusts.

    c. If the person loses consciousness, lower the person to the floor and begin Procedure 16-2, beginning with step 6.

7. The person should be evaluated by a doctor following the choking incident.

8. Record your observations and actions according to your facility's policy.

PROCEDURE 16-2
Relieving a Foreign-Body Airway Obstruction in Unconscious Adults and Children Older than 1 Year

Why you do it: If breathing and circulation are not restored, the person will die.

1. **Responsiveness:** Check the person's state of consciousness by gently shaking or tapping her. Quickly check to see if the person is breathing (at least 5 seconds, but no more than 10 seconds).
2. Stay with the person and call for help. Have the person who is helping you activate the facility's emergency response system.
3. Check for a pulse (no more than 10 seconds). If there is no pulse, go on to step 6.

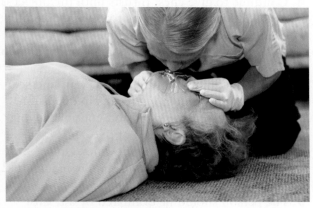

STEP 4 ■ Rescue breathing.

4. **Rescue breathing:** If you feel a definite pulse, open the airway, using a head tilt-chin lift, and deliver one breath into the person's mouth through a ventilation barrier device. Deliver enough air into the person to make the person's chest rise.
5. If the chest does not rise, repeat the head tilt-chin lift and give a second breath. If you are unable to ventilate the person after two attempts, promptly begin chest compressions.
6. **Chest compressions.** If the person does not have a pulse, or if you are unable to ventilate the person after two attempts, begin chest compressions. To give chest compressions:
   a. Kneel beside the person.
   b. Place the heel of your hand closest to the person's head on his sternum (breastbone) and place your other hand on top and interlock your fingers.
   c. Position your body forward so that your shoulders are over the center of the person's chest and your arms are straight. You will want to compress straight down and up. Do not rock back and forth.
   d. **Push hard, push fast:** Compress the chest at a rate of at least 100 compressions per minute with a depth of at least 2 inches for adults and approximately 2 inches for children. Allow the chest to recoil completely after each compression.
7. After you have given 30 chest compressions, quickly open the person's mouth wide and look for the object. If you see an object that can easily be removed, remove it with your fingers.
8. Perform the head tilt-chin lift maneuver. Blow one breath into the person's mouth through a ventilation barrier device. If the air does not go in, repeat the head tilt-chin lift maneuver and attempt one breath again.
9. If the breath does not go in, continue with the chest compressions, object check, and ventilation attempt cycle until the obstruction has been relieved or advanced help arrives.
10. Repeat the chest compression–object check–rescue breathing sequence until the object is expelled, rescue breathing is successful, or other trained personnel arrive and take over.

PROCEDURE 16-3
Performing Chest-Thrusts in Conscious Adults and Children Older Than 1 Year

Why you do it: If the object is not removed from the airway, allowing air to get to the lungs, the person will die.

IF THE PERSON IS CONSCIOUS

1. Stand behind the person and place your arms under the person's armpits and around her chest.

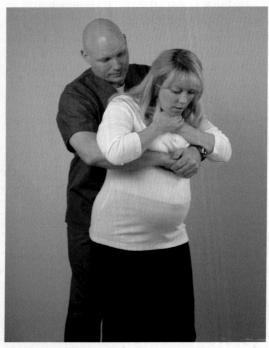

STEP 2 ■ Place your fist over the person's sternum.

2. Make a fist with one hand and place the thumb of the fist against the center of the person's sternum. Be sure that your thumb is centered on the sternum, not on the lower tip of the sternum (the xiphoid process) and not on the ribs.
3. Give up to five quick chest thrusts by grasping your fist with your other hand and pressing inward five times. Each thrust should compress the chest at least 2 inches.
4. Continue to give chest thrusts until the object is expelled, the person begins to cough forcefully, or the person loses consciousness.
   a. If the object is expelled, stay with the person, and follow the nurse's directions.
   b. If the person begins to cough, wait and see whether the coughing results in expulsion of the object. If it does not, continue giving chest thrusts in groups of five.
   c. If the person loses consciousness, lower the person to the floor and begin Procedure 16-2, beginning with step 6.
5. The person should be evaluated by a doctor following the choking incident.
6. Record your observations and actions according to facility policy.

WHAT DID YOU LEARN?

Multiple Choice

Select the single best answer for each of the following questions.

1. A person with an airway obstruction will usually:
   a. Have a seizure
   b. Vomit
   c. Be able to speak and breathe normally
   d. Clutch at his/her throat

2. In the Guidelines for BLS, the "C" stands for:
   a. Cardiac
   b. Consciousness
   c. Compressions
   d. Check for bleeding

3. Where do you place your fist while clearing an obstructed airway in a conscious adult?
   a. On the person's back
   b. Above the person's navel
   c. On the person's chest
   d. Below the person's navel

4. If a person with an obstructed airway is coughing but able to breathe, you should:
   a. Administer oxygen
   b. Use a finger sweep to remove the object that is obstructing the person's airway
   c. Perform abdominal thrusts
   d. Stay with the person and allow him to continue coughing

5. Which is a sign or symptom of shock?
   a. Low blood pressure
   b. A weak, rapid pulse
   c. Cool, clammy, pale skin
   d. All of the above

6. Which of the following actions should you take to assist a person who is having a seizure?
   a. Protect the person's head by placing a pillow underneath it
   b. Clear the area by moving furniture out of the way
   c. Avoid placing anything in the person's mouth
   d. All of the above

7. Which of the following best describes the recovery position?
   a. Positioned on the back
   b. Positioned on the abdomen
   c. Sitting with the head between the knees
   d. Lying on the side

Matching

Match each word with its definition.

_____ 1. Aspiration
_____ 2. Seizure
_____ 3. Syncope
_____ 4. Disoriented
_____ 5. Cardiac arrest
_____ 6. Hemorrhage
_____ 7. Respiratory arrest
_____ 8. Unresponsive

a. The heart stops beating

b. Fainting

c. Unable to answer basic questions about person, place, or time; a state of confusion

d. Breathing has stopped

e. The state of being unconscious and unable to be aroused

f. Severe, uncontrolled bleeding

g. The accidental inhalation of foreign material into the lungs

h. Generalized and violent contraction and relaxation of the body's muscles

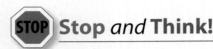 **Stop** *and* **Think!**

You work as a nursing assistant in a nursing home. One of your responsibilities is to check on the residents while the nurses are attending the change-of-shift report. You enter Mrs. Oblonsky's room and find her on the floor. She has no roommate, so no one witnessed what happened. It does not appear that Mrs. Oblonsky fell out of bed. Her color is pale, and her lips are turning blue. What do you do first?

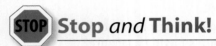 **Stop** *and* **Think!**

One of your responsibilities is to oversee the residents of the long-term care facility where you work while they are in the recreation room. Today, the residents are gathered and getting ready for an activity. Everyone is busy talking, selecting teams, and generally having fun. Everyone, that is, except for Mr. Grant. Normally outgoing and friendly, today Mr. Grant is just sitting in his wheelchair, staring into space without moving. You speak to Mr. Grant and notice that he seems confused and is having difficulty forming his words. The left side of his mouth looks droopy and he's drooling a bit. These observations may be signs of what emergency situation? What should you do?

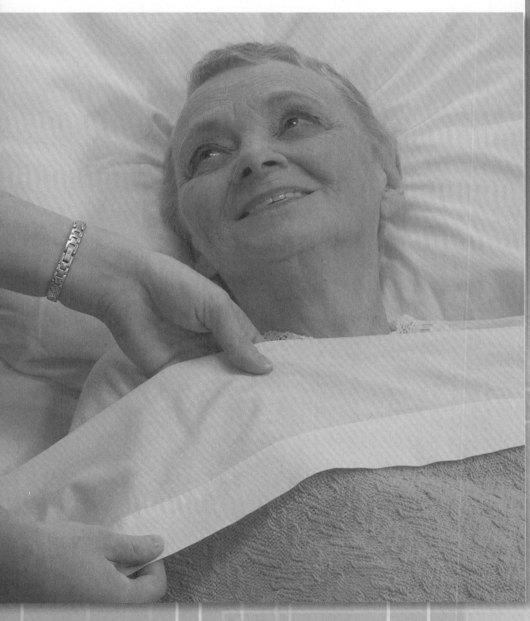

Basic Patient and Resident Care

In Unit 5, we will explore the skills and responsibilities that form the basis for the daily care you will provide for your patients and residents.

Assisting With Repositioning and Transferring

Many of your patients or residents will have limited ability to change position in bed or move from the bed to a chair. As a nursing assistant, assisting patients and residents with movement will be a major part of your daily routine.

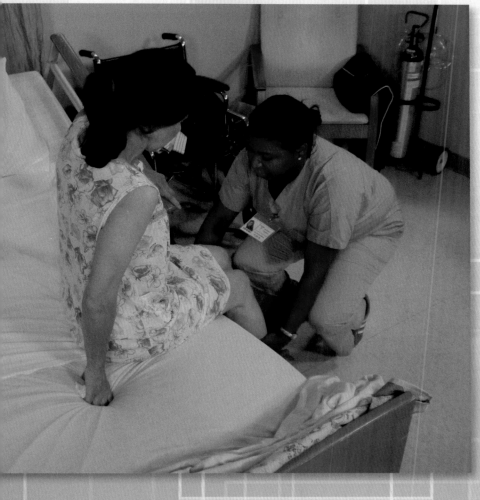

Photo: *A nursing assistant helps a resident to transfer out of bed.*

Assisting With Repositioning

What will you learn?

When you are finished with this section, you will be able to:

1. Explain complications that can occur as a result of immobility and list signs and symptoms of these complications.
2. Describe the benefits of proper body alignment and explain how to check for proper body alignment in a person who is lying on his back, side, or abdomen.
3. Describe six basic body positions that are used when a person must remain in bed or seated for a long period of time.
4. Demonstrate how to move a person to the side of the bed.
5. Demonstrate how to move a person up in bed.
6. Demonstrate how to turn a person onto her side.
7. Demonstrate how to logroll a person.
8. Define the words **body alignment**, **supportive devices**, **shearing**, **friction**, and **lift (draw) sheet**.

Changing position frequently helps us to stay comfortable while we are sitting or lying down. It also prevents complications that can result from spending long periods of time in the same position (Fig. 17-1). Some of your patients or residents may not be able to reposition themselves easily without your help. Weakness, pain, disability, and coma (a state of unconsciousness) are all reasons why a person might need help with repositioning. When you are assisting a person with repositioning, take the opportunity to observe for signs and symptoms of complications of immobility.

Promoting Good Body Alignment

Six basic positions are used when a person must remain in bed or seated for a long period of time (Table 17-1). After moving a person into one of these positions, you must ensure that the person is in good **body alignment** (Fig. 17-2). Good body alignment:

- Is most comfortable for the patient or resident
- Relieves strain on muscles and joints
- Promotes good heart and lung function
- Helps to prevent contractures and pressure ulcers

Sometimes **supportive devices** (Fig. 17-3) are needed to keep the person in good body alignment. Make sure that you ask the nurse or physical therapist about the proper use of any supportive devices for your patients or residents.

Body alignment positioning of the body so that the spine is not twisted or crooked

Supportive devices devices used when positioning a person to help the person maintain proper body alignment, such as rolled sheets, towels, or blankets, and devices designed specifically for the purpose of offering support

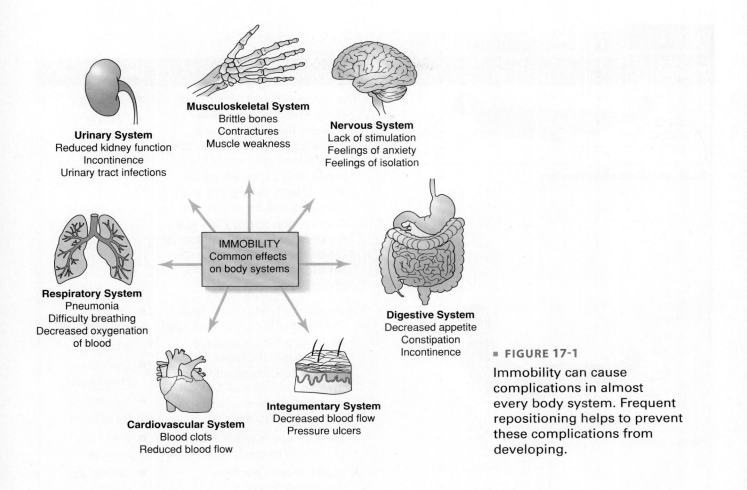

Urinary System
Reduced kidney function
Incontinence
Urinary tract infections

Musculoskeletal System
Brittle bones
Contractures
Muscle weakness

Nervous System
Lack of stimulation
Feelings of anxiety
Feelings of isolation

IMMOBILITY
Common effects
on body systems

Respiratory System
Pneumonia
Difficulty breathing
Decreased oxygenation
of blood

Digestive System
Decreased appetite
Constipation
Incontinence

Cardiovascular System
Blood clots
Reduced blood flow

Integumentary System
Decreased blood flow
Pressure ulcers

■ **FIGURE 17-1**

Immobility can cause complications in almost every body system. Frequent repositioning helps to prevent these complications from developing.

Preventing Shearing and Friction Injuries

Patients and residents who are being moved in bed are at risk for **shearing** and **friction** injuries if they are not moved gently and carefully. The injuries caused by shearing and friction forces can start the process of skin breakdown, which can lead to pressure ulcers. The risk of shearing and friction injuries can be minimized by rolling or lifting, instead of pulling or dragging, a person who needs to be repositioned. A **lift (draw) sheet** is often used to lift or roll a person during repositioning procedures to help prevent shearing and friction injuries.

Techniques Used for Repositioning

General guidelines for repositioning a person are given in Guidelines Box 17-1. Specific techniques used when repositioning a person are described in Procedures 17-1 through 17-5.

Shearing the force created when something or someone is pulled across a surface that offers resistance

Friction the force created when two surfaces (such as a sheet and a person's skin) rub against each other

Lift (draw) sheet a small, flat sheet that is placed over the middle of the bottom sheet, covering the area of the bed from above the person's shoulders to below his or her buttocks

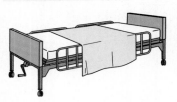

(text continued on page 366)

TABLE 17-1   Six Basic Positions

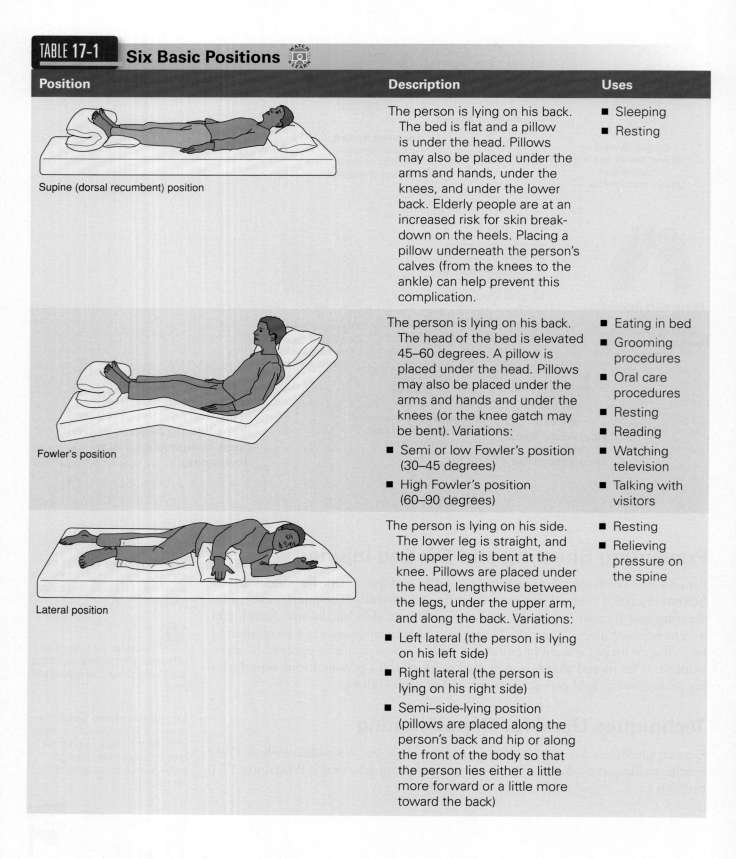

Position	Description	Uses
Supine (dorsal recumbent) position	The person is lying on his back. The bed is flat and a pillow is under the head. Pillows may also be placed under the arms and hands, under the knees, and under the lower back. Elderly people are at an increased risk for skin breakdown on the heels. Placing a pillow underneath the person's calves (from the knees to the ankle) can help prevent this complication.	■ Sleeping ■ Resting
Fowler's position	The person is lying on his back. The head of the bed is elevated 45–60 degrees. A pillow is placed under the head. Pillows may also be placed under the arms and hands and under the knees (or the knee gatch may be bent). Variations: ■ Semi or low Fowler's position (30–45 degrees) ■ High Fowler's position (60–90 degrees)	■ Eating in bed ■ Grooming procedures ■ Oral care procedures ■ Resting ■ Reading ■ Watching television ■ Talking with visitors
Lateral position	The person is lying on his side. The lower leg is straight, and the upper leg is bent at the knee. Pillows are placed under the head, lengthwise between the legs, under the upper arm, and along the back. Variations: ■ Left lateral (the person is lying on his left side) ■ Right lateral (the person is lying on his right side) ■ Semi–side-lying position (pillows are placed along the person's back and hip or along the front of the body so that the person lies either a little more forward or a little more toward the back)	■ Resting ■ Relieving pressure on the spine

Position	Description	Uses
 Prone position	The person is lying on his abdomen with his head turned to one side. The arms are bent at the elbows, and the hands are placed on either side of the head, palms facing down. Small pillows are placed under the head, under the lower abdomen and pelvis, and under the person's lower legs.	■ Relieving pressure on the hips and spine
 Sims' position	The person is lying on his side, almost prone. The head is turned to one side. The knee on that side is bent sharply and supported by a pillow. The corresponding arm is bent at the elbow with the hand in front of the face, palm down. The lower leg is straight, and the lower arm extends out from the side with the palm turned upward.	■ Receiving an enema ■ Having a rectal temperature taken ■ Relieving pressure on the tailbone and hip bone
 Sitting position	The feet are flat on the floor or wheelchair footrests. The knees are bent approximately 90 degrees. The calves of the legs do not touch the chair. The buttocks and back rest against the back of the chair. Pillows are placed under paralyzed arms and hands.	■ Sitting in a chair or a wheelchair

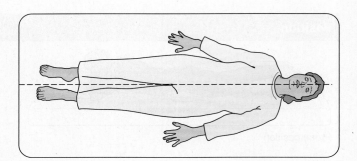

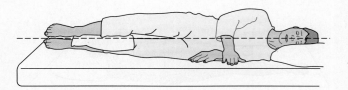

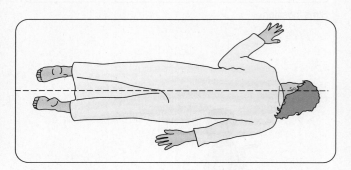

■ FIGURE 17-2

When a person is in proper body alignment, an imaginary straight line can be drawn connecting the person's nose, breastbone (sternum), and pubic bone, whether the person is lying on her back, on her side, or on her abdomen.

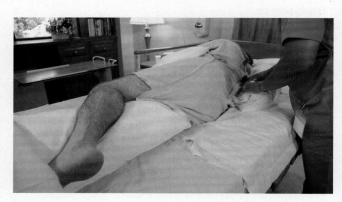

■ FIGURE 17-3

Some people require extra support to maintain proper body alignment. This support can be achieved by using pillows; a rolled-up towel, sheet, or blanket; or a supportive device made especially for this purpose.

GUIDELINES BOX 17-1 Guidelines for Repositioning a Person

What you do	Why you do it
Plan how you will reposition the person and get help from others if necessary.	*Depending on the person's medical condition or size, extra equipment or people may be necessary. Planning ahead helps to ensure that the procedure will be carried out efficiently and with the most consideration for the person's safety and comfort.*
Know the specific positioning guidelines for each person in your care. Refer to the person's care plan or ask the nurse as necessary.	*Depending on the person's medical condition, some positions may be required and others may not be allowed. Failure to follow your patient's or resident's specific positioning guidelines can cause the person injury or discomfort.*
Reposition the person at least every 2 hours or according to the person's care plan.	*Regular repositioning is necessary to prevent complications of immobility, such as pressure ulcers.*
Explain the procedure to the person, even if she is unconscious.	*Understanding how the procedure is done builds trust and helps the person feel like an active participant. Although it may seem that an unconscious person would be unaware of being moved, the person may be aware on some level that someone is doing something to her. Telling the person what you are doing reassures the person and helps the person to feel safe.*
Make sure that you allow the person to assist in the repositioning to the full extent of her ability.	*This promotes independence and self-confidence.*
Provide for the person's modesty by keeping her body covered.	*Keeping the person's body covered preserves the person's dignity.*
Take care to protect any tubes or drains from being pulled out while the person is being repositioned.	*The person experiences pain not only when the tube or drain is pulled out initially but also when it has to be reinserted.*
Use good body mechanics when helping to reposition a person.	*Using good body mechanics will protect you, as well as the patient or resident, from injury.*
Use a gentle touch to avoid injury to delicate skin and fragile bones. Use a lift sheet to reposition the person whenever possible.	*A lift sheet allows you to lift the person (instead of dragging her across the sheets). This helps to prevent shearing and friction injuries.*
Avoid moving or lifting someone by holding onto her arm or leg.	*You could pull the arm or leg out of its socket or stretch the joint beyond its range of motion.*

(*box continues on page 366*)

GUIDELINES BOX 17-1 Guidelines for Repositioning a Person (continued)

What you do	Why you do it
After repositioning a person, make sure that the bed linens are free of wrinkles and that the person's clothing is not twisted or wrinkled up underneath the person.	*Lying on wrinkled bed linens or clothing can lead to skin breakdown. Skin breakdown increases the person's risk of getting a pressure ulcer.*
Gently move the person's clothing aside to check the person's skin, especially on the part of the body the person was just lying on.	*Reddened or pale skin can be a sign that a pressure ulcer is starting.*

Concerns for Long-Term Care

Many people who reside in a long-term care setting will only need minimal assistance with moving and repositioning in bed or a chair. Some residents only need to be reminded to change position at regular intervals. Even though it may be faster to reposition the resident yourself, make sure that you encourage the person to do as much as he can. For example, if the person is able to reach across and grasp the side rail of the bed with his hand while you help him roll onto his side, it will help to promote his independence and prevent loss of function.

It is also important to remember that an elderly person's skin is fragile and can be easily torn or bruised during routine care. Always use a lift sheet when moving a resident up in bed or during repositioning to help prevent injuries from shearing and friction. Use a gentle touch and move the person slowly and smoothly. After repositioning, always check underneath the person to make sure that there are no wrinkles in his bedding or clothing. Lying for a while on wrinkled sheets or clothes can cause the skin to begin to break down, especially for an elderly person.

Putting it all together!

- Some patients or residents may be unable to change positions without help. This is uncomfortable, and the person is at risk for developing serious complications, including pressure ulcers, contractures, pneumonia, and blood clots. You can help to prevent your patients and residents from developing complications of immobility by assisting them with repositioning every 2 hours or according to the care plan.
- Check the person's skin every time you reposition him. Reddened areas that do not return to their normal color; pale, white, or shiny areas; and hot, reddened painful areas in the lower legs could be complications of immobility and must be reported to the nurse.

- The basic positions that are used when a person must stay in bed or in a chair for long periods of time include supine, Fowler's, lateral, prone, Sims', and sitting. Proper positioning helps to ensure proper body alignment, which promotes comfort, relieves strain on the muscles and joints, promotes good heart and lung function, and helps to prevent contractures and pressure ulcers.

- Using proper technique when repositioning a person in bed can help to prevent shearing and friction injuries to the skin.

Assisting With Transferring

What will you learn?

When you are finished with this section, you will be able to:

1. Discuss safety measures related to assisting with transferring.
2. Demonstrate how to apply a transfer belt.
3. Demonstrate how to assist a person to sit on the edge of the bed ("dangle"), and explain why it is important to allow a person time to do this before getting out of bed.
4. Demonstrate how to transfer a person from a bed to a wheelchair and back again.
5. Demonstrate how to transfer a person from a bed to a stretcher and back again.
6. Demonstrate how to transfer a person using a mechanical lift.
7. Define the words **transfer**, **weight-bearing ability**, and **transfer (gait) belt**.

A person's ability to **transfer** is affected by the person's **weight-bearing ability**. Factors such as leg or hip surgery, arthritis, and paralysis can affect a person's ability to bear weight. People who have trouble bearing weight may need help from you to transfer.

When assisting a person out of bed into a standing position, it is important to give the person time to "dangle," or sit on the edge of the bed. When a person has been resting in bed, especially for a long time, sitting up and then standing too quickly can cause blood to flow away from the head. This can lead to dizziness or fainting. Dangling allows time for the heart and blood vessels to make up for the change in position and prevents the person from becoming dizzy or losing consciousness. The procedure for assisting someone to dangle is given in Procedure 17-6.

Most health care facilities require nursing assistants to use a **transfer (gait) belt** when helping a weak or unsteady person to stand, walk, or transfer. The transfer belt is put around the person's waist. When using a transfer belt, remember:

- Some patients or residents may have medical conditions that make it dangerous to use a transfer belt on them. Transfer belts should not be used on people who have just had abdominal surgery or on people with certain heart disorders. Make sure to check the nursing care plan or ask the nurse for specific directions.

Transfer move from one place to another, for example, from the bed to a wheelchair

Weight-bearing ability the ability to stand on one or both legs

Transfer (gait) belt a webbed or woven belt with a buckle that is used to assist a weak or unsteady person with standing, walking, or transferring

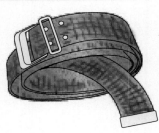

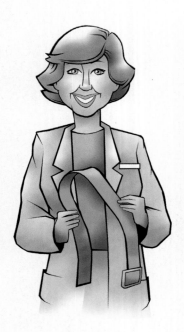

Remember that a person who needs your help during a transfer may feel weak and shaky. The person may be frightened. Always explain the transfer procedure to the person, and allow the person to assist as much as possible. Encouragement and reassurance from you, along with firm, steady assistance, will help your patient or resident to gain confidence in his abilities and learn to trust that you will be there to offer help as necessary.

■ A transfer belt is only an assist device and should never be used to "lift" a person who is unable to bear weight. A person who is unable to bear weight should be moved with a mechanical lift device.

The procedure for applying a transfer belt is given in Procedure 17-7.

Transfer-Assist Devices

The use of assist devices when transferring, lifting, and repositioning patients and residents is an effective way to help prevent work-related injuries for the health care worker. When used correctly, these devices not only help protect you from injury, they are safer for those you care for also. Many of these devices help patients and residents to move and reposition themselves with minimal assistance. This helps to promote their independence and, because they are more likely to continue to use their muscles and joints during the process, prevent complications of immobility.

There are many different types of devices that will be used to assist with moving and transferring people in a health care setting. For example:

■ *Lift sheets* are a simple, yet effective way to help move and reposition a person in bed.

■ *Side rails* on a person's bed can give a person something to hold onto when repositioning in bed or to steady himself when standing up.

■ *Stand-assist devices* attach to the side of the bed or are placed beside the person's bed and allow a person to grasp it to steady himself while he stands, either alone or with your assistance.

■ *Powered stand-assist devices* can be used for a patient or resident who can bear weight on at least one leg and is cooperative. The device mechanically lifts the person and then can be wheeled to a chair or the toilet where she is then lowered into a sitting position (Fig. 17-4).

■ *Lateral transfer-assist devices*, such as a sliding board (Fig. 17-5), allow a person who has good upper-body strength to slide across from a bed to a chair, or from a wheelchair to the toilet, often with minimal assistance. Other types of lateral transfer-assist devices can be used to move a dependent patient or resident from a bed to a stretcher. These devices, such as transfer boards or roller boards, significantly reduce the friction between a person and the sheet during lateral transfers.

■ *Mechanical lift devices* are used to lift a person from one place to another when he is unable to bear weight, is weak or unsteady, or large in size.

Accidents are common during transferring, for both the nursing assistant and the person being transferred. For example, trying to transfer a person into or out of a wheelchair with unlocked or poorly locked wheels is a common cause of accidents. When assisting with transferring, always follow the safety measures summarized in Guidelines Box 17-2. Specific techniques used when assisting a person with transferring are described in Procedures 17-8 through 17-12.

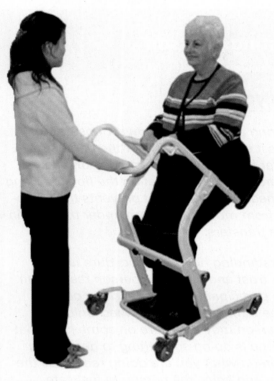

■ **FIGURE 17-4**
Stand-assist devices are used to assist people into a standing position.

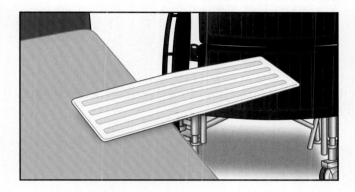

■ **FIGURE 17-5**
Sliding boards allow a person with good upper-body strength to move from one surface to another.

GUIDELINES BOX 17-2   Guidelines for Assisting a Person With Transferring

What you do	Why you do it
Plan the transfer and get help from others if necessary.	*Depending on the person's medical condition or size, extra equipment or people may be necessary. Planning ahead helps to ensure that the procedure will be carried out efficiently and with most consideration for the person's safety and comfort. As a general rule, if a caregiver is required to lift more than 35 pounds of a patient's or resident's weight, assistive devices and assistance from another caregiver should be used.*
Make sure you are aware of what the recommended transfer method is for the person. Ask the nurse or check the person's care plan if you are unsure.	*A person's medical condition may require the use of special equipment, or some equipment may not be allowed because of the person's medical condition.*
Make sure that equipment is in good working condition.	*Making sure that the equipment is in good working condition helps to prevent accidents and injury.*

(*box continues on page 370*)

GUIDELINES BOX 17-2 **Guidelines for Assisting a Person With Transferring** (continued)

What you do	Why you do it
Make sure that beds are lowered to their lowest position and wheels are locked on beds, stretchers, and wheelchairs.	Lowering the bed to the lowest position makes it easier and safer for the person to transfer because the lowest position allows the person to put her feet on the floor. Locking the wheels on equipment prevents the equipment from moving out from under the person as she transfers.
Explain the procedure to the person, even if she is unconscious.	Understanding how the procedure is done builds trust and helps the person feel like an active participant. An unconscious person may be transferred using a mechanical lift. The person may be aware on some level that someone is doing something to her. Telling the person what you are doing reassures the person and helps the person to feel safe.
Check the person's clothing and shoes. Clothing should fit. Shoes should provide good foot support and have nonskid soles.	Long or loose clothing and shoes that do not provide enough support or have slippery soles could lead to tripping.
Use a transfer belt on the person according to your facility policy and the person's care plan.	The transfer belt gives you a safe place to grasp and support the person during the transfer.
Make sure that front swivel wheels on wheelchairs face forward in line with the back wheels.	Having front wheels facing forward makes the wheelchair more stable and less likely to tip over.
Plan the transfer so that the person is leading with her strongest side, if possible.	Doing so allows the person to bear weight in the direction she is going.
Make sure that footrests on a wheelchair are removed or folded back to the side of the chair.	Keeping the footrests out of the way can help prevent the person from tripping over them during a transfer or bumping into them and receiving an injury.
Allow the person to assist in the transfer to the full extent of her ability.	This promotes independence and self-confidence.
Use good body mechanics. Keep your body close to the person and bend at the knees.	Using good body mechanics will protect you, as well as the patient or resident, from injury.

What you do (continued)	**Why you do it** (continued)
Do not allow a person to hold onto you during a transfer. Instead, have an unsteady person grasp the arm of the chair or a transfer bar for support.	*If the person stumbles or falls while holding onto you, you could be injured.*
Do not place your hands under a person's arms to help support her.	*If the person stumbles or falls, the person may be injured when you lift up as she is falling down.*
Do not use a mechanical lift until you have been taught specifically how to use that lift.	*Lifts from different manufacturers may vary greatly in their procedures for use.*
Before using a mechanical lift, always make sure that the person you need to transfer weighs less than the weight limit specified on the lift.	*Exceeding the mechanical lift's weight limit can cause injury to the person, to you, or to both.*

Putting it all together!

- Nursing assistants are responsible for helping patients and residents to transfer from one place to another many times throughout the day.
- Allowing a person who has been lying down in bed to "dangle" before standing up can help to prevent a fall.
- Transfer belts give you a safe place to grasp and support the person when assisting with a transfer. Transfer belts are used according to facility policy and the person's care plan.
- Advance planning and proper technique help to ensure a safe transfer.
- The use of transfer-assist devices is safer for both the health care worker and the patient or resident.

PROCEDURE 17-1
Moving a Person to the Side of the Bed (One Assistant)

Why you do it: Moving a person to the side of the bed is a necessary first step in many procedures, such as the procedures for turning a person onto his side, assisting a person to sit on the edge of the bed, or assisting a person to get out of bed.

GETTING READY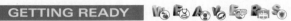

1. Complete the "Getting Ready" steps.

PROCEDURE

2. Make sure that the bed is positioned at a comfortable working height, usually elbow height of caregiver (to promote good body mechanics), and that the wheels are locked.

3. Place the pillow at the head of the bed, on its edge against the headboard. This gets the pillow out of the way.

4. If the side rails are in use, lower the side rail on the working side of the bed. The side rail on the opposite side of the bed should remain up. Lower the head of the bed so that the bed is flat (as tolerated). Fanfold the top linens to the foot of the bed.

5. Stand at the side of the bed with your feet spread about 12 inches apart and with your knees slightly bent to protect your back.

6. Gently slide your hands under the person's head and shoulders and move the person's upper body toward you.

7. Gently slide your hands under the person's torso and move the person's torso toward you.

8. Gently slide your hands under the person's hips and legs and move the person's lower body toward you.

9. Now, position the person as planned (for example, in the prone or lateral position).

10. Reposition the pillow under the person's head and straighten the bottom linens. Draw the top linens over the person. Raise the head of the bed as the person requests.

11. Make sure that the bed is lowered to its lowest position and that the wheels are locked. If the side rails are in use, return them to the raised position.

FINISHING UP

12. Complete the "Finishing Up" steps.

WHAT YOU DOCUMENT

- The position the person was placed in
- Any special support devices used
- Personal care given
- Appearance of skin, especially over bony prominences

PROCEDURE 17-2
Moving a Person to the Side of the Bed (Two Assistants)

Why you do it: This method of moving a person to the side of the bed is safer for both you and the person if the person is large, very ill or injured, or uncooperative. Using a lift sheet also helps to prevent shearing and friction injuries.

GETTING READY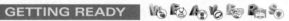

1. Complete the "Getting Ready" steps.

SUPPLIES

- lift sheet (if one is not already on the bed)

PROCEDURE

2. Make sure that the bed is positioned at a comfortable working height, usually elbow height of caregiver (to promote good body mechanics), and that the wheels are locked.
3. Place the pillow at the head of the bed, on its edge against the headboard. This gets the pillow out of the way.
4. If the side rails are in use, lower the side rails. Lower the head of the bed so that the bed is flat (as tolerated). Fanfold the top linens to the foot of the bed.
5. If the lift sheet is already on the bed, make sure that it is positioned so that it is under the person's shoulders and hips. (If a lift sheet is not already on the bed, position one under the person's shoulders and hips.)

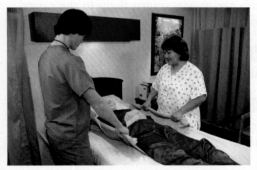

STEP 6 ■ Stand opposite your co-worker.

6. Stand at the side of the bed, opposite your co-worker, with your feet spread about 12 inches apart and with your knees slightly bent to protect your back.
7. Grasp the edge of the lift sheet and roll it over as close to the person's body as possible. This

will provide for a better grip. (Your co-worker does the same.)

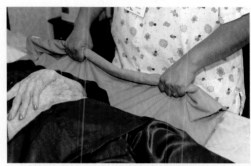

STEP 8 ■ Grasp the rolled lift sheet with both hands, palms and fingers facing down.

8. Grasp the rolled edge of the lift sheet with both hands, palms and fingers facing down. One hand should be level with the person's shoulders, and the other should be level with his or her hips.
9. On the count of "three," slowly and carefully lift up on the lift sheet in unison and move the person to the side of the bed.
10. Now, position the person as planned (for example, in the prone or lateral position).
11. Reposition the pillow under the person's head and straighten the bottom linens. Draw the top linens over the person.
12. Make sure that the bed is lowered to its lowest position and that the wheels are locked. If the side rails are in use, return them to the raised position.

FINISHING UP

13. Complete the "Finishing Up" steps.

WHAT YOU DOCUMENT

- The position the person was placed in
- Any special support devices used
- Personal care given
- Appearance of skin, especially over bony prominences

PROCEDURE 17-3
Moving a Person up in Bed (Two Assistants)

Why you do it: Gravity causes a person who is sitting in bed to slide down over time, leading to discomfort and interfering with the person's ability to breathe. Helping the person to move up in bed promotes comfort and makes it easier for the person to breathe. In order to move a dependent person up in bed safely, you will need to have another person assist you. This is not a one-person task! Using a lift sheet also helps to prevent shearing and friction injuries.

GETTING READY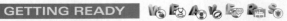

1. Complete the "Getting Ready" steps.

SUPPLIES

■ lift sheet (if one is not already on the bed)

PROCEDURE

2. Make sure that the bed is positioned at a comfortable working height, usually elbow height of caregiver (to promote good body mechanics), and that the wheels are locked.

3. Place the pillow at the head of the bed, on its edge against the headboard. This gets the pillow out of the way. It also pads the headboard in case you move the person up a little too much or too fast!

4. If the side rails are in use, lower the side rails. Lower the head of the bed so that the bed is flat (as tolerated). Fanfold the top linens to the foot of the bed.

5. If the lift sheet is already on the bed, make sure that it is positioned so that it is under the person's shoulders and hips. (If a lift sheet is not already on the bed, position one under the person's shoulders and hips.)

6. Stand at the side of the bed, opposite your co-worker, with your feet spread about 12 inches apart and with your knees slightly bent to protect your back.

7. Grasp the edge of the lift sheet and roll it over as close to the person's body as possible. This will provide for a better grip. (Your co-worker does the same.)

8. Grasp the rolled edge of the lift sheet with both hands, palms and fingers facing down. One hand should be level with the person's shoulders, and the other should be level with his or her hips. If the person is able to assist, have him bend his knees and push during the move upward.

9. On the count of "three," slowly and carefully lift up on the lift sheet in unison and move the person toward the head of the bed. Avoid dragging the person across the bottom linens.

10. Reposition the pillow under the person's head and straighten the bottom linens. Draw the top linens over the person. Raise the head of the bed as the person requests.

11. Make sure that the bed is lowered to its lowest position and that the wheels are locked. If the side rails are in use, return them to the raised position.

FINISHING UP

12. Complete the "Finishing Up" steps.

WHAT YOU DOCUMENT

■ Amount of assistance needed
■ Personal care given

PROCEDURE 17-4
Turning a Person Onto His or Her Side

Why you do it: The lateral position is part of the cycle of positions for people who are unable to reposition themselves. The person is moved from the supine position to the lateral position, then back to the supine position, and then to the lateral position on the other side.

GETTING READY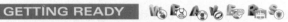

1. Complete the "Getting Ready" steps.

SUPPLIES

- additional pillows or other supportive devices (if not already in the room)

PROCEDURE

2. Make sure that the bed is positioned at a comfortable working height, usually elbow height of caregiver (to promote good body mechanics), and that the wheels are locked.

3. Place the pillow at the head of the bed, on its edge against the headboard. This gets the pillow out of the way.

4. If the side rails are in use, lower the side rail on the working side of the bed. The side rail on the opposite side of the bed should remain up. Lower the head of the bed so that the bed is flat (as tolerated). Fanfold the top linens to the foot of the bed.

5. If the lift sheet is already on the bed, make sure that it is positioned so that it is under the person's shoulders and hips. (If a lift sheet is not already on the bed, position one under the person's shoulders and hips.)

6. Stand at the side of the bed with your feet spread about 12 inches apart and with your knees slightly bent to protect your back.

7. Move the person to the side of the bed opposite the side to which he or she will be turned.

8. Cross the person's arm that is nearest you over the person's chest. If the person is able to assist, have him or her reach over and grasp the side rail on the side of the bed toward which he or she is turning.

9. Roll the person onto his or her side:
   a. **To roll the person away from you:** Making sure that the side rail is raised on the side in which the person is being rolled toward, roll the lift sheet close to the person's body and grasp with one hand near the person's

shoulder and the other hand near the person's hips. Gently roll the person away from you, toward the opposite side of the bed.
   b. **To roll the person toward you:** Raise the side rail and move to the other side of the bed. Lower that side rail. Reaching across the person, roll the lift sheet close to the person's body and grasp with one hand near the person's shoulder and the other hand near the person's hips. Gently roll the person toward you.

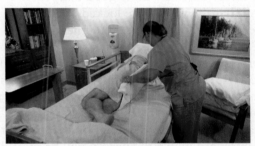

STEP 9 ■ Gently roll the person away from you, toward the opposite side of the bed.

10. Reposition the pillow under the person's head and straighten the bottom linens. Support the person by placing a pillow lengthwise between the person's legs. The person's lower leg should be straight, and the upper leg should be slightly bent at the knee. Place additional pillows under the person's upper arm, and behind his or her back. Draw the top linens over the person.

11. Make sure that the bed is lowered to its lowest position and that the wheels are locked. If the side rails are in use, return them to the raised position.

FINISHING UP

12. Complete the "Finishing Up" steps.

WHAT YOU DOCUMENT

- Position the person was placed in
- Any special support devices used
- Personal care given
- Appearance of skin, especially over bony prominences

PROCEDURE 17-5
Logrolling a Person (Three Assistants)

Why you do it: Logrolling is done whenever it is necessary to move a person who has had back surgery or an injury to the neck or spine. The person is rolled in one fluid motion so that the head, torso, and legs move as one unit and the body is kept in alignment.

GETTING READY

1. Complete the "Getting Ready" steps.

SUPPLIES

- lift sheet (if one is not already on the bed)

PROCEDURE

2. Make sure that the bed is positioned at a comfortable working height, usually elbow height of caregiver (to promote good body mechanics), and that the wheels are locked.
3. Keep the pillow in place underneath the person's head to keep the neck aligned.
4. If the side rails are in use, lower the side rails. Lower the head of the bed so that the bed is flat (as tolerated). Fanfold the top linens to the foot of the bed.
5. Stand with another assistant on the side of the bed toward which the person will be moved. The third assistant stands on the opposite side of the bed. Stand facing the bed with your feet spread about 12 inches apart and with your knees slightly bent to protect your back. One assistant is aligned with the person's head and shoulders; the other is aligned with the person's hips and legs. The third assistant is on the opposite side of the bed.
6. Roll the lift sheet close to the person's sides and grasp it. Lifting in unison, gently move the person toward the side of the bed opposite to that which the person will be turned.
7. Place a pillow lengthwise between the person's legs and fold the person's arms across his chest.
8. The two assistants on the side of the bed toward which the person is being moved should roll the lift sheet in close to the person's body. The third assistant should gently support the person's head during the move to prevent twisting of the person's neck. That assistant should grasp the lift sheet with her lower hand near the person's shoulders. The other assistant

on that side of the bed should grasp the lift sheet near the person's hips and place the lower hand behind the person's knees. The third assistant will assist from behind the person.

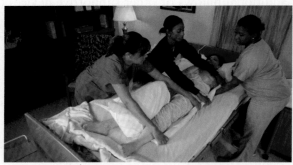

STEP 8 ■ Reach over the person and grasp the lift sheet.

9. On the count of "three," roll the person as a unit toward the side of the bed with the two assistants in a single movement, being sure to keep the person's head, spine, and legs aligned.

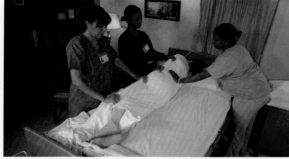

STEP 9 ■ On the count of "three," roll the person in one fluid movement.

10. Reposition the pillow under the person's head and straighten the bottom linens. Make sure that the person is in straight alignment. Support the person by bolstering his back with pillows. The pillow between the person's legs should remain in place, and additional pillows or folded towels should be used to support the person's arms. Draw the top linens over the person.

11. Make sure that the bed is lowered to its lowest position and that the wheels are locked. If the side rails are in use, return them to the raised position.

FINISHING UP

12. Complete the "Finishing Up" steps.

WHAT YOU DOCUMENT

- Position the person was placed in
- Number of people assisting
- Any special positioning or support devices used
- Personal care given
- Appearance of skin, especially over bony prominences

PROCEDURE 17-6

Assisting a Person With Sitting on the Edge of the Bed ("Dangling")

Why you do it: Allowing a person time to "dangle" before getting out of bed reduces the person's risk of falling due to dizziness or loss of consciousness.

GETTING READY

1. Complete the "Getting Ready" steps.

PROCEDURE

2. Make sure that the bed is lowered to its lowest position and that the wheels are locked.

3. If the side rails are in use, lower the side rail on the working side of the bed. The side rail on the opposite side of the bed should remain up. If the person uses the side rail as an assistive device to sit, leave the top half of the side rail in the up position. Fanfold the top linens to the foot of the bed.

4. Help the person into a side-lying position, facing you.

5. Raise the head of the bed into a sitting position.

6. Gently slide one arm behind the person's upper back. Slide the other arm under her knees and rest your hand on the side of her thigh.

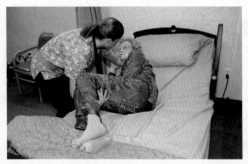

STEP 6 ■ Slide one arm behind the person's upper back. Slide the other arm under her knees.

7. With a single smooth movement, slide the person's legs over the side of the bed while moving her head and shoulders upward so that she is sitting on the edge of the bed.

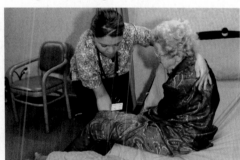

STEP 7 ■ Help the person to sit on the edge of the bed.

8. Have the person put her hands on the edge of the bed, alongside each thigh, for support or raise the upper section of the side rails for her to hold on to. Watch for signs of dizziness or fainting. If the person feels faint, help her to lie down and call for the nurse.

9. Allow the person to "dangle" her legs over the side of the bed for the specified period of time, and then either take her vital signs (if indicated), help her to lie back down, or assist her to a standing position. Stay with her during the entire time.

FINISHING UP

10. Complete the "Finishing Up" steps.

WHAT YOU DOCUMENT

- How long the person dangled
- How much assistance was needed
- How the person tolerated dangling

PROCEDURE 17-7
Applying a Transfer (Gait) Belt

Why you do it: The transfer belt gives you a safe place to grasp and support the person when assisting the person with standing, transferring, or walking.

GETTING READY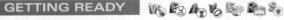

1. Complete the "Getting Ready" steps.

SUPPLIES

- transfer belt

PROCEDURE

2. If the person is in bed, make sure that the bed is lowered to its lowest position and that the wheels are locked. If the side rails are in use, lower the side rail on the working side of the bed. The side rail on the opposite side of the bed should remain up. Fanfold the top linens to the foot of the bed. Assist the person to sit on the edge of the bed.

3. Apply the belt around the person's waist, over her clothing. Buckle the belt in the front by threading the tongue of the belt through the side of the buckle that has "teeth" first, and then placing the tongue of the belt through the other side of the buckle.

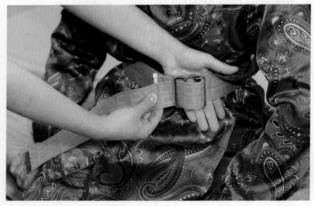

STEP 3 ▪ Thread the tongue of the belt through the side of the buckle that has "teeth" first.

4. Before tightening the belt, turn it so that the buckle is off-center in the front or to the side.

5. Tighten the belt and check for fit. The belt should be snug, but you should be able to slip your fingers between the belt and the person's waist. When applying a transfer belt to a woman, make sure that her breasts are not trapped underneath the belt.

6. Use an underhand grasp when holding the belt to provide greater safety.

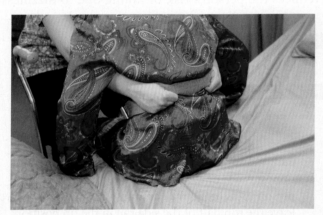

STEP 6 ▪ Use an underhand grasp to hold the belt.

FINISHING UP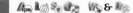

7. When the person has finished transferring and is ready to return to bed, reverse the procedure.

8. Complete the "Finishing Up" steps.

WHAT YOU DOCUMENT

- That a transfer belt was used
- The nature of the transfer (for example, from bed to wheelchair, wheelchair to toilet, to ambulate)
- How the person tolerated the transfer (any complaints of dizziness, pain, or other discomfort)

PROCEDURE 17-8
Transferring a Person From a Bed to a Wheelchair (One Assistant)

Why you do it: Wheelchairs are used to transport people who are unable to walk. Using proper technique helps to keep both you and the person safe during the transfer from bed to wheelchair.

GETTING READY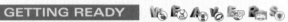

1. Complete the "Getting Ready" steps.

SUPPLIES

- wheelchair
- lap blanket (optional)
- person's robe
- person's slippers or shoes
- transfer belt

PROCEDURE

*Note: This technique can be used with two assistants, having one on either side of the patient or resident during the transfer.

2. Determine the person's strongest side, and then place the wheelchair alongside the bed. (You may need to move other items of furniture or equipment out of the way so that you can maneuver safely.) Position the wheelchair so that the person will move toward the chair "strong side first." Whenever possible, position the wheelchair so that it is against a wall or a solid piece of furniture so that it will not slide backward during the transfer.

3. Lock the wheelchair wheels, and either remove the footrests or swing them to the side.

4. Fanfold the top linens to the foot of the bed.

5. Make sure that the bed is lowered to its lowest position and that the wheels are locked. Raise the head of the bed as tolerated. If the person uses the side rail to assist herself to sit up or stand, leave the top half of the rail in the up position.

6. Help the person to move toward the side of the bed where the wheelchair is located.

7. Assist the person to dangle.

8. Allow the person to rest on the edge of the bed. The person should be sitting squarely on both buttocks, with her knees apart and both feet flat on the floor (to offer a broad base of support). The person's arms should rest alongside her thighs. Watch for signs of dizziness or fainting. Position yourself in front of the person so that you can offer assistance in case she loses balance.

9. Help the person to put her shoes or slippers on and help her to get into a robe. Apply a transfer belt.

10. Help the person to stand. (If the person uses a stand-assist device, have them grasp this to come to a standing position.)
    a. Stand facing the person.

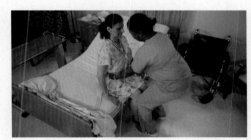

STEP 10 ■ Help the person to stand. Brace the person's knees with your knees, and the person's feet with your feet.

b. Have the person put her hands on the edge of the bed, alongside each thigh.

c. Make sure that the person's feet are flat on the floor.

d. Have the person lean forward.

e. Grasp the transfer belt at each side, using an underhand grasp. (If you are not using a transfer belt, pass your arms under the person's arms and rest your hands on her upper back.)

f. Position your feet alongside the person's feet, flexing your knees. Place your shins against the person's shins to block the person's feet and keep her knees from buckling as she stands up.

g. Have the person push down on the bed with her hands or grasp the stand-assist device and stand on the count of "three." Assist the

(procedure continues on page 380)

PROCEDURE 17-8 (continued)
Transferring a Person From a Bed to a Wheelchair (One Assistant)

person into a standing position by pulling on the transfer belt as you straighten your knees. (If you are not using a transfer belt, assist the person into a standing position by gently pulling her up and forward as you straighten your knees.) Remember to keep your back straight.

11. Support the person in the standing position by holding the transfer belt or by keeping your hands on her upper back. Continue to block the person's feet and knees with your feet and knees.

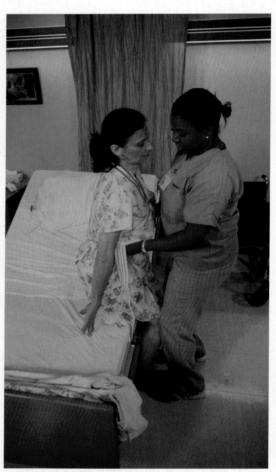

STEP 11 ▪ Support the person in the standing position.

12. Help the person to turn by pivoting on the stronger leg toward the chair. This will allow the person to grasp the far arm of the wheelchair.

13. Continue to assist the person with turning until she is able to grasp the other armrest. The backs of the person's legs should touch the edge of the chair.

14. Lower the person into the wheelchair by bending your hips and knees.

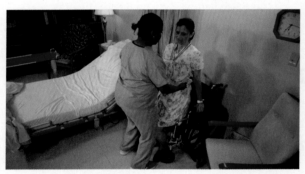

STEP 14 ▪ Lower the person into the wheelchair by bending your hips and knees.

15. Make sure that the person's buttocks are at the back of the chair. Make sure that the person is comfortable and in good body alignment.

16. Remove the transfer belt.

17. Position the person's feet on the footrests of the wheelchair. Buckle the wheelchair safety belt (if ordered) and cover the person's lap and legs with a lap blanket, if desired. Make sure that the lap blanket does not drag on the floor.

FINISHING UP

18. Position the wheelchair according to the person's preference.

19. Complete the "Finishing Up" steps.

WHAT YOU DOCUMENT

▪ Whether or not a transfer belt was used
▪ How the person tolerated the transfer

PROCEDURE 17-9
Transferring a Person From a Wheelchair to a Bed

Why you do it: Wheelchairs are used to transport people who are unable to walk. Using proper technique helps to keep both you and the person safe during the transfer from wheelchair to bed.

GETTING READY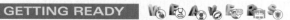

1. Complete the "Getting Ready" steps.

SUPPLIES

- transfer belt

PROCEDURE

2. Make sure that the bed is lowered to its lowest position and that the wheels are locked. Raise the head of the bed, fanfold the top linens to the foot of the bed, and raise the opposite side rail. (You may need to move other items of furniture or equipment out of the way so that you can maneuver safely.)

3. Position the wheelchair close to the side of the bed so that the person's strong side is next to the bed. Lock the wheelchair wheels, and either remove the footrests or swing them to the side.

4. Remove the person's lap blanket (if one was used) and release the wheelchair safety belt, if in use. Apply a transfer belt.

5. Stand facing the person with your feet spread about 12 inches apart and with your knees slightly bent to protect your back. With your back straight, slide the person to the front of the wheelchair seat.

6. Grasp the transfer belt (or pass your arms under the person's arms, placing your hands on her upper back). Position your feet alongside the person's feet, flexing your knees. Place your shins against the person's shins to block the person's feet and keep her knees from buckling as she stands up.

7. Have the person place her hands on the arm-rests of the wheelchair and press down as you assist her to stand by pulling on the transfer belt as you straighten your knees. (If you are not using a transfer belt, assist the person into a standing position by gently pulling her up and forward as you straighten your knees.) Remember to keep your back straight. Alternatively, a person who requires less assistance can make use of a stand-assist device to stand while you offer support.

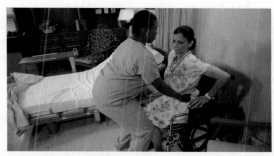

STEP 7 ■ Help the person to stand.

8. Slowly help the person to turn toward the bed by pivoting on her strong leg. Help the person to sit on the edge of the bed.

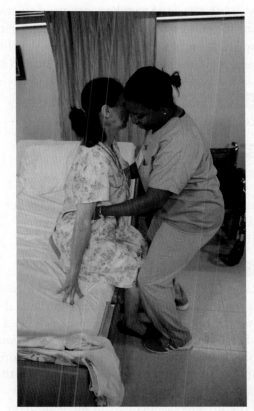

STEP 8 ■ Help the person to sit on the edge of the bed.

(procedure continues on page 382)

PROCEDURE 17-9 (continued)
Transferring a Person From a Wheelchair to a Bed

9. Remove the transfer belt and the person's robe and slippers, if appropriate.
10. Move the wheelchair out of the way.
11. Place one of your arms around the person's shoulders and one arm under her legs. Swing the person's legs onto the bed.
12. Help the person to move to the center of the bed and position her comfortably.
13. Straighten the bottom linens and make sure that the person is comfortable and in good body alignment. Draw the top linens over the person.
14. If the side rails are in use, return them to the raised position.

FINISHING UP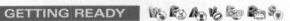

15. Complete the "Finishing Up" steps.

WHAT YOU DOCUMENT

- How long the person has been in the chair
- Whether or not a transfer belt is used
- Position the person was placed in once in bed
- Any personal care given
- Appearance of skin, especially on buttocks
- How the person tolerated the transfer

PROCEDURE 17-10
Transferring a Person From a Bed to a Stretcher (Three Assistants)

Why you do it: Stretchers are used to transport people to other parts of the facility for surgery or diagnostic testing. Critically ill and comatose people are also transported on stretchers. Using proper technique helps to keep both you and the person safe during the transfer from bed to stretcher.

GETTING READY

1. Complete the "Getting Ready" steps.

SUPPLIES

- stretcher
- lift sheet (if one is not already on the bed)
- lateral-assist device (transfer board or roller board)
- blanket

PROCEDURE

2. Raise the bed so that it is level with the height of the stretcher. Lower the head of the bed so that the bed is flat. Make sure that the bed wheels are locked. Lower the side rails. Fan-fold the top linens to the side of the bed opposite the stretcher and cover the person with the blanket.
3. If the lift sheet is already on the bed, make sure that it is positioned so that it is under the person's shoulders and hips. (If a lift sheet is not already on the bed, position one under the person's shoulders and hips.)
4. Two assistants should stand on the stretcher side of the bed. A third assistant should stand on the side of the bed without the stretcher. Have the person fold her arms across her chest. Rolling and grasping the lift sheet close to the person's body, the assistants should move the person toward the side of the bed where the stretcher will be.
5. Position the stretcher alongside the bed. Place the transfer-assist device on the stretcher. Lock the stretcher wheels and move the stretcher safety belts out of the way.
6. The assistant on the side opposite the stretcher reaches across the person and, using the lift sheet, slightly rolls the person over toward her so that the other two assistants can place the lateral-transfer device across the space between the stretcher and the bed, slightly underneath the person. The person is then gently rolled back onto her back.

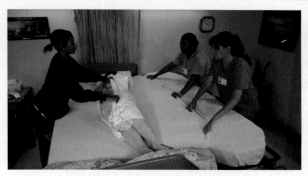

STEP 6 ■ Place the lateral-transfer device across the space between the stretcher and the bed.

7. Each assistant now grasps the lift sheet, and on the count of three, gently slides the person across the lateral-assist device onto the stretcher.

8. Once the person is centered on the stretcher, remove the transfer device. Unlock the stretcher wheels and move it away from the side of the bed.

9. Position the person on the stretcher and make sure that he or she is in good body alignment.

Reposition the pillow under the person's head and cover the person with a blanket for modesty and warmth. Buckle the stretcher safety belts across the person and raise the side rails on the stretcher. Raise the head of the stretcher as the person requests.

FINISHING UP

10. Transport the person to the appropriate site. A person on a stretcher should always be transported "feet first." Remain with the person; never leave someone alone on a stretcher.

11. Complete the "Finishing Up" steps.

WHAT YOU DOCUMENT

■ The time of the transfer
■ Number of people assisting
■ Transfer aids used (drawsheet, roller board, mechanical lift)
■ Use of side rails/safety strap on stretcher
■ Where the person is being transported

PROCEDURE 17-11

Transferring a Person From a Stretcher to a Bed (Three Assistants)

Why you do it: Stretchers are used to transport people to other parts of the facility for surgery or diagnostic testing. Critically ill and comatose people are also transported on stretchers. Using proper technique helps to keep both you and the person safe during the transfer from stretcher to bed.

GETTING READY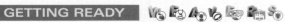

1. Complete the "Getting Ready" steps.

SUPPLIES

■ lift sheet (if one is not already on the stretcher)
■ lateral-assist device (transfer board or roller board)

PROCEDURE

2. Raise or lower the bed so that it is level with the height of the stretcher. Lower the head of the bed so that the bed is flat. Place the

transfer-assist device on the bed. Make sure that the bed wheels are locked. Lower the side rails. Fanfold the top linens to the side of the bed opposite the stretcher.

3. If the lift sheet is already on the stretcher, make sure that it is positioned so that it is under the person's shoulders and hips. (If a lift sheet is not already on the stretcher, position one under the person's shoulders and hips.)

4. Unbuckle the stretcher safety belts and lower the side rails on the stretcher.

5. Position the stretcher against the bed and lock the stretcher wheels.

(procedure continues on page 384)

PROCEDURE 17-11 (continued)
Transferring a Person From a Stretcher to a Bed (Three Assistants)

6. Two assistants stand at the far side of the bed facing the third assistant, who is positioned along the outside edge of the stretcher. (Some facilities allow the assistants on the far side of the bed to kneel on the bed to complete the transfer; follow your facility's policy.)

7. Grasp the edge of the lift sheet and roll it over as close to the person's body as possible. This will provide for a better grip.

8. The assistant on the stretcher side will reach across the person and, using the lift sheet, roll the person up slightly while the other two assistants place the transfer-assist device across the space between the stretcher and the bed, partially underneath the person. Roll the person back onto her back.

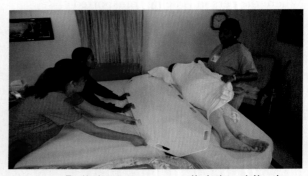

STEP 8 ▪ Roll the person up slightly while the 2 other assistants place the transfer-assist device across the space between the stretcher and the bed.

9. Grasping the lift sheet close to the person's body, on the count of "three," all three assistants slowly and carefully pull the lift sheet in unison and move the person to the bed. Move the stretcher away from the bed and remove the transfer-assist device from the bed.

10. Help the person to move to the center of the bed and, if desired, remove the lift sheet by turning the person first to one side, then the other. Position the person comfortably.

11. Straighten the bottom linens and make sure that the person is comfortable and in good body alignment. Draw the top linens over the person.

12. Make sure that the bed is lowered to its lowest position and that the wheels are locked. If the side rails are in use, return them to the raised position.

FINISHING UP

13. Complete the "Finishing Up" steps.

WHAT YOU DOCUMENT

- The time of the transfer
- Number of people assisting
- Transfer aids used
- Position the person placed in once in bed
- Personal care given

PROCEDURE 17-12
Transferring a Person Using a Mechanical Lift (Two Assistants)

Why you do it: Using a mechanical lift to move a person who is helpless or very heavy is safer for both you and the person.

GETTING READY

1. Complete the "Getting Ready" steps.

SUPPLIES

- wheelchair or chair
- mechanical lift
- sling in proper size
- lap blanket (optional)
- lap restraint (if ordered)

PROCEDURE

2. Make sure that the bed is positioned at a comfortable working height, usually elbow height of caregiver (to promote good body mechanics), and that the wheels are locked. Move other equipment or furniture out of the way to clear room for the lift and the wheelchair or chair.
3. If the side rails are in use, lower the side rails.
4. Fanfold the top linens to the foot of the bed.
5. Center the sling under the person. If the sling is for use with more than one patient or resident, place a cover or pad on the sling. (To get the sling under the person, move the person as if you were making an occupied bed.) The sling should be positioned evenly underneath the person, from shoulders to mid-thigh.

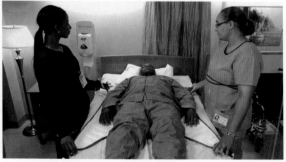

STEP 5 ■ Center the sling under the person.

6. Move the chair or wheelchair to the side of the bed. Lock the wheels.
7. Roll the base of the lift underneath the side of the bed nearest the chair. Center the frame over the person and lock the wheels of the lift.

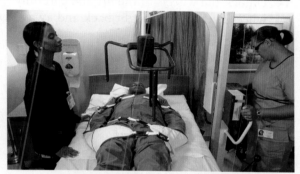

STEP 7 ■ Move the lift into position over the person.

8. Widen the legs of the lift to provide a solid base of support. The legs must be locked in this position.
9. Lower the arms of the lift down toward the person, close enough to attach the sling to the frame.
10. Fasten the sling to the straps or chains of the lift. Make sure that the hooks face away from the person.

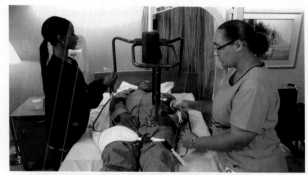

STEP 10 ■ Fasten the sling to the lift according to the manufacturer's instructions.

11. Attach the sling to the swivel bar with the short straps attached to the top of the sling and the long straps attached to the bottom of the sling.
12. Have the person cross his arms across his chest. Check to make sure that all tubes and drains are free and will not be pulled out during the transfer.

(procedure continues on page 386)

PROCEDURE 17-12 (continued)
Transferring a Person Using a Mechanical Lift (Two Assistants)

13. With an assistant standing on each side of the lift, raise the lift until the person and the sling are about 6 inches above the bed.
14. Unlock the wheels of the lift and carefully wheel the person straight back and away from the bed.
15. Have your co-worker support the person's legs as you move the lift into position over the wheelchair.

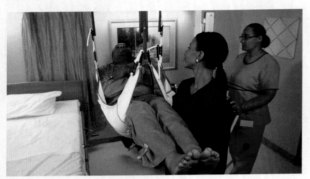

STEP 15 ■ A co-worker supports the person's legs as you move him into position over the wheelchair.

16. Position the person over the chair with the base of the lift straddling the chair.
17. Gently lower the person into the wheelchair. Make sure that the person's buttocks are at the back of the chair.

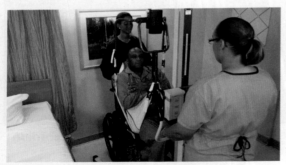

STEP 17 ■ Gently lower the person into the wheelchair.

18. Lower the swivel bar so that you can unhook the sling. Leave the sling under the person unless it is needed for use with another patient or resident prior to moving this person back into bed.
19. Make sure that the person's buttocks are at the back of the chair. Make sure that the person is comfortable and in good body alignment.
20. Position the person's feet on the footrests of the wheelchair. Buckle the wheelchair safety belt (or place a lap restraint, if ordered). Cover the person's lap and legs with a lap blanket, if desired. Make sure that the lap blanket does not drag on the floor.

FINISHING UP

21. Position the wheelchair according to the person's preference.
22. Follow the "Finishing Up" steps.
23. When the person is ready to return to bed, reverse the procedure.

WHAT YOU DOCUMENT

- Type of mechanical lift used
- Number of people assisting
- Where the person was transferred to (wheelchair, geri-chair, bathtub, stretcher)
- Any special positioning aids used
- How the person tolerated transfer

WHAT DID YOU LEARN?

Multiple Choice

Select the single best answer for each of the following questions.

1. Which of the following describes good standing posture when helping to reposition or transfer a person?
   a. Feet 12 inches apart
   b. Abdominal muscles relaxed
   c. Arms out straight
   d. Feet close together

2. When assisting a person to move to the head of the bed, you should:
   a. Face the head of the bed
   b. Unlock the bed wheels
   c. Place a pillow under the person's head
   d. Place the foot that is farthest away from the bed edge behind the other foot

3. Which person is likely to need help moving and turning in bed?
   a. A person who can get out of bed
   b. A person who has Alzheimer's disease
   c. A sleeping person
   d. An unconscious person

4. To transfer a person correctly from a bed to a stretcher, you must:
   a. Use a mechanical lift
   b. Get help from at least five co-workers
   c. Use good body mechanics
   d. Raise the far side rail of the stretcher first

5. When moving and positioning people, you should:
   a. Avoid friction and shearing
   b. Use good body mechanics
   c. Use pillows and rolled towels to maintain the position
   d. All of the above

6. When transferring a person from one place to another, you should:
   a. Use a transfer belt (unless the person has a condition that prevents the use of a transfer belt)
   b. Adjust the bed to the lowest possible height
   c. Lock the brakes of the bed, wheelchair, or stretcher
   d. All of the above

7. A person in the prone position is lying on his:
   a. Right side
   b. Left side
   c. Abdomen
   d. Back

8. When moving a person by yourself and the person is wearing a transfer belt:
   a. Lift from the side
   b. Use an underhand grasp
   c. Use an overhand grasp
   d. Stand behind the person

9. A nurse asks you to place a patient in the semi-Fowler's position while his tube feeding is running. You know the head of the bed should be elevated:
   a. 90 degrees
   b. 60 degrees
   c. 30 degrees
   d. 15 degrees

10. A mechanical lift can be used to:
    a. Move a patient or resident who is very heavy
    b. Move a patient or resident who is very weak
    c. Help a nursing assistant carry out her duties without injuring herself
    d. All of the above

11. When transferring a person from a bed to a stretcher, you should position the bed:
    a. At its lowest level
    b. Level with the stretcher
    c. In the high Fowler's position
    d. In the supine position

12. A person who cannot reposition himself independently is at risk for developing:
    a. Pressure ulcers
    b. Blood clots
    c. Pneumonia
    d. All of the above

13. Why is it important to ensure that your patients or residents are in good body alignment every time you reposition them?
    a. Good body alignment is most comfortable for the patient or resident
    b. Good body alignment helps prevent complications, such as pressure ulcers and contractures
    c. Good body alignment helps the person to breathe easier and improves blood flow to tissues
    d. All of the above

14. What technique would you use to move Rosemary, a 15-year-old patient who has just had spinal surgery?
    a. Logrolling
    b. A mechanical lift
    c. Dangling
    d. Turning

15. Sitting a person on the side of the bed prior to walking is called:
    a. Fowler's
    b. Proning
    c. Dangling
    d. Supining

 Stop *and* **Think!**

Cynthia, a new nursing assistant, has been assigned to take care of Mrs. Adkins. Mrs. Adkins weighs more than 250 pounds and has had a stroke, so she is paralyzed completely on her left side. Cynthia has to transfer Mrs. Adkins from her bed to a wheelchair so that she can go to the shower room. What steps should Cynthia take to ensure a safe transfer for Mrs. Adkins?

 Stop *and* **Think!**

You have been assigned to the north hall and have five residents you must awaken and dress for breakfast. You walk into Mr. Clark's room and announce cheerfully that it is time to get up for breakfast. Mr. Clark is a very large man, with many medical problems. Although he can sit up and get out of bed, he tends to be unsteady on his feet. How would you go about getting Mr. Clark up and dressed?

Assisting With Exercise

Physical activity has many positive effects, even in very old people. Regular exercise keeps the body healthy, reduces the effects of many chronic illnesses (such as diabetes), and delays or decreases the effects of aging. Your patients or residents may need your help to exercise. In this chapter, you will learn about two forms of exercise that nursing assistants often assist patients and residents with: walking and range-of-motion exercises.

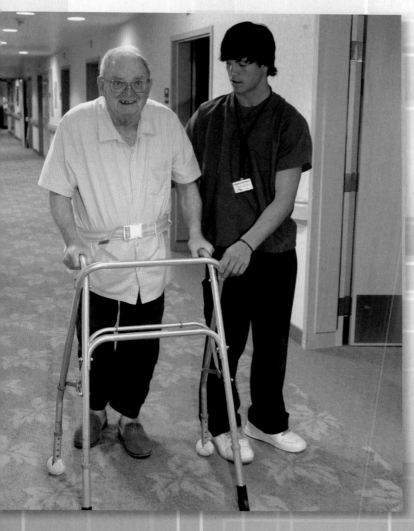

Photo: *A nursing assistant helps a resident to walk (ambulate) down the hall. Walking is an important form of exercise for patients and residents.*

Assisting With Walking (Ambulation)

Tell the Nurse!

Problems with walking (ambulation)

- The person complains of dizziness, shortness of breath, chest pain, a rapid heart beat (palpitations), or sudden head pain

- The person complains of pain when he tries to bear weight, and this is new

- You observe any changes in the person's usual grip, strength, or ability

- A usually cooperative person refuses to participate ("I just don't feel like it today")

- An assistive device is in need of repair, or the person is not using it correctly

What will you learn?

When you have finished with this section, you will be able to:

1. Discuss the benefits of walking.
2. Describe how to help a person to walk safely.
3. Describe assistive devices that a person may use when walking and explain how to use these devices properly.
4. Demonstrate how to assist a person with walking.
5. State observations that you may make when assisting a person with walking that should be reported to the nurse.

It is important to encourage people who are able to walk (either with or without assistance) to walk on a regular basis. Walking helps to:

- Prevent complications of immobility (see Chapter 17, Fig. 17-1)
- Improve a person's appetite
- Prevent constipation
- Promote rest and sleep

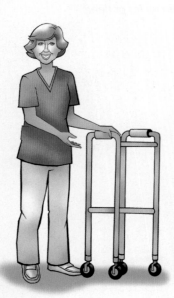

Encouraging and assisting patients and residents to walk enhance their quality of life by providing both physical and emotional benefits. Walking helps a person to remain independent for as long as possible by preventing complications of immobility. If the person is weak or unsteady, your encouragement and assistance can help the person to gain confidence in her abilities. Independence and self-confidence are important for a person's self-esteem.

Your patient or resident may use an assistive device when walking, such as a walker, cane, or crutches (Table 18-1). Because these devices are specially fitted to each person, they should not be shared.

Procedure 18-1 explains how to assist a person with walking. Safety guidelines for assisting a person with walking are summarized in Guidelines Box 18-1.

Concerns for Long-Term Care

Long-term care facilities are often understaffed, creating an increased workload for the nursing assistants who work there. There are so many residents who need assistance getting to the dining hall or to the activities room and only one you! Although using a wheelchair to transfer a resident may be quicker or easier for you, it can result in unnecessary dependence and a decline in the resident's overall abilities. Walking helps to preserve mobility, improves heart and lung function, and promotes digestion. Walking can also stimulate and help preserve a resident's mental functioning.

TABLE 18-1   Assistive Devices for Walking (Ambulating)

Device	Who Uses It	How It Is Used
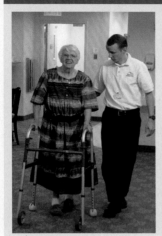 **Walker**	People who can bear weight but may be weak or unsteady	**Proper fit:** Handgrips level with the person's hips **Proper technique:** The person grasps the top of the frame, lifts the walker up, and places it squarely on the ground 10 to 18 inches in front of her body. The tips of the walker are placed flat on the floor. Using the top of the frame for support, the person moves one leg forward and then the other, stepping into the frame of the walker. The process is then repeated. The person can use the top of the frame for support between steps if necessary.
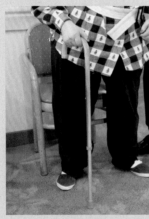 **Cane** (may have one tip, three tips, or four tips)	People who can bear weight but are weak on one side	**Proper fit:** Handle level with the person's hip **Proper technique:** The person holds the cane on her strong side, placing it in front of the body and using it to support her weight while moving. The tip of the cane is placed flat on the floor. If the person is using a three- or four-tipped cane, all of the tips are placed flat on the floor at the same time. The weaker leg is moved forward first, followed by the stronger leg. The nursing assistant stands slightly behind and to the side of the person, on the person's weak side.
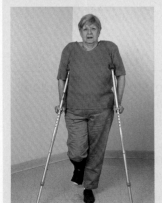 **Crutches**	People who cannot bear full weight on one leg	**Proper fit:** Top of the crutches rest against the person's sides, not underneath the arms **Proper technique:** The person supports her weight with hands on the handgrips (not under the arms). The tips of the crutches are placed flat on the floor. The nurse or physical therapist will teach the person how to move using the crutches.

GUIDELINES BOX 18-1   Guidelines for Assisting a Person With Walking (Ambulation)

What you do	Why you do it
Request help from a co-worker as necessary when you must assist a weak, unsteady, or uncooperative person with walking.	*A person who is weak, unsteady, or uncooperative is likely to fall, injuring both of you. Having help from a co-worker makes a fall less likely.*
Allow the person to "dangle" for the specified amount of time before assisting the person to stand up.	*Allowing a person time to "dangle" before getting out of bed reduces the person's risk of falling due to dizziness or loss of consciousness.*
Use a transfer belt on the person according to your facility's policy and the person's care plan.	*The transfer belt gives you a safe place to grasp and support the person.*
Use correct body mechanics.	*Using good body mechanics will protect you, as well as the patient or resident, from injury.*
Watch the person for fatigue or discomfort.	*A person who is tired or uncomfortable is at greater risk for tripping or fainting.*
Check the person's clothing and shoes. Clothing should fit. Shoes should provide good foot support and have nonskid soles.	*Long or loose clothing and shoes that do not provide enough support or have slippery soles could lead to tripping.*
Check assistive devices to ensure that they are in good condition. Tips on canes and walkers should not be cracked, worn, or missing.	*The tips on canes and walkers provide traction. If they are cracked or worn, they can slip, causing the person to fall.*
Ensure that the person is using assistive devices correctly.	*Using an assistive device correctly reduces the person's risk of slipping and falling.*

 Putting it all together!

- Walking helps patients and residents to remain as independent as possible for as long as possible by providing the health benefits of exercise and preventing complications of immobility.
- Falls are common when assisting a person to walk. Following safety guidelines is important to help prevent accidents.
- Many patients or residents use assistive devices for walking, such as walkers, canes, or crutches. Checking to make sure that the assistive device is in good working order and that the person is using it properly can help to prevent accidents.

Assisting With Range-of-Motion Exercises

What will you learn?

When you have finished with this section, you will be able to:

1. Explain the benefits of range-of-motion exercises for people with limited mobility.
2. Describe the three types of range-of-motion exercises and the nursing assistant's role in assisting with each.
3. List and demonstrate the words used to describe joint movement.
4. Demonstrate how to assist a person with range-of-motion exercises.
5. Define the word **range of motion**.

Normal activities, such as dressing, grooming, walking, and eating, usually put all of our joints through their complete **range of motion** several times each day. Regular movement reduces aches and pains and helps to keep our joints flexible and our muscles strong. However, some of your patients or residents will have limited mobility. These patients or residents may not be able to do all of the activities that would normally exercise their joints and muscles. These patients or residents may need your help with range-of-motion exercises to help keep their joints and muscles functioning.

Range-of-motion exercises are usually performed at least twice a day, often along with other personal care activities, such as bathing and dressing. The exercises can be done while the person is in bed or sitting down. Depending on the person's needs, only one, some, or all of the joints may be put through their range of motion.

There are three types of range-of-motion exercises. These types differ according to how much assistance you must provide.

- **In active range-of-motion exercises,** the patient or resident performs the exercises independently. You may only need to provide encouragement and directions.

- **In active-assistive range-of-motion exercises,** the patient or resident performs the exercises with some help. For example, the person may be able to lift his arm out to the side, but you will need to help him to complete the movement of bringing the arm up near his head.

- **In passive range-of-motion exercises,** you will move the patient's or resident's joints through the exercises. Passive range-of-motion exercises are done for people who are unable to move on their own (for example, paralyzed or unconscious people).

Table 18-2 reviews words that are used to describe joint movement. Procedure 18-2 explains how to assist a patient or resident with passive range-of-motion exercises. Because range-of-motion exercises can hurt the person if they are not done properly, always follow the general guidelines for assisting a person with range-of-motion exercises given in Guidelines Box 18-2.

Range of motion the complete extent of movement that a joint is normally capable of without causing pain

TABLE 18-2 Words Used to Describe Movement

	Word	Definition
	Flexion	Bending of a joint
	Extension	Straightening of a joint
	Abduction	Moving a body part away from the midline of the body
	Adduction	Moving a body part toward the midline of the body
	Rotation	Twisting or turning of a joint
	Supination	Rotation of the palm so that it is facing up or forward
	Pronation	Rotation of the palm so that it is facing down or backward
	Eversion	Rotation of the sole of the foot outward
	Inversion	Rotation of the sole of the foot inward
	Dorsiflexion	Bending the foot upward at the ankle by pulling the toes toward the head
	Plantar flexion	Flexing the arch of the foot by pointing the toes downward

GUIDELINES BOX 18-2 Guidelines for Assisting With Range-of-Motion Exercises

What you do	Why you do it
Make sure to check the person's care plan, or ask the nurse before performing range-of-motion exercises.	There may be some exercises that the person is not allowed to do or certain body parts that should not be exercised for medical reasons. The care plan will also change as the person's physical condition and abilities change.
Use good body mechanics.	Using good body mechanics saves energy and prevents muscle strain and injury.
Remove pillows and other positioning devices.	Pillows and positioning devices can prevent a person from achieving full range of motion of the joint.
Position the person so that each joint can be moved through all of the usual positions.	Positioning the person in a position that will allow each joint to be moved through all of its usual positions saves time (because the person will not have to be repositioned in between exercises) and helps to ensure that all of the exercises will be completed.
Move through the exercises in a systematic way (for example, from the head down).	Developing a routine helps to ensure that you do not forget an exercise.
Unless instructed otherwise, perform the same exercise on each corresponding body part (for example, do the same thing for the right arm that you do for the left).	Exercising corresponding joints equally ensures that both sides of the body remain equally strong and flexible.
Support each joint as you exercise it.	Support reduces discomfort and strain on the joint.
Do not push a joint past its point of resistance.	Each joint has a limit to its range of motion. Attempting to exceed this limit can lead to joint pain and injury.
Watch the person's face for signs of pain or discomfort (for example, grimacing or wincing).	A person may not be able to tell you if what you are doing hurts.
Avoid exercising a painful joint.	Exercising a painful joint can cause additional injury.
If you notice sudden, continuous contractions of the muscle (spasticity), take a break or move the limb more slowly to allow the muscle to recover. Applying gentle pressure to the muscle can also relieve spasticity.	Spasticity is a sign that the muscle is working too hard. It may also be a sign that the person is in pain or that the joint's range of motion has been exceeded.

(*box continues on page 396*)

GUIDELINES BOX 18-2 Guidelines for Assisting With Range-of-Motion Exercises (continued)

What you do	Why you do it
Expect the person's respiratory rate and heart rate to increase during the exercise. If these vital signs do not return to their normal resting rates after the activity ends, report this to the nurse immediately.	*During activity, the tissues require more oxygen and nutrients, so the heart and lungs work harder to supply the tissues. However, once the activity ends, the heart rate and respiratory rate should return to normal because the tissues' demand for oxygen and nutrients will be less.*
Encourage the person to help with the exercises as much as possible.	*Active participation increases the person's sense of independence and improves function.*

 Putting it all together!

- Range-of-motion exercises are used to preserve joint and muscle function in people who have conditions that limit use of their joints and muscles.

- Depending on the person's situation, range-of-motion exercises may be active, active-assistive, or passive, depending on how much assistance the person needs to do them.

- Because range-of-motion exercises can cause pain or injury if they are not done properly, it is important to follow the person's care plan and any specific instructions provided by the nurse or physical therapist when you are assisting a person with range-of-motion exercises.

- Words used to describe joint movement include flexion and extension, abduction and adduction, rotation, supination and pronation, eversion and inversion, and dorsiflexion and plantar flexion.

CHAPTER 18 PROCEDURES

Why you do it: Assisting a person to ambulate regularly helps to meet the person's need for exercise and helps prevent complications of immobility. It also helps to keep a person as independent as possible for as long as possible.

GETTING READY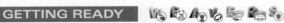

1. Complete the "Getting Ready" steps.

SUPPLIES

- transfer belt
- cane or walker (if indicated)
- person's robe
- person's slippers or shoes (nonskid soles)

PROCEDURE

2. If the person is in bed, make sure that the bed is lowered to its lowest position and that the wheels are locked.
3. Assist the person to "dangle." Check the person's pulse; a weak pulse could lead to lightheadedness. If the person's pulse is weak, stay with her and alert the nurse before attempting ambulation.
4. Help the person put her shoes or slippers on and help her into a robe. Apply a transfer belt.
5. Help the person to stand.
   a. Stand facing the person.
   b. Have the person put her hands on the edge of the bed, alongside each thigh.
   c. Make sure that the person's feet are flat on the floor.
   d. Have the person lean forward.
   e. Grasp the transfer belt at each side, using an underhand grasp. (If you are not using a transfer belt, pass your arms under the person's arms and rest your hands on her upper back.)
   f. Position your feet alongside the person's feet, flexing your knees. Place your shins against the person's shins to block the person's feet and keep her knees from buckling as she stands up.
   g. Have the person push down on the bed with her hands or grasp the stand-assist device and stand on the count of "three." Assist the person into a standing position by pulling on the transfer belt as you straighten your knees. (If you are not using a transfer belt, assist the person into a standing position by gently pulling her up and forward as you straighten your knees.) Remember to keep your back straight.
6. Have the person grasp the cane or walker, if she is using one, in order to maintain balance. The person should hold the cane on her strong side.

(procedure continues on page 398)

PROCEDURE 18-1 (continued)
Assisting a Person With Walking (Ambulating)

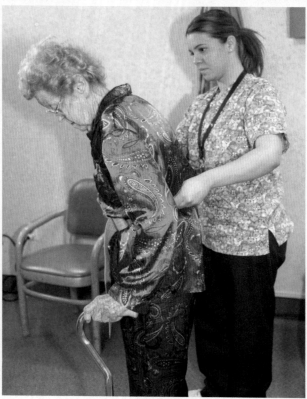

STEP 7 ▪ Grasp the transfer belt with an underhand grip from the back.

7. Help the person to walk, reminding her to keep her head up, looking forward. Stand slightly behind the person on her weaker side. Grasp the transfer belt with an underhand grip from the back. If the person is using an ambulation device, make sure that she is using it correctly.

8. After returning to the person's room, help her back into bed or a chair.

FINISHING UP

9. Complete the "Finishing Up" steps.

WHAT YOU DOCUMENT

- Date and time
- Whether or not a gait belt was used
- What ambulation devices (if any) were used
- How far or where the person ambulated
- How the person tolerated ambulating

PROCEDURE 18-2
Assisting a Person With Passive Range-of-Motion Exercises

Why you do it: Range-of-motion exercises help to keep the joints and muscles healthy in people who have a limited ability to move.

GETTING READY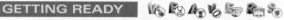

1. Complete the "Getting Ready" steps.

SUPPLIES

- bath blanket

PROCEDURE

2. Make sure that the bed is positioned at a comfortable working height (to promote good body mechanics) and that the wheels are locked. If the side rails are in use, lower the side rail on the working side of the bed. The side rail on the opposite side of the bed should remain up. Raise or lower the head of the bed to a flat or semi-Fowler's position.

3. Assist the person into the supine position.

4. Spread the bath blanket over the top linens (and the person). If the person is able, have him hold the bath blanket. If not, tuck the corners under his shoulders. Fanfold the top linens to the foot of the bed.

5. Perform each range-of-motion exercise in steps 6 through 13 according to the person's care plan, being careful to expose only the part of the body that is being exercised. Repeat each exercise three to five times, as written in the care plan.

6. If your facility permits, exercise the person's neck:

   a. Forward and backward flexion and extension (neck). Support the person's head by putting one hand under his chin and the other on the back of the head. Gently bring the head forward, as if to touch the chin to the chest, and then bring it backward, chin pointing to the sky.

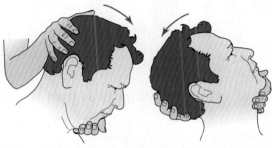

STEP 6a ■ Gently bring the head forward, then backward.

   b. Side-to-side flexion (neck). Support the person's head by putting one hand under his chin and the other near the opposite temple. Gently tilt the head toward the right shoulder and then toward the left.

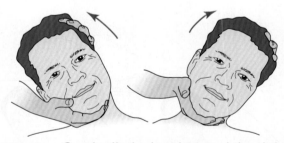

STEP 6b ■ Gently tilt the head toward the right shoulder, then the left.

(procedure continues on page 400)

PROCEDURE 18-2 (continued)

Assisting a Person With Passive Range-of-Motion Exercises

c. Rotation (neck). Support the person's head by putting one hand under his chin and the other on the back of the head. Gently move the head from side to side, as if the person were shaking his head "no."

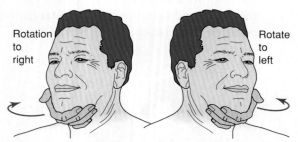

Rotation to right

Rotate to left

STEP 6c ■ Gently move the head from side to side.

7. Exercise the person's shoulder:

a. Forward flexion and extension (shoulder). Support the person's arm by putting one hand under his elbow and the other under his wrist. Keeping the person's arm straight with the palm facing down, lift the arm up so that it is alongside his ear and then return it to its original position.

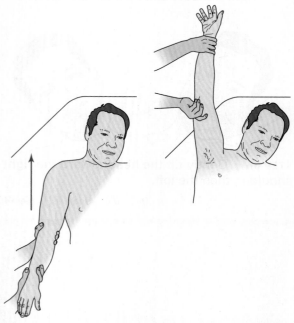

STEP 7a ■ Lift the arm up so that it is alongside the person's ear, then return it to its original position.

b. Abduction and adduction (shoulder). Support the person's arm by putting one hand under his elbow and the other under his wrist. Keeping the person's arm straight with the palm facing up, move his arm away from the side of his body and then return it to its original position.

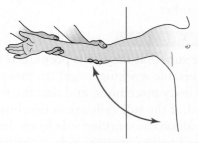

STEP 7b ■ Move the arm away from the person's side, then return it to its original position.

c. Horizontal abduction and adduction (shoulder). Support the person's arm by putting one hand under his elbow and the other under his wrist. Keeping the person's arm straight with the palm facing up, move his arm away from the side of his body. Gently bending the person's elbow, touch his hand to the opposite shoulder, then straighten the elbow and bring the arm back out to the side.

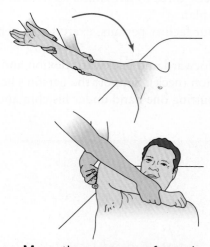

STEP 7c ■ Move the arm away from the person's side, then touch the person's hand to the opposite shoulder.

d. Rotation (shoulder). Support the person's arm by putting one hand under his elbow and the other under his wrist. Move the person's arm away from the side of his body and bend his arm at the elbow. Gently move the person's forearm up so that it forms a right angle with the mattress and then back down. This movement is similar to the motion a police officer makes when he is signaling someone to stop.

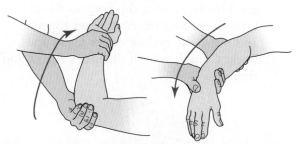

STEP 7d ▪ Move the person's forearm up, then back down.

8. Exercise the person's elbow.
   a. Flexion and extension (elbow). Support the person's arm by putting one hand under his elbow and the other under his wrist. Starting with the person's arm straight and with the palm facing up, bend his elbow so that his hand moves toward his shoulder. Then, straighten out the elbow, returning the person's hand to its original position.

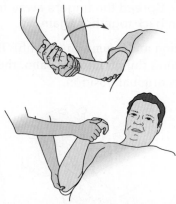

STEP 8a ▪ Bend the arm so that the hand moves toward the shoulder, then return it to its original position.

b. Pronation and supination (elbow). Support the person's arm by putting one hand under his elbow and the other under his wrist. Move the person's arm away from the side of his body and slightly bend his arm at the elbow. Gently move the person's forearm up so that it forms a right angle with the mattress. Gently turn the person's hand so that the palm is facing the end of the bed. Then turn the hand the other way so that the palm is facing the head of the bed.

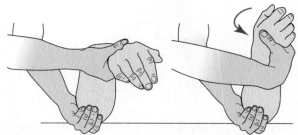

STEP 8b ▪ Turn the hand so that the palm is facing the end of the bed, then turn the hand the other way so that the palm is facing the head of the bed.

9. Exercise the person's wrist.
   a. Flexion and extension (wrist). Support the person's wrist with one hand. Use the other hand to gently bend the person's hand down and then back.

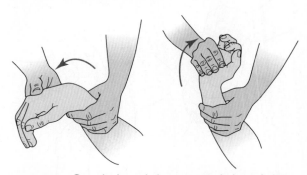

STEP 9a ▪ Gently bend the person's hand down, then back.

(procedure continues on page 402)

PROCEDURE 18-2 (continued)
Assisting a Person With Passive Range-of-Motion Exercises

b. **Radial and ulnar flexion (wrist).** Support the person's wrist with one hand. Use the other hand to gently turn the person's hand toward his thumb. Then turn the hand the other way, toward the little finger.

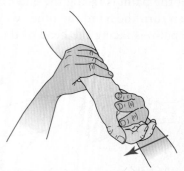

STEP 9b ■ Gently turn the person's hand one way, then the other.

10. Exercise the person's fingers and thumb.

a. **Flexion and extension (fingers and thumb).** Support the person's wrist with one hand. Using your other hand, flex the person's fingers to make a fist, tucking his thumb under the fingers. Then straighten each finger and the thumb, one by one.

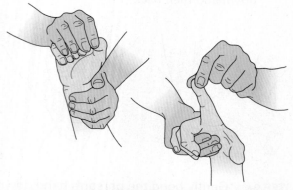

STEP 10a ■ Flex the person's fingers to make a fist, then straighten each finger and thumb, one by one.

b. **Abduction and adduction (fingers and thumb).** With one hand, hold the person's thumb and index finger together. With the other hand, move the middle finger away from the index finger. Then move the middle finger back toward the index finger and hold the middle finger, index finger, and thumb together. Next, move the ring finger away from the other two fingers and thumb, then move it back toward the group. Do the same with the little finger. Finally, reverse the process. Hold the little finger and the ring finger together and move the middle finger away and back. Complete with the index finger and thumb.

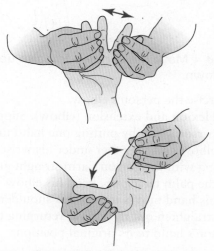

STEP 10b ■ Spread the fingers away from each other, then back together again.

c. **Flexion and extension (thumb).** Bend the person's thumb into his palm, then return it to its original position.

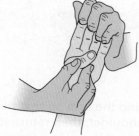

STEP 10c ■ Bend the thumb into the palm, then return it to its original position.

d. Opposition. Touch each fingertip to the thumb.

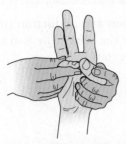

STEP 10d ▪ Touch each fingertip to the thumb.

11. Exercise the person's hip and knee.

a. Forward flexion and extension (hip and knee). Support the person's leg by putting one hand under his knee and the other under his ankle. Gently bend the person's knee, moving it toward his head. Then straighten the person's knee and gently lower the leg to the bed.

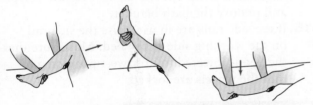

STEP 11a ▪ Gently bend the knee, moving it toward the head. Then straighten the leg and lower it to the bed.

b. Abduction and adduction (hip). Support the person's leg by putting one hand under his knee and the other under his ankle. Keeping the person's leg straight, move his leg away from the side of his body and then return it to its original position.

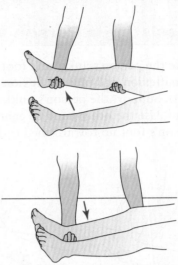

STEP 11b ▪ Move the leg away from the person's side, then return it to its original position.

c. Rotation (hip). Support the person's leg by putting one hand under his knee and the other under his ankle. Keeping the person's leg straight, gently turn the leg inward and then outward.

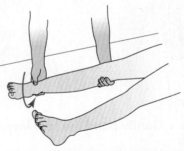

STEP 11c ▪ Gently turn the leg inward, then outward.

(*procedure continues on page 404*)

PROCEDURE 18-2 (continued)
Assisting a Person With Passive Range-of-Motion Exercises

12. Exercise the person's ankle and foot.
    a. **Dorsiflexion and plantar flexion (ankle and foot).** Support the person's ankle with one hand. Use the other hand to gently bend the person's foot up toward the head and then back.

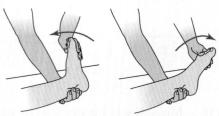

STEP 12a ▪ Gently bend the foot toward the head, then back.

    b. **Inversion and eversion (ankle and foot).** Support the person's ankle with one hand. Use the other hand to gently turn the inside of the foot inward and then outward.

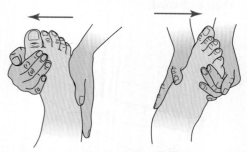

STEP 12b ▪ Gently bend the foot inward, then outward.

13. Exercise the person's toes.
    a. **Flexion and extension (toes).** Put one hand under the person's foot. Put the other hand over the person's toes. Curl the toes downward and then straighten them.

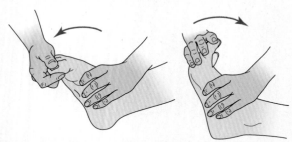

STEP 13a ▪ Curl the toes downward, then straighten them.

    b. **Abduction and adduction (toes).** Spread each toe the same way you spread each finger in step 10b.

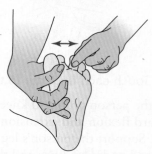

STEP 13b ▪ Spread the toes away from each other, then back together again.

14. Straighten the bed linens and make sure that the person is comfortable and in good body alignment. Draw the top linens over the person and remove the bath blanket.
15. If the side rails are in use, raise the side rail on the working side of the bed. Make sure that the bed is lowered to its lowest position and that the wheels are locked.

FINISHING UP

16. Complete the "Finishing Up" steps.

WHAT YOU DOCUMENT

- Date and time
- Body parts exercised
- Complaints of pain or discomfort
- Any decrease in the person's usual range of motion

WHAT DID YOU LEARN?

Multiple Choice

Select the single best answer for each of the following questions.

1. Mr. Davis is recovering from a stroke that left him weak on his right side. He is now ready to start walking again. Which assistive device would be best for Mr. Davis?
   a. Crutches
   b. A cane held in his right hand
   c. A walker
   d. A cane held in his left hand

2. Assisting a person to walk on a regular basis helps to do all of the following except:
   a. Improve a person's appetite
   b. Prevent complications of immobility
   c. Cause constipation
   d. Promote rest and sleep

3. A patient or resident performs the ordered range-of-motion exercises independently in which type of exercise?
   a. Active-assistive
   b. Passive
   c. Active
   d. Flexion

4. The proper height for a cane is:
   a. Handle level with the person's hip
   b. Handle level with the person's waist
   c. Handle slightly above the person's waist
   d. Handle slightly below the person's hip

Matching

Match each word used to describe movement with the appropriate picture.

_____ 1. Flexion/extension

_____ 2. Supination/pronation

_____ 3. Dorsiflexion/plantar flexion

_____ 4. Rotation

_____ 5. Abduction/adduction

_____ 6. Inversion/eversion

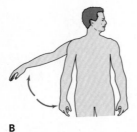

A

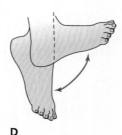

D

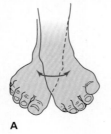

B

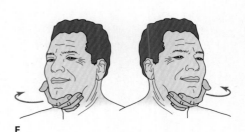

E

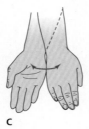

C

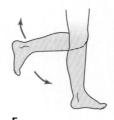

F

STOP Stop *and* Think!

You are preparing to assist Mrs. Olsen out of bed for a walk down the hall to go to BINGO. After sitting her on the side of the bed, you are assisting her with her shoes and you notice that she is pale and breathing rapidly. When you ask her if she feels dizzy, she says no. You suspect that she really is in a hurry to go to BINGO so that she can get her favorite seat. What should you do now?

Bedmaking

For someone who is tired or ill, nothing is quite as comforting as clean, crisp linens on the bed. Clean linens help your patients or residents to rest. Clean linens are also important for controlling the spread of infection and for helping to prevent pressure ulcers.

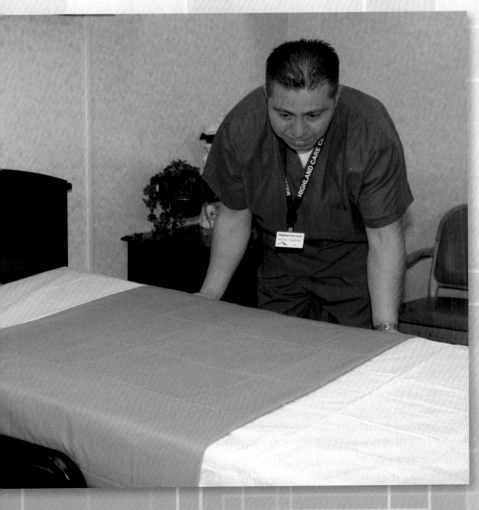

Photo: *A well-made bed is essential to a person's mental and physical well-being. Here, a nursing assistant tucks in a lift (draw) sheet.*

Linens

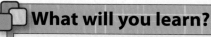

What will you learn?

When you are finished with this section, you will be able to:

1. List the different types of linens and describe their uses.
2. Describe how to handle clean and soiled linens in a way that prevents the spread of infection.
3. Define the words **bed protector** and **bath blanket**.

Types of Linens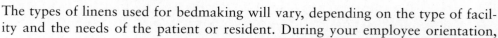

The types of linens used for bedmaking will vary, depending on the type of facility and the needs of the patient or resident. During your employee orientation, you will learn which linens to use to make the beds. Additional information specific to each patient or resident will be provided on the nursing care plan. Linens, in the order that they are put on the bed, may include the following:

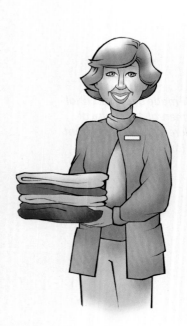

> All of us can probably remember a time when we were really sick and someone came and freshened us up and changed our sheets. Think about how loved and well cared for you felt then! That is how your patients or residents will feel when you replace their hot, wrinkled, soiled linens with cool, ironed, clean ones.

- A **mattress pad** is a thick layer of padding that is placed on the mattress to help make the bed more comfortable for the patient or resident and to protect the mattress from moisture and soiling. Mattress pads may be "fitted" (with elasticized sides that grip the sides of the mattress) or "flat." Many health care facilities now have mattresses that do not require the use of a mattress pad. The mattress is covered with a material that is resistant to liquid and easily cleaned. This material allows air to circulate so that heat does not build up underneath the person lying there. This helps to prevent skin breakdown.

- A **bottom sheet** is placed over the mattress pad. The bottom sheet may be fitted or flat.

- A **lift (draw) sheet** is a small, flat sheet that is placed over the middle of the bottom sheet. The lift sheet is used during repositioning procedures (see Chapter 17) and also as a moisture-absorbing barrier between the person's body and the mattress if a mattress pad is not being used. If the lift sheet is made of rubber, cover it with a cotton lift sheet to protect the person's skin from contact with the rubber. If a folded flat sheet is being used as a lift sheet, position the folded edge of the sheet above the person's shoulders and the loose ends below the buttocks.

Bed protector a square of quilted absorbent fabric backed with waterproof material that measures approximately 3 feet by 3 feet; used to prevent soiling of the bottom linens; sometimes called an *incontinence pad* or a *soaker pad*

- A **bed protector** is used for people who are incontinent and for people with draining wounds. The urine, feces, or wound drainage is pulled away from the person's body by the absorbent layers of the bed protector, and the waterproof layer keeps the liquid from soiling the linens underneath. Sometimes, only the bed protector needs to be changed, resulting in more efficient and economical care. Bed protectors may be disposable, or they may be laundered and reused.

- A **top sheet** is a flat sheet that covers the person.
- A **blanket** provides warmth. Blankets may be wool, cotton, or synthetic, depending on the person's preference and the climate. Because wool blankets can create static and sparks, they should be used with caution if the person is receiving oxygen therapy. Electric blankets should be checked for faulty wiring or plugs and may not be safe to use if the person is incontinent or unable to adjust the controls independently (for example, if the person is very old or very young). Electric blankets should only be used according to facility policy.
- A **bedspread** covers the bed and adds a decorative touch to the person's room. Many long-term care facilities encourage residents to use their own bedspreads from home. This practice helps residents to feel more at home in the facility.
- A **pillowcase** is used to cover the pillow and protect it from moisture and soiling.
- A **bath blanket** is not made into the bed, but because it is used during bed baths and linen changes, it is gathered along with the other linens.

Bath blanket a lightweight cotton blanket used to cover a person during a bed bath or linen change to help provide modesty and warmth

Concerns for Long-Term Care

Many long-term care facilities use flannel-type sheets to provide extra warmth, especially for elderly residents who may feel cold in bed. Residents are encouraged to use their own bedspreads, comforters, decorative pillows, and coverlets to add a "touch of home". Be sure that you handle these personal items with care when you are changing the person's bed linens.

Handling Linens

Both clean and soiled linens must be handled in a way that prevents the spread of infection (Guidelines Box 19-1).

 Putting it all together!

- Many different linens are used to make a bed. Facility policy and the patient's or resident's needs dictate which linens are used to make the bed.
- Linens that are typically used to make a bed in a health care facility include a mattress pad, a bottom sheet, a lift (draw) sheet, a bed protector, a top sheet, a blanket, a bedspread, and a pillow and pillowcase. A bath blanket is gathered along with the bed linens and is used to provide modesty and warmth during procedures that involve exposing the patient or resident by removing or folding down the top linens.
- Following standard infection control practices—such as performing proper hand hygiene before handling clean linens, holding linens away from your uniform, and wearing gloves when removing soiled linens from the bed—is important to keep yourself, your co-workers, and your patients or residents safe from infection.

GUIDELINES BOX 19-1 Guidelines for Handling Linens

What you do	Why you do it
Always perform proper hand hygiene before collecting clean linens.	*Proper hand hygiene prevents pathogens on your hands from being transferred to the clean linens.*
Do not hold linens, clean or dirty, against your uniform. 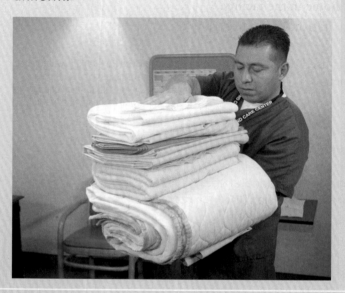	*If you hold clean linens against your uniform, pathogens on your uniform could be transferred to the linens. If you hold dirty linens against your uniform, then pathogens from the dirty linens could be transferred to your uniform.*
When collecting linens, collect only those that you will need for that person's bed. For example, if a lift sheet is not needed, do not collect one.	*Extra linens brought into a person's room are considered soiled, and therefore must not be returned to the clean linen cart or used for another person. These linens must now be laundered, which costs the facility extra money and labor and creates additional wear on the linens, shortening their lifetime of use.*
Collect linens in the order that they will be used. Once you have collected your stack of linens, flip the stack over so that the item you will need first is on the top of the stack.	*Collecting linens in the order that they will be put on the bed helps you to remember which linens you need to collect. In addition, because the linens will be arranged in order of use, you will be able to make the bed more efficiently without having to search through the stack for the proper item.*
Place clean linens on a clean surface in the room, such as the over-bed table or a chair. Do not place clean linens on the floor.	*Clean linens can become contaminated with pathogens if you place them on a "dirty" surface, such as the floor.*

What you do (continued)

Wear gloves when removing used linens from a bed. Roll the linens toward the center of the bed to confine the soiled area inside.

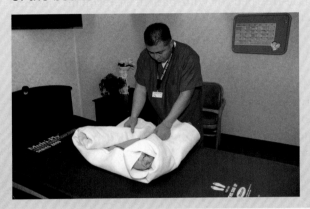

If body fluids or substances leak through the linens to the mattress or bed frame, the mattress or bed frame should be wiped with an appropriate cleaning solution before placing clean linens on the bed. Remove your gloves and perform hand hygiene before handling the clean linens.

After removing the dirty linens from the bed, place them in the linen hamper immediately. Your facility may require you to place dirty linens in a smaller linen bag before placing them in the linen hamper. Do not place dirty linens on the floor or on any other surface.

Why you do it (continued)

Any item contaminated with blood or other body substances can expose you to pathogens. Following the standard precautions and wearing proper personal protective equipment (PPE) will help to minimize your exposure. Confining the soiled area to the inside of the linens helps to ensure that other people, such as the people in the laundry, do not come in contact with the soiled area.

These infection control methods help to prevent the clean sheets from becoming contaminated.

Placing the dirty linens in the linen hamper immediately helps to control the spread of infection.

Standard Bedmaking Techniques

What will you learn?

When you are finished with this section, you will be able to:
1. Explain when a patient's or resident's linens should be changed.
2. Demonstrate how to miter a corner.
3. Demonstrate how to make an unoccupied bed.
4. Demonstrate how to make an occupied bed.
5. Define the words **mitered corner**, **closed bed**, **open bed**, **fanfolded**, and **surgical bed**.

Routine bedmaking is usually done in the morning, before visiting hours, while your patients or residents are bathing or dressing. At the minimum, the linens are changed completely according to the schedule at your facility (for example, every day or every other day). However, any time the linens become soiled or excessively wrinkled, you must remake the person's bed. Change as many of the linens as necessary to ensure a clean, dry, wrinkle-free bed for your patient or resident. General guidelines for bedmaking are given in Guidelines Box 19-2.

Mitering Corners

Mitered corner a corner that is made by folding and tucking the sheet so that it lies flat and neat against the mattress

To make a bed, you will need to know how to make a **mitered corner**. When the bottom sheet is flat (instead of fitted), mitered corners are made at the head of the bed to help secure the bottom sheet to the mattress. Mitered corners are also made at the foot of the bed to hold the top sheet, blanket, and bedspread in place. Figure 19-1 shows you how to make a mitered corner.

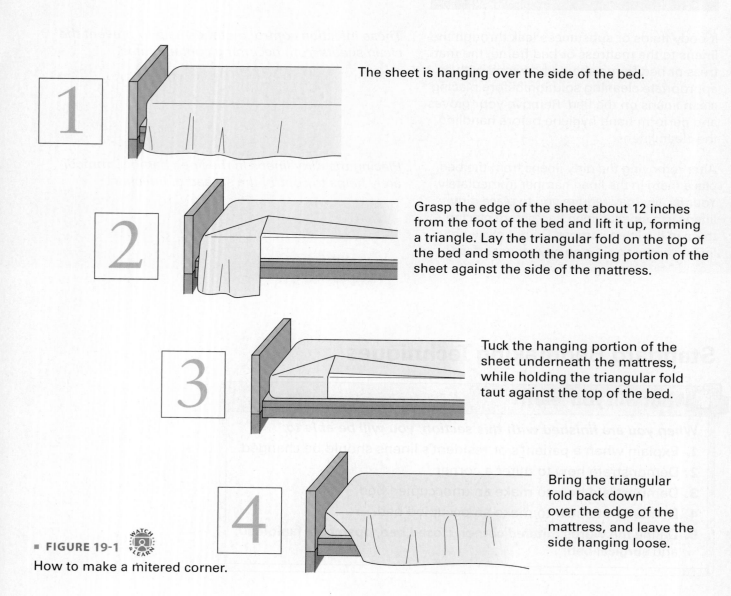

1 The sheet is hanging over the side of the bed.

2 Grasp the edge of the sheet about 12 inches from the foot of the bed and lift it up, forming a triangle. Lay the triangular fold on the top of the bed and smooth the hanging portion of the sheet against the side of the mattress.

3 Tuck the hanging portion of the sheet underneath the mattress, while holding the triangular fold taut against the top of the bed.

4 Bring the triangular fold back down over the edge of the mattress, and leave the side hanging loose.

■ **FIGURE 19-1**
How to make a mitered corner.

GUIDELINES BOX 19-2   Guidelines for Bedmaking

What you do	Why you do it
Always place linens on the bed so that the seams of the sheets face away from the person's skin.	*The seams of the sheets can rub the person's skin, causing irritation and leading to skin breakdown, which can lead to pressure ulcers.*
Bottom linens must be pulled tightly to avoid wrinkling. Layering should be kept to a minimum.	*Wrinkles and extra layers of linens can cause skin breakdown, which can lead to pressure ulcers.*
Linens should be changed whenever they become soiled or wet, regardless of the time of day.	*Besides causing discomfort, soiled or wet linens can cause skin breakdown, which can lead to pressure ulcers.*
Do not shake linens when placing them on the bed.	*Shaking linens stirs up dust from the floor. The dust then settles on surfaces in the room and can be easily transferred onto eating utensils or into a wound, causing an infection.*
When you need to change the linens on a person's bed with the person still in the bed, be sure to explain what you are doing throughout the procedure. Talk reassuringly to the person, even if the person is unconscious and you think that the person cannot hear you.	*Having the bed linens changed while still in the bed can be a very frightening experience for the patient or resident, particularly if the person is unconscious. Explaining to the person what you are doing as you are doing it can help the person feel more secure.*
When you need to change the linens on a person's bed with the person still in the bed, close the door, pull the privacy curtain, and keep the person covered with a bath blanket.	*Taking actions to protect the person's privacy and modesty will help him to feel less exposed during the procedure.*
Check the bed linens for personal items before removing the linens from the bed.	*Personal items, such as dentures, eyeglasses, or jewelry, may become lost in the bed linens. If these linens are removed from the bed, bundled up, and sent to the laundry, the mislaid personal items may not be discovered and they could be damaged in the wash cycle, or they may be lost altogether. Personal items may be expensive and inconvenient to replace. If they hold sentimental value, they may be irreplaceable.*
Disconnect the call light control and any tubes or drains that may be connected to the bed linens before removing the linens from the bed.	*Disconnecting equipment and tubes from the linens will help prevent discomfort from pulling on or possibly accidental removal of tubes and drains.*

Closed bed an empty, made bed

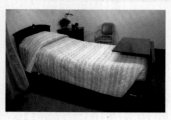

Open bed a bed ready to receive a patient or resident

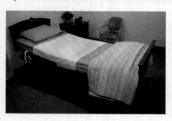

 Fanfolded adjective used to describe the top sheet, blanket, and bedspread of a closed bed when they have been turned back (toward the foot of the bed)

Surgical bed a closed bed that has been opened to receive a patient or resident who will be arriving by stretcher; the top sheet, blanket, and bedspread are folded toward the side of the bed, leaving one side open and ready to receive the person

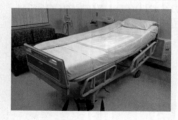

Making an Unoccupied Bed

Often, your patients or residents will be out of the bed when you change the linens. This is called making an unoccupied bed. Procedure 19-1 explains how to make an unoccupied bed.

An unoccupied bed may be either "closed" or "open":

- A **closed bed** is neatly made with the top bed linens pulled to the top of the bed.
- An **open bed** is created when the top sheet, blanket, and bedspread are **fanfolded** toward the foot of the bed. Opening the bed makes it easier for the person to get into. A **surgical bed** is a special type of open bed made to receive a person from a stretcher.

Making an Occupied Bed

Some conditions make it difficult or impossible for a person to get out of bed for a linen change. When this is the case, the linens are changed while the person is still in the bed. This is called making an occupied bed. In most facilities, the linens are changed after the person has been given a bed bath. Procedure 19-2 explains how to make an occupied bed.

Putting it all together!

- Clean, dry, wrinkle-free linens promote comfort and rest.
- Clean, dry, wrinkle-free linens help to prevent complications, such as pressure ulcers. Dampness contributes to skin breakdown, and wrinkled sheets can cause friction, both of which are factors in the development of pressure ulcers.
- Clean, dry linens are important for odor and infection control.
- Bed linens are changed according to facility policy and as often as necessary to ensure that the patient or resident has a clean, dry, wrinkle-free bed at all times.

PROCEDURES

PROCEDURE 19-1
Making an Unoccupied (Closed) Bed

Why you do it: Clean, dry, wrinkle-free linens promote comfort, help to prevent complications (such as pressure ulcers), and are important for odor and infection control.

GETTING READY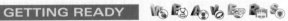

1. Complete the "Getting Ready" steps.*

SUPPLIES

- mattress pad (if necessary)
- bottom sheet
- lift (draw) sheet (if necessary)
- bed protector (if necessary)
- top sheet
- blanket
- bedspread
- pillowcase

PROCEDURE

2. Place the linens on a clean surface close to the bed (for example, the over-bed table).
3. Make sure that the bed is positioned at a comfortable working height to promote good body mechanics (usually elbow height of the caregiver) and that the wheels are locked.
4. Lower the side rails and move the mattress to the head of the bed (it may have shifted toward the foot of the bed if the occupant of the bed had the head of the bed elevated).
   Note: The mattress pad, bottom sheet, and draw sheet are positioned and tucked in on one side of the bed before moving to the other side to complete these actions. This is most efficient in terms of energy and time.
5. Place the mattress pad on the bed and unfold it so that only one vertical crease remains. Make sure that this crease is centered on the mattress.

If the mattress pad is fitted, carefully pull the corners of the near side over the corners of the mattress and smooth down the sides. If the mattress pad is flat, make sure the top of the pad is even with the head of the mattress. Open the mattress pad across the bed, taking care to keep it centered.

6. Place the bottom sheet on the bed. If the bottom sheet is fitted, carefully pull the corners of the near side over the corners of the mattress and smooth down the sides. If the bottom sheet is flat:
   a. Place the sheet so that when you unfold it, the wide hem will be at the head of the bed and the hem stitching will be against the mattress, away from the person who will be occupying the bed.
   b. Unfold the sheet so that only one vertical crease remains. Make sure that this crease is vertically centered on the mattress.

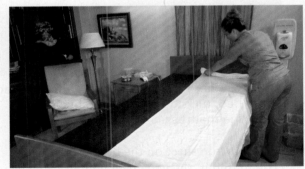

STEP 6b ■ Unfold the sheet so that only one vertical crease remains.

---

*It is assumed that the dirty linens have been removed from the bed, and the bed has been cleaned, as per facility policy, prior to beginning this procedure.

(*procedure continues on page 416*)

PROCEDURE 19-1 (continued)
Making an Unoccupied (Closed) Bed

   c. Open the sheet across the bed, taking care to keep it centered. The same length of sheet (approximately 12 to 18 inches) should hang over each side of the bed. Make sure that the lower edge of the sheet is even with the foot of the mattress.

   d. Tuck the sheet under the mattress at the head of the bed and miter the corner.

   e. Tuck the near side of the sheet underneath the mattress, working from the head of the bed toward the foot. As you tuck, make sure there are no wrinkles in the sheet and that the mattress pad remains smooth and in place.

7. Place the lift sheet on the bed so that the top of the sheet is approximately 12 inches from the head of the mattress. If you are using a plastic or rubberized lift sheet, place a cotton lift sheet on top of it. Smooth the lift sheet across the bed and tuck the near side under the mattress.

8. Now, move to the other side of the bed and repeat the process of aligning the mattress pad, mitering the corner, and tucking in the bottom sheet and lift sheet.

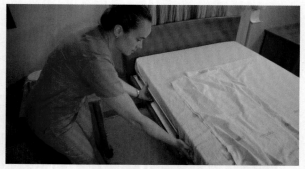

STEP 8 ■ After mitering the corner at the head of the bed, tuck the side of the sheet underneath the mattress.

9. Place the top sheet on the bed so that when you unfold it, the wide hem will be at the head of the bed and the hem stitching will be facing

upward, away from the person who will be occupying the bed.

   a. Unfold the sheet so that only one vertical crease remains. Make sure that this crease is centered vertically on the mattress.

   b. Open the sheet across the bed, taking care to keep it centered. The same length of sheet (approximately 12 to 18 inches) should hang over each side of the bed. Make sure that the top edge of the sheet is even with the head of the mattress. Pull the bottom of the sheet over the foot of the bed, but do not tuck it in yet (it will be tucked in with the blanket and bedspread).

10. Place the blanket on the bed and unfold it in the same manner as the sheet, keeping the center crease in the center of the bed. The same length of blanket (approximately 12 to 18 inches) should hang over each side of the bed. Make sure that the top edge of the blanket is approximately 6 to 8 inches from the head of the mattress. Pull the bottom edge of the blanket over the sheet at the foot of the bed, but do not tuck anything in yet.

11. Place the bedspread on the bed and unfold it in the same manner as the sheet, keeping the center crease in the center of the bed. The sides of the bedspread should be even and cover all of the other bed linens. Make sure that the top of the bedspread is even with the head of the mattress, unless the pillow is to be tucked under the bedspread (in which case you will need to allow more length at the top). Pull the bottom of the bedspread over the blanket and sheet at the foot of the bed.

12. Together, tuck the bedspread, the blanket, and the top sheet under the foot of the mattress. Make a mitered corner at the foot of the bed on both sides.

13. Fold the upper 6 inches of the top sheet and blanket down over the spread to make a cuff.

14. Rest the pillow on the bed. Grasping the closed end of the pillowcase, turn the pillowcase

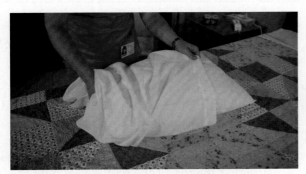

STEP 14 ■ Grasp the pillow through the pillowcase and pull the pillowcase down over the pillow.

inside out over your hand and arm. Grasp the pillow through the pillowcase and pull the pillowcase down over the pillow. Make sure that any tags or zippers are on the inside of the pillowcase.

15. Place the pillow on the bed with the open end of the pillowcase facing away from the door.

FINISHING UP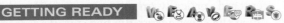

16. Complete the "Finishing Up" steps.

PROCEDURE 19-2
Making an Occupied Bed

Why you do it: Clean, dry, wrinkle-free linens promote comfort, help to prevent complications (such as pressure ulcers), and are important for odor and infection control.

GETTING READY

1. Complete the "Getting Ready" steps.

SUPPLIES

- gloves
- bath blanket
- mattress pad (if necessary)
- bottom sheet
- lift (draw) sheet
- bed protector (if necessary)
- top sheet
- blanket
- bedspread
- pillowcase

PROCEDURE

2. Place the linens on a clean surface close to the bed (for example, the over-bed table). Make sure to position the table holding the linens

close enough to the bed that you don't have to step away from the bedside to reach it.

3. Make sure that the bed is positioned at a comfortable working height to promote good body mechanics (usually elbow height of the caregiver) and that the wheels are locked.

4. Disconnect the call light control and any tubes or drains from the bed linens. Check the bed for dentures or any other personal items.

5. Lower the head of the bed so that the bed is flat (as tolerated).

6. Put on the gloves (the linens may be wet or soiled).

7. Remove the bedspread and blanket from the bed. If they are to be reused, fold them and place them on a clean surface, such as a chair.

8. Loosen the top sheet at the foot of the bed and spread a bath blanket over the top sheet (and the person).

(*procedure continues on page 418*)

PROCEDURE 19-2 (continued)
Making an Occupied Bed

9. If the person is able, have her hold the bath blanket. If not, tuck the corners under the person's shoulders. Remove the top sheet by pulling it out from underneath the bath blanket, being careful not to expose the person.

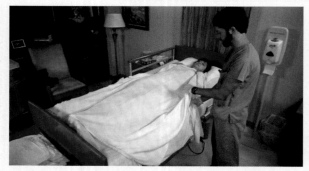

STEP 9 ■ Remove the top sheet by pulling it out from underneath the bath blanket.

10. Place the top sheet in the linen hamper or linen bag.
11. If the side rails are in use, lower the side rail on the working side of the bed. The side rail on the opposite side of the bed should remain up. Turn the person onto her side so that she is facing away from you. Reposition the pillow under the person's head, and adjust the bath blanket to keep the person covered.
12. Loosen the lift sheet, bottom sheet, and (if necessary) the mattress pad.
13. Fanfold the bottom linens toward the person's back, tucking them slightly underneath her.*

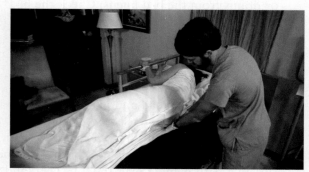

STEP 13 ■ Fanfold the bottom linens toward the person's back.

*If the linens are wet or soiled, make sure that you change your gloves before handling the clean linens.

14. Straighten the mattress pad (if it is not being changed). If the mattress pad is being changed, place the clean mattress pad on the bed and unfold it so that only one vertical crease remains. Make sure that this crease is centered vertically on the mattress. If the mattress pad is fitted, carefully pull the corners of the near side over the corners of the mattress and smooth down the sides. If the mattress pad is flat, make sure that the top of the pad is even with the head of the mattress. Fanfold the opposite side of the mattress pad close to the patient or resident tucking them underneath the old linens.
15. Place the clean bottom sheet on the bed. If the bottom sheet is fitted, carefully pull the corners over the corners of the mattress and smooth down the sides. If the bottom sheet is flat:
   a. Place the sheet so that when you unfold it, the wide hem will be at the head of the bed and the hem stitching will be against the mattress, away from the person who will be occupying the bed.
   b. Unfold the sheet so that only one vertical crease remains. Make sure that this crease is centered vertically on the mattress.
   c. Open the sheet across the bed, taking care to keep it centered. The same length of sheet (approximately 12 to 18 inches) should hang over each side of the bed. Make sure that the lower edge of the sheet is even with the foot of the mattress. Fanfold the opposite side of the sheet close to the patient or resident tucking it underneath the old linens.

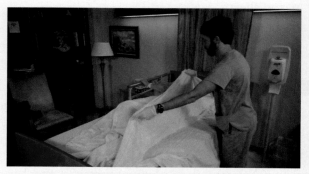

STEP 15c ■ Open the sheet across the bed, taking care to keep it centered.

d. Tuck the sheet under the mattress at the head of the bed and miter the corner.

e. Tuck the near side of the sheet underneath the mattress, working from the head of the bed toward the foot. As you tuck, make sure that there are no wrinkles in the sheet and that the mattress pad remains smooth and in place.

16. Place the lift sheet on the bed so that the top of the sheet is approximately 12 inches from the head of the mattress. If you are using a plastic or rubberized lift sheet, place a cotton lift sheet on top of it. Fanfold the opposite side of the lift sheet close to the patient or resident tucking it underneath the old linens. Smooth the lift sheet across the bed and tuck the near side under the mattress.

17. Raise the side rail on the working side of the bed. Help the person to roll toward you, over the folded linens. Reposition the pillow under the person's head and adjust the bath blanket to keep the person covered.

18. Move to the other side of the bed and lower the side rail.

19. Loosen and remove the soiled bottom linens and place them in the linen hamper or linen bag. Change your gloves if they become soiled.

20. Now, repeat the process of aligning the mattress pad, mitering the corner, and tucking in the bottom sheet and lift sheet.

21. Help the person to move to the center of the bed and position her comfortably. Raise the side rail on the working side of the bed.

22. Change the pillowcase and place the pillow under the person's head.

23. Place the clean top sheet over the person (who is still covered with the bath blanket), being careful not to cover her face. The sheet should be placed so that when you unfold it, the wide hem will be at the head of the bed and the hem stitching will be facing upward, away from the person who will be occupying the bed.

a. Unfold the sheet so that only one vertical crease remains. Make sure that this crease is centered vertically on the mattress.

b. Open the sheet across the bed, taking care to keep it centered. The same length of sheet (approximately 12 to 18 inches) should hang over each side of the bed.

c. If the person is able, have her hold the top sheet. If not, tuck the corners under her shoulders. Remove the bath blanket by pulling it out from underneath the top sheet, being careful not to expose the person. Place the bath blanket in the linen hamper or linen bag.

24. Place the blanket and then the bedspread over the top sheet. Together, tuck the bedspread, the blanket, and the top sheet under the foot of the mattress. Make a mitered corner at the foot of the bed on both sides.

25. Make a toe pleat by grasping the top sheet, the blanket, and the bedspread over the person's feet and pulling the linens straight up. The toe pleat allows the person to move her feet and helps to relieve pressure on the feet from tightly tucked linens.

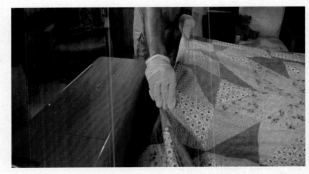

STEP 25 ■ Make a toe pleat by pulling straight up on the top linens.

26. Lower the bed to its lowest position and make sure that the wheels are locked. Raise the head of the bed as the person requests.

27. Remove your gloves, dispose of them in a facility-approved waste container, and perform hand hygiene.

FINISHING UP

28. Complete the "Finishing Up" steps.

WHAT DID YOU LEARN?

Multiple Choice

Select the single best answer for each of the following questions.

1. What is a lift (draw) sheet?
   a. A fitted bottom sheet
   b. A half-sized sheet that is placed over the middle of the bottom sheet and has varied uses, including repositioning and lifting a person in bed
   c. A half-sized sheet that is placed over the middle of the top sheet and used to make toe pleats
   d. A sheet used to add a decorative touch to the person's room

2. What is a bed that has a person in it called?
   a. An open bed
   b. A closed bed
   c. A surgical bed
   d. An occupied bed

3. When you are handling linens, always remember to:
   a. Shake the bedspread to remove dust
   b. Place the dirty linens on the floor, to get them out of your way
   c. Hold the linens away from your body
   d. All of the above

4. What personal protective equipment (PPE) should be worn when removing used bed linens?
   a. Gloves
   b. A gown
   c. Eye goggles
   d. No PPE is necessary

5. When are bed linens changed?
   a. When they become wet or soiled
   b. According to facility policy
   c. When they become excessively wrinkled
   d. All of the above

6. Mrs. Owens is returning to her room following a diagnostic procedure. She will be arriving on a stretcher. What sort of bed should you make?
   a. An open bed
   b. A closed bed
   c. A surgical bed
   d. An occupied bed

 Stop *and* Think!

Barbara is a nursing assistant on 3 West. She has already changed the bed linens twice during her shift for one of her patients, Mrs. Bridges. Mrs. Bridges is receiving chemotherapy for cancer, and one of the side effects of the medication is uncontrollable diarrhea. Now Mrs. Bridges' call light is on again. When Barbara goes to check on her, she discovers that Mrs. Bridges has soiled the bed again. Barbara tells Mrs. Bridges she will be right back and leaves to get supplies from the linen closet. What are some items that Barbara should collect, along with clean sheets?

Measuring and Recording Vital Signs, Height, and Weight

Vital signs provide essential information about a person's health. The vital signs are body temperature, pulse, respirations, and blood pressure. Many members of the health care team depend on your ability to measure and record vital signs, height, and weight accurately. In this chapter, you will learn how to take these measurements, as well as what findings should be reported to the nurse immediately.

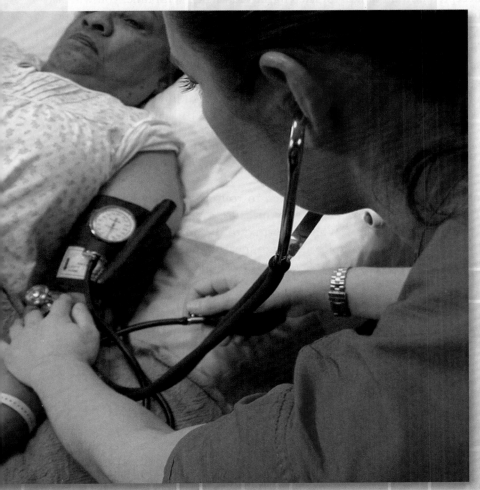

Photo: *A nursing assistant takes a resident's blood pressure.*

Introduction to Vital Signs

What will you learn?

When you are finished with this section, you will be able to:

1. Discuss factors that can cause changes in a person's vital signs.
2. Understand the importance of accurately measuring and recording vital signs.
3. Discuss the importance of reporting any changes in a person's vital signs to the nurse immediately.
4. Define the word **vital signs**.

Vital signs certain key measurements that provide essential information about a person's health

Vital signs reflect functions that the body controls automatically, such as:

- The internal temperature of the body
- How fast the heart beats
- How fast a person breathes

There are accepted normal ranges for each of the vital signs. With time, you will also come to know what is "normal" for each of your patients or residents. What is normal for a person depends on the person's age, gender, race, and other factors, such as medical conditions that the person may have or medications that the person is taking.

A person's vital sign measurements may change several times over the course of a day while still staying within the range of "normal." However, a major or long-lasting change in these measurements may be a sign of illness or injury. Other factors that can cause a person's vital sign measurements to change include:

- Pain
- Strong emotions (such as anxiety, fear, or excitement)
- Exercise

The nursing care plan will tell you when to routinely measure each patient's or resident's vital signs. However, you may measure a person's vital signs whenever you feel that it is necessary. When reporting to the nurse, it is often useful to provide objective data (for example, vital sign measurements) along with subjective data (for example, the patient's or resident's complaint of pain, dizziness, or nausea).

If you measure a person's vital signs and get a measurement that is abnormal, you should take the measurement again to make sure that it is accurate and then report your findings to the nurse immediately. If you are having trouble measuring a patient's or resident's vital signs, you should ask for help from the nurse or another nursing assistant.

Putting it all together!

- Vital signs provide essential information about a person's health. The vital signs are body temperature, pulse, respiration, and blood pressure.

- As a nursing assistant, you must be familiar with accepted normal ranges for all of the vital signs. In addition, you must come to recognize what is "normal" for each of the patients or residents in your care.

- Many factors can affect vital sign measurements, including illness, pain, emotions, and activity. Significant or long-lasting changes in vital signs could be an early indication that something is wrong, and they need to be reported to the nurse immediately.

- Measuring, reporting, and recording vital sign measurements accurately are critical because many people rely on this information to make important decisions about the patient's or resident's care.

Body Temperature

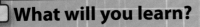

What will you learn?

When you are finished with this section, you will be able to:

1. List common sites used for measuring a person's body temperature and the advantages and disadvantages of each site.
2. State the normal range for an adult's temperature and findings that should be reported to the nurse immediately.
3. Demonstrate the proper use of a glass thermometer and an electronic thermometer.
4. Demonstrate how to measure an oral temperature, a rectal temperature, an axillary temperature, a tympanic temperature, and a temporal temperature.
5. Define the word **fever**.

Measuring the Body Temperature

The body temperature is simply a measurement of how hot the body is. The body temperature can be measured from many different areas of the body (Table 20-1). Where the body temperature is measured depends on facility policy and the needs of the patient or resident. Procedures 20-1 through 20-5 explain how to measure an oral temperature, a rectal temperature, an axillary temperature, a tympanic temperature, and a temporal temperature. Because the method used to measure the temperature affects the accuracy of the measurement, you should note which method was used when you record the temperature, per your facility's policy. For example, many facilities use "O" for oral, "R" for rectal, "A" for axillary, and "T" for tympanic or temporal.

(text continued on page 426)

TABLE 20-1 Sites for Measuring Body Temperature

Site	Devices Used to Take Temperature	Advantages	Disadvantages	Do Not Use This Method if the Person:
Mouth (oral temperature)	Oral glass thermometer Oral electronic thermometer	■ Fast ■ Causes patient or resident minimal discomfort	■ Measurement may not be as accurate as with some other methods ■ If a person eats, drinks, smokes, or chews gum within 15 minutes of having an oral temperature taken, the measurement may not be accurate	■ Is unconscious ■ Is unable to keep the mouth closed ■ Is unable to breathe through the nose ■ Is likely to bite the thermometer ■ Is coughing or sneezing ■ Has recently had mouth surgery or an injury to the mouth ■ Is receiving oxygen by a face mask
Rectum (rectal temperature)	Rectal glass thermometer Rectal electronic thermometer	■ Measurement is more accurate than with some other methods	■ Can be uncomfortable and embarrassing for the patient or resident	■ Has hemorrhoids, rectal bleeding, or a disease involving the rectum ■ Has diarrhea ■ Has had rectal surgery ■ Has certain heart conditions

Site	Devices Used to Take Temperature	Advantages	Disadvantages	Do Not Use This Method if the Person:
Armpit (axillary temperature)	Axillary glass thermometer Axillary electronic thermometer	■ Causes patient or resident minimal discomfort	■ Slow ■ Provides least accurate measurement of body temperature	■ Has recently had chest or breast surgery that affects both sides of the body
Ear (tympanic temperature)	Tympanic thermometer	■ Fast ■ Causes patient or resident minimal discomfort ■ Provides very accurate measurement	■ If the person has been sleeping with one side of his head against a pillow, use the other ear for taking the temperature	■ Has an ear infection ■ Has excessive build-up of cerumen (ear wax)
Forehead (temporal temperature)	Temporal artery thermometer (Courtesy of Exergen Corporation, 2004)	■ Fast ■ Causes patient or resident no discomfort ■ Provides very accurate measurement	■ If a person is sweating, it can cause a false low temperature reading ■ If a person has anything covering the forehead (hair, a wig, a hat, or bandages), a false high temperature reading can result	■ Not applicable; safe for use with everyone

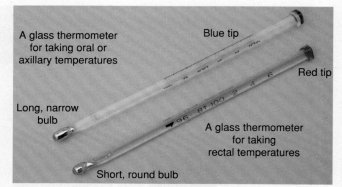

■ **FIGURE 20-1**

Glass thermometers may vary slightly in appearance depending on their intended use.

The body temperature is measured in either degrees Fahrenheit (°F) or degrees Celsius (°C), using a thermometer. Many different types of thermometers are used to measure the body temperature (see Table 20-1).

Using a Glass Thermometer

Glass thermometers consist of a glass bulb attached to a thin glass tube that is marked with a temperature scale and filled with a liquid substance (Fig. 20-1). In past years, glass thermometers contained mercury, a toxic substance. Because of the dangers associated with breakage and spilled mercury, most health care settings do not use glass thermometers at all. Some settings still use glass thermometers, but have switched to using newer models, which contain a substance that behaves the same way as mercury but is less toxic. The liquid inside the thermometer expands with heat and moves up the glass tube, showing the temperature on the scale (Fig. 20-2). Before you use a glass thermometer, the liquid must be "shaken down" to below the 94° mark on a Fahrenheit thermometer or the 34° mark on a Celsius thermometer (Fig. 20-3). To read a glass thermometer, hold it horizontally by the stem at eye level and rotate it until the line of liquid becomes visible (Fig. 20-4). It will show up as a thin silvery or red line. The temperature measurement is the reading at the end of the line farthest away from the bulb.

In most facilities that use glass thermometers, each patient or resident has his own thermometer, which is kept in a case at the person's bedside. Because glass thermometers are not disposable, they must be cleaned properly after each use, according to facility policy. The thermometer is washed with cool water and soap

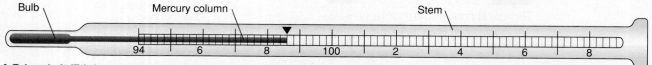

A **Fahrenheit (F°) thermometer** is scaled from 94°F to 108°F. Each long line indicates 1 degree and each short line indicates $^2/_{10}$ (0.2) of a degree. This thermometer is reading 98.6°F.

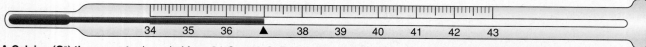

A **Celsius (C°) thermometer** is scaled from 34°C to 43°C. Each long line indicates 1 degree and each short line indicates $^1/_{10}$ (0.1) of a degree. This thermometer is reading 37°C.

■ **FIGURE 20-2**

Temperature scales on glass thermometers.

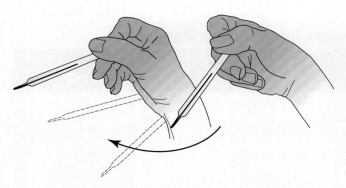

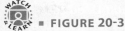 **FIGURE 20-3**

A glass thermometer is "shaken down" before use by holding the thermometer firmly by the stem and snapping your wrist downward.

(never hot water, which can cause the thermometer to shatter), rinsed with cool water, and placed in a disinfectant solution. The disinfectant solution is rinsed off the thermometer before the thermometer is used again.

If a glass thermometer breaks while you are cleaning it (or at any other time), avoid touching the liquid and the broken glass and prevent others from doing so as well. Glass thermometers are still sometimes used in the home health care setting and some states are still requiring nursing assistants to learn how to use glass thermometers to take a person's temperature.

Using an Electronic Thermometer

Electronic thermometers are powered by batteries, and the temperature is displayed on a screen on the front of the instrument. A probe is placed in the patient's or resident's mouth, rectum, or armpit to measure the temperature. The probe is color coded (blue for oral and axillary use, red for rectal use). Before use, the probe is covered with a disposable sheath.

Tympanic and temporal artery thermometers are special types of electronic thermometers (see Table 20-1). A tympanic thermometer is placed in the person's ear canal, where it rests near the eardrum (tympanic membrane). A temporal artery thermometer is swept across the person's forehead.

Normal and Abnormal Findings

Table 20-2 shows normal adult temperature ranges, depending on the method used to measure the temperature. **Fever** can be a sign of illness or infection and should be reported to the nurse right away. Be aware that an elderly person's temperature

Fever a body temperature that is higher than normal

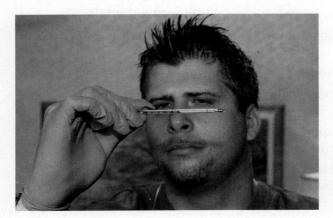

 FIGURE 20-4

Reading a glass thermometer.

TABLE 20-2	Normal Adult Temperature Ranges		
Method Used to Obtain Temperature	Fahrenheit (°F)	Celsius (°C)	
Oral	97.6 to 99.6	36.5 to 37.5	
Rectal	98.6 to 100.6	37 to 38.1	
Axillary	96.6 to 98.6	36 to 37	
Tympanic	98.6	37	
Temporal	99.6	37.5	

Tell the Nurse!

Problems with body temperature

- The person's temperature is higher than normal
- The person's temperature is lower than normal
- You have difficulty taking and reading the person's temperature

may actually decrease, or only slightly increase, in response to illness or infection. For this reason, even a very slight change in an older person's temperature should be reported to the nurse.

Putting it all together!

- Body temperature is a measure of how hot the body is.
- A glass or electronic thermometer is used to measure the body temperature. Tympanic thermometers and temporal artery thermometers are special types of electronic thermometers.
- A person's temperature may be measured in the mouth, rectum, ear, armpit, or forehead. When recording a temperature measurement, it is important to also record where the temperature was measured.
- A change in a person's temperature (either higher or lower than normal) must be reported to the nurse right away.

Pulse

What will you learn?

When you are finished with this section, you will be able to:

1. Describe what qualities should be noted when taking a person's pulse.
2. List common sites used for taking a person's pulse.
3. Demonstrate the proper way to measure and record a radial pulse and an apical pulse.
4. State the normal range for an adult's pulse rate and the findings that should be reported to the nurse immediately.
5. Define the words **pulse rate**, **pulse rhythm**, **pulse amplitude**, **stethoscope**, and **pulse deficit**.

Each time the heart beats, it sends a wave, or *pulse*, of blood through the arteries. The pulse, a throbbing sensation just underneath the skin, can be felt by placing your fingers gently over an artery that runs close to the surface of the skin, such as the carotid artery in the neck or the radial artery in the wrist. By feeling for and counting the pulse, we are able to tell:

■ How fast the heart is beating (the **pulse rate**)

■ How regularly the heart is beating (the **pulse rhythm**)

■ How strongly the heart is beating (the **pulse amplitude** or pulse character)

Measuring the Pulse

Radial Pulse

The radial pulse is measured by placing your middle two or three fingers over the patient's or resident's radial artery (located on the inside of the wrist) and counting the number of pulses that occur in either 30 seconds or 1 minute. If a person's pulse is irregular, always count it for the full minute. Procedure 20-6 describes how to measure a radial pulse.

Apical Pulse

The apical pulse is measured by listening over the apex (lower tip) of the heart with a **stethoscope**. The stethoscope allows you to hear, rather than feel, each beat of the person's heart. The apex of the heart is located approximately 2 inches below the left nipple (see Chapter 16, Fig. 16-4). Procedure 20-7 describes how to measure an apical pulse.

The apical pulse rate and the radial pulse rate should be the same in any single person. Occasionally, however, the heart does not pump strongly enough to send enough blood through the arteries with each beat. This means that although each beat of the heart may be heard over the apex of the heart using a stethoscope, it may not be felt in the wrist. The **pulse deficit** is measured by having one member of the nursing team measure the person's apical pulse while another team member measures the person's radial pulse. The two counts are then compared to determine the pulse deficit. For example, if the apical pulse is 84 beats per minute and the radial pulse is 80 beats per minute, the difference between the apical pulse and the radial pulse (that is, the pulse deficit) is 4 beats per minute (84 − 80 = 4). When there is a pulse deficit, the apical pulse rate will always be higher than the radial pulse rate because it is easier to hear a heartbeat at the source than to feel it.

Normal and Abnormal Findings

The normal adult pulse rate is between 60 and 100 beats per minute. The pulse rhythm should be smooth and regular, with the same amount of time in between each pulsation. Each pulsation should be strong, and easy to feel. Pulses that are difficult to feel may be described as "weak" or "thready." A weak or thready pulse usually means that the heart is having trouble circulating blood throughout the body. Any change in pulse rate, rhythm, or amplitude should be reported to the nurse immediately.

Pulse rate the number of pulsations that can be felt over an artery in 1 minute; an indication of the heart rate

Pulse rhythm the pattern of the pulsations and the pauses between them

Pulse amplitude the force or quality of the pulse

Stethoscope a device that amplifies sound and transfers it to the listener's ears

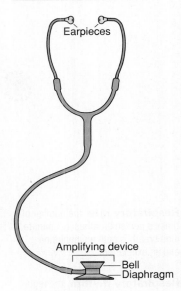

Earpieces

Amplifying device

Bell
Diaphragm

Pulse deficit the difference between the apical pulse rate (the pulse that is measured by listening over the apex of the heart with a stethoscope) and the radial pulse rate (the pulse that is measured by placing the middle two or three fingers over the radial artery, located on the inside of the wrist)

Tell the Nurse!

Problems with pulse

- The person's pulse rate is higher than normal
- The person's pulse rate is lower than normal
- The person's pulse rhythm is irregular
- The pulse is weak or "thready"
- You have difficulty taking the person's pulse

Putting it all together!

- The pulse reflects the rate, rhythm, and strength of the heartbeat. A steady, strong, regular heartbeat is necessary to ensure that all of the tissues get the oxygen and nutrients they need.
- The pulse can be measured by feeling the radial artery (in the wrist) or by listening to the apical pulse (in the chest) with a stethoscope. Be sure to note the pulse rhythm and amplitude, as well as the rate.
- The following should be reported to the nurse immediately: a pulse rate that is either slow (less than 60 beats per minute) or fast (more than 100 beats per minute), an irregular pulse, or a weak or "thready" pulse.

Respiration

What will you learn?

When you are finished with this section, you will be able to:

1. Describe what qualities should be noted when measuring a person's respirations.
2. Demonstrate the proper way to measure and record a person's respirations.
3. State the normal range for an adult's respiratory rate and findings that should be reported to the nurse immediately.
4. Define the words **respiratory rate**, **respiratory rhythm**, **depth of respiration**, and **dyspnea**.

Respiration is the process of breathing. The chest rises each time we inhale and falls each time we exhale. One respiration is one inhalation and one exhalation. By looking at and counting a person's respirations, we are able to tell:

- How fast the person is breathing (the **respiratory rate**)
- How regularly the person is breathing (the **respiratory rhythm**)
- How deeply the person is breathing (the **depth of respiration**)

Respiratory rate the number of times a person breathes in 1 minute (one breath is both an inhalation and an exhalation)

Respiratory rhythm the regularity with which a person breathes

Depth of respiration the quality of each breath

Measuring Respiration

The respiratory rate is measured by watching the rise and fall of the person's chest and counting the number of respirations that occur in either 30 seconds or 1 minute. Because a person's breathing may change if the person knows she is being watched, a more accurate measurement may be obtained if you measure the respiratory rate right after you measure the person's pulse, with your fingers still on the person's wrist as if you were still counting the pulse. If the person's respirations are irregular, always count them for the full minute. Procedure 20-8 describes how to measure a person's respiratory rate.

Normal and Abnormal Findings

The normal adult respiratory rate is between 12 and 20 breaths per minute. The chest should rise and fall evenly on both sides in a regular rhythm. Breathing should be quiet and easy. **Dyspnea** or any change in respiratory rate, rhythm, or depth should be reported to the nurse immediately.

Putting it all together!

- The respiratory rate, rhythm, and depth show us how well the person is breathing, or taking oxygen in and getting rid of carbon dioxide.
- When measuring a person's respiration, remember that one respiration equals both an inhalation and an exhalation. Be sure to note the respiratory rhythm and depth of respiration, as well as the rate.
- Dyspnea or any change in respiratory rate, rhythm, or depth should be reported to the nurse immediately.

Blood Pressure

What will you learn?

When you are finished with this section, you will be able to:

1. Identify the parts of a sphygmomanometer and demonstrate how to use this tool to measure a person's blood pressure.
2. State the normal range for an adult's blood pressure and findings that should be reported to the nurse immediately.
3. Define the words **systolic pressure**, **diastolic pressure**, **sphygmomanometer**, **hypertension**, **hypotension**, and **orthostatic hypotension**.

The blood pressure is the pressure that the blood puts on the arterial walls. Blood pressure is considered a vital sign because it gives us important information about a person's health and risk for disease. If the blood pressure is too low, the tissues of the body do not receive enough oxygen and nutrients. If the blood pressure is too high, it forces the heart to do extra work and places too much strain on other vital organs and the blood vessels.

Measuring Blood Pressure

Blood pressure is measured in millimeters of mercury (mm Hg) and is recorded as a fraction. The **systolic pressure**, which is higher, is recorded first, followed by the **diastolic pressure**, which is lower. For instance, if a person's systolic measurement is 110 mm Hg and the diastolic measurement is 72 mm Hg, then the blood pressure would be recorded as 110/72 mm Hg.

Dyspnea labored or difficult breathing

Systolic pressure the pressure that the blood exerts against the arterial walls when the heart muscle contracts; the first blood pressure measurement that is recorded

Diastolic pressure the pressure that the blood exerts against the arterial walls when the heart muscle relaxes; the second blood pressure measurement

TABLE 20-3	Blood Pressure Cuff Sizes
Arm Measurement (cm)	Size of Cuff to Use
13 to 20	Child
24 to 32	Adult
32 to 42	Large Adult
42 to 50	Thigh

Sphygmomanometer a device used to measure blood pressure

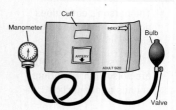

The most common method of measuring a person's blood pressure is by using a manually operated **sphygmomanometer** and a stethoscope. A manual sphygmomanometer consists of the following:

- A cuff (a flat, cloth-covered inflatable pouch)
- A bulb, which is squeezed or pumped to fill the cuff with air
- A manometer (the gauge that measures the air pressure in the cuff)

You must use the correct size of cuff for your patient or resident (Table 20-3). Two tubes are attached to the cuff; one tube is attached to the bulb used to inflate the pouch, and the other tube is attached to the manometer. The manometer may be either aneroid or mercury (Fig. 20-5). Long dashes mark increments of 10 mm Hg and the short dashes in between mark increments of 2 mm Hg.

The most common place to measure a person's blood pressure is in the brachial artery. The cuff is wrapped around the person's upper arm, and the diaphragm of the stethoscope is placed at the inner aspect of the elbow, over the brachial artery. The cuff is inflated, increasing the pressure that the cuff places on the brachial artery and cutting off the blood flow. Then the air is slowly released from the cuff, lowering the pressure on the artery. When the pressure in the cuff is equal to or slightly lower than the systolic pressure in the artery, blood will suddenly begin to flow through the brachial artery and you will start hearing the pulse. Normally, you are not able to hear the brachial pulse, but under pressure, you can. When you hear the first sound of the pulse, note the reading on the manometer. This is your systolic pressure. Now continue to listen to the pulse. When the pressure inside the cuff is less than the lowest arterial pressure, or diastolic pressure, the sound of

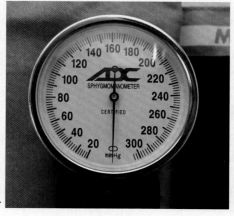

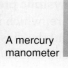

■ **FIGURE 20-5**
Manometers.

An aneroid manometer

A mercury manometer

the pulse will stop because the artery is no longer under pressure. When you hear the last sound of the pulse, note the reading on the manometer. This is your diastolic pressure. Procedure 20-9 explains how to measure a blood pressure step by step. Guidelines for taking a blood pressure are given in Guidelines Box 20-1.

GUIDELINES BOX 20-1 Guidelines for Taking a Person's Blood Pressure

What you do	Why you do it
Allow the person time to relax for at least 5 minutes prior to taking the blood pressure.	*Recent exercise and emotions (such as fear) can cause a blood pressure reading to be falsely elevated.*
Make sure the manometer is properly calibrated (that is, it reads "0" when there is no air in the cuff).	*A manometer that is not properly calibrated will not give an accurate pressure reading.*
Use a cuff that is properly sized for the patient or resident.	*A cuff that does not fit will not allow you to accurately measure the person's blood pressure. A cuff that is too small will result in a high reading, while a cuff that is too large will result in a low reading.*
Make sure the cuff fits snugly around the person's arm before inflating it.	*A cuff that is too loose can cause the skin to "pinch" under the cuff when the cuff is inflated, damaging the skin.*
Do not place the cuff over a person's clothing.	*Clothing will make it harder to hear the sounds of the brachial pulse.*
Have the patient or resident assume a comfortable lying or sitting position with the forearm supported at the level of the heart and the palm of the hand facing upward.	*If the upper arm is positioned below the level of the heart, the blood pressure measurement will read too high. If the upper arm is above the level of the heart, the measurement will read too low.*
Do not take a blood pressure on an arm where an intravenous (IV) line is placed or on an arm that is injured or in a cast.	*Inflating the cuff can cause pain and swelling, and it may dislodge an IV line if one is present.*
In a person who has had a mastectomy, do not take a blood pressure on the arm that is on the same side of the body as the breast that was removed.	*Some people who have mastectomies also have the lymph nodes in the armpit removed, which disrupts fluid flow from the tissues in the hand and lower arm. This can lead to an inaccurate blood pressure reading.*
Do not take a blood pressure on an arm that is used for hemodialysis access.	*Pressure from the blood pressure cuff can cause the fistula or shunt used for dialysis to clot or be damaged.*
Do not partially deflate the cuff and then reinflate it while taking a blood pressure measurement. If you make a mistake, release all of the air from the cuff and wait at least 1 minute before trying again.	*Not only is partially deflating and then reinflating the cuff uncomfortable for the patient or resident, it will result in an inaccurate reading.*

(*box continues on page 434*)

GUIDELINES BOX 20-1 Guidelines for Taking a Person's Blood Pressure (continued)

What you do	Why you do it
If you are unable to hear the sounds of the brachial pulse, make sure the room is quiet and check your equipment: ■ Make sure the diaphragm of the stethoscope is active by gently tapping on it. ■ Make sure the diaphragm of the stethoscope is placed directly over the brachial pulse. ■ Make sure the earpieces of the stethoscope are seated properly in your ears.	*Most difficulties with measuring blood pressure result from operator error. However, if you have checked your equipment and you still cannot hear the sounds of the brachial pulse, notify the nurse immediately. The person may have severe hypotension.*

Learning to measure blood pressures takes time and practice. At first, you will need to concentrate on how to operate the equipment and control the rate at which the air leaves the cuff. Next, you will need to become familiar with the sounds that you will hear as the cuff deflates and learn to recognize the beginning and ending sounds. Each person's blood pressure will sound slightly different. In some people, the blood pressure is easy to measure. In others, measuring the blood pressure will challenge even the most experienced nursing assistant. As with any skill you will learn, if you have difficulty taking a person's blood pressure or if you are unsure of a reading you get, always ask for a second opinion or help from another nursing assistant or a nurse.

The facility where you work may use automated (electronic) sphygmomanometers instead of manual ones. Some automated models feature automatic inflation and deflation of the cuff, while others require the cuff to be manually inflated but will deflate automatically. The blood pressure is displayed digitally (Fig. 20-6). If a person has an irregular heart rate, tremors, or is unable to remain still, an electronic blood pressure device may not be able to be used. Many electronic blood pressure devices also measure the pulse, oxygen saturation, and temperature.

Tell the Nurse!

Problems with blood pressure

■ The person's blood pressure is higher than normal

■ The person's blood pressure is lower than normal

■ You have difficulty measuring the person's blood pressure

Normal and Abnormal Findings

Accepted normal ranges for the systolic pressure are between 90 and 120 mm Hg, and for the diastolic pressure, between 60 and 80 mm Hg. Normally, a person's blood pressure moves up and down within the range of normal during the course of a day. For example:

■ Blood pressure readings are usually lowest in the morning, and can increase by as much as 10 mm Hg later in the day.

■ Blood pressure is generally slightly higher when a person is lying down as compared to when he is sitting or standing.

■ Blood pressure readings are usually slightly higher after a meal. Wait for at least an hour after mealtime to take a routine blood pressure.

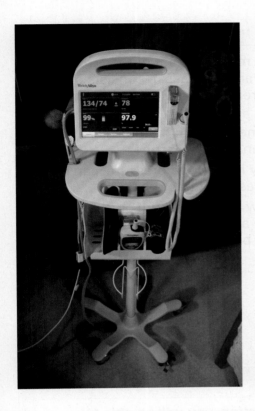

■ FIGURE 20-6
Automatic BP machine being used showing digital display of the person's BP.

■ Exercise will temporarily increase the systolic blood pressure.

■ Stress, anxiety, fear, and pain will also temporarily raise a person's blood pressure.

Hypertension is blood pressure that is consistently too high. Hypertension is often called the "silent killer" because a person with this condition does not feel ill, yet is at great risk for serious complications (such as a heart attack, stroke, or kidney failure) as a result of it. If one of your patients or residents who has been diagnosed with hypertension is not taking her medicine as ordered, you should report this to the nurse immediately.

Hypotension is blood pressure that is consistently too low. Some patients or residents may experience **orthostatic hypotension**, which is related to changing position. For these patients or residents, sitting on the edge of the bed before standing up ("dangling") is especially important to prevent a fall.

Hypertension high blood pressure; a blood pressure that is consistently greater than 140 mm Hg (systolic) and/or 90 mm Hg (diastolic)

Hypotension low blood pressure; a blood pressure that is consistently lower than 90 mm Hg (systolic) and/or 60 mm Hg (diastolic)

Orthostatic hypotension a sudden decrease in blood pressure that occurs when a person stands up from a sitting or lying position

> ### Concerns for Long-Term Care
>
> Normal ranges for vital signs vary somewhat in healthy older adults. In elderly persons who have chronic health conditions or take multiple medications, vital sign measurements may vary significantly from person to person. Older adults also have an increased tendency for their pulse rates and blood pressure measurements to fluctuate in response to postural changes (moving from supine to sitting or standing) and other factors, such as physical exertion or illness.
>
> Normal pulse rates for healthy older adults are slightly lower than for younger adults, but older adults are more likely to have irregular rhythms. Blood pressure is likely to increase, especially if the elderly person has arteriosclerosis. Respiratory changes in the older adult can increase the respiratory rate, especially with mild exertion or exercise. If the person has a history of cigarette smoking, his resting respiratory rate may be significantly higher.

Putting it all together!

- A person's blood pressure is a measurement of the force of the blood pushing against the arterial walls. It consists of a systolic and a diastolic measurement and is recorded as a fraction.
- Blood pressure is most often measured in the brachial artery using a sphygmomanometer and a stethoscope.
- Hypertension, or a consistently high blood pressure, can have serious long-term consequences if not treated.
- Orthostatic hypotension, or low blood pressure on changing positions, affects many people and is the reason people are encouraged to sit for a minute before standing up from a lying position.

Height and Weight

What will you learn?

When you are finished with this section, you will be able to:

1. Explain why accurately measuring a person's weight is important.
2. Demonstrate the proper way to measure a person's height and weight using an upright scale.
3. Demonstrate the proper way to measure a person's weight using a chair scale.

A person's height is measured only when the patient or resident is admitted to the facility. A person's weight is measured when the person enters the facility and before he leaves the facility. It may also be necessary to measure a person's weight at regular intervals throughout the person's stay at the facility, according to his care plan. A person may be weighed regularly for the following reasons:

- Changes in weight allow the health care team to evaluate the person's nutritional status. For example, the goal may be for the patient to gain weight or to lose it.
- Changes in weight can be a sign of how well the person's heart and kidneys are working. If the heart or kidneys are not working well, the person will retain fluid, which will cause an increase in weight.
- Changes in weight can indicate disease. For example, a sign of some types of cancer is major, unexplained weight loss.

■ Many medications are prescribed according to body weight. If a person gains or loses a great deal of weight, it may be necessary to adjust the person's medication doses.

Height is measured in feet (') and inches (") or in centimeters (cm). Weight is measured in pounds (lbs) or kilograms (kg). Scales may be mechanical or digital. If you are using a mechanical scale to measure a person's weight, you must slide weights along a bar by hand until the bar is balanced. If you are using a digital scale, you simply turn the scale on. The digital scale measures the person's weight automatically and displays it on a screen.

■ An **upright scale** is used to obtain height and weight measurements for a person who is able to stand on her own. Procedure 20-10 describes how to use an upright scale to measure a person's height and weight.

■ A **chair scale** is used to obtain a weight measurement for a person who cannot stand independently but is able to get out of bed. The chair scale may be a chair-like device, or it may be a platform that accommodates a person in a wheelchair. Procedure 20-11 describes how to use a chair scale.

■ A **tape measure** and a **sling scale** are used to measure the height and weight of a person who is totally bedridden (Fig. 20-7). Some specialty beds, such as those used for critically ill people, have built-in digital scales.

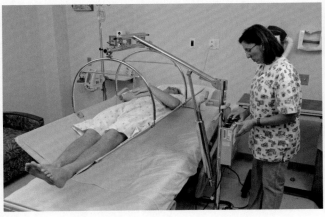

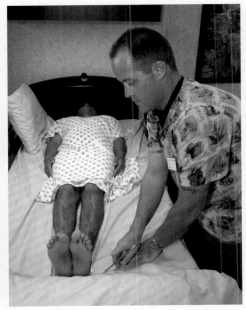

A   B

■ FIGURE 20-7

(A) A sling scale is used to obtain weight measurements for a person who cannot get out of bed. **(B)** The person's height is measured using a tape measure.

Putting it all together!

- Routine weight measurements may be necessary to monitor a person's medical condition or make sure that the person is taking the proper dose of a medication.
- A variety of devices, including upright scales, chair scales, and sling scales, can be used to measure a person's weight, depending on the person's situation.

PROCEDURES

PROCEDURE 20-1
Measuring an Oral Temperature (Glass or Electronic Thermometer)

Why you do it: A change in a person's normal temperature may be a sign of illness. Taking an oral temperature is fast and causes the patient or resident minimal discomfort.

GETTING READY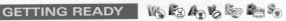

1. Complete the "Getting Ready" steps.

SUPPLIES

If using a glass thermometer:

- paper towels
- tissues
- thermometer sheath
- oral glass thermometer

If using an electronic thermometer:

- probe sheath
- electronic thermometer with oral (blue) probe

PROCEDURE

2. Ask the person if she has eaten, consumed a beverage, chewed gum, or smoked within the last 15 minutes. If so, wait 15 to 30 minutes before proceeding (or follow facility policy).
3. Prepare the thermometer.
   a. **Glass thermometer:** Run cool water over the thermometer to rinse away the disinfectant. Dry the thermometer with a paper towel and inspect it for cracks or chips. Carefully shake down the glass thermometer so that the indicator material is below the 94° mark (if using a Fahrenheit thermometer) or the 34° mark (if using a Celsius thermometer). Cover the end of the glass thermometer with the thermometer sheath.
   b. **Electronic thermometer:** Cover the electronic probe with the probe sheath. Turn the thermometer on and wait until the "ready" sign appears on the display screen.

4. Ask the person to open her mouth. Slowly and carefully insert the thermometer, placing the tip under the person's tongue and to one side.
5. Ask the person to gently close her mouth around the thermometer without biting down. If necessary, hold the thermometer in place. Ask the person to breathe through her nose.

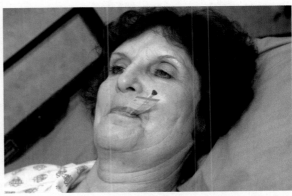

STEP 5 ■ The person breathes through her nose while holding the thermometer in her mouth.

6. Leave the thermometer in place for the specified amount of time:
   a. **Glass thermometer:** 3 to 5 minutes (or follow facility policy)
   b. **Electronic thermometer:** until the instrument blinks or beeps (usually just a few seconds)
7. Ask the person to open her mouth. Remove the thermometer from the person's mouth.

(procedure continues on page 440)

PROCEDURE 20-1 (continued)
Measuring an Oral Temperature (Glass or Electronic Thermometer)

8. Read the temperature measurement.
   a. **Glass thermometer:** Using a tissue, remove the thermometer sheath from the glass thermometer, being careful not to touch the bulb end of the thermometer. Dispose of the tissue and the thermometer sheath in a facility-approved waste container. Hold the thermometer horizontally by the stem at eye level while facing a light source. Rotate the thermometer until you can see the level of the indicator material. Read the temperature.
   b. **Electronic thermometer:** Read the temperature on the electronic thermometer's display screen. Remove the probe sheath from the probe by pushing the button on the top of the probe. Direct the probe sheath into a facility-approved waste container.
9. Prepare the thermometer for its next use.
   a. **Glass thermometer:** Shake down the glass thermometer, clean it according to facility policy, and return it to its disinfectant-filled case.

   b. **Electronic thermometer:** Replace the probe into the electronic thermometer. (Always read the temperature before placing the probe in the instrument because this action clears the display screen.) Turn the instrument off if it does not automatically turn itself off. Place the thermometer in its charger.

FINISHING UP

10. Complete the "Finishing Up" steps.

WHAT YOU DOCUMENT

- The date and time
- The person's temperature
- The method "O" for oral

Report an abnormal temperature to the nurse immediately.

PROCEDURE 20-2
Measuring a Rectal Temperature (Glass or Electronic Thermometer)

Why you do it: A change in a person's normal temperature may be a sign of illness. The rectal temperature measurement is a very accurate measurement of the body's temperature.

GETTING READY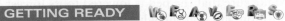

1. Complete the "Getting Ready" steps.

SUPPLIES

- gloves
- paper towels
- tissues
- lubricant jelly

If using a glass thermometer:
- thermometer sheath
- rectal glass thermometer

If using an electronic thermometer:
- probe sheath
- electronic thermometer with rectal (red) probe

PROCEDURE

2. Make sure that the bed is positioned at a comfortable working height (to promote good body mechanics) and that the wheels are locked.
3. Prepare the thermometer.
   a. **Glass thermometer:** Run cool water over the thermometer to rinse away the disinfectant. Dry the thermometer with a paper towel and inspect it for cracks or chips. Carefully shake down the glass thermometer so that the indicator material is below the 94° mark (if using a Fahrenheit thermometer) or the 34° mark (if using a Celsius thermometer). Cover the end of the glass thermometer with the thermometer sheath.
   b. **Electronic thermometer:** Cover the electronic probe with the probe sheath. Turn the thermometer on and wait until the "ready" sign appears on the display screen.
4. Place the thermometer on a clean paper towel on the over-bed table. Open the lubricant package and squeeze a small amount of lubricant onto the paper towel. Lubricate the tip of the thermometer to ease insertion.

5. If the side rails are in use, lower the side rail on the working side of the bed. The side rail on the opposite side of the bed should remain up. Lower the head of the bed so that the bed is flat (as tolerated).
6. Ask the person to lie on his side, facing away from you, in Sims' position. Help the person into this position, if necessary.
7. Fanfold the top linens to below the person's buttocks. Adjust the person's hospital gown or pajama bottoms as necessary to expose the person's buttocks.
8. Perform hand hygiene and put on the gloves.
9. With one hand, raise the person's upper buttock to expose the anus. Suggest that the person take a deep breath and slowly exhale as the thermometer is inserted. Using your other hand, gently and carefully insert the lubricated end of the thermometer into the person's rectum (not more than 1 inch for adults, or 1/2 inch for children). Never force the thermometer into the rectum. If you are unable to insert the thermometer, stop and call the nurse.

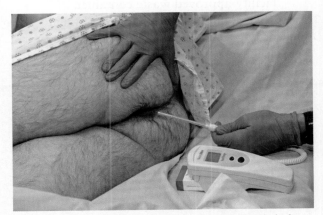

STEP 9 ▪ Gently and carefully insert the lubricated end of the thermometer into the person's rectum.

(procedure continues on page 442)

PROCEDURE 20-2 (continued)
Measuring a Rectal Temperature (Glass or Electronic Thermometer)

10. Hold the thermometer in place for the specified amount of time:
    a. **Glass thermometer:** 3 to 5 minutes (or follow facility policy)
    b. **Electronic thermometer:** until the instrument blinks or beeps (usually just a few seconds)
11. Remove the thermometer from the person's rectum. Wipe the person's anal area with a tissue to remove the lubricant, and adjust the person's hospital gown or pajama bottoms as necessary to cover the buttocks.
12. Read the temperature measurement.
    a. **Glass thermometer:** Using a tissue, remove the thermometer sheath from the glass thermometer, being careful not to touch the bulb end of the thermometer. Dispose of the tissue and the thermometer sheath in a facility-approved waste container. Hold the thermometer horizontally by the stem at eye level while facing a light source. Rotate the thermometer until you can see the level of the indicator material. Read the temperature.
    b. **Electronic thermometer:** Read the temperature on the electronic thermometer's display screen. Remove the probe sheath from the probe by pushing the button on the top of the probe. Direct the probe sheath into a facility-approved waste container.
13. Remove your gloves and dispose of them according to facility policy. Perform hand hygiene.

14. Help the person back into a comfortable position, straighten the bottom linens, and draw the top linens over the person. Raise the head of the bed, as the person requests.
15. Make sure that the bed is lowered to its lowest position and that the wheels are locked. If the side rails are in use, return the side rails to the raised position.
16. Prepare the thermometer for its next use.
    a. **Glass thermometer:** Shake down the glass thermometer, clean it according to facility policy, and return it to its disinfectant-filled case.
    b. **Electronic thermometer:** Replace the probe into the electronic thermometer. (Always read the temperature before placing the probe in the instrument because this action clears the display screen.) Turn the instrument off if it does not automatically turn itself off. Place the thermometer in its charger.

FINISHING UP
17. Complete the "Finishing Up" steps.

WHAT YOU DOCUMENT
- The date and time
- The person's temperature
- The method "R" for rectal

Report an abnormal temperature to the nurse immediately.

PROCEDURE 20-3
Measuring an Axillary Temperature (Glass or Electronic Thermometer)

Why you do it: A change in a person's normal temperature may be a sign of illness. The axillary method is used when other methods cannot be used.

GETTING READY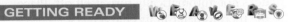

1. Complete the "Getting Ready" steps.

SUPPLIES

- paper towels
- tissues

If using a glass thermometer:
- thermometer sheath
- oral glass thermometer

If using an electronic thermometer:
- probe sheath
- electronic thermometer with oral (blue) probe

PROCEDURE

2. Ask the person if she has bathed or applied deodorant or antiperspirant within the last 15 minutes. If so, wait 15 to 30 minutes before proceeding (or follow facility policy).
3. Prepare the thermometer.
   a. **Glass thermometer:** Run cool water over the thermometer to rinse away the disinfectant. Dry the thermometer with a paper towel and inspect it for cracks or chips. Carefully shake down the glass thermometer so that the indicator material is below the 94° mark (if using a Fahrenheit thermometer) or the 34° mark (if using a Celsius thermometer). Cover the end of the glass thermometer with the thermometer sheath.
   b. **Electronic thermometer:** Cover the electronic probe with the probe sheath. Turn the thermometer on and wait until the "ready" sign appears on the display screen.
4. Assist the person with removing her arm from the sleeve of her hospital gown or pajama top in order to expose the axilla. The thermometer must be placed directly in contact with the skin.
5. Pat the axilla (underarm area) gently with a paper towel.
6. Ask the person to lift her arm slightly. Position the tip of the thermometer in the center of the axilla and ask the person to hold the thermometer in place by holding her arm close to the body (or by grasping the arm with the opposite hand).

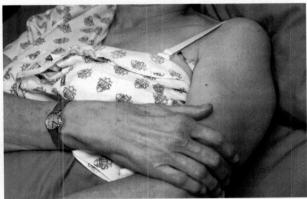

STEP 6 ▪ The person holds the thermometer in place by grasping her arm with the opposite hand.

7. Leave the thermometer in place for the specified amount of time:
   a. **Glass thermometer:** 10 minutes (or follow facility policy)
   b. **Electronic thermometer:** until the instrument blinks or beeps (usually just a few seconds)
8. Ask the person to lift her arm slightly. Remove the thermometer.
9. Read the temperature measurement.
   a. **Glass thermometer:** Using a tissue, remove the thermometer sheath from the glass thermometer, being careful not to touch the bulb end of the thermometer. Dispose of the tissue and the thermometer sheath in a facility-approved waste container. Hold the thermometer horizontally by the stem at eye level while facing a light source. Rotate the thermometer until you can see the level of the indicator material. Read the temperature.

(procedure continues on page 444)

PROCEDURE 20-3 (continued)
Measuring an Axillary Temperature (Glass or Electronic Thermometer)

b. Electronic thermometer: Read the temperature on the electronic thermometer's display screen. Remove the probe sheath from the probe by pushing the button on the top of the probe. Direct the probe sheath into a facility-approved waste container.

10. Help the person back into her hospital gown or pajama top.

11. Prepare the thermometer for its next use:

    a. Glass thermometer: Shake down the glass thermometer, clean it according to facility policy, and return it to its disinfectant-filled case.

    b. Electronic thermometer: Replace the probe into the electronic thermometer. (Always read the temperature before placing the probe in the instrument because this action clears the display screen.) Turn the instrument off, if it does not automatically turn itself off. Place the thermometer in its charger.

FINISHING UP

12. Complete the "Finishing Up" steps.

WHAT YOU DOCUMENT

- The date and time
- The person's temperature
- The method "A" for axillary

Report an abnormal temperature to the nurse immediately.

PROCEDURE 20-4
Measuring a Tympanic Temperature (Tympanic Thermometer)

Why you do it: A change in a person's normal temperature may be a sign of illness. Taking a tympanic temperature is fast and causes the patient or resident minimal discomfort.

GETTING READY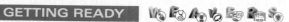

1. Complete the "Getting Ready" steps.

SUPPLIES

- tympanic probe sheath (cover)
- tympanic thermometer

PROCEDURE

2. If the person wears a hearing aid, remove it carefully and wait 2 minutes before taking the person's temperature. If the person has been sleeping or lying on his or her side with the ear against the pillow, use the ear that was not against the pillow for the temperature.

3. Inspect the ear canal for excessive cerumen (ear wax). If you see excessive wax build-up in the ear canal, gently wipe the ear canal with a warm, moist washcloth.

4. Cover the cone-shaped end of the thermometer with the probe sheath. Turn the thermometer on and wait until the "ready" sign appears on the display screen.

5. Stand slightly to the front of, and facing, the person. To straighten the ear canal (which will ease insertion of the thermometer), grasp the top portion of the person's ear and gently pull:
   a. Up and back (in an adult)
   b. Straight back (in a child)

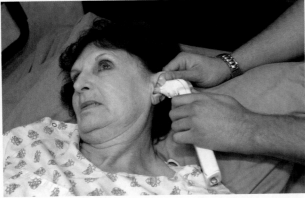

STEP 5a ▪ In an adult, grasp the top portion of the person's ear and gently pull up and back to insert the thermometer.

6. Insert the covered probe into the person's ear canal, pointing the probe down and toward the front of the ear canal (pretend that you are aiming for the person's nose). This will seal off the ear canal by seating the probe properly, leading to a more accurate temperature reading.

7. To take the temperature, press the button on the instrument. Keep the button depressed and the probe in place until the instrument blinks or beeps (usually 1 second).
8. Remove the probe and read the temperature on the display screen.
9. Remove the probe sheath from the probe by pushing the button on the side of the instrument. Direct the probe sheath into a facility-approved waste container.
10. If your facility requires a tympanic temperature to be taken in both ears, repeat the procedure, using a clean probe cover for the other ear.
11. Turn the instrument off if it does not automatically turn itself off. Place the thermometer in its charger.

FINISHING UP

12. Complete the "Finishing Up" steps.

WHAT YOU DOCUMENT

- The date and time
- The person's temperature
- The method "T" for tympanic

Report an abnormal temperature to the nurse immediately.

PROCEDURE 20-5
Measuring a Temporal Artery Temperature

Why you do it: A change in a person's normal temperature may be a sign of illness. Taking a temporal artery temperature is fast and accurate, and causes the patient or resident minimal discomfort.

GETTING READY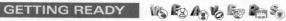

1. Complete the "Getting Ready" steps.

SUPPLIES

- temporal artery thermometer
- probe cover

PROCEDURE

2. Brush the person's hair aside if it is covering the temporal artery area. Anything covering the area, such as hair, a wig, a hat, bandages, or where the person's head was resting against the pillow can result in a false high reading.
3. Apply the probe cover.
4. Hold the thermometer like a remote control device, with your thumb on the red "ON" button. Place the probe on the center of the forehead and hold the body of the thermometer sideways.

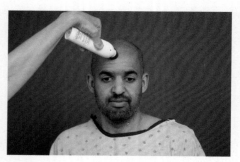

STEP 4

5. Press the ON button and keep it pressed throughout the measurement.
6. Slowly slide the thermometer straight across the forehead, midline, to the hairline. The thermometer will make a clicking noise.

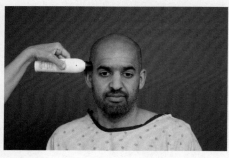

STEP 6

7. With the ON button still pressed, lift the thermometer up from the forehead and touch it to the neck, just behind the ear lobe in the little depression. This is a double check for the thermometer.

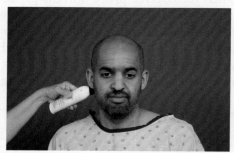

STEP 7

8. Release the ON button and read the temperature measurement.
9. Remove the probe cover by holding the thermometer over a facility-approved waste container and gently push the probe cover with your thumb.
10. Turn the thermometer off if it does not automatically turn itself off.

FINISHING UP

11. Complete the "Finishing Up" steps.

WHAT YOU DOCUMENT

- The time and date
- The person's temperature
- The method—temporal artery

Report an abnormal temperature to the nurse immediately.

PROCEDURE 20-6
Taking a Radial Pulse

Why you do it: A change in a person's normal pulse rate, rhythm, or amplitude may be a sign of illness. Taking the pulse at the radial artery is easiest for the patient or resident.

GETTING READY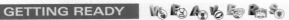

1. Complete the "Getting Ready" steps.

SUPPLIES

- watch with second hand

PROCEDURE

2. Rest the person's arm on the over-bed table or on the bed. Locate the radial pulse in the person's wrist using your middle two or three fingers. (TIP: The radial pulse will be on the person's "thumb" side.)
3. Note the strength and regularity of the pulse. Look at your watch and wait until the second hand gets to the "12" or "6." When the second hand reaches the "12" or the "6," begin counting the pulse.
   a. If the pulse rhythm is regular, count the number of pulses that occur in 30 seconds and multiply the result by 2 to arrive at the pulse rate.
   b. If the pulse rhythm is irregular, count the number of pulses that occur in 60 seconds. Counting each pulse that occurs over the course of 1 full minute is the only way to obtain a truly accurate pulse rate when the pulse is irregular.

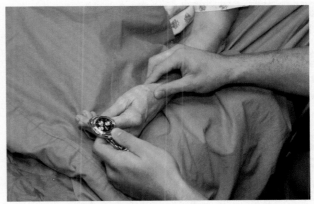

STEP 2 ■ Locate the radial pulse in the person's wrist using your middle two or three fingers.

FINISHING UP

4. Complete the "Finishing Up" steps.

WHAT YOU DOCUMENT

- The date and time
- The pulse rate
- The pulse rhythm
- The pulse amplitude

Report an abnormal pulse rate, rhythm, or amplitude to the nurse immediately.

PROCEDURE 20-7
Taking an Apical Pulse

Why you do it: An apical pulse is taken when a person has a weak or irregular pulse that may be difficult to feel in the radial artery. An apical pulse may also be used to measure heart rate in infants and in people with known heart disease.

GETTING READY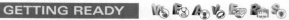

1. Complete the "Getting Ready" steps.

SUPPLIES

- alcohol wipes
- dual-sided stethoscope
- watch with second hand

PROCEDURE

2. Help the person to a semi-sitting position by raising the head of the bed.
3. Using alcohol wipes, clean the earpieces, the diaphragm, and the bell of the stethoscope. Place the earpieces in your ears.
4. Place the diaphragm (or the bell, if the person is a child or infant) of the stethoscope under the person's clothing, on the apical pulse site (located approximately 2 inches below the person's left nipple). The diaphragm or bell must be placed directly on the person's skin because clothing will distort the sound.
5. Using two fingers, hold the diaphragm or bell firmly against the person's chest. Look at your watch and wait until the second hand gets to the "12" or "6." When the second hand reaches the "12" or the "6," begin counting the heartbeat.
6. Count the number of heartbeats that occur in 60 seconds. Each time the heart beats, you will hear two sounds, best described as a "lubb" and a "dupp." Both sounds make up one beat of the heart and should be counted as such.

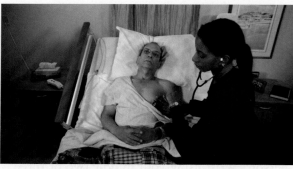

STEP 5 ■ Hold the diaphragm or bell firmly against the person's chest.

7. After 60 seconds, remove the diaphragm of the stethoscope from the person's chest. Adjust the person's clothing as necessary and help the person back into a comfortable position. Lower the head of the bed, as the person requests.
8. Using alcohol wipes, clean the earpieces, the diaphragm, and the bell of the stethoscope.

FINISHING UP

9. Complete the "Finishing Up" steps.

WHAT YOU DOCUMENT

- The date and time
- The pulse rate
- The pulse rhythm
- The pulse amplitude
- The method "A" for apical

Report an abnormal pulse rate, rhythm, or amplitude to the nurse immediately.

PROCEDURE 20-8
Counting Respirations

Why you do it: A change in a person's normal respiratory rate, rhythm, or depth of breathing may be a sign of illness.

GETTING READY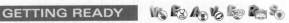

1. Complete the "Getting Ready" steps.

SUPPLIES

- watch with second hand

PROCEDURE

2. Look at your watch and wait until the second hand gets to the "12" or "6." When the second hand reaches the "12" or the "6," look at the person's chest (or place your hand near the person's collarbone or on his side) and begin counting each rise and fall of the chest as one breath.
   a. If the respiratory rhythm is regular, count the number of breaths that occur in 30 seconds and multiply the result by 2 to arrive at the respiratory rate.
   b. If the respiratory rhythm is irregular, count the number of breaths that occur in 60 seconds. Counting each respiration that occurs over the course of 1 full minute is the only way to obtain a truly accurate respiratory rate when the person's breathing is irregular.

FINISHING UP

3. Complete the "Finishing Up" steps.

WHAT YOU DOCUMENT

- The date and time
- The respiratory rate
- The respiratory rhythm
- Any abnormal sounds (wheezing, congestion)

Report abnormal respirations to the nurse immediately.

PROCEDURE 20-9
Measuring Blood Pressure

Why you do it: Blood pressure measurements allow health care workers to monitor existing problems and possibly even prevent future ones.

GETTING READY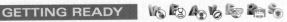

1. Complete the "Getting Ready" steps.

SUPPLIES

- alcohol wipes
- sphygmomanometer
- stethoscope

PROCEDURE

2. Assist the person into a sitting or lying position. Position the person's arm so that the forearm is level with the heart and the palm of the hand is facing upward. Assist the person with rolling up her sleeve so that the upper arm is exposed.

3. Using alcohol wipes, clean the earpieces, the diaphragm, and the bell of the stethoscope.
4. Stand no more than 3 feet away from the manometer. If it is not mounted on the wall, stand a mercury manometer upright on a flat surface, at eye level. Lay an aneroid manometer on a flat surface directly in front of you or leave it attached to the blood pressure cuff.
5. Squeeze the cuff to empty it of any remaining air. Turn the valve on the bulb clockwise to close it; this will cause the cuff to inflate when you pump the bulb.
6. Locate the person's brachial artery in the antecubital space by placing your fingers at the inner aspect of the elbow.

(*procedure continues on page 450*)

PROCEDURE 20-9 (continued)
Measuring Blood Pressure

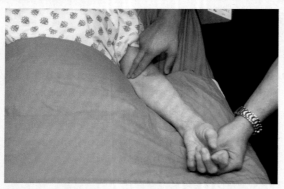

STEP 6 ■ Locate the person's brachial artery in the antecubital space (inner aspect of the elbow).

7. Place the arrow mark on the cuff over the brachial artery. Wrap the cuff around the person's upper arm so that the bottom of the cuff is at least 1 inch above the person's elbow. The cuff must be even and snug.

8. Place the stethoscope earpieces in your ears.

9. Pump the bulb until the pressure in the cuff is 30 mm Hg higher than the systolic pressure. There are two ways to do this:

   Method "A." Hold the bulb in one hand and position the diaphragm of the stethoscope over the brachial artery with the other hand. Inflate the cuff until you hear the pulse stop and then inflate the cuff 30 mm Hg more.

   Method "B." Hold the bulb in one hand and feel for the person's radial pulse (in her wrist) with the other hand. Inflate the cuff until you are no longer able to feel the radial pulse and then inflate the cuff 30 mm Hg more.

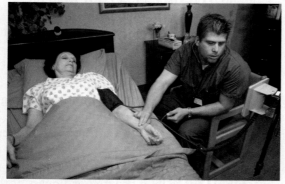

STEP 9 ■ Hold the bulb in one hand and feel for the person's radial pulse (in the wrist) with the other hand.

10. Position the diaphragm of the stethoscope over the brachial artery (or continue to hold it there if you used method "A" to inflate the cuff).

11. Turn the valve on the bulb slightly counter-clockwise to allow air to escape from the cuff slowly.

12. Note the reading on the manometer where the first sound of the brachial pulse is heard. This is the systolic reading.

13. Continue to deflate the cuff. Note the reading on the manometer where the last sound of the brachial pulse is heard. This is the diastolic reading.

14. Deflate the cuff completely and remove it from the person's arm. Remove the stethoscope from your ears.

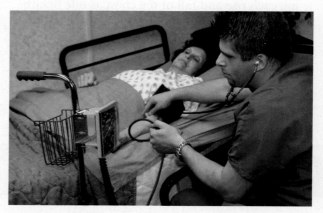

STEP 12 ■ With the diaphragm of the stethoscope over the person's brachial artery, allow the air to leave the cuff slowly while listening for the beginning and ending sounds of the brachial pulse and watching the manometer.

15. Return the sphygmomanometer to its case or wall holder.

16. Using alcohol wipes, clean the earpieces, the diaphragm, and the bell of the stethoscope.

FINISHING UP

17. Complete the "Finishing Up" steps.

WHAT YOU DOCUMENT

- The date and time
- The person's blood pressure

Report an abnormal blood pressure to the nurse immediately.

PROCEDURE 20-10
Measuring Height and Weight Using an Upright Scale

Why you do it: An upright scale is used to measure the height and weight of a person who can stand independently. A person's weight is often used to calculate medication doses. In some cases, a change in a person's weight might indicate that the person's condition is getting worse or that it is getting better.

GETTING READY

1. Complete the "Getting Ready" steps.

SUPPLIES

- upright scale

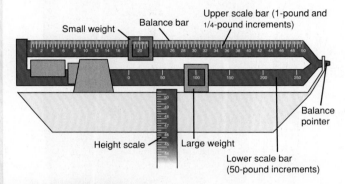

Small weight · Balance bar · Upper scale bar (1-pound and 1/4-pound increments) · Balance pointer · Height scale · Large weight · Lower scale bar (50-pound increments)

PROCEDURE

2. Ask the person to urinate. If necessary, assist the person to the bathroom or offer the bedpan or urinal.

3. Move the weights all the way to the left of the balance bar.

4. Help the person onto the scale platform so that she is facing the balance bar. Once the person is on the scale platform, do not allow her to hold on to you or to the scale.

5. Move the large weight on the lower scale bar to the right to the weight closest to the person's prior weight. For example, if the person weighed 155 pounds the last time you weighed her, you would move the large weight to the "150" mark.

6. Move the small weight on the upper scale bar to the right until the balance pointer is centered between the two scale bars.

7. Read the numbers on the upper and the lower scale bars where each weight has settled and add these two numbers together. This is the person's weight.

8. Have the person carefully turn around to face away from the scale bar. Slide the height scale

up so that you can pull out the height rod, which extends from the top of the height scale. Be careful not to hit the person in the head with the height rod.

9. Slide the height rod down so that it lightly touches the top of the person's head. Read the number at the point where the height rod meets the height scale. This is the person's height.

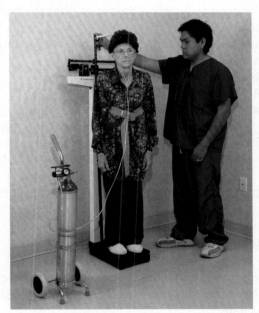

STEP 9 ■ Slide the height rod down so that it lightly touches the top of the person's head.

10. Hold the height rod in your hand, and help the person step down from the scale.

11. Assist the person back to her room.

FINISHING UP

12. Complete the "Finishing Up" steps.

WHAT YOU DOCUMENT

- The date and time
- The person's weight
- The person's height

Report a change in the person's weight to the nurse.

PROCEDURE 20-11
Measuring Weight Using a Chair Scale

Why you do it: A chair scale is used to measure the weight of a person who cannot stand independently but is able to get out of bed. A person's weight is often used to calculate medication doses. In some cases, a change in a person's weight might indicate that the person's condition is getting worse or that it is getting better.

GETTING READY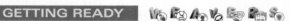

1. Complete the "Getting Ready" steps.

SUPPLIES

- transfer belt
- wheelchair*

PROCEDURE

2. Ask the person to urinate. If necessary, assist the person to the bathroom or offer the bedpan or urinal.
3. Assist or wheel the person to the scale, using a transfer belt, a wheelchair, or both.
4. Reset the scale to "0" by turning it on.
5. Help the person onto the scale.
   a. If a regular chair scale is being used, help the person to sit in the chair on the scale. Make sure that the person is seated properly, with her buttocks against the back of the chair and feet on the footrests.
   b. If a wheelchair scale is being used, roll the occupied wheelchair onto the platform and lock the wheels.
6. Read the weight on the display screen. If a wheelchair scale is being used, you must subtract the weight of the unoccupied wheelchair from this figure to determine the person's weight.
7. Help the person off of the scale.
   a. If a regular chair scale is being used, assist the person out of the chair and back into a wheelchair if one was used for the transfer.

---

*If you will be using a wheelchair scale to weigh the person, take the empty wheelchair to the scale and weigh it before taking it to the person's room. Be sure to write down the weight of the empty wheelchair.

STEP 6 ■ Read the weight on the display screen.

   b. If a wheelchair scale is being used, unlock the wheels and roll the wheelchair off the platform.
8. Assist the person back to her room.

FINISHING UP

9. Complete the "Finishing Up" steps.

WHAT YOU DOCUMENT

- The date and time
- The person's weight

Report a change in the person's weight to the nurse.

WHAT DID YOU LEARN?

Multiple Choice

Select the single best answer for each of the following questions.

1. A stethoscope is used to determine the:
   a. Brachial pulse rate
   b. Carotid pulse rate
   c. Apical pulse rate
   d. Popliteal pulse rate

2. The pressure exerted by the blood flowing through the arteries when the heart muscle relaxes is called the:
   a. Diastolic pressure
   b. Pulse pressure
   c. Pulse deficit
   d. Systolic pressure

3. The most common site for counting the pulse is the:
   a. Brachial artery
   b. Radial artery
   c. Carotid artery
   d. Apex of the heart

4. When counting respirations, you should:
   a. Have the person exercise first to get a true reading
   b. Count five respirations and then check your watch
   c. Count one inhalation and one expiration as one respiration
   d. Have the person count respirations while you take his pulse

5. You are using a glass Fahrenheit thermometer. When you shake it down, the liquid indicator should be below the:
   a. 98.6°F mark
   b. Arrow
   c. 100°F mark
   d. 94°F mark

6. Which of the following can cause an inaccurate oral temperature reading?
   a. The person exercised vigorously 15 minutes prior to having her temperature taken
   b. The nursing assistant failed to shake down the glass thermometer
   c. The person drank a cup of hot coffee 10 minutes prior to having her temperature taken
   d. All of the above

7. One of your patients, Ms. Jones, has a temperature of 98.8°F, a pulse rate of 80 beats/minute, and a respiratory rate of 30 breaths/minute. Which finding should be reported to the nurse immediately?
   a. Ms. Jones' respiratory rate
   b. Ms. Jones' pulse rate
   c. Ms. Jones' temperature
   d. None of these findings need to be reported to the nurse

8. What should you observe when taking a person's pulse?
   a. The rhythm and regularity of the pulse
   b. The number of beats per minute
   c. The strength of the pulse
   d. All of the above

9. If you notice a significant change in a person's vital signs, what should you do?
   a. Record the change with a special notation to indicate that the reading was different
   b. Mention the change to the nurse at the end of your shift
   c. Tell the patient or resident about the change
   d. Report the change to a nurse immediately

10. Which instrument is used to measure blood pressure?
    a. A temporal artery thermometer
    b. A sphygmomanometer
    c. An upright scale
    d. A watch with a second hand

11. Which one of the following conditions would prevent you from taking an oral temperature?
    a. The person has diarrhea
    b. The person has just had a mastectomy
    c. The person is unconscious
    d. The person is a 10-year-old child

Stop and Think!

It is almost time for your shift to end, and you are having trouble getting a blood pressure reading on Mr. Hayes. You really need to leave work on time today because your spouse is out of town and your daughter will be waiting for you to pick her up at school. Mr. Hayes is looking and acting the same way he always does, so you have no reason to think that his blood pressure would be different today than it is any other day. Would it be acceptable to just copy yesterday's blood pressure measurement? Why or why not? If not, what could you do to make sure that you still get out of work on time?

Assisting With Hygiene

Good personal hygiene is very important for both physical and emotional health. In this chapter, you will learn how to assist your patients or residents with caring for their teeth and keeping their skin clean, two activities that are key to maintaining personal hygiene.

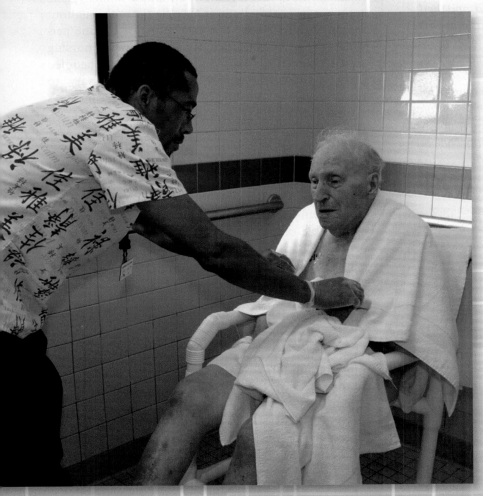

Photo: A nursing assistant assists a resident in the tub room, following a shower.

Introduction to Personal Hygiene

What will you learn?

When you are finished with this section, you will be able to:

1. Explain why good personal hygiene is important.
2. Explain what routine care is provided as part of early morning care, morning (A.M.) care, afternoon care, and evening (hour of sleep, hs) care.
3. Understand why it is important to respect a person's preferences with regard to personal hygiene practices whenever possible.
4. Define the word **PRN (as-needed) care**.

PRN (as-needed) care personal hygiene care that is provided whenever a patient or resident needs it, throughout the day or night

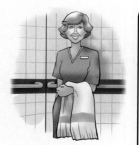

If you had always bathed in the evening, before bed, and then after entering a nursing home were told you had to bathe in the morning, how would you feel? Patients and residents may not be able to follow their normal routines when they are being cared for in a health care setting. This can be very upsetting. Looking for ways to accommodate each of your patient's or resident's personal preferences while still following the rules of the facility shows the person that you care about him as an individual.

Good personal hygiene:

- Helps to keep the skin and mucous membranes healthy
- Helps a person to feel attractive to others by preventing breath and body odors
- Helps a person to feel relaxed and well cared for

In many health care facilities, routine personal hygiene activities are carried out at specific times throughout the day (Table 21-1). The scheduling of routine personal care promotes efficiency and allows the nursing staff to plan these activities around other scheduled activities. Sometimes, however, it is necessary to break from the schedule in order to meet a person's needs. This is called providing **PRN (as-needed) care**. For example, PRN care is given any time there is wetness or soiling of the skin, clothing, or bedding.

The amount of assistance each resident or patient will need with personal hygiene activities will vary according to the person's abilities. Allowing a person to perform as much of her personal hygiene routine as possible on her own encourages feelings of independence and self-worth. It also provides a form of exercise, increasing the person's muscle tone, mobility, and circulation.

Concerns for Long-Term Care

When assisting a resident in the long-term care setting with personal care, it is important to allow the resident to do as much for himself as possible, even if it takes longer to complete the task. Provide assistance, as needed, to fill in for what the resident is not able to do. Participating in self-care helps the resident to attain or maintain his highest level of function and well-being. This is important for the resident's self-esteem and also for meeting OBRA requirements.

Many long-term care facilities have established "bathing teams" in order to more efficiently utilize bathing space and personnel. Two or more nursing assistants may be assigned to assist all residents who are scheduled for baths and showers as part of the day's routine care. This allows the nursing assistant to be able to spend more "personal" time with each resident. You may be helping a resident finish her morning shower by helping to apply lotion to her back while your teammate is changing the linens on her bed and tidying up her personal space in her room.

As a result of the culture change movement that is happening in long-term care right now, many facilities are changing their policies to allow residents to have more control over their daily lives. Upon admission, residents are asked about their preferences for care, and these preferences are accommodates as much as possible within the daily routines of the facility.

TABLE 21-1 Routine Scheduling of Personal Care

Type of Care	Definition	Related Activities
Early morning care	Care provided after a person wakes up to prepare him for breakfast or early testing or treatment	■ Toileting ■ Washing the face and hands ■ Providing oral care (including inserting dentures if necessary) ■ Brushing and combing the hair ■ Dressing
Morning (A.M.) care	Care provided in the morning to ready the person for the day, such as completion of personal hygiene and grooming activities and bedmaking	■ Toileting ■ Providing oral care ■ Bathing ■ Dressing ■ Assisting with grooming (shaving, brushing and combing the hair, putting on make-up) ■ Housekeeping (tidying the room, bedmaking)
Afternoon care	Care provided before and after lunch and dinner; general "freshening up"	■ Toileting ■ Washing the face and hands ■ Providing oral care
Evening (hour of sleep, hs) care	Care provided in preparation for sleep	■ Toileting ■ Washing the face and hands ■ Providing oral care ■ Bathing (if not done as part of morning care) ■ Changing into pajamas ■ Straightening linens

Putting it all together!

- Personal hygiene helps to keep a person healthy, both physically and emotionally. Healthy skin and mucous membranes are the body's first line of defense against infection. Good personal hygiene is also important for a person's self-esteem.
- To promote efficiency, routine personal hygiene activities are usually carried out at specific times throughout the day. In addition, assistance with personal hygiene is provided any time the patient or resident needs it. Wet or soiled skin, clothing, or bedding needs immediate attention.
- When possible, adjustments are made to the schedule to accommodate personal preferences (for example, bathing in the evening instead of in the morning).
- Encourage your patients or residents to do as much for themselves as possible. This promotes feelings of independence and self-worth.

Assisting With Oral Care

What will you learn?

When you are finished with this section, you will be able to:

1. Describe the benefits of good oral hygiene.
2. State observations that you may make when assisting a patient or resident with oral hygiene that should be reported to the nurse.
3. Describe situations that may require a person to need more frequent oral hygiene.
4. Discuss actions that promote the safe handling of a person's dentures.
5. Demonstrate proper technique for providing oral care for a person with natural teeth.
6. Demonstrate proper technique for providing oral care for a person with dentures.
7. Demonstrate proper technique for providing oral care for an unconscious person.
8. Define the word **edentulous**.

A clean, healthy mouth feels good, makes food taste better, and contributes to overall health. Poor oral hygiene can cause gum disease, dental cavities, tooth loss, and bad breath.

A person who has lost one or more natural teeth may have dental implants (prosthetic teeth that are surgically placed in the jaw bone), dentures (prosthetic teeth that can be taken in and out), or a combination of these. A person may have a partial denture or a full denture. Partial dentures are used when only some teeth are missing. Full dentures are used when a person is missing all of his top teeth or all of his bottom teeth. A person who has no teeth at all is said to be **edentulous.**

Oral care is usually provided when the person wakes up, before and after meals, and before bed. People who are unable or not allowed to take food or fluids by mouth will need oral care every 1 or 2 hours to keep their mouths fresh and moist. Some medications and health problems can cause a person to have a dry mouth. These patients or residents will also need more frequent oral care.

Most people can manage their own oral care, with assistance as needed. Occasionally a person will be too ill or weak to provide oral care for himself, and you will have to provide this care. Because the gums sometimes bleed as a result of routine oral care, always use standard precautions when assisting a patient or resident with oral care. Use droplet precautions as well if the patient or resident is known to have an infection caused by exposure to droplets released from the mouth or nose.

Providing Oral Care for a Person With Natural Teeth

Natural teeth are best cleaned with a toothbrush and toothpaste, followed by flossing. Toothbrushes should have soft bristles and be small enough to reach all of the teeth. Electric toothbrushes are simple to use and effective, especially for people who have limited strength or use of their hands. Brushing alone is not enough to remove food between the teeth, so flossing once a day is recommended as part of good oral hygiene. Many people like to use a mouthwash after brushing and flossing to complete their oral care routine. Procedure 21-1 describes how to assist a person with brushing and flossing the teeth.

Providing Oral Care for a Person With Dentures

Dentures take the place of a person's natural teeth, allowing the person to chew her food properly. Dentures that do not fit properly or that hurt the mouth when worn are not very useful for chewing. Proper care of the gums and dentures helps to keep the dentures fitting properly and comfortably.

Some people wear their dentures all of the time. Others may leave their dentures out at night or only wear them for meals. Personal preference for wearing dentures should be respected. Remember that people are more likely to wear their dentures if they are kept clean.

General guidelines for caring for dentures are given in Guidelines Box 21-1. Procedure 21-2 describes how to provide oral care for a person who wears dentures.

Edentulous without teeth

Tell the Nurse!

Assisting with oral care

- Dry, red, cracked, or bleeding lips
- Cold sores on the lips or mucous membranes
- Red, irritated, swollen, or bleeding gums
- Cracked, chipped, or broken teeth; loose teeth; blackened teeth (possibly a sign of decay)
- Chipped, cracked, or poorly fitting dentures
- Red sores or canker sores inside the mouth; white spots inside the mouth; any areas of pus or infection
- Bad breath that does not improve after oral care
- Fruity-smelling breath (possibly a sign of diabetes mellitus)
- A red or swollen tongue or a white coating on the tongue
- Complaints of pain or sensitivity

GUIDELINES BOX 21-1   Guidelines for Caring for Dentures

What you do	Why you do it
Handle a person's dentures with care.	Dentures are expensive and difficult to replace.
When a person is not wearing her dentures, store them in a denture cup filled with lukewarm water or a denture solution.	The water or solution prevents the dentures from drying out and warping. If the dentures warp, they will not fit properly.
When cleaning dentures, use lukewarm (not hot) water.	Hot water can damage the dentures.
When cleaning dentures, line the sink with a washcloth or paper towels.	The washcloth or towels help to prevent breaking or chipping of the denture if you accidentally drop it into the sink.
Use a denture brush (or a soft toothbrush) and denture cleaner to clean dentures. Do not use toothpaste.	The use of regular toothpaste is not recommended because the abrasives in the toothpaste can scratch and damage the denture surfaces.
Have the person rinse her dentures after eating.	Rinsing the dentures after eating removes food trapped between the gums and dentures. Trapped food can cause discomfort and promotes the growth of bacteria.
Allow the person to rinse with water or mouthwash or use a moist, foam-tipped applicator to clean the surfaces inside the person's mouth before placing the person's dentures in her mouth.	Placing the dentures inside the mouth is more difficult when the mouth and the dentures are dry. In addition, the moisture helps to create the suction that is needed to hold the dentures in place.
Label the person's denture cup with the person's name and room number.	Putting the person's name and room number on the denture cup helps to prevent the dentures from being misplaced.

Providing Oral Care for an Unconscious Person

A person who is unconscious needs frequent mouth care to keep the mucous membranes of the mouth moist and healthy. An unconscious person breathes with his mouth open, which can lead to drying and cracking of the lips and tongue. Cracked, dry lips are very uncomfortable and they create a portal of entry for microbes.

General guidelines for providing oral care for a person who is unconscious are given in Guidelines Box 21-2. Procedure 21-3 describes how to provide oral care for a person who is unconscious.

GUIDELINES BOX 21-2 Guidelines for Providing Oral Care for a Person Who Is Unconscious

What you do	Why you do it
Turn the person on his side so that fluids run out of the mouth, not back toward the throat.	*Turning the person onto his side helps to prevent aspiration (the accidental inhalation of foreign material into the airway). Aspiration can lead to complications such as choking or pneumonia.*
Never place your fingers in the person's mouth.	*An unconscious person may bite down involuntarily and without warning.*
Explain what you are doing throughout the procedure, even though the person may not seem to be able to hear you or respond to you.	*The person may be aware on some level that someone is doing something to him. Telling the person what you are doing reassures the person and helps the person to feel safe.*
Apply lip lubricant to the person's lips as needed.	*This helps to prevent drying and cracking of the lips, which is uncomfortable for the person and can lead to infection.*

 Putting it all together!

- Oral care involves caring for the teeth, gums, lips, and mucous membranes of the mouth.
- Oral care is important to prevent gum disease, dental cavities, and tooth loss. Painful or missing teeth can make it difficult for a person to chew food properly.
- A clean, healthy mouth provides a line of defense against infection, prevents bad breath, makes food taste better, and promotes comfort.
- Natural teeth should be brushed and flossed daily.
- Proper care of dentures helps to ensure a comfortable fit, which makes chewing easier. Dentures must be handled with care because they are expensive and difficult to replace.
- An unconscious person needs frequent oral care to prevent cracking of the lips and tongue. The person should be turned on her side to prevent aspiration during oral care.
- Standard precautions are taken when providing oral care because contact with body fluids is possible.

Assisting With Perineal Care

What will you learn?

When you are finished with this section, you will be able to:

1. Explain why perineal care is an essential part of daily hygiene.
2. State observations that you may make when assisting a patient or resident with perineal care that should be reported to the nurse.
3. Discuss sensitivity issues that you should be aware of when assisting with perineal care.
4. Demonstrate proper technique for providing perineal care for a male patient or resident.
5. Demonstrate proper technique for providing perineal care for a female patient or resident.
6. Define the word **perineal care (peri-care)**.

Perineal care (peri-care)
cleaning the perineum and anus, as well as the vulva (in women) and the penis (in men)

The parts of the body that are cleaned during **perineal care (peri-care)** are shown in Figure 21-1. Male patients or residents may be circumcised or uncircumcised (Fig. 21-2).

Providing good perineal care is important for two main reasons:

■ **Prevention of infection.** Because many microbes live in our digestive tracts and are passed from the body in the feces, there are always large numbers of microbes in and around the anus. If this area is not kept clean, it provides the perfect environment for these microbes to grow and cause an infection, especially if they enter the urinary system.

■ **Prevention of skin breakdown and odor.** The skin surrounding the perineum, vulva, and penis is delicate and contains many folds. Feces, urine, and other body

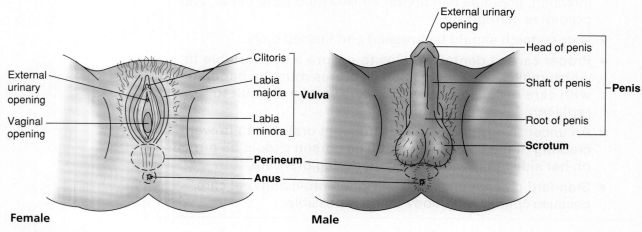

■ **FIGURE 21-1**

The parts of the body that are cleaned during perineal care.

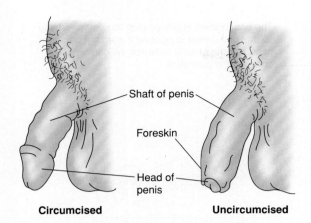

Circumcised   Uncircumcised

- Shaft of penis
- Foreskin
- Head of penis

■ **FIGURE 21-2**

Male patients or residents may have a circumcised or uncircumcised penis. Circumcision is often performed on male infants for religious or cultural reasons. During a circumcision, the fold of loose skin that covers the head of the penis (the *foreskin*) is surgically removed.

Tell the Nurse!

Assisting with perineal care

- Any unusual redness, inflammation, or skin rashes in the perineal area
- Any unusual discharge from the vagina or penis
- Any bleeding from the vagina (especially in a postmenopausal woman) or the anus
- Any abnormal odor

fluids can become trapped in these folds. This can lead to skin irritation and odor if the area is not properly cleaned.

Perineal care is routinely done at least once daily, as part of the bath. People with diarrhea or who are incontinent of urine or feces will need more frequent perineal care. For these patients or residents, a barrier cream or ointment may be applied after perineal care to help protect the skin from contact with urine or feces. Many facilities use pre-moistened disposable cloths ("perineal wipes") for routine perineal care. These wipes contain a soapless cleanser as well as antibacterial and skin-soothing ingredients that help to keep the skin healthy. However, if the perineal area is heavily soiled (for example, with large amounts of stool), soap and warm water should be used to provide perineal care.

Patients or residents who can manage their own perineal care should be encouraged to do so to the best of their ability. A person who is unable to provide for his self-care will need your help. Be sure to provide for the person's modesty during the procedure by closing the door and the curtain and draping the person with a bath blanket (Fig. 21-3). Sometimes stimulation of the penis during washing will cause a male patient or resident to become aroused during the procedure. Acting in a professional manner will help to ease embarrassment on the part of the patient or resident.

General guidelines for providing perineal care are given in Guidelines Box 21-3. Procedure 21-4 describes how to assist with perineal care for a female patient or resident, and Procedure 21-5 describes how to assist with perineal care for a male patient.

Having to help another person with perineal care may seem unpleasant or embarrassing to you. But think of it this way—what if you were sick or injured to the point that you had wet yourself or had a bowel movement in the bed? Think of how wonderful it would feel to have someone clean you up, help you change your clothes, and give you fresh bed linens. You would feel clean and cared for.

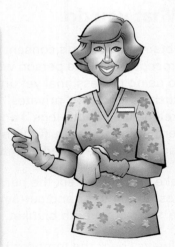

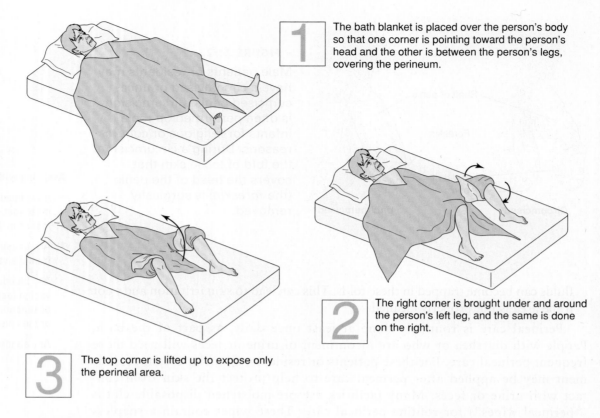

1 | The bath blanket is placed over the person's body so that one corner is pointing toward the person's head and the other is between the person's legs, covering the perineum.

2 | The right corner is brought under and around the person's left leg, and the same is done on the right.

3 | The top corner is lifted up to expose only the perineal area.

■ **FIGURE 21-3**

How to drape the person with a bath blanket during perineal care.

GUIDELINES BOX 21-3   Guidelines for Providing Perineal Care

What you do	Why you do it
Obtain the person's consent before beginning the procedure. Tell the person what you are going to do using professional yet understandable words (such as "crotch," "privates," "bottom," or "the area between your legs") and ask the person's permission to begin. If there is a language barrier, you may need an interpreter.	*To prevent misunderstandings, it is important for the person to understand where you are going to be touching him and why.*
Take care to protect the person's modesty by closing the door and curtain and draping the person with a bath blanket.	*Receiving perineal care can be very embarrassing. Properly draping the person may help the person to feel less "exposed."*
Always check the temperature of the water using a bath thermometer. The water temperature should be between 110°F (43.3°C) and 115°F (46.1°C).*	*Water that is too cold is uncomfortable, and water that is too hot could burn the person.*

What you do (continued)	**Why you do it** (continued)
Follow standard precautions when providing perineal care.	*Providing perineal care places you at risk for exposure to urine, feces, and other body fluids (for example, blood, vaginal secretions, semen).*
Perineal care is the last part of a person's bathing routine. Washcloths, towels, and the water in the wash basin (if a bed bath is being given) are discarded and not used on any other body parts after the perineal care is completed.	*The anus is a source of pathogens. To prevent spread of these pathogens to other parts of the body, where they may gain access and cause infection, the perineal area is washed last.*
The vulva (in women) or the penis (in men) is cleaned before the perineum.	*Because the anus opens onto the perineum, the perineum is often contaminated with microbes from the digestive tract. Therefore, this area is washed last to prevent microbes from the digestive tract from being introduced into the vagina or urethra, where they can cause infection.*
When you are assisting an uncircumcised man with perineal care, pull the foreskin back to clean the head of the penis. After cleaning and rinsing the penis, always remember to pull the foreskin back up over the end of the penis.	*Pulling the foreskin back allows you to clean and rinse the head of the penis thoroughly. Pulling the foreskin back into place after the head of the penis is cleaned prevents the foreskin from forming a band around the penis, which can cause pain and swelling.*
Rinse the skin thoroughly to remove all soap.	*The skin in the perineal area is very delicate. Soap is drying and can irritate the skin if not rinsed away.*
Gently pat the skin dry. Do not rub vigorously. Dry the skin thoroughly.	*The skin in the perineal area is very delicate. Vigorously rubbing the skin with a towel is uncomfortable for the person and can create friction, which in turn can cause skin breakdown. Moisture in areas where skin comes in contact with skin can also lead to skin breakdown.*
Remove your gloves and perform hand hygiene before touching clean clothing or linens.	*Gloves worn while providing perineal care are considered contaminated.*

*The water in the basin can be slightly hotter (110°F [43.3°C]) than the water in a tub or shower (105°F [40.5°C]) because it cools off quickly and the person will not be immersed in it.

Putting it all together!

- Perineal care involves cleansing of the perineum, the anus, the vulva (in women), and the penis (in men).
- Good perineal care can help prevent infection, skin breakdown (which can lead to pressure ulcers), and odor.
- Because receiving assistance with perineal care is embarrassing for most people, take extra care to preserve the person's

modesty. A professional attitude also helps to ease the patient's or resident's embarrassment.

- Standard precautions should be taken when providing perineal care because contact with body fluids is likely.
- Always wash toward the anus, away from the external urinary opening. This helps to prevent the spread of microbes from the anus into the urethra (and vagina, in women), where they could cause infection.

Assisting With Bathing

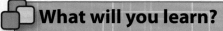

What will you learn?

When you are finished with this section, you will be able to:

1. Explain how bathing benefits a person's health.
2. State observations that you may make when assisting a patient or resident with bathing that should be reported to the nurse.
3. Describe supplies that are used for bathing.
4. Discuss sensitivity issues that you should be aware of when assisting with bathing.
5. Discuss safety issues related to assisting with a tub bath or shower.
6. Demonstrate proper technique for assisting a patient or resident with a tub bath or shower.
7. Demonstrate proper technique for assisting a patient or resident with a bed bath.

Bathing serves many purposes. The act of bathing:

- Helps a person feel relaxed and refreshed
- Cleans the skin and eliminates body odors
- Exercises muscles that might otherwise not be used
- Stimulates blood flow to the skin, which helps to prevent skin breakdown
- Gives the nursing assistant a chance to observe for skin problems and to communicate and bond with the patient or resident

The frequency and method of bathing are determined by many factors, including:

- Personal choice
- The person's culture or religion (certain cultural and religious beliefs may discourage bathing during certain times or may promote bathing as part of a ceremony or religious service)
- The person's state of health
- The person's level of activity and the weather
- The person's ability to care for herself
- Facility policy

TABLE 21-2	Supplies for Bathing	
Product	**Description**	**Use**
Soap	Available in liquid or cake form	▪ Cleans the skin of dirt, oil, microbes, and sweat
No-rinse cleansers	Available in liquid form or on premoistened disposable cloths	▪ Cleans, moisturizes, and protects the skin ▪ Rinsing is not necessary ▪ Some products are specific for the perineal area
Bath oils	Added to bath water	▪ Softens and scents the skin ▪ Use with caution because the oil can make the inside of the bathtub slippery
Lotions and creams	May be scented or unscented	▪ Creates a moisture barrier to prevent drying and chapping of the skin
Body powder	May be scented or medicated	▪ Helps to absorb moisture and sweat and reduces friction between skin surfaces that touch
Deodorants and antiperspirants	Available in spray, stick, or cream form	▪ Helps to prevent perspiration and body odor

Supplies for Bathing

Various supplies are used for bathing and skin care (Table 21-2). The type of products used will differ according to the condition of the person's skin and personal choice. Always ask new patients or residents if they have particular preferences in skin care products or if there are any products that cause problems for them.

In addition to skin care products, many types of linens are used for bathing. A bath blanket is used to preserve a person's modesty during a bed bath. A washcloth is wrapped around the hand to form a "mitt" for cleansing the body (Fig. 21-4). A towel is used to dry the body and can also be used to help preserve the person's modesty. A clean gown, pajamas, or change of clothes should be available for the person to put on after the bath.

Giving a Complete Bath

During a complete bath, the entire body is washed. A complete bath may be given in a tub or shower or in bed.

Assisting With Shower or Tub Baths

Patients who are able to get out of bed to bathe will take a shower or a tub bath. In many facilities, shower stalls are large enough for a shower chair to fit inside, allowing a weak or unsteady

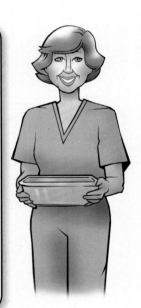

When assisting a patient or resident with personal hygiene, think about how you would feel if you were in that person's situation. You might feel embarrassed because you have to rely on someone else to help you with one of life's most basic tasks. You might also feel exposed because another person (possibly of the opposite sex) is seeing and touching your body. Acknowledge your patient's or resident's feelings by providing as much privacy as possible during the procedure and by maintaining a professional attitude at all times.

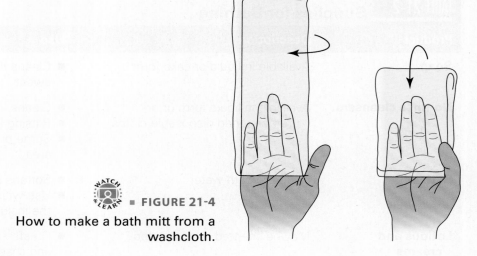

■ **FIGURE 21-4**
How to make a bath mitt from a washcloth.

person to sit down while taking a shower (Fig. 21-5). Facility bath tubs often have special modifications that make it easier for the person to get into and out of the tub safely (Fig. 21-6). Many modern tub and shower units also have controls that pre-set the water temperature, ensuring that it is not too hot or too cold. General guidelines for assisting a person with bathing are given in Guidelines Box 21-4. Procedure 21-6 describes how to assist with a tub bath or shower.

Assisting With a Bed Bath

When a patient or resident is too weak or ill to take a shower or tub bath, bath supplies and a basin of warm water are brought to the bedside, and the person is assisted with bathing in bed. Many facilities use "bag baths" as a quick and efficient

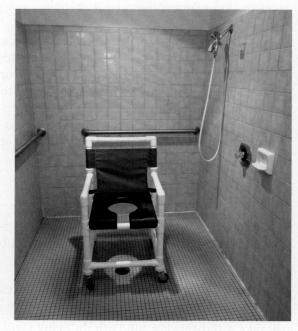

■ **FIGURE 21-5**

Shower stalls in health care facilities are usually wide enough to accommodate a shower chair. Use of a shower chair helps to reduce the risk of falling.

(text continued on page 471)

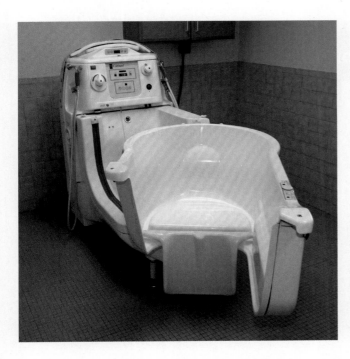

■ **FIGURE 21-6**

Bathtubs in health care facilities often have special modifications that make it easier for the person to get into and out of the tub safely. On this model, the front of the tub swings open.

GUIDELINES BOX 21-4   Guidelines for Assisting With Bathing

What you do	Why you do it
Follow the nursing care plan when determining what type of bath the person is to receive.	*Some bathing methods may not be allowed because of a person's medical condition.*
Before beginning the bath, explain to the person how the bathing procedure will be carried out (and how the person can assist in the process). In addition, explain the benefits of bathing (such as comfort and healthy skin).	*Explaining the details of the bathing process may help to relieve the person's fears (for example, about potential exposure) and will help the person to see how he can participate in the process. Explaining the procedure is particularly important for people with memory problems, who may find the bathing experience very frightening because they cannot remember what bathing is or why it is important.*
Collect all necessary equipment, linens, bath products, and clothing before beginning the bath. If the person will be taking a tub bath, check the tub room for cleanliness and prepare the tub before bringing the person into the room.	*Being prepared and having all necessary supplies and equipment at hand will allow the bath to proceed efficiently. Efficiency is necessary to protect the person's modesty and to prevent chills.*
Close all doors and windows in the room and make sure that the blinds are down or the curtains are drawn.	*Closing doors and windows eliminates drafts in the room, which could cause the person to become chilled. In addition, closing doors and covering the windows protect the person's modesty and privacy.*

(*box continues on page 470*)

GUIDELINES BOX 21-4 **Guidelines for Assisting With Bathing** (continued)

What you do	Why you do it
If non-skid strips are not in place, make sure to place a nonskid mat in the bathtub or on the shower floor. Encourage the person to use handrails. Provide a shower chair for people who are weak or unsteady.	*These measures help to protect the person from falling.*
Always keep the bathroom door unlocked.	*Because you should never leave a person alone in the bathtub or shower, if you need help for any reason, you will have to call for someone to come to you. This person will need to be able to access the bathroom without your help.*
Always check the temperature of the water using a bath thermometer. The water temperature should be at 105°F (40.5°C). Elderly people may require a slightly cooler water temperature, especially in a whirlpool tub. Make sure that you check for specific temperatures in the person's care plan.	*Water that is too cold is uncomfortable, and water that is too hot could scald the person.*
When assisting a person to and from the tub room, always make sure that she is adequately covered.	*The person's privacy and modesty must be protected at all times.*
Always help the person into and out of the bathtub or shower.	*A wet bathroom floor can be slippery and can place the person at risk for falling.*
Follow standard precautions when bathing a person.	*Bathing a person places you at risk for coming into contact with non-intact skin or body fluids.*
Wash from the cleanest to the dirtiest areas.	*This approach prevents contamination of clean areas.*
Touch the person's body gently yet deliberately, using long, firm strokes.	*A gentle yet firm touch conveys to the person that this is a routine procedure being carried out by a professional, ensures that the skin is properly cleaned, and stimulates skin circulation.*
Rinse the skin thoroughly to remove all soap.	*Soap is drying and can irritate the skin if not rinsed away.*
Gently pat the skin dry. Do not rub vigorously. Dry the skin thoroughly, especially in areas where skin touches skin (for example, underneath the breasts and between the legs).	*The skin, especially that of elderly people, is fragile. Vigorously rubbing the skin with a towel is uncomfortable for the person and can create friction, which in turn can cause skin breakdown. Moisture in areas where skin comes in contact with skin can also lead to skin breakdown.*

alternative to a traditional bed bath. With this method, a pouch containing 8 to 10 disposable cloths that are premoistened with a soapless cleanser is warmed in the microwave. A different cloth is used to clean each main body part. Another way of giving a bed bath is to moisten a fan-folded bath blanket and two washcloths with a solution of warm water and soapless cleanser. The moistened bath blanket is placed over the person and then covered with a dry bath blanket. The person's body is massaged through the blanket layers to cleanse the skin. The washcloths are used to cleanse the person's face and the perineal area. Procedure 21-7 describes how to assist with a bed bath.

Partial Baths

During a partial bath, only the face, hands, axillae (armpits), back, buttocks, and perineal area are washed. A partial bath provides many of the same health benefits as a complete bath and achieves the same goals of odor and infection control. A partial bath can be done at the sink or at the bedside.

As a person ages, the skin becomes dryer and more fragile. Frequent bathing can increase the skin's dryness, leading to itching, cracking, and injury. For this reason, many residents of long-term care facilities receive complete baths or showers only two or three times weekly, with partial baths in between. A partial bath may also be given when a complete bath or shower is not allowed for medical reasons or when a patient or resident simply does not feel up to a complete bath or shower.

Putting it all together!

- Bathing helps to prevent skin breakdown (which can lead to pressure ulcers), infection, and odor. Bathing also helps a person to feel relaxed and refreshed.
- Bathing may be accomplished in a bathtub or shower, at the sink, or in bed. A partial or complete bath may be given, depending on the person's needs.
- Assisting your patients or residents with bathing provides an excellent opportunity for you to observe the patient's or resident's skin and body for any changes that should be reported to the nurse.
- Allowing the patient or resident to choose the bath and skin care products he would like to use is an important part of respecting that person's individuality.
- Because receiving assistance with bathing is embarrassing for most people, take extra care to preserve the person's modesty. A professional attitude also helps to ease the patient's or resident's embarrassment.
- Standard precautions should be taken when assisting with bathing because contact with body fluids is likely.

PROCEDURES

PROCEDURE 21-1
Brushing and Flossing the Teeth

Why you do it: Brushing and flossing the teeth help to keep the teeth and gums healthy, make the mouth feel better and food taste better, and prevent bad breath.

GETTING READY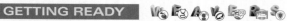

1. Complete the "Getting Ready" steps.

SUPPLIES

- gloves
- paper towels
- straw (optional)
- cup of cool water
- emesis basin
- toothbrush
- toothpaste
- dental floss
- lip lubricant (optional)
- mouthwash (optional)
- towel and washcloth

PROCEDURE

2. Clean the surface of the over-bed table and cover with paper towels. Place the oral care supplies on the over-bed table. Fill a paper cup with water.
3. Make sure that the bed is positioned at a comfortable working height (to promote good body mechanics) and that the wheels are locked.
4. If the side rails are in use, lower the side rail on the working side of the bed. The side rail on the opposite side of the bed should remain up.
5. Raise the head of the bed as tolerated. Place a towel under the person's chin.
6. Perform hand hygiene and put on the gloves.
7. Wet the toothbrush. Put a small amount of toothpaste on the toothbrush.
8. Brush the person's teeth as follows:
   a. Position the toothbrush at a 45° angle to the gums, against the outer surface of the top teeth. Starting at the back of the mouth, brush the outer surface of each tooth using a gentle circular motion. Repeat for the lower teeth. Allow the person to spit toothpaste into the emesis basin as necessary.

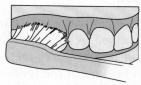

STEP 8a ■ Clean the outer surfaces of the teeth.

   b. Position the toothbrush at a 45° angle to the gums, against the inner surface of the top teeth. Starting at the back of the mouth, brush the inner surface of each tooth using a gentle circular motion. Repeat for the lower teeth.

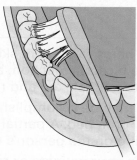

STEP 8b ■ Clean the inner surfaces of the teeth.

   c. Brush the chewing surfaces of the upper and lower teeth using a gentle circular motion.

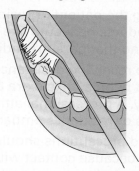

STEP 8c ■ Clean the chewing surfaces of the teeth.

   d. Brush the tongue.

9. Offer the person the cup of water (and a straw, if desired) and ask her to rinse her mouth completely. Hold the emesis basin underneath the person's chin so that she can spit the water into the basin.

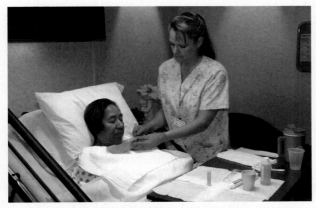

STEP 9 ■ Hold the emesis basin underneath the person's chin so that she can spit.

10. Place the emesis basin on the over-bed table and dry the person's mouth and chin thoroughly using the washcloth.

11. Cut a piece of dental floss measuring about 18 inches. Wrap the dental floss around the middle finger of each hand. Hold the dental floss between your thumb and index finger on each hand and stretch it tight.

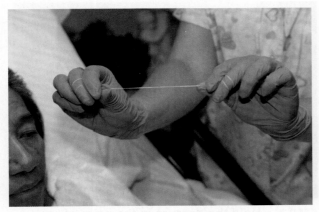

STEP 11 ■ Hold the dental floss between your thumb and index finger on each hand and stretch it tight.

12. Insert a segment of dental floss between two teeth, starting with the back upper teeth. Move

the floss up and down gently, and then remove the dental floss from the person's mouth. Advance the floss a bit by releasing it from one middle finger and wrapping it around the other, and move on to the next two teeth. Use a new strand of dental floss as necessary. Offer the person the glass of water (and the straw, if desired) to rinse as necessary. Floss all of the person's teeth.

13. Offer the person the cup of water (and the straw, if desired) and ask her to rinse her mouth completely. Hold the emesis basin underneath the person's chin so that she can spit the water into the basin.

14. Place the emesis basin on the over-bed table and dry the person's mouth and chin thoroughly using the washcloth.

15. Pour a small amount of mouthwash (approximately ¼ cup) into the cup and help the person to rinse, as the person requests.

16. Apply lip lubricant to the lips, as the person requests. Remove your gloves, perform hand hygiene, and put on a clean pair of gloves.

17. If the side rails are in use, return the side rails to the raised position. Lower the head of the bed as the person requests. Make sure that the bed is lowered to its lowest position and that the wheels are locked.

18. Gather the soiled linens and place them in the linen hamper or linen bag. Dispose of disposable items in a facility-approved waste container. Clean equipment and return it to the storage area.

19. Remove your gloves, dispose of them in a facility-approved waste container, and perform hand hygiene.

FINISHING UP

20. Complete the "Finishing Up" steps.

WHAT YOU DOCUMENT

- The date and time
- Level of assistance needed
- Any unusual observations

PROCEDURE 21-2

Providing Oral Care for a Person With Dentures

Why you do it: Proper care of the gums and dentures helps to keep the mouth healthy and the dentures fitting properly and comfortably. It also makes the mouth feel better and food taste better and prevents bad breath.

GETTING READY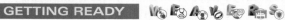

1. Complete the "Getting Ready" steps.

SUPPLIES

- gloves
- paper towels
- gauze squares (4″ × 4″)
- straw (optional)
- toothpaste and dental floss (if the person has any natural teeth)
- soft bristle toothbrush or foam-tipped applicators
- emesis basin
- cup with cool water
- denture cup
- denture brush or toothbrush
- denture cleaner
- denture solution (optional)
- mouthwash (optional)
- lip lubricant (optional)
- towel
- washcloth

PROCEDURE

2. Clean the surface of the over-bed table and cover with paper towels. Place the oral care supplies on the over-bed table.
3. Make sure that the bed is positioned at a comfortable working height (to promote good body mechanics) and that the wheels are locked. Raise the head of the bed as tolerated. Place a towel across the person's chest.
4. Perform hand hygiene and put on the gloves.
5. Ask the person to remove his dentures and place them in the emesis basin. If the person needs assistance with removing his dentures:
   a. Ask the person to open his mouth.
   b. Holding a gauze square between your thumb and index finger, grasp the upper denture, moving it up and down slightly to break the seal. Ease the denture down, forward, and out of the mouth. Place the denture in the emesis basin.
   c. Holding a gauze square between your thumb and index finger, grasp the lower denture. Turn the denture slightly, lifting it out of the mouth. Place the denture in the emesis basin.
6. Take the emesis basin, the washcloth, the denture cup, the denture brush or toothbrush, and the denture cleaner to the sink. Line the sink with the washcloth to provide extra cushioning. Fill the sink partially with lukewarm water. Do not place the dentures in the sink.
7. Wet the denture brush or the toothbrush. Put a small amount of denture cleaner on the denture brush or toothbrush. Working with one denture at a time, hold the denture in the palm of your hand and brush it on all surfaces until it is clean. Rinse the denture thoroughly under lukewarm running water and place it in the denture cup. Repeat with the other denture.

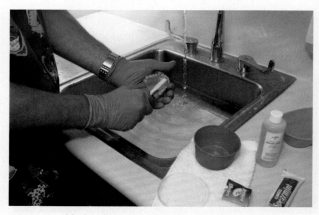

STEP 7 ■ Hold the denture in the palm of your hand, and brush it on all surfaces until it is clean.

8. If the dentures are to be stored, fill the denture cup with lukewarm water, a mixture of one part mouthwash to one part lukewarm water, or a denture solution so that the dentures are covered. Put the lid on the denture cup. Return the denture cup to the person's bedside table, making sure that it is within easy reach.

9. If the dentures are to be reinserted in the person's mouth, take the emesis basin, the denture cup, and the toothbrush to the over-bed table. If the side rails are in use, lower the side rail on the working side of the bed. The side rail on the opposite side of the bed should remain up.

   a. Offer the person the cup of water (and a straw, if desired) and ask him to rinse his mouth completely. Some people may wish to use mouthwash instead of water. Hold the emesis basin underneath the person's chin so that he can spit the water or mouthwash into the basin.

   b. Place the emesis basin on the over-bed table and dry the person's mouth and chin thoroughly using a face towel.

   c. Gently clean the person's gums and tongue and the insides of the cheeks with the toothbrush or a foam-tipped applicator moistened with water or mouthwash. Use fresh applicators as needed. If the person has any remaining natural teeth, assist with brushing and flossing those teeth.

   d. Ask the person to insert his dentures. If the person needs assistance with inserting his dentures:

   ■ Ask the person to open his mouth.
   ■ Gently lift the person's upper lip up. Grasp the upper denture between your thumb and index finger and insert it in the person's mouth. Press gently on the denture to be sure that it is seated properly.

   ■ Gently pull the person's lower lip down. Grasp the lower denture between your thumb and index finger and insert it in the person's mouth.

   e. Return the denture cup to the person's bedside table, making sure that it is within easy reach.

10. Dry the person's mouth and chin thoroughly using a towel. Apply lip lubricant to the lips, as the person requests. Remove your gloves, perform hand hygiene, and put on a clean pair of gloves.

11. Reposition the person comfortably and lower the head of the bed if necessary. If the side rails are in use, return the side rails to the raised position. Make sure that the bed is lowered to its lowest position and that the wheels are locked.

12. Gather the soiled linens and place them in the linen hamper or linen bag. Dispose of disposable items in a facility-approved waste container. Clean equipment and return it to the storage area.

13. Remove your gloves, dispose of them in a facility-approved waste container, and perform hand hygiene.

FINISHING UP

14. Complete the "Finishing Up" steps.

WHAT YOU DOCUMENT

■ The date and time
■ Amount of assistance needed
■ Any unusual observations

PROCEDURE 21-3
Providing Oral Care for an Unconscious Person

Why you do it: An unconscious person breathes through the mouth, causing the lips and mucous membranes to dry out. Frequent mouth care keeps the mucous membranes of the mouth moist and healthy and promotes comfort.

GETTING READY

1. Complete the "Getting Ready" steps.

SUPPLIES

- gloves
- paper towels
- sponge-tipped applicators
- padded tongue blade
- cup with appropriate solution (cool water, saline, mouthwash)
- emesis basin
- toothbrush and toothpaste (if the person has natural teeth)
- lip lubricant
- saline (optional)
- mouthwash (optional)
- towel and washcloth

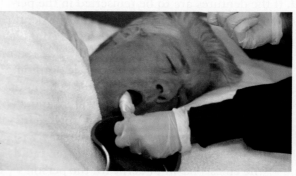

STEP 8 ■ Clean the inside of the person's mouth, using a padded tongue blade to keep the mouth open.

PROCEDURE

2. Clean the surface of the over-bed table and cover it with paper towels. Place the oral care supplies on the over-bed table.

3. Make sure that the bed is positioned at a comfortable working height (to promote good body mechanics) and that the wheels are locked. If the side rails are in use, lower the side rail on the working side of the bed. The side rail on the opposite side of the bed should remain up.

4. Position the person onto his or her side, with the head tilted forward.

5. Place a towel across the pillow underneath the person's face and spread across his or her chest. Position the emesis basin on the towel underneath the person's chin.

6. Perform hand hygiene and put on the gloves.

7. Open the person's mouth by gently applying pressure to the lower jaw in front of the mouth. Be gentle; do not force the mouth open. Insert the tongue blade between the upper and lower teeth at the back of the mouth to hold the person's mouth open.

8. Clean the inside of the mouth:

　a. If the person has natural teeth, they should be gently brushed as described in Procedure 21-1.

　b. If the person is edentulous, gently clean the person's gums and tongue and the insides of the cheeks with the toothbrush or a foam-tipped applicator moistened with water, saline, or mouthwash. Use fresh applicators as needed.

Note: Do not use a foam-tipped applicator for people who may bite it. Pieces can be aspirated by the person if they remain in the mouth.

9. Dry the person's mouth and chin thoroughly using a washcloth. Apply lip lubricant to the lips. Reposition the person comfortably. Remove your gloves, perform hand hygiene, and put on a clean pair of gloves.

10. If the side rails are in use, return the side rails to the raised position. Make sure that the bed is lowered to its lowest position and that the wheels are locked.

11. Gather the soiled linens and place them in the linen hamper or linen bag. Dispose of disposable items in a facility-approved waste container. Clean the over-bed table per facility policy. Clean equipment and return it to the storage area.

12. Remove your gloves, dispose of them in a facility-approved waste container, and perform hand hygiene.

FINISHING UP

13. Complete the "Finishing Up" steps.

WHAT YOU DOCUMENT

- Date and time
- Type of care given (teeth brushed, mouth swabbed, etc.)
- Any unusual observations

PROCEDURE 21-4
Providing Female Perineal Care

Why you do it: Proper perineal care helps to prevent skin breakdown (which can lead to pressure ulcers), infection, and odor.

GETTING READY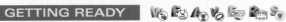

1. Complete the "Getting Ready" steps.

SUPPLIES

- gloves
- paper towels
- bed protector
- bath thermometer
- wash basin
- bedpan
- soap, no-rinse cleansing solution, or commercially packaged disposable cleaning cloths
- bath blanket
- washcloths
- towel
- clean clothing
- clean linens (if necessary)

PROCEDURE

2. Clean the surface of the over-bed table and cover with paper towels. Place the wash basin, cleansing solution or soap, washcloths, towels, and bed protector on the over-bed table. Other clean linens and clothing (if needed) can be placed on a nearby clean bedside table or chair.

3. Make sure that the bed is positioned at a comfortable working height (to promote good body mechanics) and that the wheels are locked.

4. Perform hand hygiene and put on the gloves.

5. Because bathing often stimulates the urge to urinate, offer the bedpan. If the person uses the bedpan, empty and clean it before proceeding with the perineal care. Remove your gloves and dispose of them in a facility-approved waste container. Perform hand hygiene and put on a clean pair of gloves.

6. Lower the head of the bed to a flat position (as tolerated).

7. Fill the wash basin with warm water (110°F [43.3°C] to 115°F [46.1°C] on the bath thermometer). If using a liquid no-rinse cleansing solution that is added to water, add the proper amount of the cleanser to the basin of water. Place the basin on the over-bed table. If using commercially packaged no-rinse disposable products, you will not need a basin of water unless the disposable cloths need to be placed in water to activate them.

8. If the side rails are in use, lower the side rail on the working side. The side rail on the opposite side of the bed should remain up.

9. Spread the bath blanket over the top linens (and the person). If the person is able, have her hold the bath blanket. If not, tuck the corners under the person's shoulders. Fanfold the top linens to the foot of the bed.

10. Assist the person with undressing.

11. Ask the person to open her legs and bend her knees, if possible. If she is not able to bend her knees, help her spread her legs as much as possible. (If a person is unable to spread her legs enough to expose the perineal area, you may position her onto her side with her knees bent forward to expose the perineum for cleaning.)

12. Position the bath blanket over the person so that one corner can be wrapped under and around each leg.

13. Position the bed protector under the person's buttocks to keep the bed linens dry.

14. Lift the corner of the bath blanket that is between the person's legs upward, exposing only the perineal area.

15. Wash and rinse the groin area.

16. Form a mitt around your hand with one of the washcloths. Wet the mitt with warm, clean water and apply soap or no-rinse cleansing solution. If you are using the prepackaged disposable cleaning cloths, the steps of the procedure will remain the same. You will use a clean disposable cloth for each area you clean.

(procedure continues on page 478)

PROCEDURE 21-4 (continued)
Providing Female Perineal Care

17. Using the other hand, separate the labia. Clean the vulva by placing your washcloth-covered hand at the top of the vulva and stroking downward to the anus. Use a different part of the washcloth for each stroke. Repeat until the area is clean.

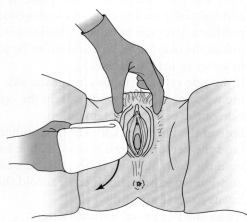

STEP 17 ■ Clean the vulva by placing your washcloth-covered hand at the top of the vulva and stroking downward to the anus.

18. Rinse the vulva and perineum thoroughly (if using a no-rinse product, omit this step):
    Form a mitt around your hand with a clean, wet washcloth. Using the other hand, separate the labia. Rinse the vulva by placing your washcloth-covered hand at the top of the vulva and stroking downward to the anus. Use a different part of the washcloth for each stroke. Repeat until the area is free of soap.

19. Dry the perineal area thoroughly using a towel.

20. Turn the person onto her side so that she is facing away from you. Help the person toward the working side of the bed so that her buttocks are within easy reach. Adjust the bath blanket to keep the person covered.

21. Form a mitt around your hand with one of the washcloths. Wet the mitt with warm, clean water and apply soap or no-rinse cleansing solution.

22. Using the other hand, separate the buttocks. Place your washcloth-covered hand at the front

of the anal area and stroke toward the back. First clean one side, then the other side, and finally the middle, using a different part of the washcloth each time, until the anal area is clean.

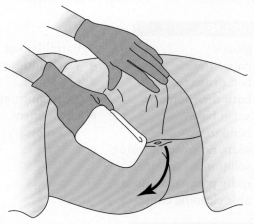

STEP 22 ■ Clean the anal area by placing your washcloth-covered hand at the front of the body and stroking toward the back.

23. Rinse (if necessary) and dry the anal area thoroughly. Remove the bed protector from underneath the person.

24. Remove your gloves and dispose of them in a facility-approved waste container. Perform hand hygiene and put on a clean pair of gloves.

25. Assist the person into the supine position. Reposition the pillow under her head. Remove the bath blanket and help the person into the clean clothing.

26. If the bedding is wet or soiled, change the bed linens.

27. If the side rails are in use, return the side rail to the raised position. Raise the head of the bed as the person requests. Make sure that the bed is lowered to its lowest position and that the wheels are locked.

28. Gather the soiled linens and place them in the linen hamper or linen bag. Dispose of disposable items in a facility-approved waste container. Clean the over-bed table per facility policy. Clean equipment and return it to the storage area.

29. Remove your gloves, dispose of them in a facility-approved waste container, and perform hand hygiene.

FINISHING UP

30. Complete the "Finishing Up" steps.

WHAT YOU DOCUMENT

- Date and time
- Presence of urine or stool
- Level of assistance needed
- Condition of skin

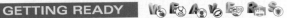

PROCEDURE 21-5
Providing Male Perineal Care

Why you do it: Proper perineal care helps to prevent skin breakdown (which can lead to pressure ulcers), infection, and odor.

GETTING READY

1. Complete the "Getting Ready" steps.

SUPPLIES

- gloves
- paper towels
- bed protector
- bath thermometer
- wash basin
- bedpan or urinal
- soap, no-rinse cleansing solution, or commercially packaged
- disposable cleansing cloths
- bath blanket
- washcloths
- towel
- clean clothing
- clean linens (if necessary)

PROCEDURE

2. Clean the surface of the over-bed table and cover with paper towels. Place the wash basin, toiletries, clean clothing, and clean linens on the over-bed table.

3. Make sure that the bed is positioned at a comfortable working height (to promote good body mechanics) and that the wheels are locked.

4. Perform hand hygiene and put on the gloves.

5. Because bathing often stimulates the urge to urinate, offer the bedpan or urinal. If the person uses the bedpan or urinal, empty and clean it before proceeding with the perineal care. Remove your gloves and dispose of them in a facility-approved waste container. Perform hand hygiene and put on a clean pair of gloves.

6. Lower the head of the bed to a flat position (as tolerated).

7. Fill the wash basin with warm water (110°F [43.3°C] to 115°F [46.1°C] on the bath thermometer). If using a no-rinse cleansing solution, add the appropriate amount to the water in the basin. Place the basin on the over-bed table. If using commercially packaged no-rinse disposable products, you will not need a basin of water unless the disposable cloths need to be placed in water to activate them.

8. If the side rails are in use, lower the side rail on the working side. The side rail on the opposite side of the bed should remain up.

9. Spread the bath blanket over the top linens (and the person). If the person is able, have him hold the bath blanket. If not, tuck the corners under the person's shoulders. Fanfold the top linens to the foot of the bed.

10. Assist the person with undressing.

11. Ask the person to open his legs and bend his knees, if possible. If he is not able to bend his knees, help him spread his legs as much as possible.

12. Position the bath blanket over the person so that one corner can be wrapped under and around each leg.

13. Position the bed protector under the person's buttocks to keep the bed linens dry.

(procedure continues on page 480)

PROCEDURE 21-5 (continued)
Providing Male Perineal Care

14. Lift the corner of the bath blanket that is between the person's legs upward, exposing only the perineal area.
15. Wash and rinse the groin area.
16. Form a mitt around your hand with one of the washcloths. Wet the mitt with warm, clean water and apply soap or the no-rinse cleansing solution. If you are using the prepackaged disposable cleaning cloths, the steps of the procedure will remain the same. You will use a clean disposable cloth for each area you clean.
17. Using the other hand, hold the penis slightly away from the body.
    a. If the person is circumcised: Place your wash-cloth-covered hand at the tip of the penis and wash in a circular motion, downward to the base of the penis. Repeat, using a different part of the washcloth each time, until the area is clean. Rinse and dry the tip and the shaft of the penis thoroughly (if using a no-rinse cleansing solution, omit the rinse):

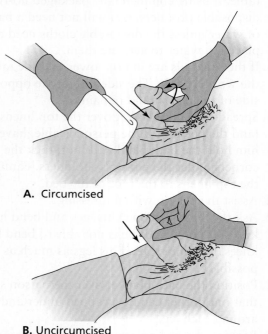

A. Circumcised

B. Uncircumcised

STEP 17 ■ To wash the penis, pass the wash-cloth in a circular motion, moving from the tip of the penis to the base. **(A)** Circumcised penis; **(B)** uncircumcised penis.

Form a mitt around your hand with a clean, wet washcloth. Using the other hand, hold the penis slightly away from the body. Place your washcloth-covered hand at the tip of the penis and wipe in a circular motion, downward to the base of the penis. Repeat, using a different part of the washcloth each time, until the area is rinsed. Dry the penis thoroughly.

    b. If the person is uncircumcised: Retract the foreskin by gently pushing the skin toward the base of the penis. Place your washcloth-covered hand at the tip of the penis and wash in a circular motion, downward to the base of the penis. Repeat using a different part of the washcloth each time until the area is clean. Rinse and dry the tip and shaft of the penis thoroughly before gently pulling the foreskin back into its normal position.
18. Form a mitt around your hand with one of the washcloths. Wet the mitt with warm, clean water and apply soap or no-rinse cleansing solution. Wash the scrotum and perineum. Rinse (if necessary) and dry the scrotum and perineum thoroughly.
19. Turn the person onto his side so that he is facing away from you. Help the person toward the working side of the bed so that his buttocks are within easy reach. Adjust the bath blanket to keep the person covered.
20. Form a mitt around your hand with one of the washcloths. Wet the mitt with warm, clean water and apply soap or no-rinse cleaning solution.
21. Using the other hand, separate the buttocks. Place your washcloth-covered hand at the front of the body and stroke toward the back. First clean one side, then the other side, and finally the middle, using a different part of the washcloth each time, until the anal area is clean.
22. Rinse (if necessary) and dry the anal area thoroughly. Remove the bed protector from underneath the person.

23. Remove your gloves and dispose of them in a facility-approved waste container. Perform hand hygiene and put on a clean pair of gloves.

24. Assist the person into the supine position. Reposition the pillow under the person's head. Remove the bath blanket and help the person into the clean clothing.

25. If the bedding is wet or soiled, change the bed linens.

26. If the side rails are in use, return the side rail to the raised position. Make sure that the bed is lowered to its lowest position and that the wheels are locked.

27. Gather the soiled linens and place them in the linen hamper or linen bag. Dispose of disposable items in a facility-approved waste container. Clean the over-bed table per facility policy. Clean equipment and return it to the storage area.

28. Remove your gloves, dispose of them in a facility-approved waste container, and perform hand hygiene.

FINISHING UP

29. Complete the "Finishing Up" steps.

WHAT YOU DOCUMENT

- Date and time
- Presence of urine or feces
- Level of assistance needed
- Condition of skin

PROCEDURE 21-6
Assisting With a Tub Bath or Shower

Why you do it: Cleansing of the skin helps to prevent skin breakdown (which can lead to pressure ulcers), infection, and odor. A shower or tub bath allows for thorough cleaning and rinsing of the skin.

GETTING READY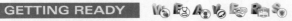

1. Prepare the tub room. If permanent non-skid strips are not present, place a nonskid mat on the floor of the tub or shower. If the person will be taking a tub bath, fill the tub halfway with warm water (105°F [43.3°C] on the bath thermometer) or as indicated on the person's care plan. Obtain a shower chair if necessary and place it in the shower. Place a towel on the chair in the tub room where the person will sit while drying off.

2. Complete the "Getting Ready" steps.

SUPPLIES

- gloves
- bath thermometer
- soap or no-rinse cleansing solution
- washcloths
- towels
- lotion (optional)
- powder (optional)
- deodorant or antiperspirant (optional)
- clean clothing

PROCEDURE

3. Ask the person if she needs to use the bathroom before bathing.

4. Assist the person to the tub room.

5. If the person will be taking a tub bath, check the temperature of the water and make sure that the nonskid mat is secure. If the person will be taking a shower, turn on the water and adjust the temperature until the water is comfortable.

6. Assist the person with undressing. Assist the person into the bathtub or shower.

7. If the person is able to bathe herself, either partially or completely:
   a. Place bathing supplies within easy reach.
   b. Many facilities require you to remain in the room while the person bathes or showers. If facility policy permits you to leave the room, explain how to use the call-light control and ask the person to signal when bathing is complete or when she has done

(procedure continues on page 482)

PROCEDURE 21-6 (continued)
Assisting With a Tub Bath or Shower

as much as she can on her own and needs help completing the bath. Stay nearby and check on the person every 5 minutes. The person should not remain in the bathtub or shower for longer than 20 minutes. Return when the person signals. Remember to knock before entering.

8. If the person is unable to bathe herself or requires assistance:

   a. Perform hand hygiene and put on the gloves. Form a mitt around your hand with one of the washcloths.

   b. If necessary, ask the person what parts of the body were not washed. Assist the person as needed with completing the bath. Wash the cleanest areas first and the dirtiest areas last:

   - **Eyes.** Wet the mitt with warm, clean water. Do not use soap around the eyes. Ask the person to close her eyes. Place your washcloth-covered hand at the inner corner of the eye and stroke gently outward, toward the outer corner. Use a different part of the washcloth for each eye.

   - **Face, neck, and ears.** Ask the person if you should use soap on the face. Rinse the washcloth and apply soap, if requested. Wash the face, neck, and ears, moving from the top of the head to the bottom (so that the nose and mouth are washed last). Rinse thoroughly.

   - **Arms and axillae (armpits).** Rinse the washcloth and apply soap. Place your washcloth-covered hand at the shoulder and stroke downward, toward the hand, using long, firm strokes. Wash the hand. If necessary, assist the person with raising her arm so that you can wash the axilla. Repeat for the other arm and axilla.

   - **Chest and abdomen.** Using long, firm strokes, wash the person's chest and abdomen.

   - **Legs and feet.** Place your washcloth-covered hand at the top of the thigh and stroke downward, toward the foot, using long, firm strokes. Wash the foot. Repeat for the other leg.

   - **Back and buttocks:** Wash the person's back and buttocks, moving from top to bottom and using long, firm strokes.

   - **Perineal area:** Complete perineal care.

9. Make sure that soap is thoroughly rinsed from all parts of the body.

10. Remove your gloves and dispose of them in a facility-approved waste container. Perform hand hygiene and put on a clean pair of gloves.

11. If the person is taking a tub bath, drain the water and carefully assist the person out of the tub and into the towel-covered chair. If the person is taking a shower, turn the water off and assist the person into the towel-covered chair.

12. Wrap a towel around the person. Using another bath towel, help the person to dry off, patting the skin dry. Take care to ensure that areas where "skin meets skin" are dried thoroughly (for example, in between the toes and underneath the breasts).

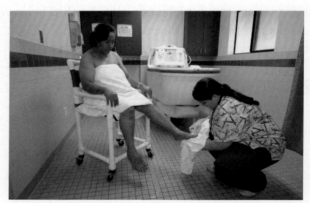

STEP 12 ■ Help the person to dry off, taking extra care to dry areas where "skin meets skin."

13. Help the person to apply lotion, powder, deodorant, antiperspirant, or other personal care products as the person requests.

14. Help the person into the clean clothing. If the person is wearing nightwear, help her into a robe. Help the person into her slippers.

15. Remove your gloves, dispose of them in a facility-approved waste container, and perform hand hygiene.

16. Assist the person back to her room.

FINISHING UP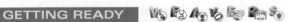

17. Complete the "Finishing Up" steps.
18. Gather the soiled linens and place them in the linen hamper or linen bag. Dispose of disposable items in a facility-approved waste container. Clean equipment and return it to the storage area.
19. Clean the tub room and shower chair (if used), if housekeeping is not responsible for this task at your facility.

WHAT YOU DOCUMENT

- Date and time
- Type of bath/shower given
- Level of assistance needed
- Any unusual observations

PROCEDURE 21-7
Giving a Complete Bed Bath

Why you do it: Cleansing of the skin helps to prevent skin breakdown (which can lead to pressure ulcers), infection, and odor. A bed bath is given when a person is too weak or ill to take a shower or tub bath.

GETTING READY

1. Complete the "Getting Ready" steps.

SUPPLIES

- gloves
- paper towels
- bed protectors
- oral hygiene supplies (see Procedures 21-1 through 21-3)
- bath thermometer
- wash basin
- bedpan or urinal
- soap, no-rinse cleansing solution, or commercially prepared disposable cleansing cloths
- lotion (optional)
- powder (optional)
- deodorant or antiperspirant (optional)
- washcloths
- towels
- bath blanket
- clean clothing
- clean linens (if necessary)

PROCEDURE

2. Clean the surface of the over-bed table and cover with paper towels. Place the wash basin, toiletries, bed protectors, washcloths and towels on the over-bed table. Place additional linens and clean clothing on a nearby clean bedside table or chair.

3. Make sure that the bed is positioned at a comfortable working height (to promote good body mechanics) and that the wheels are locked.
4. Perform hand hygiene and put on the gloves.
5. Because bathing often stimulates the urge to urinate, offer the bedpan or urinal. If the person uses the bedpan or urinal, empty and clean it before proceeding with the bath. Remove your gloves and dispose of them in a facility-approved waste container. Perform hand hygiene and put on a clean pair of gloves.
6. Assist the person with oral care.
7. Remove the bedspread and blanket from the bed. If they are to be reused, fold them and place them on a clean surface, such as the chair.
8. Spread the bath blanket over the top linens (and the person). If the person is able, have him hold the bath blanket. If not, tuck the corners under the person's shoulders. Fanfold the top linens to the foot of the bed.
9. Assist the person with undressing.
10. Lower the head of the bed so that the bed is flat (as tolerated). Position the pillow under the person's head.

(*procedure continues on page 484*)

PROCEDURE 21-7 (continued)
Giving a Complete Bed Bath

11. Fill the wash basin with warm water (110°F [43.3°C] to 115°F [46.1°C] on the bath thermometer). If using a no-rinse cleansing solution, add the appropriate amount to the water in the basin. Place the basin on the over-bed table. If using commercially packaged no-rinse disposable products, you will not need a basin of water unless the disposable cloths need to be placed in water to activate them.

12. If the side rails are in use, lower the side rail on the working side of the bed. The side rail on the opposite side of the bed should remain up.

13. Place a towel over the person's chest to keep the bath blanket dry.

14. To keep the bath water from becoming soapy too quickly, you can use two washcloths—one with soap, for washing; and one without soap, for rinsing. If using the commercially prepared disposable cleansing cloths, the steps of the procedure will remain the same. You will use a new cloth for each area and will omit the rinsing step. Form a mitt around your hand with one of the washcloths. Wet the mitt with warm, clean water. Ask the person to close his eyes. Place your washcloth-covered hand at the inner corner of the eye and stroke gently outward, toward the outer corner. Use a different part of the washcloth for each eye. Using a towel, dry the person's eyes.

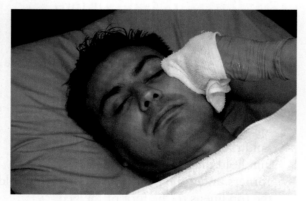

STEP 14 ■ Wash the person's eyes, moving from the inside corner toward the outer corner.

15. Ask the person if you should use soap on the face. Rinse the washcloth and apply soap, if requested. Wash the face, neck, and ears, moving from the top of the head to the bottom (so that the nose and mouth are washed last). Using the clean washcloth, rinse thoroughly (if necessary), and pat the person's face, neck, and ears dry with a towel.

16. Place a bed protector under the person's far arm, to keep the linens dry. Form a mitt around your hand with the washcloth. Wet the mitt and apply soap. Place your washcloth-covered hand at the shoulder and stroke downward, toward the hand, using long, firm strokes. Wash the hand by placing it in the basin of water to soak for a moment. If necessary, assist the person with raising his arm so that you can wash the axilla. Rinse thoroughly (if necessary), and pat the person's arm, hand, and axilla dry with a towel. Remove the bed protector from underneath the person's arm.

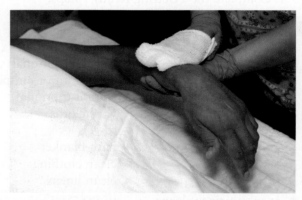

STEP 16 ■ Wash the person's arm, moving from the shoulder to the wrist.

17. Repeat for the other arm.

18. Place a towel horizontally across the person's chest. (The person is now covered with both a bath blanket and a towel.) With the towel in place, fold the bath blanket down to the person's waist. Wet the mitt and apply soap. Reach under the towel and wash the person's chest, using long, firm strokes. Using the clean washcloth, rinse thoroughly (if necessary), and pat the person's chest dry with a towel.

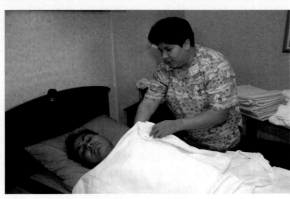

STEP 18 ▪ Reach under the towel and wash the person's chest.

19. With the towel still in place, fold the bath blanket down to the pubic area. Form a mitt around your hand with the washcloth. Wet the mitt and apply soap. Reach under the towel and wash the person's abdomen, using long, firm strokes. Rinse thoroughly (if necessary) and pat the person's abdomen dry with a towel.

20. Replace the bath blanket by unfolding it back over the towel and the person's body. Slide the towel out from underneath the bath blanket.

21. Change the water in the wash basin if it is cool or soapy. (If the side rails are in use, raise the side rails before leaving the bedside.)

22. Fold the bath blanket so that the far leg is completely exposed. Place a bed protector under the person's far leg to keep the linens dry. Wet the mitt and apply soap. Place your washcloth-covered hand at the top of the thigh and stroke downward, toward the foot, using long, firm strokes. Rinse thoroughly (if necessary) and pat the person's leg dry with a bath towel.

23. Put the wash basin on the bed protector and place the person's foot in the basin. Wash the entire foot, including between the toes, with the soapy washcloth. Rinse thoroughly (if necessary) and pat the person's foot dry with a towel. Be sure to dry between the toes. Remove

the wash basin. Remove the bed protector from underneath the person's leg.

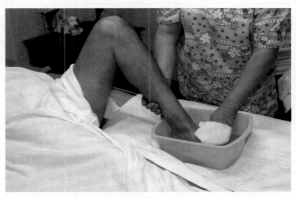

STEP 23 ▪ Put the wash basin on the bed protector and place the person's foot in the basin.

24. Repeat for the other leg and foot.

25. Change the water in the wash basin. (If the side rails are in use, raise the side rails before leaving the bedside.)

26. Turn the person onto his or her side so that he or she is facing away from you. Help the person toward the working side of the bed so that his back is within easy reach. Adjust the bath blanket to keep the front of the person covered (exposing only the back and buttocks). Place a bed protector on the bed alongside the person's back to keep the linens dry.

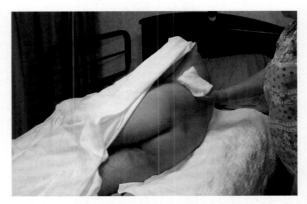

STEP 26 ▪ Wash the person's back and buttocks using long, firm strokes.

(*procedure continues on page 486*)

PROCEDURE 21-7 (continued)
Giving a Complete Bed Bath

27. Form a mitt around your hand with the washcloth. Wet the mitt and apply soap. Wash the person's back first and then the buttocks, moving from top to bottom and using long, firm strokes. Rinse thoroughly (if necessary) and pat the person's back and buttocks dry using a bath towel. At this point, a back massage may be given.

28. If the person is able to perform perineal care, assist the person into Fowler's position and adjust the over-bed table so that the bathing supplies are within easy reach. Place the call-light control within easy reach and ask the person to signal when perineal care is complete. If the person is unable to perform perineal care, assist the person onto his back and complete perineal care.

29. Remove your gloves and dispose of them in a facility-approved waste container. Perform hand hygiene and put on a clean pair of gloves.

30. Help the person to apply lotion, powder, deodorant, antiperspirant, or other personal care products as the person requests.

31. Help the person into the clean clothing.

32. If the bedding is wet or soiled, change the bed linens.

33. Carry out range-of-motion exercises as ordered.

34. If the side rails are in use, return the side rails to the raised position. Raise or lower the head of the bed as the person requests. Make sure that the bed is lowered to its lowest position and that the wheels are locked.

35. Gather the soiled linens and place them in the linen hamper or linen bag. Dispose of disposable items in a facility-approved waste container. Clean the over-bed table per facility policy. Clean equipment and return it to the storage area.

36. Remove your gloves, dispose of them in a facility-approved waste container, and perform hand hygiene.

FINISHING UP

37. Complete the "Finishing Up" steps.

WHAT YOU DOCUMENT

- Date and time
- Bathing products used (bag bath, no-rinse cleanser, etc.)
- Level of assistance needed
- Condition of skin, especially over pressure points

WHAT DID YOU LEARN?

Multiple Choice

Select the single best answer for each of the following questions.

1. As a safety measure, when you give oral care to an unconscious person, you should position the person in which position?
   a. Lateral position
   b. Sims' position
   c. Fowler's position
   d. Prone position

2. Why do you line the sink with a washcloth when cleaning a person's dentures?
   a. To ensure that you always have a wet washcloth handy when you need one
   b. To protect the sink from scratches
   c. To guard against breaking the dentures
   d. To prevent contamination of the dentures

3. Which one of the following is within the range of appropriate temperatures for bath water?
   a. 98°F (36.6°C)
   b. 212°F (100°C)
   c. 120°F (48.9°C)
   d. 105°F (40.5°C)

4. When giving a complete bed bath, you should:
   a. Position yourself on one side of the bed and stay there
   b. Use the same water throughout the bath to minimize trips to the sink
   c. Avoid washing the person's perineal area because the person may be embarrassed
   d. Keep the person covered as much as possible

5. When assisting a man with perineal care, you should always:
   a. Hold the penis at a 90° angle to the body
   b. Wash from the base of the penis toward the tip
   c. Pull the foreskin back if the man is uncircumcised
   d. Clean the scrotum first

6. When assisting a person with a shower, you should:
   a. Use a bath blanket to prevent falls
   b. Run the water until the temperature reaches 125°F (51.6°C)
   c. Wear waterproof personal protective equipment (PPE) to protect yourself from getting wet
   d. Use a shower chair if the person is weak or unsteady

7. Which one of the following actions must be taken to keep the skin healthy?
   a. Use strong soap to kill all the germs on the skin
   b. Rinse the skin well and dry it thoroughly, especially in areas where "skin meets skin"
   c. Apply generous amounts of powder after the bath
   d. Rub the skin vigorously with the washcloth

8. How are natural teeth brushed?
   a. Using a circular motion
   b. For at least 10 minutes on each side
   c. Using an "up and down" motion
   d. All of the above

9. When assisting a woman with perineal care, you should always:
   a. Gently yet thoroughly dry the perineal area and vulva
   b. Clean the rectal area last
   c. Move the washcloth in a downward direction, from front to back
   d. All of the above

10. What is the first thing you should do before assisting a person with a tub bath?
    a. Gather the necessary supplies
    b. Make sure that the tub is clean
    c. Check the temperature of the water
    d. Check the nursing care plan to make sure that the person is allowed to have a tub bath

11. Which of the following observations made while assisting with oral care would you report to the nurse?
    a. Lips that are dry, cracked, swollen, or blistered
    b. Irritations, sores, or white patches in the mouth or on the tongue
    c. Bleeding, swelling, or redness of the gums
    d. All of the above

Matching

Match each type of care with its appropriate description.

_____ **1.** Perineal care (peri-care)

_____ **2.** Evening (hour of sleep, hs) care

_____ **3.** PRN (as-needed) care

_____ **4.** Morning (A.M.) care

_____ **5.** Afternoon care

_____ **6.** Early morning care

a. Care provided before and after lunch and dinner

b. Care provided after a person wakes up to prepare him or her for breakfast or early testing or treatment

c. Care that is provided at any time of the day or night, when the person's condition warrants it

d. Care provided to ready the person for the day; includes completion of personal hygiene and grooming activities and bedmaking

e. Care that is routinely provided at bedtime

f. Cleaning of the perineum, the anus, and the vulva or penis

 Stop *and* **Think!**

Mrs. Davis is a resident at your facility, which specializes in caring for people with Alzheimer's disease. As Mrs. Davis's disease has progressed, she has become progressively more lax about matters related to personal hygiene. She dislikes bathing, and if you do not remove her soiled clothes from her room, she will continue to wear them every day. Today Mrs. Davis is scheduled to have a shower, and as you might have predicted, she tells you that she "will not take a shower today." What should you do?

Stop *and* **Think!**

Mrs. Visknaya is from Russia and came to the United States to live near her daughter. She speaks very little English and understands even less. A male nursing assistant, Josh, has been assigned to care for Mrs. Visknaya today because Juanita, who usually cares for Mrs. Visknaya, is home sick with the flu. Josh comes to Mrs. Visknaya's room and announces with a big smile that it is "time for your bath." He explains the procedure to her, and she smiles back and nods her head. Unfortunately, she doesn't understand a word he is saying! When it comes time during the bath to assist Mrs. Visknaya with her perineal care, Josh lifts the corner of the bath blanket and attempts to separate Mrs. Visknaya's legs, and she starts to scream. What, if anything, did Josh do wrong? What could have been done to prevent this situation?

Preventing Pressure Ulcers and Assisting With Wound Care

Many of your patients or residents will be at risk for developing pressure ulcers. Preventing pressure ulcers is a major concern of the nursing team because pressure ulcers are painful, hard to treat, and potentially fatal. In this chapter, you will learn about your role in preventing pressure ulcers. Pressure ulcers are just one type of wound you may see when you are caring for patients and residents. In this chapter, you will also learn about how the health care team cares for people with wounds and your role in assisting the nurse with wound care.

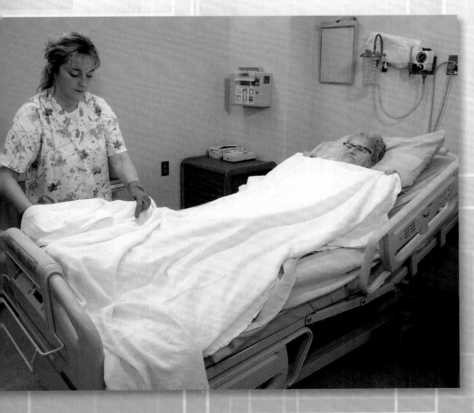

Photo: *A nursing assistant makes an occupied bed. Providing clean, wrinkle-free linens is just one way that nursing assistants help to prevent their patients or residents from developing pressure ulcers.*

Preventing Pressure Ulcers

What will you learn?

When you are finished with this section, you will be able to:

1. Explain how pressure ulcers form.
2. Discuss what conditions may increase a person's risk of developing a pressure ulcer.
3. Describe why preventing pressure ulcers is so important.
4. Describe changes in the skin that could be an early sign of a pressure ulcer.
5. Describe how nursing assistants help to prevent residents and patients from developing pressure ulcers.
6. Describe special equipment that may be used to help prevent pressure ulcers.
7. Define the words **pressure ulcer** and **pressure points**.

How Pressure Ulcers Form

Pressure ulcer a difficult-to-heal (and possibly even fatal) sore that forms when part of the body presses against a surface (such as a mattress or chair) for a long period of time; also known as pressure sores and decubitus ulcers

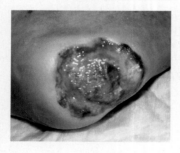

Pressure points bony areas where pressure ulcers are most likely to form; include the heels, ankles, knees, hips, toes, elbows, shoulder blades, ears, the back of the head, and along the spine

Many patients and residents are not able to change position easily due to weakness, disability, or illness. This inability to change position without help places the person at high risk for developing a **pressure ulcer**. Pressure ulcers form when **pressure points** press against a mattress, chair, or other surface (Fig. 22-1). The pressure squeezes the tissues in between the bone and the surface the person is lying or sitting on. As a result, blood flow to the tissues decreases. The tissues do not receive enough nutrients and oxygen, and they die. The dead tissue peels off or breaks open, creating an open sore or ulcer. Pressure ulcers develop in stages (Box 22-1).

The longer a person remains in one position, the more likely that person is to develop a pressure ulcer. Many people with limited mobility also have other risk factors for developing a pressure ulcer, such as:

- **Old age.** The skin of an older person is fragile and thin, with less blood flow.
- **Poor nutrition and lack of fluids.** For skin to remain healthy, good nutrition and adequate fluid intake are essential.
- **Moisture.** Prolonged contact with water, urine, feces, or sweat causes the epidermis to soften and break down (leading to "skin breakdown"). Patients and residents who are obese are at an increased risk of skin breakdown because of their skin folds, which can trap moisture.
- **Cardiovascular or respiratory problems.** People with cardiovascular or respiratory problems are at high risk for developing pressure ulcers because their medical condition prevents their tissues from receiving the full amount of oxygen and nutrients.
- **Friction and shearing injuries.** Friction (rubbing) and shearing (pulling) forces can injure the skin and lead to skin breakdown. Friction and shearing forces are described in more detail in Chapter 17.

Because a pressure ulcer can have such serious consequences for a person, OBRA expects that the health care team will do everything possible to prevent patients and residents from getting pressure ulcers. The nurse is responsible for assessing each

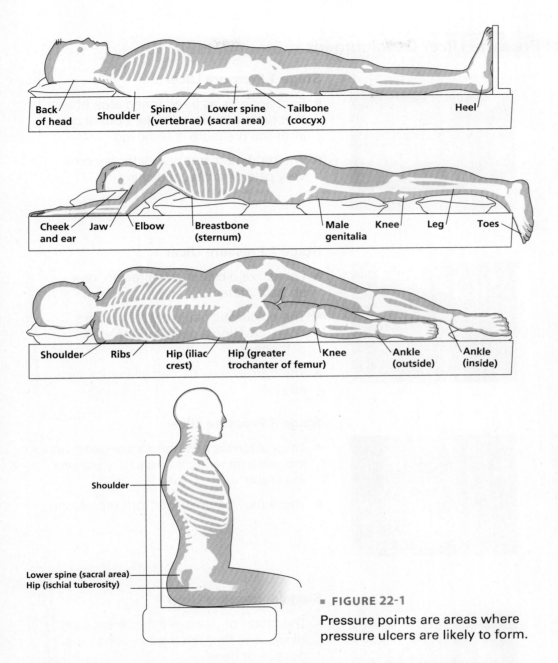

Back of head — Shoulder — Spine (vertebrae) — Lower spine (sacral area) — Tailbone (coccyx) — Heel

Cheek and ear — Jaw — Elbow — Breastbone (sternum) — Male genitalia — Knee — Leg — Toes

Shoulder — Ribs — Hip (iliac crest) — Hip (greater trochanter of femur) — Knee — Ankle (outside) — Ankle (inside)

Shoulder

Lower spine (sacral area)
Hip (ischial tuberosity)

■ **FIGURE 22-1**

Pressure points are areas where pressure ulcers are likely to form.

resident's risk for developing pressure ulcers when the resident is admitted to the long-term care facility. The nurse also documents any existing pressure ulcers. OBRA expects the health care team to maintain or improve the person's condition. This means that the health care team works to heal existing pressure ulcers and takes measures to prevent new pressure ulcers from forming. Nursing assistants help the health care team to achieve these goals by carefully following the person's care plan.

Concerns for Long-Term Care

Many residents of long-term care facilities develop pressure ulcers while being treated in the hospital for an acute illness or injury. They then return to the long-term care facility with a pressure ulcer *and* the other condition to recover from.

BOX 22-1 Stages of Pressure Ulcer Development

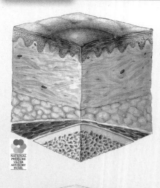

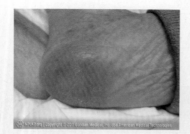

Stage 1 Pressure Ulcer

- First appears as a reddened area of skin that does not return to the normal color after the pressure is removed

- The reddened area may later become very pale or white, and shiny

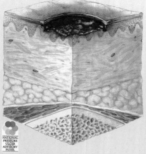

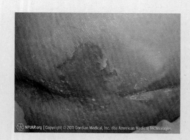

Stage 2 Pressure Ulcer

- Looks like a blister, an abrasion, or a shallow crater

- The epidermis peels away or cracks open, creating a portal of entry for pathogens

- The dermis may be partially worn away as well

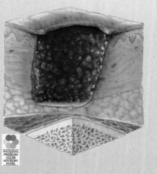

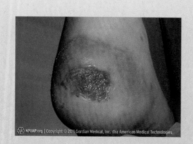

Stage 3 Pressure Ulcer

- The epidermis and dermis are gone, and the subcutaneous fat may be visible in the crater

- There may be drainage from the wound

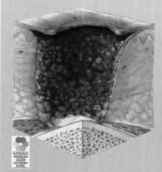

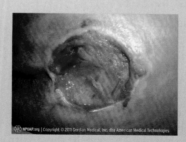

Stage 4 Pressure Ulcer

- The crater of damaged tissue extends all the way through the tissues to the muscle or bone

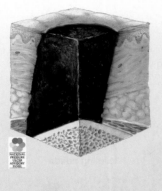

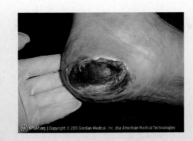

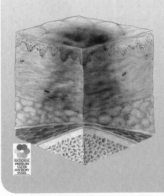

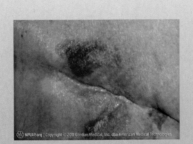

Unstageable

- There is loss of the epidermis, dermis, and subcutaneous tissue

- The full extent or depth of the ulcer is covered by *slough* (soft, moist, light-colored dead tissue) or *eschar* (tough, dry, leathery, dark-colored dead tissue)

- The ulcer will need to be cleaned and dead tissue removed to determine the true stage

Suspected Deep Tissue Injury

- The damaged underlying tissue has intact skin that is purple or maroon colored or a blood-filled blister

- The area may be painful and can be either firm or mushy, warm or cool

- May be difficult to detect in people with dark skin

The Nursing Assistant's Role in Preventing Pressure Ulcers

Pressure ulcers are very painful and difficult to treat. Ultimately, they can cause a person to die. For these reasons, every effort must be made to prevent a pressure ulcer from forming. As a nursing assistant, there are many things that you can do to help keep a person's skin healthy (Fig. 22-2). General guidelines for preventing pressure ulcers are given in Guidelines Box 22-1.

Special Equipment for Preventing Pressure Ulcers

Special devices may be used to help prevent pressure ulcers from forming.

- **Elbow pads and heel booties** help to prevent the skin from rubbing against sheets or other surfaces (Fig. 22-3).

- **A bed cradle** is used to keep the top sheet, the blanket, and the bedspread off the patient's or resident's feet (Fig. 22-4). Sometimes, just the pressure of the top linens on the feet is enough to start the process of skin breakdown that leads to pressure ulcers.

- **A footboard** is a padded board that is placed upright at the foot of the bed (Fig. 22-5). The person's feet rest flat against the footboard, helping to keep the feet in proper alignment.

Tell the Nurse!

Pressure ulcers

- A reddened area does not return to its normal color within 5 minutes after the pressure is relieved

- A previously reddened area is hot to the touch or painful

- A previously reddened area is now pale, white, or shiny

- A pressure ulcer has changed in size or depth

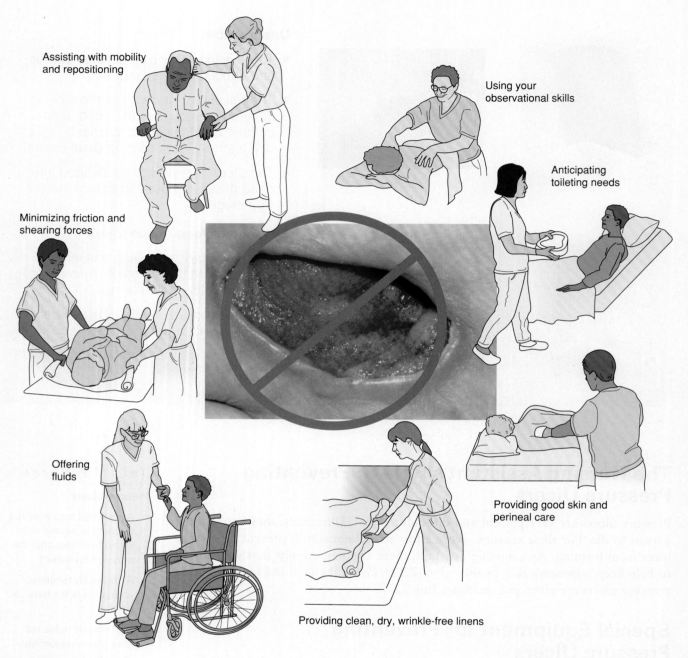

Assisting with mobility and repositioning

Using your observational skills

Anticipating toileting needs

Minimizing friction and shearing forces

Offering fluids

Providing good skin and perineal care

Providing clean, dry, wrinkle-free linens

■ **FIGURE 22-2**

There are many things you can do to help prevent a person from getting a pressure ulcer.

- **A pressure-relieving** mattress may be placed on top of the regular mattress to help prevent skin breakdown in patients and residents who must stay in bed for long periods of time. Pressure-relieving mattresses may be made of foam or gel, or filled with air or water. Smaller gel pads are also available for wheelchair seats.

- **A special bed** may be used for some patients or residents (Fig. 22-6).

(*text continued on page 498*)

GUIDELINES BOX 22-1 Guidelines for Preventing Pressure Ulcers

What you do	Why you do it
Reposition a person who must stay in bed or in a wheelchair at least every 2 hours, or according to the person's care plan.	*Regular repositioning prevents any one part of the person's body from being under pressure for too long. A person who has additional risk factors for developing a pressure ulcer may need to be repositioned even more often.*
Take the bedpan out from underneath the person as soon as the person is finished using it.	*The bedpan places pressure on the person's lower spine, one of the pressure points.*
Check the patient's or resident's skin for changes at every opportunity, including when you are assisting the person with repositioning, bathing, and dressing and when you are changing wet or soiled linens or giving a back massage. Report red, pale, white, or shiny areas over pressure points right away.	*Redness over a pressure point that does not go away after 5 minutes or an area over a pressure point that was previously red but now is pale, white, or shiny could be a sign of a stage 1 pressure ulcer. Early recognition and treatment of a pressure ulcer is important so that measures can be taken to prevent the pressure ulcer from getting worse.*
Provide good skin care. When bathing a person, clean the skin gently and thoroughly and rinse off the soap well. Make sure that the skin is dried well and use lotion to keep the skin healthy and soft. Thoroughly clean and dry areas where skin touches skin, such as under the breasts or other skin folds, and apply a light dusting of powder to keep the skin dry.	*Keeping the skin clean and dry is essential to preventing skin breakdown and pressure ulcer development.*
Provide good perineal care, especially if the person is incontinent of urine or feces.	*Urine and feces are irritating to the skin and can lead to skin breakdown. Prompt, thorough perineal care keeps the skin clean and dry, which is essential to preventing skin breakdown and pressure ulcer development.*
Assist the person to the bathroom (or provide a bedpan or urinal) frequently. Check on incontinent people every hour or so.	*Contact with wet and soiled clothing or linens can cause skin breakdown, leading to pressure ulcers. Anticipating toileting needs helps to prevent patients and residents from soiling themselves. Checking on incontinent patients and residents frequently allows you to detect and change wet and soiled clothing or linens promptly.*
Ask patients or residents who can walk to take a walk with you every 2 hours. Remind paralyzed patients or residents to change positions in the wheelchair or move to the bed for a while.	*Exercise and movement promote blood flow to the tissues and prevent the person from staying in any one position for too long a time.*

(box continues on page 496)

GUIDELINES BOX 22-1   Guidelines for Preventing Pressure Ulcers (continued)

What you do	Why you do it
Make sure that the bed linens are clean, dry, and wrinkle-free at all times.	*Soiled, wet, or excessively wrinkled linens can lead to skin breakdown and pressure ulcers.*
Provide frequent back massage.	*Back massage helps to stimulate blood flow to the skin and gives you a chance to check the person's skin for red, pale, white, or shiny areas.*
Minimize skin injury caused by friction or shearing. Use lift devices and lift sheets when moving and repositioning people. Use devices such as elbow pads and heel booties according to the person's care plan. Avoid raising the head of the bed more than 30 degrees.	*Friction and shearing forces damage the skin and underlying tissues and can put the person at risk for a pressure ulcer. Lift devices and lift sheets help reduce friction by allowing you to lift or roll, instead of drag, the person. Elbow pads and heel booties reduce friction by preventing the skin from rubbing against sheets and other surfaces. Raising the bed no more than 30 degrees helps prevent shearing, which occurs when the person slides down in the bed.*
Offer refreshing drinks frequently. Encourage your patients and residents to eat well.	*Good nutrition and adequate fluid intake help to keep the skin healthy.*
Use pressure-reducing devices according to the person's care plan.	*These devices help to distribute the person's body weight more evenly, preventing any one area from bearing most of the pressure.*
Place a pillow under a person's calves when he is in the supine position.	*Placing a pillow under the calves to "float" the heels above the surface of the bed when the person is in the supine position relieves pressure on the heels.*

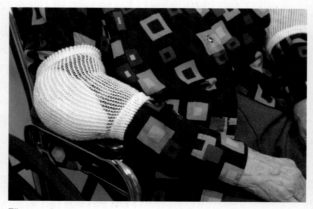

Elbow pads

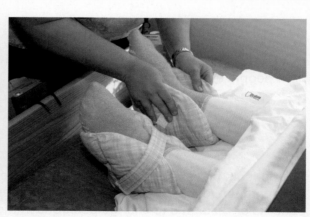

Heel booties

■ FIGURE 22-3

Devices such as elbow pads and heel booties help to prevent the skin from rubbing against sheets and other surfaces.

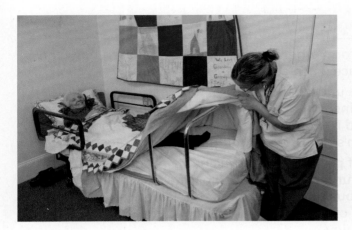

■ **FIGURE 22-4**

A bed cradle prevents the top linens from putting pressure on the person's feet.

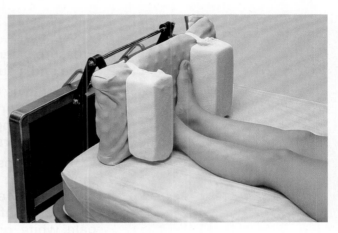

■ **FIGURE 22-5**

A footboard is placed against the end of the bed to keep the person's feet in proper alignment.

(Courtesy of the Posey Company.)

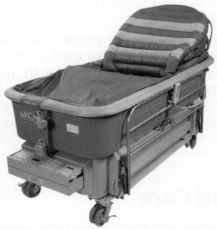

An **airflow bed** supports the person on a fabric-covered layer of tiny beads. The beads are kept constantly in movement by a current of air. The moving beads create a fluid-like effect, much like a waterbed but without the water, that helps to prevent pressure ulcers by relieving pressure on pressure points. In addition, the circulating air keeps the person's skin dry.

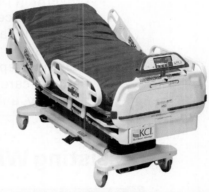

An **alternating pressure bed** supports the person on a series of compartments that fill with air and then deflate on a rotating basis. The moving areas of inflation shift the areas of pressure from place to place, helping to improve blood flow to the skin and underlying tissues and helping to prevent pressure ulcers.

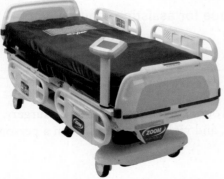

The XPRT Pulmonary Therapy Surface offers rotational, percussion and vibration therapies. These beds help to prevent pressure ulcers and pulmonary complications by automatically repositioning people who may be difficult to reposition often, such as people with traumatic injuries.

■ **FIGURE 22-6**

Specialty beds for preventing pressure ulcers.

Photograph used with permission of Stryker Corporation.

Putting it all together!

- Pressure ulcers form when soft tissues are squeezed between bone and a surface, such as a mattress or chair.

- Immobility is the underlying cause of all pressure ulcers. Several factors, including old age, poor nutrition, and moisture trapped in the folds of the skin, can increase an immobile person's risk of developing a pressure ulcer.

- Warning signs of pressure ulcers include a reddened area that does not return to its normal color after the pressure is relieved, a previously reddened area that is now hot to the touch or painful, or a previously reddened area that is now pale, white, or shiny.

- Pressure ulcers develop in stages. The sooner a pressure ulcer is recognized, the better, because then measures can be taken to prevent the pressure ulcer from getting worse. Nursing assistants are often the first members of the health care team to notice a change in a patient's or resident's skin that could be the beginning of a pressure ulcer.

- Preventing pressure ulcers is extremely important because pressure ulcers are very painful, very hard to treat, and potentially fatal. Nursing assistants do many things to prevent patients and residents from developing pressure ulcers, including repositioning, observing, providing good skin and perineal care, changing wet and soiled linens and clothing promptly, and encouraging exercise.

Assisting With Wound Care

 What will you learn?

When you are finished with this section, you will be able to:

1. State observations that you may make related to wound care that should be reported to the nurse.
2. Demonstrate proper technique for assisting a nurse with a dressing change.
3. Define the word **wound**.

Wound an injury that results in a break in the skin (and usually the underlying tissues as well)

A pressure ulcer is a type of **wound**. Wounds can also be caused by surgery, trauma (such as car accidents, burns, or falls), and violence (such as when a person is shot or stabbed).

Wound Healing

The skin is the body's first line of defense against infection. A wound creates an opening that allows microbes to enter the body, putting the person at risk for infection.

The wound must heal so that the skin is once again intact and able to protect the person. Several factors can delay healing:

- Multiple injuries
- Chronic illness
- A weakened immune system
- Very old or very young age
- Poor nutrition

The health care team does many things to help support the wound healing process. As a nursing assistant, your duties related to wound care will vary, depending on where you work. Your daily responsibilities, even if they are not directly related to wound care, will give you many chances to observe your patients or residents for problems with wound healing.

Wound Drains

As part of the healing process, some wounds produce a lot of fluid, or drainage. Fluid that is allowed to collect in a wound can delay the healing process. Wound drains may be used to remove fluids from the wound (Fig. 22-7). Vacuum-assisted closure (VAC) therapy may be used to help promote healing of complicated or chronic wounds (Fig. 22-8).

When repositioning a person with a drain, take care not to pull on the drain tubing. Pulling on the drain tubing could pull the drain out of the wound. The loss of the drain will allow fluid to collect in the wound until the doctor can replace the drain. Fluid in the wound delays wound healing.

Wound Dressings

Sometimes dressings are applied to wounds to prevent microbes from gaining access to the body, to keep the wound dry during procedures such as bathing, or to absorb drainage from the wound.

Many dressings are secured with tape (Fig. 22-9). Tape can be adhesive, paper, plastic, or elastic. The type of tape used depends on the location of the wound and the needs of the person. When a wound is draining heavily and the dressing must be changed often, a Montgomery tie may be used instead of tape (see Fig. 22-9).

Tell the Nurse!

Wound care

- Complaints of increased pain or discomfort
- Increased redness, swelling, or warmth around the wound
- Foul-smelling wound drainage
- Wound drainage that has changed in appearance or amount
- A loose, wet, or excessively soiled dressing
- Drain tubing that has been pulled out or that has become disconnected
- Fever
- VAC Therapy System that is not functioning properly

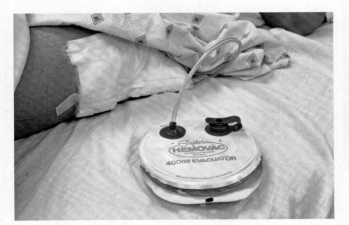

■ FIGURE 22-7

Many different types of wound drains are used. A Hemovac drain is shown here. With this type of drain, the drainage tube is placed in the wound and attached to a suction device, which draws the fluid out of the wound.

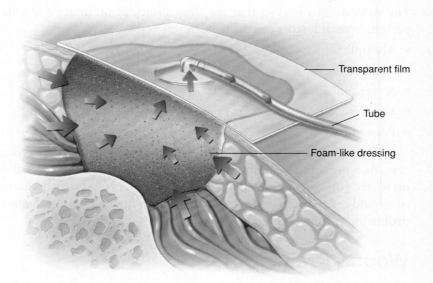

Transparent film

Tube

Foam-like dressing

A

■ **FIGURE 22-8**

Vacuum-assisted closure (VAC) Therapy is often used to promote healing of complicated or chronic wounds. **(A)** The wound is filled with a foam-like dressing. A tube is inserted into the foam, and then the area is sealed with a transparent film. When the pump is turned on, it creates suction, which draws fluid out of the wound and stimulates blood flow and the growth of new tissue. **(B)** The V.A.C. ATS Therapy System.
(Courtesy of KCL Licensing, Inc. 2010.)

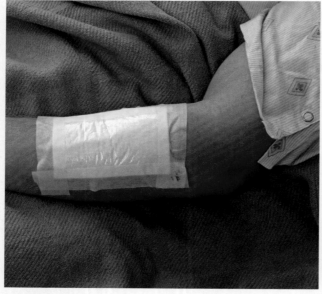

B

Dressing secured with tape

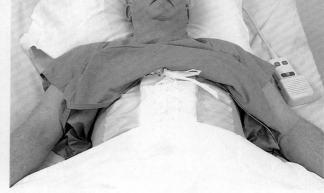

Montgomery tie

■ **FIGURE 22-9**

Wound dressings can be secured using tape or ties.
Montgomery tie, © B. Proud.

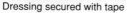

The adhesive is applied and then left in place. The ties secure the dressing and can be easily untied when a new dressing is needed. Because there is no need to remove the tape to change the dressing, Montgomery ties help to protect the person's skin from damage caused by the frequent removal and reapplication of tape.

Depending on where you work, assisting the nurse with dressing changes may be in your scope of practice. Procedure 22-1 explains how to assist a nurse with a dressing change.

Putting it all together!

- A wound is a break in the skin. Underlying tissues are usually affected as well.
- A break in the skin puts the person at risk for infection. Drains and dressings may be used to prevent infection and help a wound to heal.
- Nursing assistants have many chances to notice and report signs and symptoms that suggest that a wound has become infected or is not healing well, such as a foul-smelling discharge or excessive drainage or bleeding. Nursing assistants may also assist with dressing changes in some facilities.

PROCEDURE 22-1
Assisting the Nurse With a Dressing Change

Why you do it: Helping the nurse with a dressing change minimizes the chance that the nurse's hands or other surfaces will become contaminated by the drainage on the soiled dressing. It also helps to ensure that the new dressing remains free of pathogens that could contaminate the wound.

GETTING READY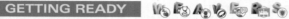

1. Complete the "Getting Ready" steps.

SUPPLIES

- gloves
- gown (if necessary)
- mask (if necessary)
- paper towels or a bed protector
- plastic bag
- tape or Montgomery ties
- dressing
- scissors

PROCEDURE

2. Clean the over-bed table and cover it with paper towels or the bed protector. Place the dressing supplies on the over-bed table. Fold the top edges of the plastic bag down to make a cuff. Place the cuffed bag on the over-bed table.

3. Make sure that the bed is positioned at a comfortable working height (to promote good body mechanics) and that the wheels are locked. If the side rails are in use, lower the side rail on the working side of the bed. The side rail on the opposite side of the bed should remain up.

4. Help the person to a comfortable position that allows access to the wound.

5. Fanfold the top linens to the foot of the bed. Adjust the person's hospital gown or pajamas as necessary to expose the wound.

6. Put on the mask, gown, or both, if necessary. Perform hand hygiene and put on the gloves.

7. The nurse will remove the old dressing. The nurse may ask you to take the old dressing and place it in the cuffed plastic bag. Be careful to keep the soiled side of the dressing out of the

person's sight. Do not let the dressing touch the outside of the plastic bag.

8. Remove your gloves, dispose of them in a facility-approved waste container, and perform hand hygiene.

9. Wait while the nurse inspects the wound and measures it, if necessary.

10. Put on a clean pair of gloves.

11. Assist as the nurse applies a new dressing.

    a. Open the wrapper containing the dressing and hold it open so that the nurse can remove the dressing. Do not touch the dressing. Dispose of the wrapper in a facility-approved waste container.

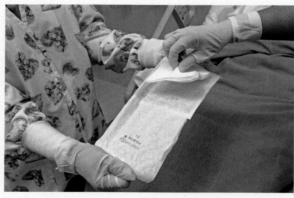

STEP 11a ■ Hold the wrapper open so that the nurse can remove the dressing.

    b. If the dressing will be secured with tape, cut four pieces of tape for securing the dressing. For a 4 × 4 dressing, each piece of tape should measure 8 inches long. Hang the tape from the edge of the over-bed table.

c. If the nurse asks you to, use the tape strips to secure the dressing by placing one piece of tape along each side of the dressing. Center each piece of tape equally over the dressing and the person's skin.

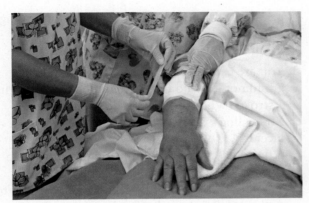

STEP 11c ■ The dressing is secured by placing one piece of tape along each side.

12. Remove your gloves (and gown and mask, if using) and dispose of them in a facility-approved waste container. Perform hand hygiene.

13. Re-cover the wound with the hospital gown or pajamas. Help the person back into a comfortable position, straighten the bottom linens, and draw the top linens over the person.

14. Make sure that the bed is lowered to its lowest position and that the wheels are locked. If the side rails are in use, return the side rail to the raised position on the working side of the bed.

15. Dispose of disposable items in a facility-approved waste container. Clean equipment and return it to the storage area.

FINISHING UP

16. Complete the "Finishing Up" steps.

WHAT YOU DOCUMENT

- Date and time
- Appearance of the wound
- Amount, color, and characteristics of any wound drainage
- Type of dressing applied

WHAT DID YOU LEARN?

Multiple Choice

Select the single best answer for each of the following questions.

1. Where are pressure ulcers most likely to form?
   a. On the heels, ankles, and toes
   b. On the elbows and shoulder blades
   c. On the spine
   d. All of the above

2. Why is it important to prevent pressure ulcers from forming?
   a. Pressure ulcers are disgusting to see
   b. People who have pressure ulcers require more care than people who do not, and this is expensive for the facility
   c. Pressure ulcers are difficult to treat and can lead to a person's death
   d. Pressure ulcers interfere with the skin's ability to make vitamin D

3. What is the underlying cause of all pressure ulcers?
   a. Continuous pressure applied to one area
   b. Poor nutrition
   c. Incontinence
   d. All of the above

4. Which of the following factors can increase a person's risk of getting a pressure ulcer?
   a. Advanced age
   b. Incontinence
   c. Poor nutrition
   d. All of the above

5. Mr. Underwood has developed a white, shiny area on his left hip about the size of a quarter. Yesterday, this same area was red and hot to the touch. If you were Mr. Underwood's nursing assistant, what would be your biggest concern?
   a. That Mr. Underwood has the chickenpox
   b. That Mr. Underwood has a stage 1 pressure ulcer

   c. That Mr. Underwood's wound is not healing properly
   d. That Mr. Underwood has jaundice

6. You are caring for Mrs. Kling, a 93-year-old grandmother who has limited mobility following a stroke. What should you do to minimize Mrs. Kling's chances of developing a pressure ulcer?
   a. Dry Mrs. Kling's skin thoroughly after each bath
   b. Reposition Mrs. Kling regularly, according to the nursing care plan
   c. Encourage Mrs. Kling to eat well
   d. All of the above

7. What do you call a metal frame that is placed between the bottom and top sheets to keep the bed linens from resting on the person's feet?
   a. A bed board
   b. A pressure-relieving mattress
   c. A bed cradle
   d. A footboard

8. Why is it important to keep the skin healthy?
   a. The skin protects the body from pathogens and helps to maintain the body's fluid balance
   b. The skin protects the body from sunburn
   c. It is easier to detect signs of disease in a person with healthy skin
   d. Keeping the skin healthy helps to prevent wrinkles in old age

 Stop *and* **Think!**

Richard is providing care to Mr. O'Meara, who has just been transferred to Willow Wood Care Center. Mr. O'Meara is confined to a wheelchair. While giving Mr. O'Meara a back massage as part of evening care, Richard notices a reddened area at the base of Mr. O'Meara's spine. What are the possible explanations for this finding? Discuss measures that Richard can take to help keep Mr. O'Meara from developing a pressure ulcer.

Assisting With Grooming

Grooming helps a person maintain a neat and attractive appearance. Grooming activities include caring for the hands and feet, dressing, washing and styling the hair, shaving, caring for vision and hearing aids, and applying make-up. In this chapter, you will learn how to help your patients or residents with their grooming activities.

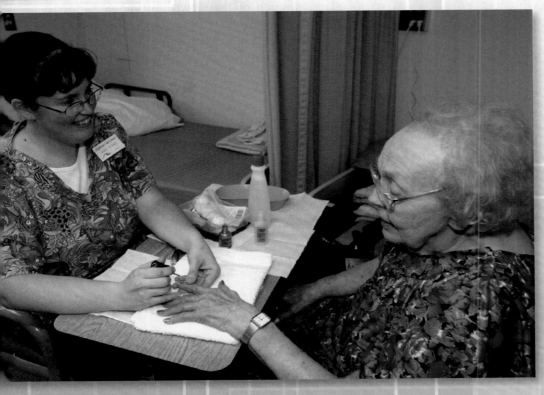

Photo: *A nursing assistant assists a resident with hand care. Grooming practices help people to feel more attractive and confident.*

Introduction to Grooming

What will you learn?

When you are finished with this section, you will be able to:

1. Explain why it is important to respect a person's preferences with regard to grooming habits whenever possible.
2. Explain how assisting a person with grooming can benefit the person emotionally.

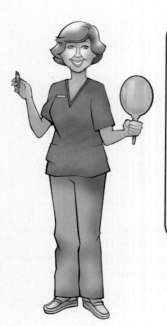

Helping a person to keep up with his or her normal personal grooming routine has an enormous impact on the person's continued well being. Taking the time to keep a man's moustache trimmed "just right" or help a woman to apply her favorite shade of lipstick lets the person know that you care about him or her as a unique individual. This idea is at the heart of holistic care.

Grooming helps us to feel attractive to others. A person's grooming practices are influenced by the person's cultural and religious beliefs, upbringing, and feelings about his or her own sexuality. Because the way we look influences how we feel about ourselves, it is important to respect your patients' or residents' preferences when assisting them with grooming.

Illness or disability can affect a person's ability to complete his or her grooming routine. Helping your patients or residents with grooming is important because it helps them to feel good about themselves. The amount of help each patient or resident will need from you will vary. Encourage your patients and residents to complete as much of their own grooming as possible (Fig. 23-1). Many patients or residents can use assistive devices (see Chapter 9) to complete grooming tasks independently. Maintaining as much independence as possible is important for the person's self-esteem.

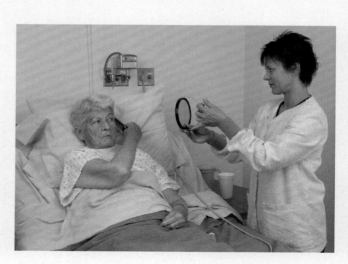

■ **FIGURE 23-1**

To foster independence and self-esteem, encourage your patients or residents to do as much as possible for themselves, while you stand by ready to offer assistance as needed.

Putting it all together!

- Grooming practices help people feel more attractive and confident.
- A person's grooming practices are influenced by the person's culture, religion, upbringing, and feelings about his or her sexuality. Respecting your patient's or resident's personal preferences is very important when assisting with grooming.
- People in health care facilities may need assistance to complete their daily grooming routines, but it is important to allow your patients or residents to do as much as possible on their own.

Assisting With Hand Care

What will you learn?

When you are finished with this section, you will be able to:

1. Understand the importance of proper hand care.
2. State observations that you may make when assisting a patient or resident with hand care that should be reported to the nurse.
3. Demonstrate proper technique for assisting with hand care.
4. Define the word **hangnails**.

Hand care is important to keep the skin of the hands healthy and the fingernails neat. Dry, chapped skin causes discomfort and creates a portal of entry for microbes. Long, rough fingernails place the person at risk for accidentally scratching herself, especially if the person is disoriented.

Assisting with hand care gives you a chance to spend "quality time" with the patient or resident and to observe for signs of health. Nailbeds should be pink with no gap between the nail and the nailbed. The cuticles should be smooth and unbroken, with no **hangnails**.

Hand care is often done immediately following a bath because the warm water helps make the nails soft and flexible. The nails are trimmed with clippers, not scissors, to a length no shorter than even with the ends of the fingers (Fig. 23-2).

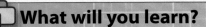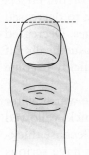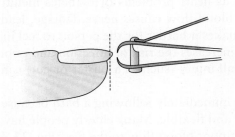

Tell the Nurse!

Hand care

- Very pale or blue nailbeds
- Bruised nailbeds
- Unusually yellow or white nails
- Unusually thick nails
- Broken nails or nails that have been cut too short (especially if there is also bleeding or tenderness)
- Torn, red, or swollen cuticles
- Rashes

Hangnails broken pieces of cuticle

- **FIGURE 23-2**
If you are allowed to trim patients' or residents' nails, cut the nails straight across, using nail clippers. Be careful not to cut too close to the skin.

In some states and facilities, trimming a patient's or resident's nails is outside the scope of practice for nursing assistants, so be sure to follow your facility's policy. After trimming, the nails are filed into an oval shape using an emery board. Hangnails may need to be trimmed with cuticle scissors so that they do not rub or snag on clothing or linens. Procedure 23-1 describes how to assist a patient or resident with hand care.

Putting it all together!

- Routine hand care keeps the skin and nails clean and healthy.
- Nailbeds should be pink. The cuticles should be smooth and unbroken.
- Assisting with hand care gives you a chance to spend quality time with your patients or residents. It also gives you a chance to observe for potential health problems.

Assisting With Foot Care

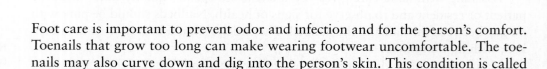

What will you learn?

When you are finished with this section, you will be able to:

1. List changes that occur in a person's feet as a result of aging or illness.
2. State observations that you may make when assisting a patient or resident with foot care that should be reported to the nurse.
3. Demonstrate proper technique for assisting with foot care.
4. Define the word **podiatrist**.

Tell the Nurse!

Foot care

- Very pale or blue nailbeds
- Bruised nailbeds
- Unusually yellow or white nails
- Unusually thick nails
- Broken nails or nails that have been cut too short (especially if there is also bleeding and tenderness)
- Cracks in the skin
- Peeling of the skin between the toes or on the soles of the feet
- Ingrown toenails
- Any unusual odors
- Complaints of itching or burning
- Any blisters, redness, or tenderness on the feet

Foot care is important to prevent odor and infection and for the person's comfort. Toenails that grow too long can make wearing footwear uncomfortable. The toenails may also curve down and dig into the person's skin. This condition is called *ingrown toenails*.

Assisting with foot care gives you a chance to observe the person's feet for problems. Many patients and residents have decreased blood flow to their feet because of disorders (such as heart problems or diabetes mellitus) or the effects of normal aging. Reduced blood flow causes nerve damage, leading to decreased sensation in the feet. This makes it harder for the person to feel injuries. Decreased blood flow to the feet also increases the risk of infection and poor tissue healing if an injury does occur. A small injury (such as a blister or cut) can quickly become very serious.

Foot care is often done immediately following a bath because the warm water helps to make the nails soft and flexible. Many elderly people have thick, yellowed toenails as a result of age or poor blood flow to the feet (Fig. 23-3). Because thickened toenails may be difficult to trim and an accidental injury can have serious

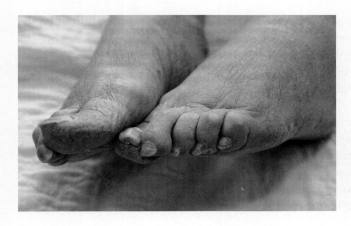

■ FIGURE 23-3
Many elderly people have thick, yellowed toenails as a result of age or poor circulation.

consequences, many health care facilities require a nurse or **podiatrist** to trim patients' or residents' toenails. If your facility policy allows you to trim your patients' or residents' toenails, use clippers and cut the toenails straight across. Never try to trim or file corns or calluses. File the nails after trimming to remove rough edges. Applying foot powder or lotion after foot care is refreshing and comforting. Procedure 23-2 describes how to assist a patient or resident with foot care.

Podiatrist a doctor who specializes in care of the feet

Putting it all together!

- Care of the feet is essential for good grooming as well as good health. Foot care helps to prevent odor and infection, and it gives you a chance to observe for potential health problems.
- People who have disorders that decrease the blood flow to the feet are especially at risk for developing serious infections from seemingly small injuries.
- Trimming patients' and residents' toenails is usually beyond the nursing assistant's scope of practice.

Assisting With Dressing and Undressing

What will you learn?

When you are finished with this section, you will be able to:
1. Describe how to assist a person who has a weak arm or leg or an intravenous (IV) line to dress.
2. Demonstrate proper technique for assisting a person with dressing.
3. Demonstrate proper technique for changing a hospital gown.

Dressing is usually a routine part of morning and evening care. Clothing is also changed whenever it becomes wet or soiled. The type of clothing worn by people receiving health care differs according to the type of facility and the abilities of the person. Residents of long-term care facilities usually wear street clothes during the day and nightwear at night. Procedure 23-3 describes how to assist a person with dressing in street clothes or nightwear. A person who is too ill to get out of bed may wear a hospital gown or nightwear day and night. Procedure 23-4 describes how to change a hospital gown.

Many of your patients or residents will have a weak side (for example as a result of a stroke). Some may have recently had surgery on an arm or leg, or have a cast. Others will have an intravenous (IV) line. When you are helping these patients or residents to dress, work with the affected side first (Fig. 23-4). When you are helping them to undress, work with the unaffected side first.

General guidelines for assisting a person with dressing and undressing are given in Guidelines Box 23-1.

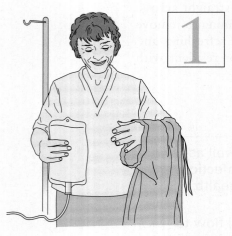

Put the IV bottle and tubing through the sleeve of the gown first, and place the IV bag on the hook.

Gently thread the sleeve down the tubing and gently bring the person's arm through the sleeve of the gown.

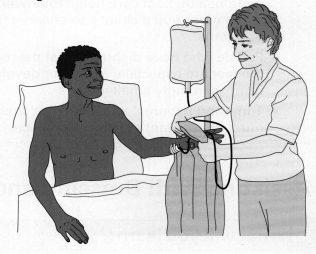

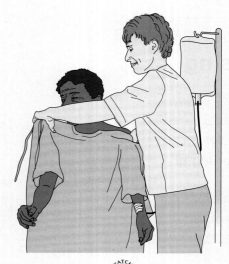

Bring the gown across the person's chest and guide the other arm through the other sleeve.

■ **FIGURE 23-4**

How to help a person who has an intravenous (IV) line in place get dressed.

GUIDELINES BOX 23-1 Guidelines for Assisting With Dressing and Undressing

What you do	Why you do it
Change clothing any time it becomes wet or soiled.	*Contact with wet or soiled clothing can cause skin breakdown, leading to pressure ulcers.*
Allow the person to choose the clothing she wishes to wear. 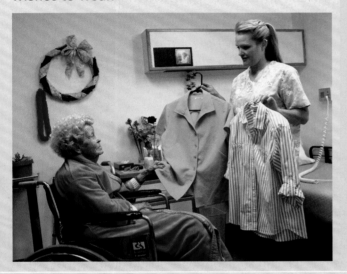	*Our choice in clothing is one way that we express "who we are" to others. Whenever possible, the patient's or resident's right to personal choice should be respected.*
If the person is not able to choose her own clothing, use good taste and common sense when choosing items for the person to wear. Consider the person's comfort, the planned activities for the day, and the temperature.	*The person should be dressed comfortably and appropriately for the day ahead.*
Allow the person to complete as much of her own dressing as possible.	*The activity puts the joints through their normal range of motion, which helps to prevent stiffness. Also, maintaining as much independence as possible is important for the person's self-esteem.*
When assisting a person with dressing or undressing, take care to protect the person's modesty by closing the door and curtain and draping the person with a bath blanket.	*Limiting the person's exposure helps to prevent the person from feeling embarrassed and from becoming chilled.*
When assisting a person with one weak side with dressing, work with the person's weak side first.	*The weak or injured arm or leg may be painful, and the person's ability to move the arm or leg may be limited. When you dress the weak limb first, you do not have to move it as much, which makes the procedure easier for the person.*

(*box continues on page 512*)

GUIDELINES BOX 23-1   Guidelines for Assisting With Dressing and Undressing (continued)

What you do	Why you do it
When assisting a person with one weak side with undressing, work with the person's strong side first.	*The weak or injured arm or leg may be painful, and the person's ability to move the arm or leg may be limited. When you undress the strong limb first, you do not have to move the weak limb as much, which makes the procedure easier for the person.*
Never remove an intravenous (IV) line from an infusion pump or disconnect IV tubing when assisting a person to dress or undress. If you are unsure about how to manage an IV line while helping a person to dress or undress, ask the nurse for help.	*IV lines are sterile on the inside. Disconnecting the line can allow microbes to enter the bloodstream, putting the person at risk for infection.*

Concerns for Long-Term Care

Comfort and ease of dressing help determine many wardrobe choices for the residents of long-term care facilities. Many residents are undergoing rehabilitation following an accident or a disabling illness, such as a stroke. The goal of rehabilitation is to return the person to the highest level of independent functioning as possible. In addition to selecting clothes that are easy to take on and off, a weak or disabled person may use one or more of the many assistive devices that are available to make dressing easier. For example, clothing that closes with a Velcro fastener instead of zippers or buttons allows a person with limited use of his or her fingers to manage dressing and toileting with little or no assistance. The use of these assistive devices can allow a person to maintain a large amount of personal independence in spite of disabilities.

Putting it all together!

- Dressing daily is necessary for warmth and modesty, and it gives people a sense of purpose. Certain conditions (such as a weak, paralyzed, or injured arm or leg or an IV line) can make dressing challenging but by no means impossible.

- For many people, dressing is a way of expressing themselves. A person's preferences regarding outfit selection should be respected whenever possible.

- Encourage your patients or residents to do as much of their own dressing as possible. The ability to do things independently is important for a person's self-esteem.

- Wet or soiled garments must be exchanged for clean, dry ones as often as necessary.

Assisting With Hair Care

What will you learn?

When you are finished with this section, you will be able to:

1. Describe the different methods used to assist a person with shampooing the hair.
2. Demonstrate proper technique for shampooing a person's hair in bed.
3. Demonstrate proper technique for combing a person's hair.
4. Describe methods used to style a person's hair.
5. State observations that you may make when assisting a patient or resident with hair care that should be reported to the nurse.

Shampooing the Hair

Hair is washed as often as necessary to keep it clean. The frequency of shampooing is determined by facility policy, the patient's or resident's personal preference, and the patient's or resident's health status. Before shampooing a person's hair, always check with the nurse or the person's care plan to find out necessary details, such as the frequency of shampoos, the method used, and the products preferred.

A person's hair can be shampooed:

- During a tub bath or shower
- At the sink
- In bed, using a shampoo cap (Fig. 23-5) or shampoo trough (Procedure 23-5)

Brushing, Combing, and Styling the Hair

Brushing, combing, and styling the hair is usually done as part of early morning care. Additional grooming may be necessary throughout the day, for example, after the person wakes up from a nap or before visiting times. Brushing, combing, and styling the hair helps to keep the hair neat and free of tangles. Grooming the hair also gives you an opportunity to observe the condition of the person's hair and scalp.

Procedure 23-6 describes how to comb a person's hair. General guidelines for assisting a person with hair care are given in Guidelines Box 23-2.

Tell the Nurse!

Hair care

- Flaking, crusting, or scaling of the scalp
- Redness, itching, or tenderness of the scalp
- Unusual hair loss, especially if it is occurring in patches
- A foul smell
- Severely matted or tangled hair
- Nits ("flakes" that cannot be brushed or shaken off the hair)

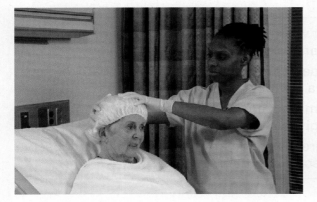

FIGURE 23-5

Shampoo caps contain a product that cleans the hair and scalp without water.

GUIDELINES BOX 23-2   Guidelines for Assisting With Hair Care

What you do	Why you do it
Allow the person to complete as much of his own hair care as possible.	*The activity puts the joints through their normal range of motion, which helps to prevent stiffness. Also, maintaining as much independence as possible is important for the person's self-esteem.*
Respect the person's preferences with regard to hairstyle and hair care products whenever possible.	*How our hair looks is one way that we express "who we are" to others. Whenever possible, the patient's or resident's right to personal choice should be respected.*
If the person spends a lot of time lying in bed, avoid placing hair accessories (such as clips, headbands, and barrettes) on the back of the head. Buns should also be avoided.	*Lying on the hair accessories or bun can cause discomfort and skin breakdown on the scalp.*
When using electrical appliances to dry and style the hair, follow the safety precautions related to the use of electrical items (see Chapter 14).	*Taking appropriate safety precautions when using electrical appliances helps to prevent electrical shocks, electrical fires, and burns.*
Use a low heat setting when using a hair dryer or curling iron.	*Low heat settings help to prevent burns to the person's scalp.*
Handle the hair gently.	*Hair, especially that of elderly people, is fragile. Handling the hair roughly can be painful for the person and can damage the hair.*
Never cut a person's hair, even if it is very matted or tangled. If you think that cutting the person's hair is the only way to remove the tangles or mats, report this need to the nurse.	*The nurse must obtain permission from the person or the person's legal guardian to cut the hair.*

Putting it all together!

- Most people feel best when their hair is clean, free of tangles, and styled in a familiar style.
- Hair may be shampooed as part of a tub or shower bath, at the sink, or in bed, using a shampoo cap or a shampoo trough.
- Regular brushing, combing, and styling keeps the hair shiny and tangle-free, and gives a neat appearance.
- Assisting with hair care gives you an excellent chance to observe for conditions of the scalp and hair.

Assisting With Shaving

What will you learn?

When you are finished with this section, you will be able to:

1. Describe the tools and supplies used for shaving.
2. Demonstrate how to safely shave a man's face.

Shaving the face is a routine grooming practice for many men. Shaving is a part of either morning or evening care, depending on the man's preference and facility policy. The frequency of shaving depends on how fast the beard grows and personal preference. A man may prefer to have a beard or mustache instead of being clean-shaven. Beards and mustaches must be kept clean and free of food and drink and will need to be combed or brushed and trimmed regularly. Be careful when shaving near the mustache or beard to avoid accidentally shaving part of the facial hair off.

Shaving the legs, underarms, or both is a routine grooming practice for many women. In addition, some women experience the growth of coarse facial hair as they age and may request your help with removing this unwanted hair. Shaving of the legs and underarms is often done as part of the bath or shower. When shaving the armpits, move in the direction that the hair grows. When shaving the legs, start at the ankle and move upward, against the direction of hair growth.

The supplies used to shave vary according to the person's preference and medical condition (Fig. 23-6):

- A safety razor has a straight blade. The hair is softened with warm water and a shaving cream, gel, or soap is applied to help the razor glide across the skin

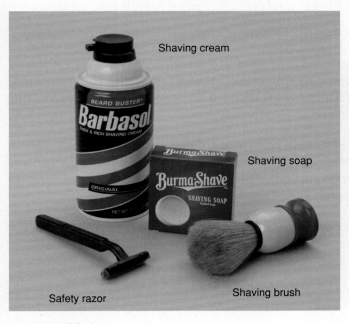

Shaving cream

Shaving soap

Safety razor

Shaving brush

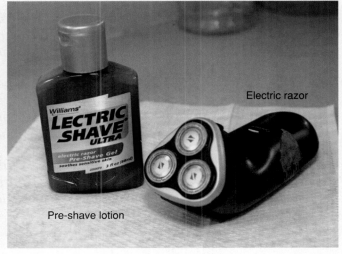

Electric razor

Pre-shave lotion

■ **FIGURE 23-6**
Shaving supplies.

more easily. A safety razor may be disposable or it may have changeable blade cartridges. Procedure 23-7 explains how to shave a person's face using a safety razor.

- An electric razor has a rotating blade. An electric razor does not require the use of water and a shaving cream, gel, or soap. Instead, a pre-shave lotion is applied to soften the hair and allow the razor to glide smoothly across the skin. People who are taking medications that decrease the blood's ability to clot should always use an electric razor because electric razors are less likely to cut or nick the skin.

General guidelines for assisting a person to shave are given in Guidelines Box 23-3.

GUIDELINES BOX 23-3   Guidelines for Assisting a Person With Shaving

What you do	Why you do it
Ask the nurse or check the nursing care plan to determine if there are any limitations or special instructions for a person's shave.	*A person may have a medical condition or be taking a medication that makes using a safety razor dangerous, due to the higher risk for cuts and nicks.*
Allow the person to complete as much of his own shave as possible.	*The activity puts the joints through their normal range of motion, which helps to prevent stiffness. Also, maintaining as much independence as possible is important for the person's self-esteem.*
When using a safety razor with changeable blades, change the blade frequently.	*Blades that become dull pull at the hair and put the person at higher risk for nicks and cuts.*
When shaving a person, always wear gloves.	*A nick or cut will put you at risk for exposure to bloodborne pathogens.*
Dispose of used blades and disposable razors in a sharps container, never a wastebasket.	*Sharps containers limit others' exposure to bloodborne pathogens by preventing accidental injuries caused by sharp contaminated objects.*
Never shave off a person's beard or moustache unless the person requests that you do so.	*A person may have a beard or moustache for cultural or religious reasons. In addition, shaving off a person's beard or moustache can significantly change the person's appearance and the way he feels about himself.*
If you accidentally cut the person during shaving, apply direct pressure to stop the bleeding and then report the incident to the nurse.	*Direct pressure will usually stop the bleeding. The nurse needs to know about any injury to a patient or resident.*

Putting it all together!

- Most men shave their faces daily, either completely or partially. Many women shave their legs, their underarms, or both.
- Supplies used for shaving vary according to personal preference and the person's medical condition.
- Standard precautions should be taken when assisting a person with shaving because contact with blood is possible.

Assisting With Vision and Hearing Accessories

What will you learn?

When you are finished with this section, you will be able to:

1. Describe how to care for eyeglasses.
2. Describe how to care for contact lenses.
3. Describe how to care for prosthetic (artificial) eyes.
4. Describe how to care for a person's hearing aid.
5. Demonstrate proper technique for inserting and removing an in-the-ear hearing aid.

Eyeglasses, contact lenses, and hearing aids help people to interact with others. Not being able to see or hear properly negatively affects a person's quality of life. A prosthetic (artificial) eye does not help the person to see, but it does contribute to the person's normal appearance. Ensuring that vision and hearing accessories are clean and in place is an important part of helping your patients or residents get ready for the day ahead.

Assisting With Eyeglasses

Eyeglasses are commonly used to correct vision. Always make sure that your patients or residents who need glasses wear them, especially if the person is confused or disoriented. Being unable to see clearly can make confusion and disorientation worse.

Clean eyeglasses with cloths or a special solution made specifically for that purpose, or with warm water (Fig. 23-7). If water or a special cleaning solution is used to clean the lenses, finish by drying them with a soft cloth or tissue. Paper towels or napkins may scratch the lenses and should not be used. When not in use, the person's eyeglasses should be stored in their case within easy reach.

Assisting With Contact Lenses

Contact lenses are made of molded plastic and fit directly on the eyeball to correct vision. Contacts may be soft or hard. How long they can be worn before taking them out depends on the type of lens. Most lenses are removed and cleaned daily.

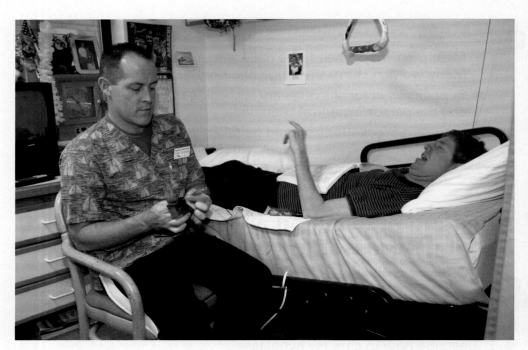

■ **FIGURE 23-7**
Take special care when handling a person's eyeglasses. They are expensive to replace.

Contact lenses must be cared for carefully to prevent infection and irritation of the eyes. Special cleaning and soaking solutions are used to clean and store the lenses. The types of solutions that are used vary according to the type of lens. Each lens is kept in its own case ("left" and "right") because the correction and size for the left and right eyes may be different. If one of your patients or residents wears contact lenses, make sure that you are familiar with the proper technique for helping the person to care for them. Report any complaints of eye irritation or discharge to the nurse immediately.

Assisting With Prosthetic Eyes

Sometimes a person's eye must be surgically removed, either because of injury or disease. A person who has had an eye removed may choose to wear a patch to cover the missing eye or may wear a prosthetic eye. Prosthetic eyes are made of ceramic or plastic and are usually designed to be very close in appearance to the person's own eye in terms of color and shape (Fig. 23-8).

Some prosthetic eyes are removable and others are permanent. If your patient's or resident's prosthetic eye is removable, you may need to help him with cleaning and storing it. A prosthetic eye is very expensive to replace and should be handled carefully. Improper handling can cause scratches or nicks on the prosthetic eye that can injure or irritate the person's eyelids. Handling the prosthetic eye with dirty hands or not cleaning it properly can result in an infection. If one of your patients or residents wears a prosthetic eye, make sure that you have been instructed in the proper way to care for it.

Assisting With Hearing Aids

It may be your responsibility to make sure that your patients or residents have their hearing aids in place because they may forget them or be physically unable to put them in and turn them on. The steps for inserting and removing an in-the-ear hearing aid are listed in Box 23-1.

Hearing aids are expensive and must be cared for carefully. General guidelines for caring for hearing aids are given in Guidelines Box 23-4.

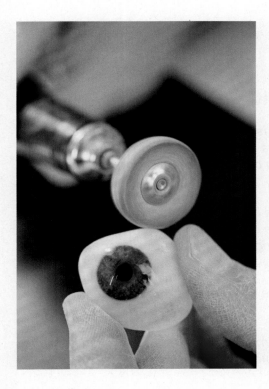

■ FIGURE 23-8
Artificial eyes are custom-made to look
very similar to the person's other eye.

BOX 23-1 **Inserting and Removing an In-the-Ear Hearing Aid**

To insert the hearing aid:

1. Perform hand hygiene.
2. Help the person into a comfortable position, with her head turned so that the ear needing the hearing aid is closest to you.
3. Inspect the ear canal for excessive wax. If you see excessive wax build-up in the ear canal, gently wipe the ear canal with a warm, moist washcloth.
4. Inspect the hearing aid, making sure it is clean and without cracks and that the batteries are inserted properly.
5. Make sure the hearing aid is turned off and the volume is low.
6. Gently insert the tapered end of the hearing aid into the ear canal. Rotate the hearing aid so that it fits into the curve of the ear. With one hand, push up and in, using your other hand to pull gently down on the person's earlobe. The hearing aid should fit snugly but comfortably, flush with the ear.
7. Turn on the control switch and adjust the volume by talking to the person as you increase the volume. Stop increasing the volume when the person can hear you.
8. Repeat for the other side if the person wears a hearing aid in both ears.
9. Perform hand hygiene.

To remove the hearing aid:

1. Perform hand hygiene.
2. Turn off the hearing aid.
3. Gently pull up on the person's ear. Lift the hearing aid up and out of the person's ear.
4. Remove the batteries or open the battery casing before storing the hearing aid in its case. This helps keep the batteries from being run down when the aid is not in use and helps to dry out any moisture that collects inside the hearing aid. Make sure the case is labeled with the person's name and store it safely.
5. Perform hand hygiene.

GUIDELINES BOX 23-4 Guidelines for Caring for Hearing Aids

What you do	Why you do it
Clean the hearing aid daily, according to the manufacturer's instructions.	*If the hearing aid is not cleaned daily, the sound passages can become blocked with cerumen (ear wax). The cerumen build-up can cause the hearing aid to stop working properly.*
Make sure that the person has a spare set of batteries on hand at all times, and replace dead batteries immediately.	*The hearing aid is battery-operated and will not work if the batteries are dead. It is inconvenient for a person who uses a hearing aid to be without it for any length of time.*
Keep hearing aids away from heat and moisture.	*Heat and moisture can damage the plastic ear mold.*
Do not use hairspray or other hair care products on a person who wears a hearing aid while the hearing aid is in place.	*The chemicals in many hair care products can damage the plastic ear mold.*
Store hearing aids at room temperature when they are not being worn.	*Hearing aids are delicate instruments. Exposure to very hot or very cold temperatures is not good for them.*
Keep replacement batteries and small hearing aids away from children and pets.	*These small objects can pose a choking hazard to children and pets. In addition, hearing aids are expensive to replace.*

 Putting it all together!

- Eyeglasses, contact lenses, and hearing aids help people to interact with others. Prosthetic eyes help a person to maintain a normal appearance. For many patients or residents, making sure hearing and vision accessories are in place is a routine grooming activity.

- Always handle your patients' or residents' eyeglasses, contact lenses, prosthetic eyes, and hearing aids with care. These items are expensive and difficult to replace. Improper handling of prosthetic eyes and contact lenses can lead to infections or injury of the eye.

PROCEDURES

PROCEDURE 23-1
Assisting With Hand Care

Why you do it: Soft, smooth skin and trimmed, filed fingernails are important for overall health and comfort.

GETTING READY

1. Complete the "Getting Ready" steps.

SUPPLIES

- gloves (if contact with broken skin is likely)
- paper towels
- orange stick
- nail clippers
- emery board (nail file)
- bath thermometer
- emesis basin
- soap
- lotion
- nail polish remover (optional)
- nail polish (optional)
- cotton balls (optional)
- washcloth
- towel

PROCEDURE

2. Make sure that the bed is lowered to its lowest position and that the wheels are locked.
3. Clean the top of the over-bed table and cover it with paper towels. Pour some liquid soap into the emesis basin and fill the basin with warm water (100°F [37.7°C] to 115°F [46.1°C] on the bath thermometer). Place the emesis basin on the over-bed table, along with the nail care supplies and clean linens.
4. If the side rails are in use, lower the side rail on the working side of the bed. The side rail on the opposite side of the bed should remain up.
5. Help the person to transfer from the bed to a bedside chair, assist the person to sit on the edge of the bed, or raise the head of the bed as tolerated.
6. Perform hand hygiene and put on the gloves if contact with broken skin is likely.
7. If the person is wearing nail polish and wants it removed, remove the nail polish by putting a small amount of nail polish remover on a cotton ball and gently rubbing each nail.

8. Help the person to position the tips of her fingers in the basin to soak. Let the person soak her fingers for about 5 minutes.

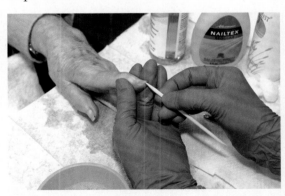

STEP 8 ■ Soak the nails to soften them.

9. Working with one hand at a time, lift the person's hand out of the basin and wash the entire hand, including between the fingers, with the soapy washcloth. Use the orange stick to gently clean underneath the person's fingernails. Rinse thoroughly and pat the person's hand dry with a towel. Be sure to dry between the fingers. Repeat with the other hand.

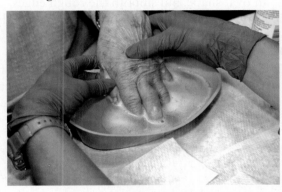

STEP 9 ■ Clean under the person's nails using the orange stick.

(*procedure continues on page 522*)

PROCEDURE 23-1 (continued)
Assisting With Hand Care

10. Remove the emesis basin and dry the person's hands thoroughly. If facility policy allows it, gently push the cuticles back with the orange stick.

11. If facility policy allows it, use the nail clippers to cut the person's fingernails. If the person's nails need to be trimmed but this task is outside of your scope of practice, report this need to the nurse.

12. Use the emery board to file the fingernails into an oval shape and smooth the rough edges.

13. Apply lotion to the person's hands and gently massage it into the skin.

14. Apply nail polish as the person requests.

15. If necessary, help the person return to bed. If the side rails are in use, return the side rails to the raised position. Lower the head of the bed as the person requests.

16. Gather the soiled linens and place them in the linen hamper or linen bag. Dispose of disposable items in a facility-approved waste container. Clean equipment and return it to the storage area.

17. Remove your gloves, dispose of them in a facility-approved waste container, and perform hand hygiene.

FINISHING UP

18. Complete the "Finishing Up" steps.

WHAT YOU DOCUMENT

- Date and time
- Type of care provided (trimming nails, filing, etc.)
- Any unusual observations (rashes, hangnails, discolored nails)

PROCEDURE 23-2
Assisting With Foot Care

Why you do it: Soft, smooth skin and trimmed, filed toenails are important for overall health and comfort.

GETTING READY

1. Complete the "Getting Ready" steps.

SUPPLIES

- gloves (if contact with broken skin is likely)
- paper towels
- bed protector
- orange stick
- nailbrush
- nail clippers
- emery board (nail file)
- wash basin
- bath thermometer
- soap
- lotion
- nail polish remover (optional)
- nail polish (optional)
- cotton balls (optional)
- washcloth
- towels
- bath blanket (if remaining in the bed)

PROCEDURE

2. Make sure that the bed is lowered to its lowest position and that the wheels are locked.

3. Clean the top of the over-bed table and cover it with paper towels. Pour some liquid soap into the wash basin and fill the basin with warm water (100°F [37.7°C] to 115°F [46.1°C] on the bath thermometer). Place the wash basin on the over-bed table, along with the nail care supplies and clean linens.

4. If the side rails are in use, lower the side rail on the working side of the bed. The side rail on the opposite side of the bed should remain up.

5. If the person is able to get out of bed, help the person to transfer from the bed to a bedside chair. If the person is not able to get out of bed, raise the head of the bed as tolerated. Fanfold the top linens to the foot of the bed. Cover the person with a bath blanket for warmth and modesty, leaving the feet exposed.

6. Perform hand hygiene and put on the gloves if contact with broken skin is likely.

7. If the person is wearing nail polish and wants it removed, remove the nail polish by putting a small amount of nail polish remover on a cotton ball and gently rubbing each nail.

8. Place a bed protector on the floor in front of the chair (if the person is out of bed) or on the bottom sheet (if the person is in bed). Place the wash basin on the bed protector.

9. Help the person to position his feet in the basin to soak. Let the person soak his feet for about 5 minutes.

10. Working with one foot at a time, lift the person's foot out of the basin and wash the entire foot, including between the toes, with the soapy washcloth. Apply soap to the nailbrush and gently scrub any rough areas. Use the orange stick to gently clean underneath the person's toenails. Rinse thoroughly and pat the person's foot dry with a towel. Be sure to dry between the toes. Repeat with the other foot.

11. If facility policy allows it, use the nail clippers to cut the person's toenails. If the person's nails need to be trimmed but this task is outside of your scope of practice, report this need to the nurse.

12. Use the emery board to smooth the rough edges of the toenails.

13. Apply lotion to the person's feet and gently massage it into the skin.

14. Apply nail polish as the person requests.

15. If necessary, help the person return to bed. If the side rails are in use, return the side rails to the raised position. Lower the head of the bed as the person requests.

16. Gather the soiled linens and place them in the linen hamper or linen bag. Dispose of disposable items in a facility-approved waste container. Clean equipment and return it to the storage area.

17. Remove your gloves, dispose of them in a facility-approved waste container, and perform hand hygiene.

FINISHING UP

18. Complete the "Finishing Up" steps.

WHAT YOU DOCUMENT

- Date and time
- Type of care provided
- Condition of skin and nails
- Presence of broken skin or rashes

PROCEDURE 23-3
Assisting a Person With Dressing

Why you do it: People who are able to be out of bed during the day usually wear regular clothing during the day and pajamas or nightgowns at night. Getting dressed in the morning helps people to feel better about themselves. Clothing must be changed every time it becomes wet or soiled.

GETTING READY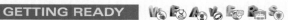

1. Complete the "Getting Ready" steps.

SUPPLIES

- gloves (if contact with broken skin is likely)
- bath blanket
- clean clothing

PROCEDURE

2. Make sure that the bed is positioned at a comfortable working height (to promote good body mechanics) and that the wheels are locked.

3. Lower the head of the bed so that the bed is flat (as tolerated). If the side rails are in use, lower the side rail on the working side of the bed. The side rail on the opposite side of the bed should remain up.

4. Perform hand hygiene and put on the gloves if contact with broken skin is likely.

5. Spread the bath blanket over the top linens (and the person). If the person is able, have her hold the bath blanket. If not, tuck the corners under the person's shoulders. Fanfold the top linens to the foot of the bed.

6. Assist the person with undressing:

   a. **Garments that fasten in the back.** Undo any fasteners, such as buttons, zippers, snaps, or ties. Gently lift the person's head and shoulders and gather the garment around the person's neck. Working with the person's strongest side first, gently remove the arm from the garment by sliding the garment down the arm. Repeat with the other arm. (If it is not possible to lift the person's head and shoulders, roll the person onto his or her side facing away from you. Working with the person's strongest side first, gently remove the arm from the garment. Roll the person onto her other side, facing you and remove the other arm from the garment.)

   Remove the garment completely by lifting it over the person's head.

   b. **Garments that fasten in the front.** Undo any fasteners, such as buttons, zippers, snaps, or ties. To remove the top, gently lift the person's head and shoulders. Working with the person's strongest side first, gently remove the arm from the garment by sliding the garment over the shoulder and down the arm. Gather the garment behind the person and remove the garment completely by sliding the other sleeve over the weak shoulder and arm. To remove the bottoms, undo any fasteners, such as buttons, zippers or snaps. Ask the person to lift her buttocks off the bed and gently slide the pants down to the ankles and over the feet. (If the person cannot raise her buttocks off the bed, help the person to roll first to her strong side, allowing you to pull the bottoms down on the weak side. Then roll the person to her weak side and finish pulling the bottoms down.)

7. Assist the person with putting on her undergarments:

   a. **Underpants.** Facing the foot of the bed, gather the underpants together at the leg opening and at the waistband. Working with one foot at a time, slip first one foot and then the other through the waistband and into the leg openings. Slide the underpants up the person's legs as far as they will go, and then ask the person to lift her buttocks off the bed. Gently slide the underpants up over the buttocks. (If the person cannot raise her buttocks off the bed, help the person to roll first to her strong side, allowing you to pull the underpants up on the weak side. Then roll the person to her weak side and finish pulling the underpants up.) Adjust the underpants so that they fit comfortably.

b. Bra. Working with the person's weak side first, slip the arms through the straps and position the straps on the shoulders so that the front of the bra is covering the person's chest. Adjust the cups of the bra over the person's breasts. Raise the person's head and shoulders and help the person to lean forward so that you can fasten the bra in the back.

c. Undershirt. Facing the head of the bed, gather the top and the bottom of the undershirt together at the neck opening. Place the undershirt over the person's head. Working with the person's weak side first, slip the arms through the arm openings. Raise the person's head and shoulders and help the person to lean forward so that you can pull the undershirt down, smoothing out any wrinkles.

8. Assist the person with putting on her outerwear:

a. Pants. Assist the person with putting on her pants by following the same procedure as that used for putting on underpants (see step 7a). Fasten any buttons, zippers, snaps, or ties.

b. Shirts and sweaters that fasten in the front. Facing the head of the bed, place your hand and arm through the wristband of the garment. Working with the person's weak side first, grasp the person's hand and slip the garment off of your hand and arm, gently guiding the person's arm into the sleeve. Pull the sleeve up, adjusting it at the shoulder. Raise the person's head and shoulders and help the person to lean forward so that you can bring the other side of the garment around the back of the person's body. Guide the person's strong arm into the sleeve of the garment. Fasten any buttons, zippers, snaps, or ties.

c. Sweatshirts and pullover sweaters. Assist the person with putting on a sweatshirt or pullover sweater by following the same procedure as that used for putting on an undershirt (see step 7c). Fasten any buttons, zippers, snaps, or ties.

d. Blouses that fasten in the back. Facing the head of the bed, place your hand and arm through the wristband of the garment. Working with the person's weak side first, grasp the person's hand and slip the garment off of your hand and arm, gently guiding the person's arm into the sleeve. Pull the sleeve up, adjusting it at the shoulder. Repeat for the other side. Raise the person's head and shoulders and help the person to lean forward so that you can bring the sides of the garment around to the back. Fasten any buttons, zippers, snaps, or ties.

9. Assist the person with putting on footwear:

a. Socks or knee-high stockings. Gather the sock or stocking, bringing the toe area and the opening together. With the toe area facing up, slip the sock or stocking over the person's foot. Smooth the heel of the sock or stocking over the person's heel, and pull the sock or stocking up into position. Adjust the sock or stocking so that it fits comfortably. Repeat for the other foot.

b. Shoes or slippers. If the shoe has laces, loosen them completely to make it easier to slip the shoe onto the foot. Guide the person's foot into the shoe or slipper. A shoehorn may be used to help ease the person's heel into the shoe. Make sure that the foot is seated properly in the shoe. Socks or stockings should not be bunched at the toe. If necessary, tie the shoe or fasten the Velcro fasteners securely.

10. If the person will be remaining in bed and the side rails are in use, return the side rails to the raised position. Raise the head of the bed as the person requests.

11. Gather the soiled garments and place them in the linen hamper or linen bag.

12. Remove your gloves, dispose of them in a facility-approved waste container, and perform hand hygiene.

FINISHING UP

13. Complete the "Finishing Up" steps.

WHAT YOU DOCUMENT

- Date and time
- Type of clothing applied
- Any abnormal observations

PROCEDURE 23-4
Changing a Hospital Gown

Why you do it: People who are too ill to get out of bed may wear a hospital gown. The gown must be changed every time it becomes wet or soiled.

GETTING READY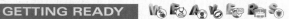

1. Complete the "Getting Ready" steps.

SUPPLIES

- gloves (if contact with broken skin is likely)
- clean hospital gown

PROCEDURE

2. Make sure that the bed is positioned at a comfortable working height (to promote good body mechanics) and that the wheels are locked.

3. Lower the head of the bed so that the bed is flat (as tolerated). If the side rails are in use, lower them on the working side of the bed. The side rails on the opposite side of the bed should remain up.

4. Perform hand hygiene and put on the gloves if contact with broken skin is likely.

5. Fanfold the bed linens toward the foot of the bed.

6. Have the person turn onto her side facing away from you so that you can untie the gown at the neck and waist. Assist the person back into the supine position.

7. Loosen the gown from around the person's body.

8. Unfold the clean gown and lay it over the person's chest.

9. Working with the person's strongest side first, remove one sleeve at a time, leaving the old gown draped over the person's body.

10. Working with the person's weakest side first, slide the arm through the sleeve of the clean gown. Repeat for the other arm.

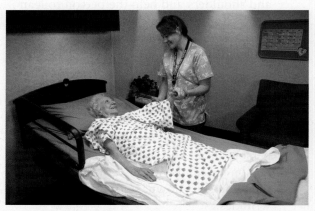

STEP 10 ■ Slide the person's arm through the sleeve of the clean gown.

11. Remove the soiled gown from underneath the clean gown and place it in the linen hamper or linen bag.

12. Have the person turn onto her side, facing away from you, so that you can tie the gown at the neck and waist. Adjust the gown so that it fits comfortably and does not have wrinkles underneath the person.

13. Pull the bed covers back up over the person.

14. If the side rails are in use, return the side rails to the raised position. Raise the head of the bed as the person requests.

15. Remove your gloves, dispose of them in a facility-approved waste container, and perform hand hygiene.

FINISHING UP

16. Complete the "Finishing Up" steps.

WHAT YOU DOCUMENT

- Date and time
- Any abnormal observations

PROCEDURE 23-5
Shampooing a Person's Hair in Bed

Why you do it: Clean hair helps a person to look and feel attractive and is important for a person's self-esteem.

 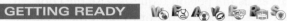

1. Complete the "Getting Ready" steps.

SUPPLIES

- gloves (if contact with broken skin is likely)
- paper towels
- bed protector
- wash basin
- water pitcher
- bath thermometer
- shampoo trough
- comb
- brush
- blow dryer (optional)
- shampoo
- conditioner (optional)
- washcloth
- towels

PROCEDURE

2. Make sure that the bed is positioned at a comfortable working height (to promote good body mechanics) and that the wheels are locked.
3. Fill the water pitcher with warm water (100°F [37.7°C] to 115°F [46.1°C] on the bath thermometer).
4. Clean the top of the over-bed table and cover it with paper towels. Place the hair care supplies and clean linens on the over-bed table.
5. Raise the head of the bed as tolerated. Comb the person's hair to remove snarls and tangles.
6. Lower the head of the bed so that the bed is flat (as tolerated). If the side rails are in use, lower the side rail on the working side of the bed. The side rail on the opposite side of the bed should remain up.
7. Perform hand hygiene and put on the gloves if contact with broken skin is likely.
8. Gently lift the person's head and shoulders and reposition the pillow under the person's

shoulders. Cover the head of the bed and the pillow with the bed protector and place the shampoo trough on the bed protector. Help the person to rest his head on the shampoo trough. Place a towel across the person's shoulders and chest.

9. Place the wash basin on the floor beside the bed to catch the water as it drains from the shampoo trough.
10. Ask the person to hold the washcloth over his eyes.
11. Holding the water pitcher in one hand, slowly pour water over the person's hair until the hair is completely wet. Use your other hand to help direct the flow of water away from the person's eyes and ears.

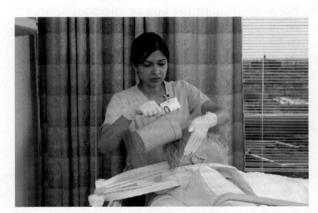

STEP 11 ■ Wet the person's hair, being careful to keep the water out of his eyes.

12. Apply a small amount of shampoo to the wet hair. Lather the hair and massage the scalp to help stimulate the circulation.
13. Using the water pitcher, rinse the hair thoroughly.

(procedure continues on page 528)

PROCEDURE 23-5 (continued)
Shampooing a Person's Hair in Bed

14. Apply conditioner, as the person requests. Rinse the hair thoroughly.

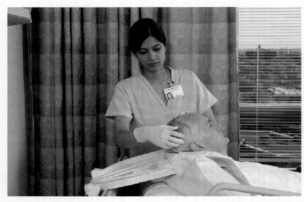

STEP 12 ■ Apply a small amount of shampoo and work it into a lather.

15. Gently lift the person's head and shoulders and remove the shampoo trough and bed protector. Wrap the person's hair in a towel.
16. Raise the head of the bed as tolerated. Gently pat the person's face, neck, and ears dry and finish towel drying the hair.
17. Replace any wet or soiled linens. (If the side rails are in use, raise the side rails before leaving the bedside to get the necessary replacement linens.)
18. If wearing gloves, remove them and perform hand hygiene. Put on a clean pair of gloves.

19. Comb the person's hair to remove snarls and tangles.
20. Dry and style the hair with the brush and blow dryer, as the person requests. Use the cool setting and take care not to burn the person's scalp or face.
21. Reposition the pillow under the person's head and straighten the bed linens. If the side rails are in use, return the side rails to the raised position. Lower the head of the bed as the person requests.
22. Gather the soiled linens and place them in the linen hamper or linen bag. Dispose of disposable items in a facility-approved waste container. Clean equipment and return it to the storage area.
23. Remove your gloves, dispose of them in a facility-approved waste container, and perform hand hygiene.

FINISHING UP

24. Complete the "Finishing Up" steps.

WHAT YOU DOCUMENT

■ Date and time
■ Type of care provided and products used
■ Any unusual observations of the hair or scalp

PROCEDURE 23-6
Combing a Person's Hair

Why you do it: Combing the hair helps to prevent tangles and gives the hair a neat appearance.

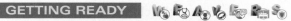

GETTING READY

1. Complete the "Getting Ready" steps.

SUPPLIES

- paper towels
- wide-toothed comb or pick
- brush
- mirror
- hair accessories (optional)
- detangler or leave-in conditioner (optional)
- towels

PROCEDURE

2. Make sure that the bed is positioned at a comfortable working height (to promote good body mechanics) and that the wheels are locked.
3. Clean the top of the over-bed table and cover it with paper towels. Place the hair care supplies and clean linens on the over-bed table.
4. Raise the head of the bed as tolerated. Gently lift the person's head and shoulders and cover the pillow with a towel. Drape another towel across the person's back and shoulders.
5. If the side rails are in use, lower the side rail on the working side of the bed. The side rail on the opposite side of the bed should remain up.
6. If the hair is tangled, work on the tangles first. Put a small amount of detangler or leave-in conditioner on the tangled hair. Begin at the ends of the hair and work toward the scalp. Hold the lock of hair just above the tangle (closest to the scalp) and use the wide-tooth comb to gently work through the tangle.
7. Using the brush and working with one 2-inch section at a time, gently brush the hair, moving from the roots of the hair toward the ends.

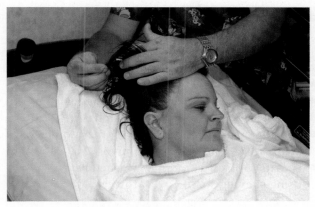

STEP 7 ■ Hold the lock of hair just above the tangle.

8. Secure the hair using barrettes, clips, or pins or braid the hair, as the person requests. Offer the person the mirror to check her appearance when you are finished. Remove the towels from the person's shoulders and the pillow.
9. Reposition the pillow under the person's head and straighten the bed linens. If the side rails are in use, return the side rails to the raised position. Lower the head of the bed as the person requests.
10. Gather the soiled linens and place them in the linen hamper or linen bag. Dispose of disposable items in a facility-approved waste container. Clean equipment and return it to the storage area.

FINISHING UP

11. Complete the "Finishing Up" steps.

WHAT YOU DOCUMENT

- Date and time
- Type of care provided
- Presence of excessive tangling or any unusual observations of the hair or scalp

PROCEDURE 23-7
Shaving a Person's Face

Why you do it: Shaving removes unwanted hair and is a routine grooming practice for many patients and residents.

 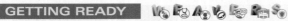

1. Complete the "Getting Ready" steps.

SUPPLIES

- gloves
- paper towels
- safety razor
- shaving cream/gel/soap
- shaving brush (if using shaving soap)
- aftershave lotion (optional)
- wash basin
- bath thermometer
- mirror
- washcloth
- towels

PROCEDURE

2. Make sure that the bed is lowered to its lowest position and that the wheels are locked. (If the person is remaining in bed, raise the level of the bed to a comfortable working height.)
3. Fill the wash basin with warm water (100°F [37.7°C] to 115°F [46.1°C] on the bath thermometer).
4. Clean the top of the over-bed table and cover it with paper towels. Place the wash basin, shaving supplies, and clean linens on the over-bed table.
5. If the side rails are in use, lower the side rail on the working side of the bed. The side rail on the opposite side of the bed should remain up.
6. Help the person to transfer from the bed to a bedside chair, assist the person to sit on the edge of the bed, or raise the head of the bed as tolerated.
7. Place a towel across the person's shoulders and chest.
8. Perform hand hygiene and put on the gloves.
9. Wet the washcloth with warm, clean water. Soften the beard by holding the washcloth against the person's face for 2 to 3 minutes.
10. Apply shaving cream, gel, or soap to the beard.
11. Shave the person's cheeks:
    a. Stand facing the person.
    b. Gently pull the skin tight and shave downward, in the direction of hair growth (that is, toward the chin). Use short, even strokes, rinsing the razor frequently in the wash basin. Repeat until all of the lather on the cheek has been removed.
    c. Repeat for the other cheek.

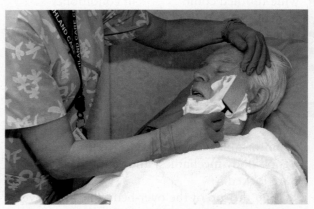

STEP 11 ■ Shave downward, in the direction of hair growth.

12. Shave the person's chin:
    a. Ask the person to "tighten the chin" by drawing the lower lip over the teeth.
    b. Shave the chin using short, even, downward strokes. Repeat until all of the lather on the chin has been removed, rinsing the razor frequently in the wash basin.
13. Shave the person's neck:
    a. Ask the person to tip his head back.
    b. Gently pull the skin tight and shave upward, in the direction of hair growth (that is, toward the chin). Use short, even strokes, rinsing the razor frequently in the wash basin. Repeat until all of the lather on the neck has been removed.
14. Shave the area between the person's nose and upper lip:
    a. Ask the person to "tighten his upper lip" by drawing the upper lip over the teeth.

b. Shave the area between the nose and the upper lip using short, even downward strokes. Repeat until all of the lather has been removed, rinsing the razor frequently in the wash basin.

15. Change the water in the wash basin. (If the side rails are in use, raise the side rails before leaving the bedside.) Form a mitt around your hand with the washcloth and wet the mitt with warm, clean water. Wash the person's face and neck. Rinse thoroughly and pat the person's face, neck, and ears dry with the face towel.

16. Apply aftershave lotion, as the person requests.

17. If you have accidentally nicked the skin and the person is bleeding, apply direct pressure with a tissue until the bleeding stops. Report the incident to the nurse.

18. If necessary, help the person return to bed. If the side rails are in use, return the side rails to the raised position.

19. Gather the soiled linens and place them in the linen hamper or linen bag. Dispose of disposable items in a facility-approved waste container. Clean equipment and return it to the storage area.

20. Remove your gloves, dispose of them in a facility-approved waste container, and perform hand hygiene.

FINISHING UP

21. Complete the "Finishing Up" steps.

WHAT YOU DOCUMENT

- Date and time
- Type of razor used
- Occurrence of cuts or nicks in the skin
- Unusual observations of the skin

WHAT DID YOU LEARN?

Multiple Choice

Select the single best answer for each of the following questions.

1. You are a nursing assistant in a long-term care facility. Which one of the following procedures may be beyond your scope of practice?
   a. Assisting a resident with bathing
   b. Polishing a female resident's fingernails
   c. Trimming the toenails of a resident with diabetes
   d. Assisting a resident with oral care

2. When helping a person to dress, which item of clothing would you put on first?
   a. Underpants
   b. Socks
   c. Slacks
   d. Sweater

3. Mrs. Dinksley, one of your residents, had a stroke that caused her left side to become weak. You are helping Mrs. Dinksley put on a cardigan sweater. Which arm should you put in the sleeve first?
   a. The left arm
   b. The right arm
   c. Either arm; it makes no difference
   d. Neither arm; Mrs. Dinksley should wear a hospital gown

4. What should you use to clean the lenses in a person's eyeglasses?
   a. Soap and a paper towel
   b. Window cleaner and a tissue
   c. A special eyeglass cleaning solution and a soft cloth
   d. A special eyeglass cleaning solution and a paper towel

5. Brushing the hair is important to:
   a. Make it grow faster
   b. Prevent tangles
   c. Keep it clean
   d. Keep it free from lice

6. When shaving a man's face with a safety razor and shaving cream, you should:
   a. Soften the beard with warm water before applying the shaving cream
   b. Apply aftershave lotion after the shave is complete if the man requests it
   c. Give the man a mirror so that he can check his appearance when you are finished
   d. All of the above

7. When shaving a man's face, you should:
   a. Apply shaving cream sparingly
   b. Use upward strokes when shaving the cheeks
   c. Apply an antiseptic to any cuts or nicks
   d. Use downward strokes to shave the chin

8. Which one of the following statements about nail care is true?
   a. Scissors are used to trim the nails.
   b. Elderly people do not need nail care because their nails do not grow as fast.
   c. Providing nail care allows you to examine the hands and feet for signs of health and disease.
   d. Nail care is an activity that can be skipped if there is not enough time.

9. Which one of the following statements about helping a resident to dress is true?
   a. Residents like staff members to decide what they are going to wear.
   b. Residents are used to being dressed in front of others.
   c. Residents care about how they look.
   d. Residents who are disabled do not need to dress in street clothes.

10. One of your residents, Mrs. Ament, has diabetes. Why is providing foot care an important part of caring for Mrs. Ament?
    a. The circulation to her feet is likely to be poor, which puts her at risk for infection and other complications.
    b. Diabetes makes the toenails grow faster.
    c. People with diabetes usually do not take good care of their feet.
    d. All of the above

11. You must remove a soiled gown from a patient who has an intravenous (IV) line. What is the best way to do this?
    a. Remove the gown from the arm with the IV first.
    b. Ask the nurse to disconnect the bag and tubing before beginning.
    c. Disconnect the bag and tubing before beginning.
    d. Remove the opposite arm from the gown first.

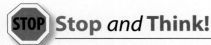 **Stop** *and* **Think!**

You have been assigned to take care of Mr. Wiseman, an Orthodox Jewish rabbi who is recovering from a stroke. As you are assisting Mr. Wiseman with his morning care, you note that his long beard is matted. You look out into the hall for a nurse. Seeing no one, you decide to trim Mr. Wiseman's beard yourself. As you are finishing up, the medication nurse arrives in the room. She says to you, "Oh, no! Didn't you realize that Mr. Wiseman's beard is part of his religion? What are we going to tell his wife?" What did you do wrong? What could you have done to prevent this mistake?

Assisting With Nutrition

Having a good meal can be one of life's pleasures. Eating meets many needs for people, both emotionally and physically. In this chapter, you will learn how to help your patients and residents to meet their nutritional needs.

Photo: *Meal time is as much about socializing as it is about eating.*

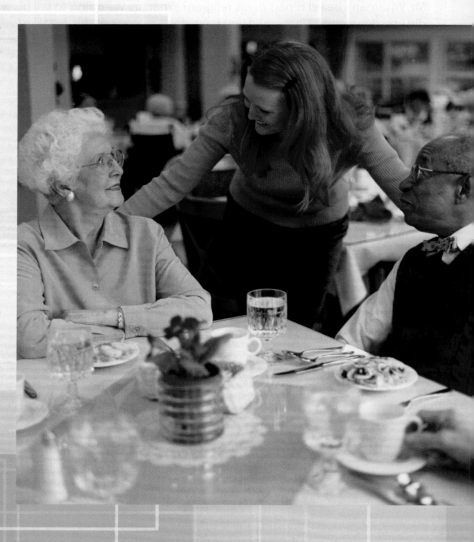

Introduction to Nutrition

What will you learn?

When you are finished with this section, you will be able to:

1. List the six general types of nutrients.
2. Describe a healthy diet.
3. Define the words **nutrition**, **nutrients**, **calories**, and **glucose**.

Nutrition involves the following steps:

- **Ingestion:** the intake of food
- **Digestion:** the breaking down of food into simple elements called **nutrients**
- **Absorption:** the transfer of these nutrients from the digestive tract into the bloodstream
- **Metabolism:** the conversion of nutrients into energy in the body's cells

There are six general types of nutrients. Three of these nutrient types (carbohydrates, proteins, and fat) supply energy to power all of the body's processes. The amount of energy a food supplies is measured in **calories**. The remaining three nutrients (minerals, vitamins, and water) regulate body processes.

- **Carbohydrates** supply us with **glucose**. Glucose is carried in the blood and rapidly absorbed by every cell in the body. The cells use glucose to "run," much like your car uses gas. Extra carbohydrates that are not used immediately as fuel are either stored in the liver or changed to fat and stored elsewhere in the body. Carbohydrates are found in bread, cereal, fruit, vegetables, and table sugar.
- **Proteins** are the "building blocks" of all of the body's cells. Protein helps the body to rebuild tissue that breaks down from normal use and to grow new tissue after illness or injury. Protein is found in foods such as milk and cheese, meat, poultry, fish, eggs, nuts, and dried peas and beans.
- **Fats** provide energy and help our bodies to function properly. For example, some vitamins must be dissolved in fat before the body can use them. Fat also protects our organs and helps us to stay warm. Fats are found in butter, cooking oils, whole milk, cheese, meat, egg yolks, nuts, shortening, and lard.
- **Vitamins** are chemicals that help to regulate the body's processes. For example, vitamin K helps the blood to clot. Other key vitamins include vitamin A, vitamin B_1 (thiamin), vitamin B_2 (riboflavin), vitamin B_3 (niacin), vitamin B_{12}, folic acid, vitamin C, vitamin D, and vitamin E. Some foods, such as milk, bread, and cereal, have vitamins added to them. Vitamins are also found in whole grains, fruits, and vegetables.
- **Minerals** help to provide structure within the body and work with vitamins to regulate body processes. Key minerals include calcium, sodium, potassium, iron, and iodine. Sources of minerals include vegetables, milk products, seafood, fruit, table salt, meat, and grains.
- **Water** is found in many foods, such as fruits and vegetables. Although water provides no calories and has no nutritional value, it is essential to life.

Nutrition the process of taking in and using food

Nutrients substances in foods and fluids that the body uses to grow, to repair itself, and to carry out processes essential for living

Calories the unit of measure used to describe the energy content of food

Glucose the body's most basic type of fuel; supplied by carbohydrates and sometimes referred to as "blood sugar"

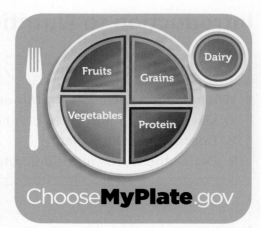

■ **FIGURE 24-1**
MyPlate.
Courtesy of USDA.

A Balanced Diet

For the best health, you must follow a diet that provides your body with a balanced amount of the essential nutrients. To help Americans plan a healthy diet, the United States Department of Agriculture (USDA) developed MyPlate (Fig. 24-1). MyPlate is part of an initiative based on the *2010 Dietary Guidelines for Americans* and replaces the earlier MyPyramid information. MyPlate was designed to remind people to eat healthfully and uses a place setting to illustrate the five food groups in the proportion they would appear on a person's plate.

Some foods contain many nutrients that our bodies need to remain healthy, but other foods have little or no nutritional value. The best way to get the nutrients you need is to eat a variety of healthy food every day. The following suggestions (Box 24-1), found at www.ChooseMyPlate.gov, are intended to help people make healthier food choices and maintain a healthy weight.

BOX 24-1 **Healthy Dietary Guidelines**

■ **Build a healthy plate**

- Make half your plate fruits and vegetables, especially vegetables that are red, orange, and dark green

- Switch to skim or 1% milk

- Make at least half your grains whole: Check the ingredients list on your food packages to make sure that they contain whole grains

- Vary your protein food choices by eating seafood two times a week, adding beans as a protein source, and keeping meat and protein portions small and lean

■ **Eat the right amount of calories for you**

- Enjoy your food, but eat less

- Cook more often at home, where you are in control of what's in your food

- When eating out, choose lower calorie menu options

- Write down what you eat to keep track of how much you eat

■ **Cut back on foods high in solid fats, added sugars, and salt**

- Choose foods and drinks with little or no added sugar by drinking water instead of sugary drinks and selecting fruit, instead of sugary desserts

- Look out for salt (sodium) in the foods you buy by comparing packing labels and choosing food with lower numbers

- Eat fewer foods that are high in solid fats and select lean cuts of meats or poultry and low-fat milk, yogurt, and cheese

■ **Be physically active your way**

- Pick activities that you like and start by doing what you can, at least 10 minutes at a time

In general, the recommendations in MyPlate apply for all healthy people older than 2 years. However, nutritional requirements vary at different times throughout a person's life. For example:

- Infants and young children have an increased need for calories and iron because they are growing rapidly.
- Teenagers experiencing "growth spurts" have increased caloric and nutritional needs.
- Pregnant and breast-feeding women need more protein and calcium.
- People who are recovering from physical trauma, such as that caused by burns or surgery, have different nutritional requirements than healthy people. Similarly, some illnesses change the nutritional requirements of the body, including chronic conditions such as diabetes, kidney disease, or alcoholism.

Nutrition labels, like the one shown in Figure 24-2, contain specific information about the food's nutritional value, approximate serving size, and any related health claims. By reading the nutrition label, you can see how the food can help you to achieve your nutrition goals for the day. Look at the label to see how big a serving size is and how many calories are contained in a serving size. The % Daily Value (DV) shows the percentage that each nutrient meets based on a 2,000 calorie/day diet.

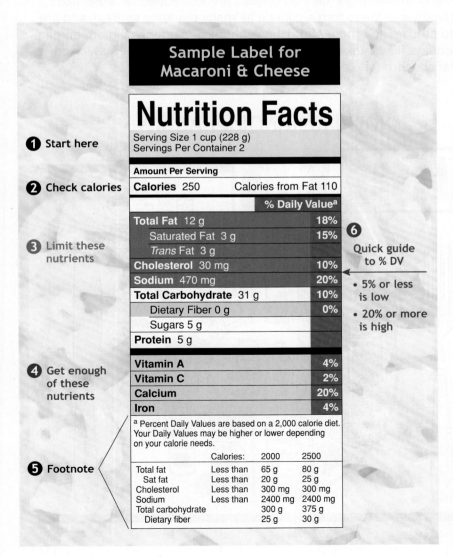

■ **FIGURE 24-2**

The law requires all packaged foods to have a nutrition label like this one.

Concerns for Long-Term Care

Older people have different nutritional requirements due to the physical changes that occur with normal aging. Older people do not need as many calories as younger people because they experience a slowdown in metabolism and are usually less physically active. Although the need for calories decreases as we age, the need for other nutrients, especially protein, increases or remains the same. Older people also may not feel thirsty as often, although the need for water and other fluids increases with age. This age-related decline in thirst can increase the person's risk of dehydration, especially during illness or periods of hot weather.

MyPlate for Older Adults was introduced in 2011 by the USDA Human Nutrition Research Center on Aging. MyPlate for Older Adults addresses the unique nutritional and physical needs associated with people 70 years and older. MyPlate for Older Adults (Fig. 24-3) contains drawings of examples of different forms of foods for each food group that are convenient, affordable, and readily available. The MyPlate for Older Adults diagram focuses on the importance of eating several servings of bright- and deep-colored fruits and vegetables each day. Icons representing frozen, dried, and low-sodium/low-sugar canned options are also added because fruits and vegetables in these forms contain as many nutrients as fresh and are easier to prepare and more affordable. Other icons on the diagram emphasize adequate fluid intake and regular physical activity, both of which are a particular concern for older people.

MyPlate for Older Adults

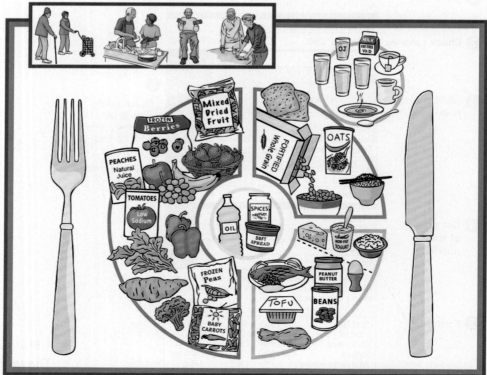

■ FIGURE 24-3
MyPlate for Older Adults.

Putting it all together!

- The body uses nutrients from the foods we eat to grow, to repair itself, and to carry out processes essential for living.
- There are six general types of nutrients. Carbohydrates, proteins, and fat supply energy. Minerals, vitamins, and water regulate body processes.
- MyPlate guidelines and nutrition labels on packaged foods can be used to plan a healthy diet.
- MyPlate for Older Adults contains dietary suggestions directed specifically for people over 70 years of age.

Factors That Affect Food Choices and Eating Habits

What will you learn?

When you are finished with this section, you will be able to:

1. Explain factors that influence a person's food preferences.
2. Define the words **appetite**, **anorexia**, and **dysphagia**.

The use of the MyPlate guidelines and nutrition labels on packaged foods can help us to make wise food choices. However, there are other factors that often affect the choices we make about what we eat and when we eat it:

- **Religion.** Dietary restrictions are a part of many religions. Some of these restrictions are specific to certain days (for example, the Roman Catholic custom of avoiding meat on Fridays during Lent). Other dietary restrictions are in effect all of the time (for example, some Jewish people keep a kosher kitchen).

- **Culture and geography.** People often like certain foods because they are associated with their culture or the area where they grew up.

- **Individual taste.** We are all unique in our likes and dislikes. For example, one person may love mushrooms on her pizza, while another person may not like them at all.

- **Finances.** Many people, especially those on a fixed income, make decisions about what they eat based on what they can afford to buy.

- **Kitchen skills.** People who do not know how to cook, do not like to cook, or do not have time to cook may choose to eat in restaurants more often. They may also rely on convenience foods and packaged foods.

Meal times can be emotionally difficult for people who are receiving health care. The person may miss her family members. Foods that the person used to love may no longer be on the person's diet. Pain, anxiety, illness, and medication side effects can cause the person to have little or no appetite. Part of providing holistic care is encouraging your patients or residents to eat adequate amounts of food, even when they have no appetite.

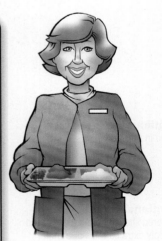

Appetite the desire for food

Anorexia loss of appetite

Dysphagia difficulty swallowing

- **Appetite. Appetite** is both physically driven (by hunger) and emotionally driven. A person who is ill or under emotional stress may experience **anorexia**.

- **Swallowing problems.** Difficulty chewing and swallowing, also called **dysphagia**, can occur as a result of many different conditions. People who have difficulty chewing or swallowing may need a modified diet that makes it easier to chew and swallow without choking. A speech-language pathologist may also work with the person on exercises and positioning techniques that can help with controlling food in the mouth and swallowing.

- **Disability.** Many people in the health care setting have temporary or permanent disabilities that may affect their ability to eat. An injury, weakness, or paralysis of the person's arm can cause the person to be totally unable to feed himself and either need to use assistive devices or be fed by another person.

- **Impaired cognitive function.** People who have dementia, certain developmental disabilities, or brain injury may not know how to or have forgotten how to feed themselves.

 Putting it all together!

- Factors such as religion, culture and geography, individual taste, and appetite affect our food choices and eating habits.

- Illness, homesickness, and other factors can cause a person in a health care facility to lose his appetite. Nursing assistants play an important role in encouraging patients and residents to eat.

Special Diets

 What will you learn?

When you are finished with this section, you will be able to:

1. List and describe common special diets.
2. Define the words **dietitian** and **nutritional supplement**.

Dietitian a person who has a degree in nutrition

Many patients and residents have special nutritional needs because of surgery, illness, or chronic health problems. Special diets are ordered by a doctor and planned by a **dietitian**. Table 24-1 gives examples of special diets that are commonly seen in health care facilities. It is important for you to become familiar with your facility's special diets and the types of food they include. That way, if a mistake is made and the wrong meal is sent for one of your patients or residents, you will be able to notice that an error has been made.

Nutritional supplement a flavored shake or drink that is used to supply extra calories or protein; often served with meals or as a snack in between meals

The dietitian also plans for **nutritional supplements** as necessary. It is usually the nursing assistant's responsibility to serve these nutritional supplements at specific times throughout the day and record that the supplements have been consumed. If the patient or resident does not consume the supplement, you should report this to the nurse.

TABLE 24-1   Examples of Special Diets

Type of Diet	Ordered for . . .	Description of Diet	Typical Foods
Regular ("house") diet	A healthy person	No restrictions on specific foods or condiments; simply a well-balanced diet	Fruits, vegetables, whole grains, milk and milk products, meat, fish, and beans
Clear liquid diet	People who are nauseated or vomiting, have just had surgery, or are recovering from an acute illness or injury	Foods and beverages that can be poured at room or body temperature and that you can see through	Water, gelatin, broth or bouillon, popsicles, clear juices, clear carbonated sodas, and coffee and tea (without cream)
Full liquid diet	People who have been on a clear liquid diet and are ready to progress to food with more nutrition	Clear liquid diet, plus any other food that can be poured at room or body temperature	Milk, plain frozen desserts (such as ice cream or frozen yogurt), egg custard, eggnog, cereal gruels, and strained soups and juices*
Mechanical diet	People who have difficulty chewing, swallowing, or digesting food	Most foods are chopped or creamed to serve Foods are not highly seasoned, are not fried, and are not high in fiber	Moist, tender meat, fish, or poultry; mashed potatoes; creamed spinach; scrambled eggs; applesauce; pudding
Pureed diet	People who have very poor dentition, are very frail, or who have end-stage disease	Food is blended to a smooth consistency, similar to that of pudding or very moist mashed potatoes	Moist foods that can be blended. Foods are not high in fiber or highly seasoned.
Carbohydrate (CHO)-controlled diet	People with diabetes mellitus	Regulates the amount of fat, carbohydrate, and protein that a person consumes to maintain blood sugar levels	Different for each person, depending on the person's specific nutritional needs
Sodium-restricted diet	People with certain types of heart disease, high blood pressure, or kidney disease	Regulates the amount of salt that a person consumes; restriction may be moderate or severe	Most foods, except those high in sodium (such as bacon, cold cuts, pickles, and salty snack foods) Foods may be prepared without any salt at all Salt substitutes may or may not be permitted
Low-cholesterol diet	People with certain types of heart disease	Foods are chosen that are lower in animal fat and prepared in ways that do not add additional fats	Fruits, vegetables, whole grains, and fat-free or low-fat milk products

*High-calorie, high-protein liquid nutritional supplements may be added if the person must remain on the full liquid diet for more than 3 days.

Putting it all together!

- People in health care settings often have special needs as far as nutrition goes. Special diets are ordered by a doctor and planned by a dietitian.
- It is important for you to be familiar with the types of special diets served in your facility so that you are able to recognize a mistake if one is made.
- Nutritional supplements should be served at the scheduled time according to the person's care plan.

Assisting With Meals

What will you learn?

When you are finished with this section, you will be able to:

1. Discuss the importance of making meals attractive and the dining experience pleasant.
2. Discuss the OBRA regulations related to meals in long-term care facilities.
3. Explain how to prepare a person for meal time.
4. Describe ways that you may need to help a person during meal time.
5. Demonstrate proper technique for feeding a person who cannot feed himself.
6. Describe how the amount of solid food eaten is recorded.
7. State observations that you may make when assisting a person to eat that should be reported to the nurse.

Meal time for people in a health care setting can be difficult for many reasons:

- Food choices may be limited, or the food may not be prepared the way the person likes it.
- Meals are usually served at specific times, not just whenever the person feels like eating.
- Meal time can be lonely, especially if the person must stay in her room to eat.
- The person may miss family members or familiar foods.
- Physical problems (such as pain or nausea) and emotional problems (such as anxiety) can affect a person's appetite.
- The person may be embarrassed if he needs help to eat.

Long-term care facilities that receive government funding must follow Omnibus Budget Reconciliation Act (OBRA) regulations pertaining to meals (Box 24-2). These regulations ensure that each resident's rights are respected. They help to ensure that meal time is as enjoyable as possible for the resident. However, even if you work in a facility that is not required to follow OBRA regulations, you must make an effort to make meal time as pleasant as possible for your patients or residents. Actions such as providing pleasant conversation

BOX 24-2 Aspects of the Resident's Dining Experience Regulated by the Omnibus Budget Reconciliation Act

- Meals must meet the individual nutritional needs of each resident.

- Food must be served at the proper temperature.*

- Food must be appealing to look at and seasoned to the individual resident's preference.

- Special diets, such as those followed for religious reasons, must be provided.

- Dining in the company of other residents is recommended.

- Residents in rehabilitation who are learning how to eat independently again must have a private area in which to eat.

*The United States Department of Agriculture (USDA) requires that hot foods be cooked to a safe internal temperature and be kept at least 140°F until being served. Bacteria that may be in the food can multiply rapidly at temperatures between 40°F and 140°F.

and making sure the person is physically comfortable help the person to relax and enjoy the meal.

Preparing for Meal Time

You will need to help your patients and residents get ready for each meal. Be sure to give people plenty of time to prepare for meals. In a long-term care facility, most residents are assisted to the dining room to eat. In a hospital, the patients usually take their meals in their rooms. The following actions are taken to help prepare a person for meal time:

- **Assist the person with toileting.** Help the person to the bathroom or offer the bedpan or urinal.

- **Assist the person with basic hygiene.** Help the person to wash his hands and face and brush his teeth. A clean, fresh mouth makes food taste better. If the person wears dentures, glasses, or a hearing aid, make sure that these items are clean and in place.

- **Position the person for eating.** Residents in long-term care facilities are walked to the dining room or taken in a wheelchair. In many facilities, the resident is helped from the wheelchair into a standard dining chair for the meal. If the person will be eating her meal in bed, smooth the bed linens and raise the head of the bed if permitted. Clear the over-bed table of clutter and wipe down the surface if necessary.

- **Provide a pleasant environment.** Make sure that any offensive or odorous items, such as bedpans or emesis basins, are removed from the room. Adjust the lighting for comfort and turn on the radio or television if the person asks you to.

- **Assist the person with putting on a clothing protector if the person desires.** A clothing protector may be used to prevent a person's clothing from being soiled by dropped food or drink. Wearing a clothing protector is a matter of personal choice, so always ask the resident or patient if it is all right for you to put the clothing protector on her before the meal. You should not refer to the clothing protector as a "bib." This can be very embarrassing and demeaning for the patient or resident.

- **Make sure that food is served at the correct temperature.** It is important to keep "hot foods hot and cold foods cold." If a person eats foods that have been allowed to sit for a while at the wrong temperature, it can allow bacteria to multiply and cause the person to become sick with a food-born illness, commonly known as food poisoning. Make sure that you serve food trays promptly when they arrive on the unit or are ready in the dining room. If a person's meal needs to be reheated in the microwave, make sure that it reaches at least 165°F.

Assisting the Person to Eat

Help the person to eat as necessary. Encourage your patients or residents to do as much for themselves as possible to help promote their independence. Assistive devices (Fig. 24-4) allow many people with physical disabilities to feed themselves with little help. You may need to help the person with opening milk cartons, removing silverware from its wrapper, buttering bread, or cutting up meat. If you need to help with seasoning food, make sure that you do it according to that person's taste. If the person has poor eyesight, you will need to tell him where items are on the tray. Describe the food and help the person to find it on the plate by referencing a clock face (Fig. 24-5).

It is also important that you wear gloves if it is necessary for you to touch a person's food with your hands. Gloves are not necessary if you are only opening juice or milk cartons or holding a spoon when feeding a dependent patient or resident. Just make sure that you only touch the person's eating utensils by the handles and

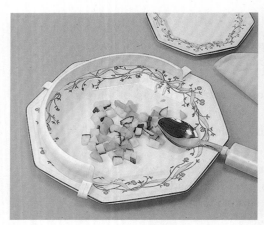

Plate guard

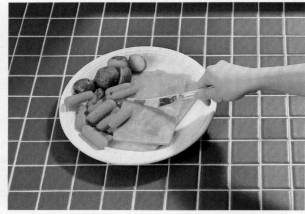

Knife with a rounded blade

■ **FIGURE 24-4**

Assistive devices can help a
person with physical disabilities
to eat independently.
(Photos courtesy of Sammons Preston Rolyan,
Bolingbrook, IL.)

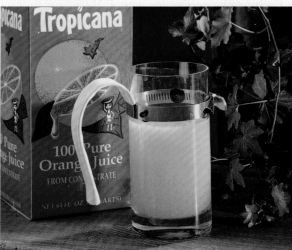

Cup holder

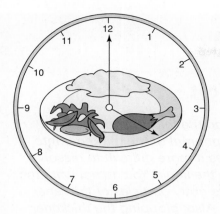

■ **FIGURE 24-5**

You can help a person with poor eyesight locate food on the plate by describing its location in terms of a clock face.

not the part that touches the food or goes into the mouth. As always, perform hand hygiene after assisting one person, before going to assist someone else.

Some people may have difficulty swallowing as the result of a stroke, injury, or dementia. These people can choke easily on liquids, so always offer liquids slowly. Sometimes the doctor will order the use of an additive that thickens the liquid, making it easier to swallow. The doctor orders a specific consistency for thickened liquids. These consistencies are:

■ **Nectar.** A nectar consistency can be poured very easily.

■ **Honey.** A honey consistency is thicker than a nectar consistency and is not as easily poured.

■ **Pudding.** A pudding consistency "plops" rather than pours from a cup. Although it is a thickened liquid, this consistency is eaten with a spoon

The nurse or therapist will show you how to use these additives to thicken liquids if this is necessary for one of your patients or residents. Guidelines for providing thickened liquids are given in Guidelines Box 24-1.

Some people may not be able to feed themselves at all. Procedure 24-1 describes how to assist a dependent person to eat.

General guidelines for assisting a person with eating are given in Guidelines Box 24-2.

GUIDELINES BOX 24-1 Guidelines for Providing Thickened Liquids

What you do

If thickened liquids have been ordered for a person, thicken all of the liquids on the person's tray, including soup.

Carefully read and follow the instructions on the thickener to prepare the desired consistency.

Why you do it

Thickened liquids have been ordered for the patient or the resident because the person has difficulty swallowing. Providing any liquid without the thickener puts the person at risk for chocking.

There are several thickeners available, and the product used in the facility can change on the basis of pricing. There may be some variation in the amount of product needed to produce a particular consistency.

(*box continues on page 546*)

GUIDELINES BOX 24-1 Guidelines for Providing Thickened Liquids (continued)

What you do	Why you do it
When adding a thickener to a liquid, use a "sprinkle and stir" technique, rather than a "plop and stir" technique.	It is better to add the thickener gradually. "Plopping" a spoonful of the thickener into the liquid makes it more difficult to dissolve the thickener in the liquid. You do not want the resident to taste gritty particles of thickener when drinking. Also, plopping the thickener into the liquid often results in the liquid becoming too thick. If the liquid becomes too thick, then the consistency will need to be adjusted by adding more liquid.
Allow the liquid to sit for a minute or two before serving to make sure it is the right consistency.	It takes a few minutes for the full effect of the thickener to take place. If you think the liquid is the right consistency and serve it right away, the liquid will continue to thicken and in a few minutes it will no longer be the consistency ordered for the person. If the liquid becomes too thick, then the consistency will need to be adjusted by adding more liquid.
Add all condiments (for example, creamer, lemon juice) to the liquid before adding the thickening product.	Adding anything to a prepared thickened liquid can change the consistency.
Do not add ice to thickened liquids.	As the ice melts, it thins down the liquid.
Check the person's hot beverages periodically for changes in consistency.	Hot beverages thicken as they cool. Some additional hot liquid may need to be added to return the beverage to the correct consistency.
Do not give the person any food item that melts at room temperature (such as gelatin or ice cream).	These kinds of foods melt in the mouth and may become too thin for the person to swallow without choking.
Do not provide the patient or resident with a bedside water pitcher.	Water must be thickened before drinking. Leaving unthickened liquid at the bedside puts the person at risk for choking. You cannot thicken the water ahead of time to leave at the bedside because the water continues to thicken as it sits.
Offer thickened beverages throughout the day.	Like all patients and residents, those on thickened liquids need to drink throughout the day to maintain adequate hydration. Because the person must depend on the staff to prepare all liquids, she cannot drink whenever she wants to, so it is important to offer beverages frequently throughout the day.

GUIDELINES BOX 24-2   Guidelines for Assisting a Person to Eat

What you do	Why you do it
Provide privacy as necessary, especially if the person is just learning how to eat independently again.	*It can be embarrassing for the person to spill food or to need help eating.*
Serve the meal as soon as it is sent up from the kitchen.	*This helps to ensure that hot foods are served hot and cold foods are served cold.*
Check that the name on the meal tray matches the name of the person who will be receiving it. Also make sure that the diet noted on the tray matches the diet that has been ordered for that person.	*Many patients or residents are on special diets for medical reasons. It is important that they receive the correct meal tray with the correct diet on it.*
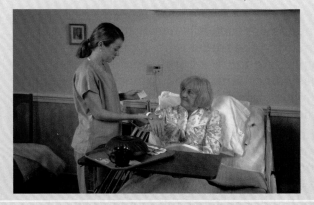	
Tell the person what foods are on the tray.	*Some of your patients or residents may not be able to see well, or they may be confused. Knowing what is on the tray helps the person to decide what he would like to eat first.*
Sit down next to the person and provide pleasant conversation throughout the meal, even if the person cannot answer you.	*Meal time is a social time in a person's day. Pleasant conversation helps the person feel less lonely, which in turn increases the person's appetite.*
Encourage the person to do as much as possible for himself during the meal. Even if the person is almost totally dependent on you to feed him, you can still try to involve him in the process as much as possible (for example, by asking the person to hold his own napkin).	*Doing as much as possible independently is important for the person's self-esteem.*
When assisting a dependent person with a meal, use a spoon, not a fork.	*The sharp tines of a fork could accidentally injure the person.*
When assisting a dependent person with a meal, offer small bites of food slowly. Give the person enough time to chew and swallow each bite.	*Some people may have difficulty chewing and swallowing as a result of a stroke, injury, or dementia. Offering small bites of food slowly helps to prevent choking.*
When assisting a dependent person with a meal, offer small sips of liquids frequently between bites.	*Liquids help to moisten the mouth, making chewing and swallowing easier. Offering small sips helps to prevent choking.*

Measuring and Recording Food Intake

You may be asked to record the amount of food that the person eats. Depending on facility policy, you may have to record the percentage of the *total meal* that was eaten (for example, the resident ate 80% of her lunch). Or you may have to record the percentage of *each food* that was eaten (for example, at dinner, the resident ate 100% of his mashed potatoes, 50% of his salad, and 75% of his chicken breast).

As a nursing assistant, you will play a key role in monitoring your patients' or residents' food intake. You will see which foods are eaten readily and which are left on the tray. By using good communication skills and open-ended questions, you can find out why a person has left food on the tray. Maybe the person is not feeling well in general. Or maybe he just does not like the food that was served. The feedback you provide to the nurse will help the health care team monitor the person's nutritional status and plan future meals for the person.

 Putting it all together!

- When our emotional needs are met, it is easier for us to meet our physical needs. Ensuring that meal time is pleasant—by helping the person to prepare for meal time, serving meals promptly, providing assistance with eating as necessary, and taking the time to talk with the person during the meal—can help to improve a person's appetite.

- OBRA sets standards for meal time in long-term care facilities. These standards help to ensure that the residents' rights are respected and that meal time is as pleasant as possible.

- Assistive devices are available to help people with physical disabilities maintain their independence when eating. A person who cannot feed herself will need to be fed. Be sensitive to your patients' or residents' feelings as you assist them with meals. Many adults feel very self-conscious about needing assistance with something as basic as eating.

- Nursing assistants are the members of the health care team who have the most contact with patients and residents during meal times. Your observations are important to help the health care team monitor the person's nutritional status and plan future meals.

Assisting With Fluids

 What will you learn?

When you are finished with this section, you will be able to:

1. Explain why water is essential for life.
2. List factors that affect the body's fluid balance.
3. Describe how to measure and record a person's fluid intake.
4. List the types of fluids that are considered "output."
5. Define the words **fluid balance**, **dehydration**, **edema**, **NPO status**, **intake and output (I&O) flow sheet**, and **graduate**.

Adequate water intake is essential for life. Water forms the basis for many important body fluids, including:

- Cytoplasm, the jelly-like substance inside the body's cells
- Plasma, the liquid part of the blood
- Urine, which carries waste products out of the body
- Sweat, which helps to keep the body cool
- Mucus, which keeps the mucous membranes moist
- Synovial fluid, which helps our joints to move smoothly

Maintaining **fluid balance** is important for health. A healthy adult needs to drink 1.5 to 3 quarts (48 to 96 ounces) of fluid each day just to keep up with the fluid that normally leaves the body in urine, feces, sweat, and the air we exhale. In situations that cause excessive amounts of fluid to leave the body, such as diarrhea, vomiting, hemorrhage, severe burns, or excessive sweating, **dehydration** can occur. Dehydration can also occur from not drinking enough water. Older people are often at risk for dehydration because they do not feel thirsty as often as younger people do. People who have difficulty communicating and people with dementia are also at risk for dehydration because they may not be able to ask for a drink.

Some medical conditions, such as kidney disease and certain types of heart disease, make it hard for the body to get rid of extra water, resulting in **edema**. For a person with edema, the doctor may restrict the person's fluid intake or order medication to help the body rid itself of the excess fluid.

Fluid balance a state where the amount of fluid taken into the body equals the amount of fluid that leaves the body

Dehydration too little fluid in the tissues of the body

Edema too much fluid in the tissues of the body

Offering Fluids

Nursing assistants are responsible for providing fresh drinking water and other fluids to patients and residents. Many of the people you care for will be allowed to have as much water as they like and should be encouraged to drink (Fig. 24-6). People are more likely to drink fluids that taste good and are served at the temperature they prefer. Remember to offer a drink regularly to people who are elderly, confined to bed, confused, or taking pain medications. These people might not remember to drink fluids often enough.

Sometimes it may be necessary to either increase or restrict a person's fluid intake. The doctor will write the order, and the nurse will give you information about the amount and type of fluids that should be offered.

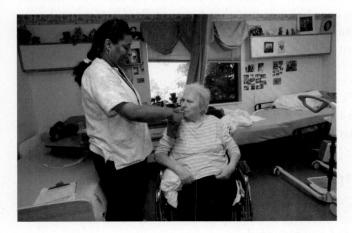

■ **FIGURE 24-6**

Water is essential to life.

- **Encouraging fluids.** If it is necessary to increase a person's fluid intake, offer small amounts of a drink that the person likes frequently through the day. Most people do not enjoy having to drink a large amount of liquid all at once.

- **Restricting fluids.** If it is necessary to restrict a person's fluid intake, make sure that you know the total amount of fluid that the person will be allowed to have during your shift. Divide that amount into small amounts that can be given throughout the day. Frequent oral care can help to keep the person comfortable and prevent "dry mouth."

- **Giving no fluids.** The doctor will place some patients or residents on **NPO status** prior to surgery or a diagnostic procedure. When a person is on NPO status, the person is not allowed to have any fluids at all, not even water or ice chips. Food, hard candy, and gum are not permitted either. Empty the person's water pitcher and store it out of sight. Gently remind visitors that the person is not allowed food or drink and suggest that they enjoy their own snacks and beverages out of sight of the person. Being on NPO status can be very uncomfortable. Frequent oral care helps to relieve some of the discomfort until the person is allowed to have fluids again.

NPO status a doctor's order specifying that a patient or resident is to have "nils per os" (nothing by mouth)

Measuring and Recording Fluid Intake and Output

Some medical conditions can make monitoring the person's fluid balance very important. For people with these conditions, an order to "maintain intake and output (I&O) measurements" will be followed. Each time the person takes in fluids or fluids leave the body, the amount is recorded on the **intake and output (I&O) flow sheet**. The amounts are totaled at the end of the shift and again at the end of the 24-hour reporting period. The amount of fluid intake can then be compared to the amount of fluid output to monitor the person's fluid balance.

Intake and output (I&O) flow sheet a document used for recording measurements of all of the fluids that enter and leave the body

Measuring Fluid Intake

Fluid intake includes all of the fluids that a person drinks, including those foods that are liquid at room or body temperature. Other fluids that are considered as part of a person's total intake include enteral (tube) feedings and intravenous (IV) fluids. The nurse is responsible for recording those amounts.

The health care facility where you work will have lists that show how much fluid is contained by the cups, glasses, and bowls that are used there. Packaged beverages will state how much fluid the package contains on the label. The amount of fluid the container or package holds is stated in terms of *fluid ounces*. In health care facilities, fluids are measured and recorded in *milliliters (mL)*. To record the amount of fluid intake, you will need to convert fluid ounces to mL. One fluid ounce is equal to 30 mL.

If the person does not consume all of the liquids that were offered, you will have to estimate the person's fluid intake (Box 24-3). When it is necessary to report the person's exact fluid intake, a **graduate** is used to measure the liquids that were not consumed, and then this measurement is subtracted from the total amount of fluids offered (Box 24-4).

Graduate a measuring device used to measure fluids

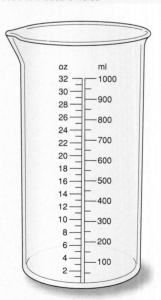

Measuring Fluid Output

Fluids that are considered "output" include urine, vomit, blood, wound drainage, and diarrhea. If the person is on I&O status, none of these fluids can be discarded until they have been measured and recorded.

BOX 24-3 Estimating Fluid Intake

Example: The person is offered an 8-ounce glass of milk and finishes half of it. There are two ways to calculate the person's approximate fluid intake.

Method A

1. Estimate how much the resident drank. In this case, he drank about half of the milk, so that would be about 4 ounces:

   8 ounces × 1/2 glass = 8 ounces ÷ 2 = 4 ounces

2. Convert the ounces consumed to mL. Remember that 1 ounce = 30 mL:

   4 ounces × 30 mL = 120 mL

Method B

1. Convert the total amount of fluid offered to mL. Remember that 1 ounce = 30 mL:

   8 ounces × 30 mL = 240 mL

2. Multiply the total ounces offered by the fraction that represents how much the person drank. In this case, the person drank 1/2 glass. Therefore,

   240 mL × 1/2 glass = 240 ÷ 2 = 120 mL

- **Urine.** You will be responsible for measuring and recording the person's urine output (see Chapter 25).
- **Vomit.** The amount can be measured using the markings on the emesis basin. If the person vomits somewhere other than into the emesis basin, then the nurse will estimate the amount of vomit.
- **Blood.** The amount of blood lost is estimated by the nurse.
- **Wound drainage.** The amount of wound drainage is either estimated by the nurse or measured in a graduate if the wound drain has a collection device.
- **Diarrhea.** The nurse will estimate the amount.

BOX 24-4 Calculating Exact Fluid Intake

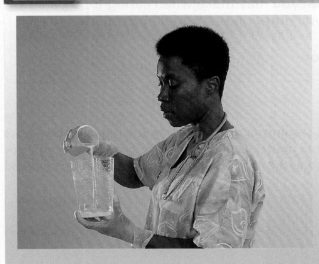

Example: At the beginning of the meal, the person's meal tray contained 150 mL of orange juice, 240 mL of milk, and 90 mL of water.

1. Calculate how much fluid was offered:

   150 mL + 240 mL + 90 mL = 480 mL

2. Pour the leftover fluids into the graduate. Note the amount of fluid contained in the graduate (let's say there are 40 mL of fluid in the graduate).

3. Subtract the amount in the graduate from the total amount offered to determine the person's fluid intake:

   480 mL − 40 mL = 440 mL

Putting it all together!

- The amount of fluids taken into the body should equal the amount of fluids that leave the body. Dehydration can occur if more fluids leave the body than enter it. Edema can occur if more fluids enter the body than leave it.

- The doctor may order a person's fluid intake to be increased or restricted. People who have no fluid restrictions should be encouraged to drink frequently.

- A person who is on NPO status is not allowed to have anything by mouth.

- In some cases, it may be important to monitor a patient's or resident's fluid balance. This is done by measuring and recording the person's fluid intake and output. Fluid "intake" includes any liquids that the person drinks, foods that become liquid at room or body temperature, tube feedings, and IV fluids. Fluid "output" includes urine, vomit, blood, wound drainage, and diarrhea.

Alternate Methods of Providing Nutrition and Fluids

What will you learn?

When you are finished with this section, you will be able to:

1. Describe why a person might have an intravenous (IV) line.
2. State observations that you may make when caring for a person with an IV line that should be reported to the nurse.
3. Discuss ways of providing nutrition for people who are unable to take food by mouth.
4. State observations that you may make when caring for a person who is receiving enteral nutrition that should be reported to the nurse.
5. Define **enteral nutrition**.

Tell the Nurse!

Problems with intravenous (IV) lines

- Disconnected tubing
- Empty fluid bag
- IV fluid is not dripping into the drip chamber
- Blood in the IV tubing
- Pain at the IV site
- Swelling or redness at the IV site

Drinking water and chewing, swallowing, and digesting food are the best ways for a person to obtain fluids and nutrients. However, some people have problems chewing, swallowing, or digesting their food and must obtain their nutrition and fluids in another way.

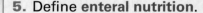

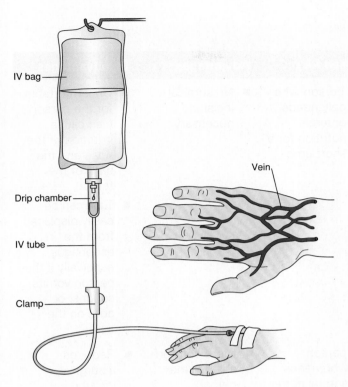

IV bag

Drip chamber

IV tube

Clamp

Vein

■ **FIGURE 24-7**

Intravenous (IV) therapy is used to give fluids. The IV fluid drips from the bag, into the tubing, and into the person's vein. The nurse uses the clamp to control the rate of flow.

Intravenous (IV) Therapy

In intravenous (IV) therapy, fluids are given through a small tube that is inserted into a vein. In addition to water, the IV fluid usually contains sugar, vitamins, and minerals. Medications may also be added to the IV fluid. Sometimes, blood is given through an IV line.

The IV tubing is connected to a bag that contains the fluid (Fig. 24-7). The fluid slowly drips through the tubing and into the vein and is absorbed into the body. Usually the IV line is inserted into one of the small veins in the arm or the back of the hand. In some cases, it may be inserted into the larger veins of the neck or upper chest.

You will not be responsible for managing IV therapy, but you may care for a person who has an IV line in place.

Enteral Nutrition

Enteral nutrition (*tube feeding*) eliminates the need for the person to chew or swallow. The formula-like fluid given through the tube provides the person with the six types of nutrients. There are many ways to access the digestive tract with the feeding tube (Table 24-2).

Nurses are responsible for feeding people who are receiving enteral nutrition. Enteral feedings may be given at scheduled times or continuously by an infusion pump. Aspiration can occur if the person regurgitates the feeding formula and it goes down the windpipe and into the lungs. To help avoid regurgitation and aspiration, the head of the bed is raised during the feeding and for a period of time afterward.

Tell the Nurse!

Problems with enteral nutrition (feeding tubes)

- Nausea, bloating, or pain during the feeding
- Coughing, gagging, or vomiting during the feeding
- A swollen abdomen
- Diarrhea
- Drainage from around the tube insertion site
- Disconnected tubing

Enteral nutrition placing food directly into a person's stomach or intestines

TABLE 24-2 Enteral Feeding Tubes

Type of Tube	Used for . . .	Advantages	Disadvantages
Nasogastric (nose to stomach) Nasointestinal (nose to intestine)	A person who only needs enteral nutrition for a short time	▪ No surgical incision necessary	▪ Uncomfortable for the person (can cause irritation of the nose and the back of the throat) ▪ Tube can be easily displaced from the esophagus, especially if the person vomits, coughs, or pulls on the tube
Gastrostomy (direct to stomach) Jejunostomy (direct to intestine)	A person who needs enteral nutrition for more than a few days	▪ More comfortable for the person ▪ Tube is less likely to become displaced	▪ Requires a surgical incision

Esophagus

Stomach

Small intestine

Putting it all together!

- When a person has difficulty with chewing or swallowing, fluids and nutrition must be given in another way.
- Intravenous (IV) therapy provides fluids through a small tube inserted into a vein. IV therapy does not provide complete nutrition.
- Enteral nutrition is provided by a tube that is placed directly into the stomach or intestines. The tube may be passed down the nose and esophagus or through a small surgical incision in the abdomen. The formula-like fluid used in enteral nutrition provides all of the nutrients the person needs.

Monitoring Blood Glucose Levels

What will you learn?

When you are finished with this section, you will be able to:

1. Demonstrate the proper technique for monitoring a person's blood glucose level.
2. Define the word **glucometer**.

You learned in Chapter 8 that diabetes control involves balancing diet, exercise, and medication. A person with diabetes needs to monitor his or her blood glucose levels regularly to make sure that the prescribed treatment is keeping the blood glucose level within the desired range. A **glucometer** is used to monitor blood glucose levels. Most glucometers use a drop of blood obtained from the person's finger (Fig. 24-8). The "finger-stick" method of monitoring blood glucose levels can be painful for the person and can also expose the health care worker to bloodborne diseases. If you are allowed to assist patients or residents with blood glucose monitoring using this method, make sure to wear gloves.

Many people with diabetes monitor their own glucose levels, but some patients or residents may need help with this. Different facilities will have different policies about who is responsible for blood glucose monitoring. You may work in a facility that allows nursing assistants to perform blood glucose monitoring. Make sure that you have been adequately trained in how to use the equipment and record your findings. A normal blood glucose level is between 70 and 120 mg/dL. A blood glucose level out of that range should be reported to the nurse immediately.

General guidelines for monitoring blood glucose levels are given in Guidelines Box 24-3. Procedure 24-2 gives step-by-step instructions for monitoring blood glucose levels.

Glucometer a type of blood glucose meter

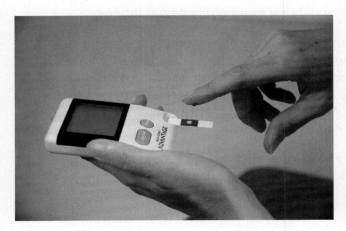

■ **FIGURE 24-8**

Most glucometers use a drop of blood obtained from the person's finger.

GUIDELINES BOX 24-3   Guidelines for Monitoring Blood Glucose Levels

What you do	Why you do it
Ensure that the blood glucose meter is properly calibrated (for example, it returns accurate readings for the testing solutions).	*A blood glucose meter that is not properly calibrated will yield inaccurate results.*
Use the testing strips specified by the manufacturer of the blood glucose meter.	*The testing strips are specific to the blood glucose meter. Using the wrong kind of testing strips will yield inaccurate test results.*
Remove the testing strip from the bottle right before you are going to use it. Replace the lid on the bottle of testing strips immediately after removing the testing strip you are going to use.	*Testing strips are sensitive to light and humidity. Exposure to light and humidity affects their quality, which in turn affects the accuracy of the test results.*
Note the expiration date on the bottle of testing strips. Do not use the testing strips past their expiration date.	*Using expired testing strips will yield inaccurate test results.*
When opening a new bottle of testing strips, write the date on the bottle.	*The testing strips are only good for 3 to 4 months after opening the bottle. The manufacturer dictates how long an opened bottle of testing strips can be kept before it must be discarded. Using old testing strips may yield inaccurate test results.*
Wear gloves when obtaining a blood glucose sample.	*Blood puts you at risk for exposure to bloodborne pathogens.*
Use a new lancet for each patient or resident.	*The lancet comes in contact with the person's blood. Using the same lancet on multiple people could put your patients or residents at risk for bloodborne illnesses or other infections.*
After use, dispose of the lancet in an approved sharps container.	*Proper disposal of sharps (such as lancets) helps limit others' exposure to bloodborne pathogens.*
Before obtaining the blood sample, have the patient or resident wash her hands with warm, soapy water.	*Washing with warm soapy water helps remove pathogens that may be on the surface of the skin, lowering the person's risk of infection. Washing with warm, soapy water also removes any sugars that might be on the surface of the skin, preventing a false high reading.*
If using an alcohol swab to cleanse the skin, allow the skin to dry completely before using the lancet.	*Alcohol can interfere with the accuracy of the test results, if not completely dried.*

What you do (continued)	**Why you do it** (continued)
Insert the lancet on the side of the fingertip instead of in the center.	*The center of the fingertip contains the highest number of nerve endings. If you obtain the blood sample from the side of the fingertip, the person will experience less pain.*
If possible, avoid taking blood from the thumb or index finger.	*The thumb and index finger are the fingers we use most frequently to perform day-to-day activities (for example, grasping small objects, buttoning a shirt). If these fingers are sore from blood glucose testing, the person will experience pain every time he tries to use the fingers.*
Wipe away the first drop of blood with gauze or a cotton ball (if recommended by the manufacturer of the blood glucose meter or your facility policy).	*Some manufacturers of blood glucose meters recommend discarding the first drop of blood because it may be mixed with serum or the cleansing agent, resulting in an inaccurate test result.*
Apply the correct amount of blood to the testing strip. The manufacturer of the blood glucose meter will specify how much blood to apply to the testing strip.	*Applying too much or not enough blood to the testing strip may result in inaccurate test results.*

Putting it all together!

- A blood glucose meter is used to monitor blood glucose levels. If monitoring blood glucose levels is part of your job description, make sure that you have been trained in the proper use of the equipment at your facility and always follow standard precautions.

PROCEDURES

PROCEDURE 24-1
Feeding a Dependent Person

Why you do it: A person who cannot feed himself will need to be fed to ensure that he receives proper nutrition. Providing companionship during the meal is just as important as providing assistance with the actual task of eating.

GETTING READY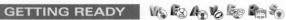

1. Complete the "Getting Ready" steps.

SUPPLIES

- gloves
- paper towels
- clothing protector
- oral hygiene supplies
- wash basin
- bedpan or urinal
- towel
- washcloth

PROCEDURE

2. Clean the surface of the over-bed table and cover it with paper towels. Place the oral hygiene supplies on the over-bed table. Fill the wash basin with warm water (110°F [37.7°C] to 115°F [46.1°C] on the bath thermometer). Place the basin on the over-bed table.

3. If the side rails are in use, lower the side rail on the working side of the bed. The side rail on the opposite side of the bed should remain up. Raise the head of the bed. Make sure that the bed is positioned at a comfortable working height (to promote good body mechanics) and that the wheels are locked.

4. Perform hand hygiene and put on the gloves.

5. Assist the person with oral hygiene.

6. Offer the bedpan or urinal. If the person uses the bedpan or urinal, empty and clean it before proceeding with the meal. Remove your gloves and dispose of them in a facility-approved waste container. Perform hand hygiene.

7. Wash the person's hands and face.

8. Clear the over-bed table, wipe the surface with a facility-approved cleaning solution, and position it over the bed at the proper height for the person.

9. Perform hand hygiene and get the meal tray from the dietary cart. (If the side rails are in use, raise the side rails before leaving the bedside.) Check the meal tray to make sure that it has the person's name on it and that it contains the correct diet for the person. Place the meal tray on the over-bed table.

10. Ask the person if he would like to use a clothing protector. Put the clothing protector on the person, if desired.

11. Uncover the meal tray and prepare the food for eating (for example, cut the meat, butter the bread, open any containers). Remember to put on gloves if you will be touching any of the food with your hands. Tell the person what is on the tray.

12. Take a seat and make sure that the bed height has been lowered so that it is at a comfortable working height.

13. Allow the person to choose what he would like to taste first. Using a spoon, offer a small bite to the person (fill the spoon no more than one-third full). Allow the person enough time to swallow the food.

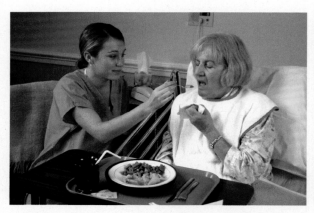

STEP 13 ▪ Using a spoon, offer a small bite to the person.

14. Offer the person something to drink every few bites. Use the napkin to wipe the person's mouth and chin as often as necessary. Allow the person to assist with the eating process to the best of his ability.

15. Continue in this manner until the person is finished. Encourage the person to finish the food on the tray, but do not force the person to eat.

16. Remove the tray and the clothing protector when the person has finished eating.

17. Perform hand hygiene and put on a clean pair of gloves. Assist the person with oral hygiene.

18. If the side rails are in use, return the side rails to the raised position. Lower the head of the bed as the person requests. Make sure that the bed is lowered to its lowest position and that the wheels are locked.

19. Gather the soiled linens and place them in the linen hamper or linen bag. Dispose of disposable items in a facility-approved waste container. Clean equipment and return it to the storage area.

20. Remove your gloves, dispose of them in a facility-approved waste container, and perform hand hygiene.

FINISHING UP

21. Complete the "Finishing Up" steps.

WHAT YOU DOCUMENT

- Date and time
- Percentage of food eaten
- Fluid intake
- Report an abnormal appetite or if the person consumes less than 70% of the meal to the nurse

PROCEDURE 24-2
Monitoring the Blood Glucose Level

Why you do it: Blood glucose monitoring is necessary for people who are at risk of having blood glucose levels that are too high or too low.

GETTING READY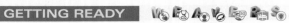

1. Complete the "Getting Ready" steps.

SUPPLIES

- blood glucose meter
- gloves
- sterile lancet
- testing strips
- cotton ball or gauze
- alcohol swab or
- wash basin and warm water
- soap
- washcloth and towel

PROCEDURE

2. Perform hand hygiene and put on your gloves.
3. Help the person to wash his hands with soap and water. Dry the person's hands with towel. Or, if your facility policy requires, use the alcohol swab to cleanse the finger. Allow the skin to dry completely.
4. Turn the blood glucose meter on and wait until the "ready" sign appears on the display screen.
5. Remove a testing strip from the bottle. Immediately replace the cap on the bottle. Make sure that the code on the testing strip matches the code on the blood glucose meter. Depending on the type of blood glucose meter you are using, you may be required to insert the testing strip into the meter at this time.
6. Gently massage the side of the finger toward the intended puncture site to encourage blood to flow to the area.
7. Prepare the lancet by removing the safety cap. Grasp the person's finger and hold the lancet at a 90° angle to the skin. Press the lancet straight down to pierce the person's skin.
8. Wipe away the first drop of blood with gauze or a cotton ball (if recommended by the manufacturer or your facility's policy).
9. Lightly stroke the finger and/or lower the hand to encourage bleeding until a drop of blood forms. Do not squeeze the finger or touch the puncture site or blood drop with your gloved hands.
10. Transfer the drop of blood by touching it to the pad on the test strip without smearing it. Make sure to apply an adequate amount of blood to the test strip.
11. Press the time button on the blood glucose meter if directed by the manufacturer.
12. Apply pressure to the puncture site using gauze or a cotton ball.
13. When testing is completed, note the blood glucose results, remove the test strip and dispose of it in a facility-approved waste container. Dispose of the lancet in a sharps container.
14. Remove your gloves and perform hand hygiene.
15. Record the reading on the blood glucose meter. Turn off the meter if it does not automatically turn itself off.

FINISHING UP

16. Complete the "Finishing Up" steps.

WHAT YOU DOCUMENT

- The date and time
- The person's blood glucose level

WHAT DID YOU LEARN?

Multiple Choice

Select the single best answer for each of the following questions.

1. When assisting a person with eating, one of the first things you should do is:
   a. Provide the person with privacy
   b. Butter the person's muffin
   c. Wash your hands and the person's hands
   d. Cut the food into large pieces

2. Mrs. Wellington is blind. Which one of the following should she have during meal time?
   a. A soft diet
   b. Help identifying the location of the food on the plate
   c. A large spoon
   d. A cup holder

3. Mr. Jones is 98 years old and has no food restrictions. However, he is missing several teeth. Which one of the following menus would be the best choice for Mr. Jones?
   a. Spare ribs, macaroni and cheese, coleslaw, and fruit cocktail
   b. Hamburger, french fries, corn on the cob, and ice cream
   c. Baked fish, mashed potatoes, spinach soufflé, and tapioca
   d. Fried chicken, baked potato, green beans, and chocolate chip cookies

4. Which one of the following lists only items that would be included in fluid intake?
   a. Orange juice, soft boiled egg, toast
   b. Milk, soup, gelatin
   c. Water, mashed potatoes, egg custard
   d. Milk, ham sandwich, ice cream bar

5. Miss Lee drank one third of an 8-ounce glass of iced tea. How many milliliters of fluid did Miss Lee drink?
   a. 60 mL
   b. 80 mL
   c. 100 mL
   d. 240 mL

6. Which one of the following lists foods that are good sources of protein?
   a. Steak, chicken, fish
   b. Spinach, carrots, beets
   c. Bread, cereal, rice
   d. Apples, oranges, bananas

7. At the beginning of your shift, you give Mr. Gibson a water pitcher containing 270 mL of water. At the end of your shift, you note that 35 mL of water is left in the pitcher. How much water did Mr. Gibson drink?
   a. 35 mL
   b. 175 mL
   c. 235 mL
   d. 140 mL

8. Which of the following lists foods that are good sources of carbohydrates?
   a. Liver, fish, chicken
   b. Cereal, fruit, bread
   c. Milk, beans, cheese
   d. Water, soda, butter

9. Which health care professional is specially trained to plan for the patient's or resident's nutritional needs and teach about good nutrition?
   a. The nurse
   b. The dietitian
   c. The nursing assistant
   d. The doctor

10. Which one of the following can affect a person's food likes and dislikes?
    a. The person's religious beliefs
    b. The person's culture
    c. Where the person lives
    d. All of the above

Matching

Match the amount of fluid in milliliters (mL) with the same amount in ounces (oz).

_____ **1.** 240 mL   **a.** 10 oz

_____ **2.** 180 mL   **b.** 5 oz

_____ **3.** 300 mL   **c.** 8 oz

_____ **4.** 30 mL   **d.** 4 oz

_____ **5.** 120 mL   **e.** 1 oz

_____ **6.** 150 mL   **f.** 6 oz

 Stop *and* **Think!**

Mrs. Giovanni was recently admitted to your long-term care facility. She is a bit underweight and her doctor wants her to consume more calories each day. The problem is Mrs. Giovanni will only eat about half of her meal at mealtime. She says, "I just get full quickly." What are some ways you may be able to help Mrs. Giovanni improve her nutritional intake?

STOP **Stop** *and* **Think!**

You work in an assisted living facility, and one of your residents, Mr. Wayne, has severe arthritis in his hands. The arthritis makes it hard for Mr. Wayne to use his silverware, but he refuses to let you help him eat. Lately, the arthritis has gotten much worse, and Mr. Wayne is having more and more difficulty eating. Most of the food winds up beside the plate instead of in his mouth, and what little food makes it to his mouth is ice-cold by the time it gets there. You know that Mr. Wayne has to eat to maintain his health. What can you do to assist Mr. Wayne in feeding himself? What member of the staff could you ask to assist you?

Assisting With Urinary Elimination

One of our most basic physical needs is the need to eliminate waste from the body. One way of eliminating waste is through urinary elimination, or the passing of urine from the body. Your patients or residents may have physical or mental difficulties that affect their ability to manage urinary elimination. As a nursing assistant, you will need to help them as necessary.

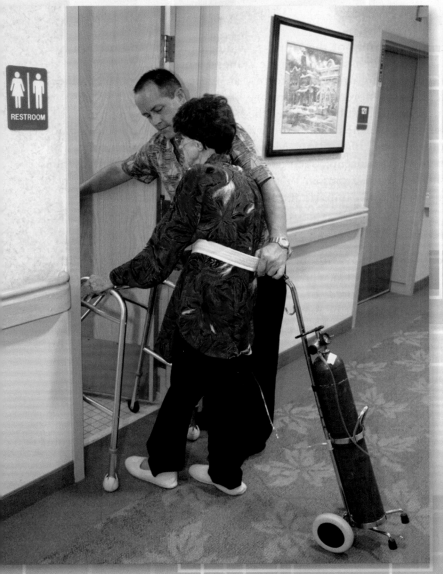

Photo: *A nursing assistant helps a resident to the bathroom.*

Introduction to Urinary Elimination

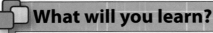

What will you learn?

When you are finished with this section, you will be able to:

1. Describe how the urinary system helps to remove waste products from the body.
2. Describe the characteristics of normal urine.
3. State observations that you may make when assisting a person with urinary elimination that should be reported to the nurse.
4. Discuss actions you can take to promote normal urinary elimination.
5. Define the words **urination**, **voiding**, **micturition**, **hematuria**, **frequency**, **urgency**, **nocturia**, and **dysuria**.

The Urinary System

The urinary system is made up of the kidneys, bladder, ureters, and urethra (see Chapter 7, Fig. 7-21). Blood passes through the kidneys, which remove waste products and excess fluid, forming urine. As it forms, the urine flows from the kidneys through the ureters and is stored in the urinary bladder. As the bladder fills, we begin to feel the urge to urinate. Urine leaves the body through the urethra.

    The process of passing urine from the body is known by several terms, including **urination**, **voiding**, and **micturition**. Many of your patients or residents will have their own terms for urinating, such as "peeing" or "passing water." When talking about urination with a patient or resident, use words that the person is familiar with. This is especially important when talking with children.

Urination the process of passing urine from the body

Voiding urination

Micturition urination

Characteristics of Urine

In healthy people, urine is clear, without cloudiness or particles. Sometimes urine that has been in a container for a while will become cloudy as it cools. Healthy urine is pale yellow, straw-colored, or dark gold (amber) in color, with a slight odor. A slight red tinge to the urine may indicate **hematuria**. This is an abnormal finding. Some foods and drugs can also affect the color and odor of urine. When you are helping a patient or resident with urination, observe the urine and report any abnormalities to the nurse. Urine with an unusual odor or appearance could be a sign of illness or infection.

Hematuria blood in the urine

Urination Habits

The frequency of voiding and the amount of urine voided each time will differ from person to person. Many factors influence a person's urination habits, including:

- The amount of fluids the person drinks
- The types of medications the person takes
- The person's age
- The person's lifelong habits

Some people void quite frequently, at the first urge, while others may hold their urine for as long as possible, even if a bathroom is readily available. You will soon become aware of the urination habits that are normal for each person in your care. This knowledge will allow you to recognize any changes that may occur. Terms used to describe changes in a person's urination habits include **frequency, urgency, nocturia**, and **dysuria**.

Promoting Normal Urinary Elimination

Being in a health care facility can change a person's normal urination habits, which can cause health problems. The most effective method of dealing with urinary problems is to prevent them from happening in the first place. There are many ways that you can help promote normal urinary function for your patients or residents (Guidelines Box 25-1).

Frequency urination that occurs more often than usual

Urgency a need to urinate immediately

Nocturia the need to get up more than once or twice during the night to urinate, to the point where sleep is disrupted

Dysuria painful or difficult urination

GUIDELINES BOX 25-1   Guidelines for Promoting Normal Urinary Elimination

What you do	Why you do it
Encourage plenty of fluids, unless a person has a medical condition that requires fluid restriction.	*Drinking plenty of fluids helps the kidneys to work properly, and regular urination flushes harmful bacteria from the bladder, helping to prevent urinary tract infections.*
Always honor a person's request for assistance with elimination as quickly as possible.	*Holding urine for too long can lead to problems with urinary elimination. It is also uncomfortable for the person.*
Encourage your patients or residents to call when they first feel the urge to void.	*Holding urine for too long can lead to problems with urinary elimination. It is also uncomfortable for the person.*
Offer your patients or residents the chance to eliminate frequently, especially if they are bed-bound or require assistance.	*Some people may find it easier to accept an offer of assistance than to ask for help.*
Always provide your patients or residents with as much privacy and comfort as safety considerations will allow.	*Many people have difficulty urinating if they think that someone else can hear them or if someone else is in the bathroom with them.*
If a person is having trouble starting the stream of urine, try turning on the faucet and allowing water to run into the sink or putting the person's fingers in a basin of warm water.	*The sound of running water, which accompanied many of our early toilet training lessons, can help a person to relax enough to start the urine stream. The sound of the running water also helps to cover up the sounds of urination, which may put some people more at ease.*

Putting it all together!

- The elimination of waste products, such as urine, from the body is one of the most basic physical needs.

- The urinary system rids the body of waste products that have been filtered from the blood.

- Normal urine is clear, pale yellow to dark gold in color, with a characteristic odor.

- Urination habits vary from person to person.

- A change in the odor or appearance of a person's urine or in the person's normal urination habits can be a sign of illness or infection and should be reported immediately.

- Normal urinary elimination can be promoted by encouraging fluids, answering the call light promptly, and providing for the person's privacy and comfort.

Assisting With Bedside Commodes, Bedpans, and Urinals

What will you learn?

When you are finished with this section, you will be able to:

1. Describe the equipment that may be used to assist people with urinary elimination.

2. Demonstrate the proper technique for assisting a person with a bedpan.

3. Demonstrate the proper technique for assisting a person with a urinal.

4. Define the words **bedside commode**, **bedpan**, **fracture pan**, and **urinal**.

Many of your patients or residents will only need a steady arm to lean on during the trip to the bathroom. The bathrooms in many health care facilities have special features that make them easier for people with physical disabilities to use (Fig. 25-1). For example, handrails attached to the walls alongside the toilet or onto the toilet itself make it easier for the person to sit down and get back up. Some toilets have higher seats, so the person does not have to bend her knees as much to sit down and get back up. Modifications like these allow many patients or residents to use the toilet in the bathroom with very little assistance from you. However, some of your patients or residents may not be able to get out of bed at all, or they may be too weak or ill to walk to the bathroom. These people need more help with elimination and need special equipment. General guidelines for assisting a person with urinary elimination are given in Guidelines Box 25-2.

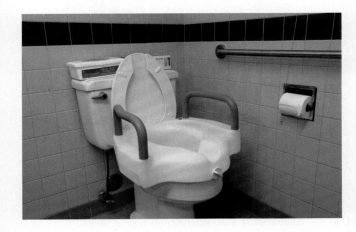

■ FIGURE 25-1
Many toilets in health care facilities have special modifications that make them easier to use.

GUIDELINES BOX 25-2 Guidelines for Assisting With Elimination

What you do	Why you do it
Always honor a person's request for assistance with elimination as quickly as possible.	*Answering call lights promptly builds trust, helps to prevent the person from accidentally soiling himself, and helps to prevent falls (for example, if a weak or unsteady person tries to make it to the bathroom unassisted). Also, it is uncomfortable for the person to "hold" urine for a long time, and doing so can change the normal elimination patterns, causing health problems.*
Provide privacy to the extent possible with regard to the safety of the person. Close the bathroom door (or close the privacy curtains and the door to the room if the person cannot use the regular toilet).	*Most people consider urination to be a very private activity. Providing as much privacy as possible helps to protect the person from feeling embarrassed and promotes normal elimination.*
If you leave the person alone, always make sure that the call light control is within easy reach of the person.	*The person will need the call light control to let you know when he is finished or if he needs help.*
Make sure the toilet paper is within easy reach of the person. If the person is unable to wipe himself, assist with this task.	*Wiping promotes comfort and helps to prevent irritation, odors, and infection.*
Be sure to provide good perineal care as necessary.	*Good perineal care promotes comfort and helps to prevent irritation, odors, and infection.*
Provide the person with the chance to wash his hands after elimination. This can be accomplished by stopping by the sink if the person is in the bathroom or by providing a warm, wet washcloth after assisting the person from the bedside commode or removing the bedpan or urinal.	*Handwashing is important for hygiene.*

(*box continues on page 568*)

GUIDELINES BOX 25-2   Guidelines for Assisting With Elimination (continued)

What you do	Why you do it
Always wear gloves when assisting a person with elimination or when handling a bedpan, bedside commode bucket, or urinal that contains urine.	*Urine is a body fluid and may contain pathogens.*
When wearing gloves while assisting a person with elimination, be sure to remove at least one glove prior to touching side rails, door knobs, or other objects in the person's room. You may need to change gloves several times while assisting a person with elimination.	*Gloves that are possibly contaminated will spread germs to other objects and surfaces that you touch.*
Before disposing of urine, observe the urine for amount and any unusual characteristics. Report and record your observations.	*Abnormalities in the urine could indicate a health problem.*
Never place a bedpan or urinal on an over-bed table or bedside table, even if the bedpan or urinal is clean. Dirty bedpans and urinals are taken to the bathroom immediately after use and cleaned and disinfected according to facility policy. Clean bedpans are either stored in a cabinet underneath the bedside table or returned to the equipment room. Clean urinals may be hung over the side rail, stored in a cabinet, or returned to the equipment room.	*The over-bed table and bedside table are considered "clean" areas. Even if the bedpan or urinal is clean, most people do not want items associated with elimination placed on surfaces where they eat or have personal items displayed.*
Disinfect equipment used for elimination carefully, according to facility policy.	*Bedpans, urinals, and bedside commode buckets can transmit pathogens and cause infection if they are not properly disinfected.*

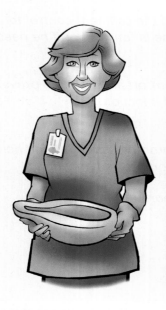

Think about how it would affect you to be a patient or a resident in a health care facility. You may have to share a bathroom, or worse yet, use a bedpan while being separated from other people in the room by only a curtain! Elimination, especially when it must take place in a fairly public way, is very embarrassing for many people. Providing as much privacy as possible and having a professional, kind, and straightforward attitude will help to ease any embarrassment your patient or resident may feel.

Bedside Commodes

For a person who is able to get out of bed but is not able to walk to the bathroom, a **bedside commode** can make toileting easier. If the person is weak or unsteady, you will need to help him get out of bed and over to the bedside commode.

Bedpans

A woman who cannot get out of bed uses a **bedpan** to urinate and for bowel movements. A man who cannot get out of bed uses a bedpan for bowel movements. A bedpan may be made from molded plastic or metal. It is

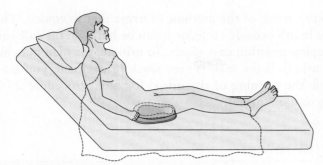

Standard bedpan: Wide end toward head of bed

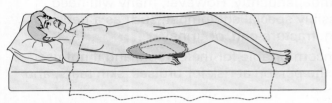

Fracture pan: Thin end toward head of bed

■ FIGURE 25-2

Positioning a bedpan.

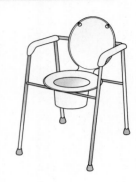

Bedside commode a device used for elimination when a person is able to get out of bed, but unable to walk to the bathroom; it consists of a chair-like frame with a toilet seat and a removable collection bucket

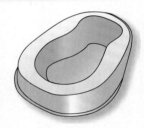

Bedpan a device used for elimination when a person is unable to get out of bed

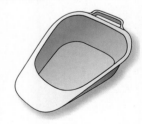

Fracture pan a wedge-shaped bedpan that is used when a person has an injury or disability that makes it too uncomfortable or dangerous to use a regular bedpan

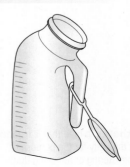

Urinal a device used for urination when a man is unable to get out of bed

positioned under the person like a regular toilet seat, with the narrow end pointed toward the foot of the bed (Fig. 25-2).

Bedpans, while sometimes necessary, must be used with extreme care. It is very easy to bruise or tear the fragile skin of an elderly or disabled person. In addition to causing immediate pain to the person, an injury like this can also lead to the formation of a pressure ulcer later on. Arthritis can make using a bedpan very painful, as can fractures of the back or legs. If a person has an injury or disability that makes it too uncomfortable or dangerous to use a regular bedpan, a special bedpan called a **fracture pan** is used. The fracture pan, which is wedge shaped, is placed underneath the person's buttocks with the thin edge toward the person's back (see Fig. 25-2).

Using a bedpan is very uncomfortable, and the discomfort alone can cause the person to have difficulty using it. To help make using a bedpan more comfortable for the person, you can do the following:

- If the facility where you work uses metal bedpans, be sure to warm the bedpan before offering it to the person. You can do this by wrapping the bedpan in a warm towel or running warm water over the seat area and then drying it before use.
- A light dusting of baby powder on the seat area of either a plastic or metal bedpan can help it to slide more easily against the person's skin.
- If the person's condition allows, raise the head of the bed to promote a more natural elimination position.
- Provide as much privacy as safely possible.

Procedure 25-1 describes how to help a person to use a bedpan.

Urinals

A man uses a **urinal** to urinate when he cannot get out of bed. The urinal fits between the man's legs. It is usually made from clear plastic and has marks on the side that make it easier to keep track of the amount of urine that is voided. The urinal is usually stored in the man's bedside table, or it can be hung on the side rail of the bed by the handle, keeping it within easy reach. To urinate, the man puts his penis in the opening of the urinal. If the man is very weak or disabled, you may need to place his penis inside the opening of the urinal for him. Procedure 25-2 describes how to help a man to use a urinal.

Putting it all together!

- Many patients or residents will be able to manage urinary elimination fairly independently. However, many will need your help and possibly special equipment, such as a bedside commode, bedpan, fracture pan, or urinal.
- Bedpans can be uncomfortable for the person, and if not used with care, can put the person at risk for bruises, skin tears, and pressure ulcers.
- A kind and professional attitude will help to ease any embarrassment the patient or resident may feel about needing assistance to urinate.
- Standard precautions should be taken when assisting a person with urination because contact with body fluids is likely.

Caring for a Person With an Indwelling Urinary Catheter

What will you learn?

When you are finished with this section, you will be able to:

1. Describe situations when an indwelling urinary catheter may need to be used.
2. Describe how to handle the catheter tubing and drainage bag when caring for a person with an indwelling urinary catheter.
3. Demonstrate the proper technique for providing routine urinary catheter care.
4. Demonstrate the proper technique for emptying a urine drainage bag.
5. State observations you may make when caring for a person with an indwelling urinary catheter that should be reported to the nurse.
6. Define the words **catheter** and **catheter care**.

Catheter a tube that is inserted into the body for the purpose of administering or removing fluids

Sometimes a person is unable to urinate using a toilet, bedpan, urinal, or bedside commode. In these situations, a urinary **catheter** is used. A urinary catheter is inserted into the bladder to allow the urine in the bladder to drain out.

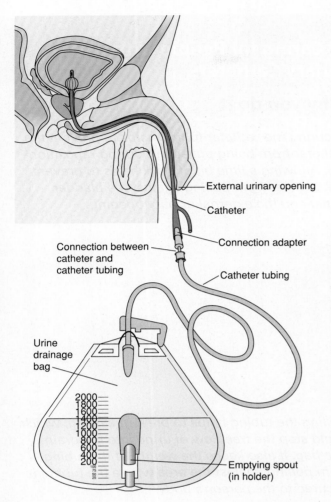

External urinary opening

Catheter

Connection adapter

Connection between catheter and catheter tubing

Catheter tubing

Urine drainage bag

2000
1800
1600
1400
1200
1000
800
600
400
200
100
75
50
25

Emptying spout (in holder)

■ **FIGURE 25-3**

The indwelling urinary catheter drainage system consists of a catheter that is connected to a urine drainage bag by way of a length of tubing. The urine drainage bag has a connection adapter, where the tubing attaches, and an emptying spout, which is unclamped to allow the urine to drain from the bag. When not in use, the emptying spout is stored in a holder that is part of the bag.

There are different types of urinary catheters. One very common type is the indwelling urinary catheter (also known as a Foley or retention catheter). An indwelling catheter is left inside the bladder to provide continuous urine drainage. It has a soft balloon that is inflated inside the bladder to keep the catheter from sliding out of the urethra. Urine collects in a drainage bag, which is attached to the indwelling catheter by a length of tubing (Fig. 25-3).

A person may need an indwelling urinary catheter for many different reasons:

■ A person is recovering from a serious illness or injury.

■ The bladder needs to be emptied before or during a surgical procedure.

■ The person is incontinent of urine and has wounds or pressure ulcers that would be made worse by contact with urine.

■ A person is unable to urinate because of an obstruction in the urethra.

Usually, inserting a urinary catheter is beyond the scope of practice for a nursing assistant. Inserting a catheter is a procedure that requires sterile technique because it involves placing a foreign object (that is, the catheter) into a person's body. If sterile technique is not used, bacteria can travel on the catheter into the person's bladder, possibly resulting in an infection. However, even if you are not responsible for catheterizing your patients or residents, you will most likely be responsible for caring for people who have indwelling catheters. General guidelines for caring for a person with an indwelling urinary catheter are given in Guidelines Box 25-3.

GUIDELINES BOX 25-3 Guidelines for Caring for People With Indwelling Urinary Catheters

What you do	Why you do it
Loosely secure the catheter tubing to the person near the insertion site, using a catheter strap or adhesive tape.	*Securing the catheter tubing helps to prevent the catheter from being pulled out during repositioning. Allowing a little bit of slack helps to prevent the catheter from pulling against the bladder outlet and the external urinary opening.*

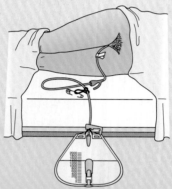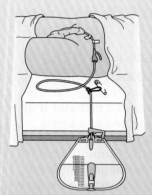

Women: taped to inner thigh   **Men:** taped to inner thigh or lower abdomen

The remaining length of tubing is gently coiled and secured to the bed linens using a plastic clip.	*Coiling the tubing helps to prevent kinking, which could stop the free flow of urine into the drainage bag. It also keeps the weight of the tubing from pulling against the area where the tubing is secured to the person's body.*
When repositioning a person who has an indwelling urinary catheter, always make sure to unclip the coiled tubing from the linens before beginning the procedure. When you are finished with the procedure, secure the coiled tubing to the linens again.	*The person needs to be able to move freely during procedures such as repositioning. If you try to move a person in the direction opposite from the length of tubing and the length of tubing is still attached to the bed linens, then the resulting opposing forces could cause the catheter to be pulled out of the person's body.*
Make sure that the person is not lying on the coiled tubing.	*This would be uncomfortable for the person. In addition, the weight of the person's body on the tubing could stop the free flow of urine into the drainage bag.*
Always make sure that the urine drainage bag is placed at a level lower than that of the person's bladder.	*Raising the urine drainage bag up higher than the bladder can cause old, contaminated urine to run back into the bladder, which can lead to infection.*

What you do (continued)

Never attach a urine drainage bag to a side rail. Instead, attach the urine drainage bag to the bed frame or to the back of the person's wheelchair.

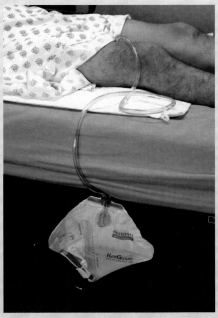

Bed frame

Why you do it (continued)

Raising the side rail would raise the urine drainage bag to a level that is higher than the person's bladder. The bed frame does not move; therefore, the level of the urine drainage bag cannot change. Attaching the urine drainage bag to the back of the wheelchair keeps it at the proper level, and also out of the way of the moving parts of the wheelchair.

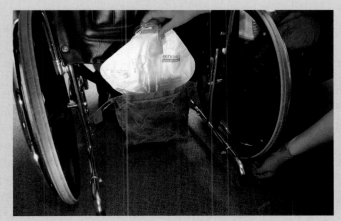

Back of wheelchair

Try to avoid disconnecting the urine drainage bag from the tubing once the catheter is in place. If you must disconnect the tubing from the bag, be sure to prevent the end of the tubing from touching anything, and wipe the exposed tubing with an antibacterial wipe before reconnecting the urine drainage bag.

Because the inside of the catheter and tubing are sterile, it is safer for the person if the bag is not disconnected from the tubing once the catheter is in place. Disconnecting the bag from the tubing can allow harmful bacteria to enter the catheter.

Keep the urine drainage bag off the floor. When emptying the urine drainage bag, be sure that the open emptying spout does not touch anything.

Bacteria can enter the closed drainage system in this manner. The presence of bacteria in the system can cause a urinary tract infection.

Always wear gloves when emptying the urine drainage bag.

Urine is a body fluid and may contain pathogens.

Empty the collecting bag using a separate graduate for each patient or resident.

Using a separate graduate for each person helps to prevent the transfer of harmful bacteria from one person to another.

Providing Catheter Care

Because bacteria can be introduced into the body both when a urinary catheter is inserted and after it is in place, urinary tract infections in catheterized people are among the most common health care–associated infections (HAIs). (Remember that an HAI is an infection acquired in the health care setting.) Because of this, the CDC has issued new guidelines regarding when and for how long indwelling catheters should be used in the health care setting. **Catheter care** is done to reduce the risk of an HAI in people with indwelling urinary catheters.

Many facilities require catheter care to be provided routinely (for example, once or twice daily) and again whenever the perineal area becomes soiled (such as when a person is incontinent of feces). Soap and water should be used when providing catheter care. The procedure for providing catheter care is given in Procedure 25-3.

Emptying Urine Drainage Bags

There are many different types of urine drainage bags used in health care settings. Some urine drainage bags have a long length of tubing that allows them to be carried or secured to a bed frame or the back of a wheelchair. Other urine drainage bags, called "leg bags," are connected to the catheter by a short length of tubing and are secured to the person's thigh with rubberized straps. Leg bags are useful because they are worn underneath a person's clothing and allow the person to move around freely.

All urine drainage bags have a connection adapter (where the catheter tubing attaches) and an emptying spout that is opened to allow urine to drain from the bag. Urine drainage bags are routinely emptied and the urine measured at the end of each shift unless ordered otherwise. Urine drainage bags should also be emptied if they become full. Leg bags need to be emptied more frequently because they are smaller and hold less urine. The procedure for emptying a urine drainage bag is given in Procedure 25-4.

 Putting it all together!

- A person who is having trouble urinating may need to have a urinary catheter placed to remove the urine from the bladder.
- An indwelling urinary catheter is a type of urinary catheter that is inserted into the bladder and left in place to provide continuous urine drainage.
- Indwelling urinary catheters are a leading cause of health care–associated infections (HAIs).
- Although inserting an indwelling urinary catheter is usually beyond the nursing assistant's scope of practice, nursing assistants are responsible for caring for people with indwelling urinary catheters.
- Proper handling of the catheter tubing is necessary to keep the patient or resident comfortable, prevent kinking of the tubing, and prevent the tubing from being pulled out of the body accidentally.
- Proper handling of the urine drainage bag and routine catheter care are necessary to prevent infection.
- Standard precautions should be taken when assisting with catheter care and emptying urine drainage bags because contact with body fluids is likely.

Caring for a Person Who Is Incontinent of Urine

What will you learn?

When you are finished with this section, you will be able to:

1. List five common types of urinary incontinence.
2. Describe how urinary incontinence can affect a person both physically and emotionally.
3. Describe the products that are available to help manage urinary incontinence and the proper use of these products.
4. Discuss how bladder training is used to assist people who are incontinent of urine.
5. Define the words **urinary incontinence**, **urinary retention**, and **condom catheter**.

Urinary incontinence may be temporary or permanent. Temporary urinary incontinence is a fairly common occurrence in health care facilities. The effects of medications, being in a strange place, reluctance to ask for help, and physical or mental disabilities can all lead to accidents. Permanent urinary incontinence can be caused by many things, including:

- Decreased muscle tone in the bladder or the muscles that support the bladder, that may occur after childbirth or from obesity
- Injuries or illnesses that affect the spinal cord, the brain, or the nerves that control the bladder function
- Dementia

Being incontinent of urine places a person at risk for developing skin problems (such as rashes and pressure ulcers) and for falling (as the person rushes to the bathroom to avoid having an accident).

> **Urinary incontinence** the inability to hold one's urine, or the involuntary loss of urine from the bladder

Concerns for Long-Term Care

Urinary incontinence can be emotionally devastating for both the incontinent person and the person's caregivers. For the person who is incontinent, having wet clothes or smelling like urine can be very embarrassing. For the caregiver, caring for a person who is incontinent of urine can be frustrating and emotionally draining. It is not uncommon to change a person's clothes or bedding, only to have the person wet herself all over again. Because caring for an incontinent person can be so emotionally trying and time-consuming, incontinence is the factor that most often leads family members to have a relative admitted to a long-term care facility. In fact, studies have shown that in the long-term care setting, as many as 90% of the residents who have dementia are incontinent of urine.

Types of Urinary Incontinence

- **Stress incontinence** is probably the most common type of urinary incontinence. In stress incontinence, urine leaks from the bladder when the person coughs, sneezes, or exerts herself. Stress incontinence can also occur if a person delays voiding and the bladder becomes too full. Stress incontinence can often be corrected with exercises or surgery.

- **Urge incontinence** is the involuntary release of urine right after feeling a strong urge to void. This type of incontinence is common in people with urinary tract infections because irritation of the bladder causes the bladder muscle to spasm, causing the bladder to empty with little warning.

- **Functional incontinence** occurs in the absence of physical or nervous system problems affecting the urinary tract. The person just cannot make it to the bathroom in enough time or wait until a bedpan or urinal is provided. Confusion, disorientation, and loss of mobility are contributing factors.

- Overflow incontinence occurs when the bladder is too full of urine. Overflow incontinence is associated with **urinary retention**. A person with overflow incontinence may "dribble" urine between visits to the bathroom.

- **Reflex incontinence** occurs when there is damage to the nerves that allow the person to control urination. The bladder fills, but the person does not feel the urge to urinate. When the bladder is completely full, it empties on its own.

Urinary retention the inability of the bladder to empty either completely during urination, or at all

Managing Urinary Incontinence

Many products are available to help manage urinary incontinence, including incontinence pads, incontinence briefs, bed protectors, and condom catheters. In addition, techniques such as bladder training may be used to help a person overcome certain types of incontinence. For some people, temporary or permanent catheterization may be needed to manage the incontinence.

Incontinence Pads, Incontinence Briefs, and Bed Protectors

Several products are available to absorb urine and hold it away from the person's skin:

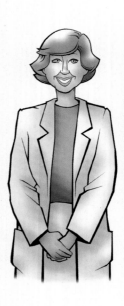

How would being incontinent of urine make you feel? Would it be embarrassing to have wet clothes or to smell like urine? Although it can be frustrating to have to change a person's clothes or bed linens several times during one shift, try to remember that the person cannot help being incontinent.

- **Incontinence pads** are placed inside a person's underpants (Fig. 25-4A).
- **Incontinence briefs** are worn instead of underpants (see Fig. 25-4B). When caring for a person who wears incontinence briefs, you should not refer to these products as "diapers." This can be very embarrassing and demeaning for the patient or resident.
- **Bed protectors** are placed on the bed to keep the bed linens and mattress dry.

Keeping the skin, clothing, and bed linens dry helps to reduce the skin problems that can occur from prolonged contact with urine. Many facilities have policies that specify that incontinence briefs are to be used only when the person is out of bed and that bed protectors are to be used when the person is in bed. Incontinence briefs tend to fit closely, which makes it difficult for air to reach the skin. Switching between

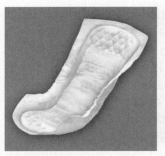

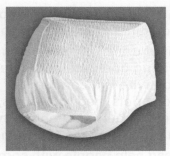

A. Incontinence pad   B. Incontinence brief

■ **FIGURE 25-4**

Incontinence pads and briefs are worn under clothing to absorb moisture and keep it away from the body. These products are very useful for active people. **(A)** DEPEND Guards for men. **(B)** DEPEND Extra Absorbency Underwear.

(Photographs courtesy of Kimberly-Clark Worldwide, Inc., Neenah, WI.)

briefs and bed protectors helps to prevent skin breakdown by allowing the skin to be exposed to the air.

Perineal care (see Chapter 21) is especially important for people who are incontinent of urine. You will be responsible for making sure that incontinence products are changed frequently and that urine is cleaned from the skin whenever the change occurs.

Condom Catheters

A **condom catheter** (also called a *Texas catheter*) is not a true catheter because it is not placed inside the body. It consists of a soft plastic or rubber sheath, tubing, and a collection bag for the urine. The sheath is placed over the penis and the collection bag is attached to the leg. The urine flows through the tubing into the collection bag, allowing the man to urinate at will.

The condom must fit the penis. It should be tight enough to prevent leaking, but not so tight that it cuts off blood flow. Many condom catheters have adhesive material on the inside of the condom that allows for a good seal. Others must be secured with elastic tape. The tape strip is applied in a spiral fashion to allow for changes in the size of the penis. Applying the tape in an overlapping, circular fashion would cut off the blood flow if the man had an erection, possibly causing permanent damage to the penis.

Use of a condom catheter requires good skin care. The penis must be cleaned, and the condom changed, daily.

Condom catheter a device used to manage urinary incontinence in men; it consists of a soft plastic or rubber sheath, tubing, and a collection bag for the urine

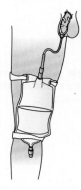

Bladder Training

Bladder training is commonly used to help people who are incontinent of urine. As part of bladder training, the person may be encouraged to use the bedpan, urinal, or commode at scheduled times. Scheduling helps to promote regular emptying of the bladder. The main goal is for the person to be able to control involuntary urination. If this is not possible, then the person may still at least be able to get to the bathroom in time to avoid accidents because he will know when voiding is due to occur. The person's care plan will note any special bladder training techniques that are being used, and the nurse will instruct you on any specific duties you will be assigned as part of that training.

Putting it all together!

- Urinary incontinence has many causes and may be temporary or permanent.
- The five main types of urinary incontinence are stress incontinence, urge incontinence, functional incontinence, overflow incontinence, and reflex incontinence.

- Being incontinent of urine is difficult emotionally for both the person who is incontinent and that person's caregiver.
- Being incontinent of urine places a person at risk for skin breakdown. Providing good perineal care is essential when caring for a person who is incontinent of urine. Incontinence pads, incontinence briefs, bed protectors, and condom catheters must be changed frequently, and urine should be cleaned from the skin whenever the change occurs.
- Bladder training can help people with some types of incontinence.

Obtaining a Urine Specimen

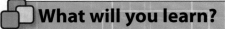

What will you learn?

When you are finished with this section, you will be able to:

1. Demonstrate proper technique for collecting a routine urine specimen.
2. Demonstrate proper technique for collecting a midstream ("clean catch") urine specimen.
3. Define the words **urinalysis** and **midstream ("clean catch") urine specimen**.

Urinalysis examination of the urine under a microscope and by chemical means

Urinalysis is a commonly used diagnostic tool in the health care setting. To perform urinalysis, a sample of the person's urine, called a urine specimen, is needed. You may be asked to help by collecting the specimen and delivering it to the laboratory. General guidelines for collecting and handling any type of specimen (for example, of urine, feces, sputum, or any other body fluid) are given in Guidelines Box 25-4.

Collecting a Routine Urine Specimen

When a routine urine specimen is needed, the person is asked to urinate directly into the specimen cup, if possible. If this is difficult for the person, he or she can urinate into a specimen collection device such as a "commode hat" (Fig. 25-5) or into a bedpan or urinal. The person must not have a bowel movement at the same time the urine is being collected or place toilet paper in the collection device because these actions will change the urinalysis results. The urine is then poured from the collection device, bedpan, or urinal into the specimen cup. The procedure for obtaining a routine urine sample is described in Procedure 25-5.

Collecting a Midstream ("Clean Catch") Urine Specimen

Midstream ("clean catch") urine specimen a method of collecting urine that prevents contamination of the urine by the bacteria that normally exist in and around the urethra

In some situations, it may be necessary to obtain a **midstream ("clean catch") urine specimen** using a sterile specimen container. This method of collecting urine is usually ordered when the doctor suspects a urinary tract infection. In this way,

GUIDELINES BOX 25-4 Guidelines for Collecting Specimens of Any Type

What you do	Why you do it
Always make sure that the specimen container is properly labeled with the person's name and room number.	*Proper identification on the specimen container is necessary to ensure that the test results are matched with the correct patient or resident. Otherwise, a person may be diagnosed with, and receive treatment for, a condition he does not have!*
Before going to collect a specimen, always ask yourself: ■ Do I have the right person? ■ Do I have the right paperwork? ■ What method is to be used to collect the specimen? ■ Do I have the right type of specimen container? ■ Is the specimen container properly labeled? ■ What is the correct date and time? ■ What storage and delivery method must I use?	*Having the answers to these questions helps to ensure that the specimen will be correctly identified, collected, and transported or stored. This reduces the risk that another specimen will need to be obtained and the test repeated.*
Make sure that the specimen is handled correctly after you obtain it. For example, some specimens may need to be delivered to the laboratory while they are still warm or placed in a special transport bag. If a specimen is not being delivered to the laboratory right away, then it needs to be stored properly until the scheduled pick-up time.	*Failing to deliver the specimen promptly (or store it properly until pick-up) can change the test results or make it impossible to use the specimen. In this case, another specimen will need to be obtained, which delays diagnosis and treatment, adds to costs, and is inconvenient for the patient or resident.*
Always remember to wear gloves when assisting with specimen collection and when handling the specimen containers.	*Specimens are body fluids and may contain pathogens.*

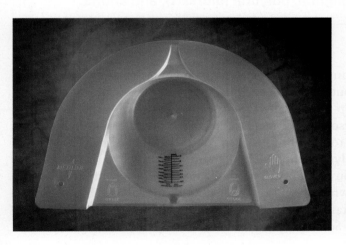

■ **FIGURE 25-5**

A collection device (sometimes called a "commode hat") is placed over the toilet seat before the person urinates.

(Photograph courtesy of Medline Industries, Inc.)

if any bacteria are found in the urine sample, the doctor knows that they are the ones most likely responsible for the infection. When a midstream ("clean catch") urine specimen is requested, the person is asked to clean the area around the urethral opening with a special cleansing wipe. The person begins to urinate, then stops, then starts again. The urine sample is collected from the restarted flow. Procedure 25-6 describes how to assist a person with obtaining a midstream ("clean catch") urine specimen.

Putting it all together!

- When handling specimens of any type, it is important to make sure that the proper method is used to collect the specimen, that the specimen is properly identified, and that the specimen is properly transported and stored.
- Methods for obtaining a urine specimen may vary, depending on the situation. Many times, a routine urine specimen will be all that is needed. A midstream ("clean-catch") urine specimen is often required when the doctor suspects a urinary tract infection. If you are unsure about what method to use to collect the specimen, ask the nurse.
- When collecting a urine specimen using either method, it is important to remind the person not to have a bowel movement or place toilet paper in the collection device.
- Standard precautions should be taken when handling a urine specimen because contact with body fluids is likely.

Measuring Urine Output

What will you learn?

When you are finished with this section, you will be able to:

1. Demonstrate methods used to measure and record urine output.
2. Define the words **oliguria**, **polyuria (diuresis)**, and **anuria**.

Oliguria the state of voiding a very small amount of urine over a given period of time (for example, voiding only 100 to 400 mL of urine over 24 hours)

Polyuria (diuresis) excessive urine output

Anuria the state of voiding less than 100 mL of urine over the course of 24 hours

Urine output is simply the amount of urine the person voids over a given period of time. A person's urine output can help to tell us how well the person's kidneys are functioning. It can also help to tell us whether or not the person is maintaining a good fluid balance. In a person who is maintaining a good fluid balance, urine output is neither too high nor too low. Terms used to describe abnormalities in urine output include **oliguria**, **polyuria (diuresis)**, and **anuria**.

Not all of the people you care for will need to have their urine output measured and recorded, but people who have illnesses or take medications that may affect their body's ability to maintain a healthy fluid balance will need to have their urine output measured regularly. Some people who are critically ill will have their urine output measured and recorded every hour, but most people in the health care setting have routine orders for their urine output to be measured and recorded each shift.

If a person uses a regular toilet, you will need to remind the person to void into a specimen collection device ("commode hat") and to call you after she has finished voiding so that you can measure and record the amount of urine. Specimen collection devices, urinals, and the drainage bags used with urinary catheters often have markings that make measuring urine output easy. If they do not, then the urine output can be measured by pouring it into a graduate. A graduate is also used to measure urine output if a person voids into a bedpan or bedside commode bucket. Remember to place the graduate on a flat surface when measuring urine so that your measurements are accurate.

If the urine output of one of your residents or patients is being monitored, you will need to keep a record of the amount of urine passed at each voiding. Some intake and output (I&O) flow sheets will have spaces to record the amount of each individual voiding, while others may only have a space to record the end-of-shift amount. To obtain the end-of-shift amount, simply add the individual amounts together and record the total in the appropriate space.

Putting it all together!

- Urine output is a key indicator of fluid balance. In a person who is maintaining a good fluid balance, urine output is neither too high nor too low.

- Monitoring a person's urine output is also a good way to determine how well the person's kidneys are working.

- Urine can be collected in a urine collection device ("commode hat"), bedpan, urinal, or urine drainage bag, depending on the situation. In some cases, it may be necessary to pour the urine into a graduate to measure it.

- Standard precautions should be taken when measuring urine output because contact with body fluids is likely.

PROCEDURES

PROCEDURE 25-1
Assisting a Person With Using a Bedpan

Why you do it: Bedpans are used for women who cannot get out of bed to urinate or have a bowel movement and for men who cannot get out of bed or have a bowel movement.

GETTING READY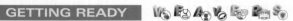

1. Complete the "Getting Ready" steps.

SUPPLIES

- gloves
- bed protector
- toilet paper
- bedpan
- bedpan cover (or paper towels)
- perineal care supplies
- washcloth
- towel

PROCEDURE

2. Make sure that the bed is positioned at a comfortable working height (to promote good body mechanics) and that the wheels are locked. If the side rails are in use, lower the side rail on the working side of the bed. The side rail on the opposite side of the bed should remain up. If necessary, lower the head of the bed so that the bed is flat (as tolerated).

3. Perform hand hygiene and put on the gloves.

4. Fanfold the top linens just far enough down to place the bedpan. Place the bed protector on the bed. Adjust the person's hospital gown or pajama bottoms as necessary to expose the person's buttocks.

5. Place the bedpan underneath the person's buttocks. This can be accomplished by either helping the person to lie on her side, facing away from you, or by asking the person to bend her knees, press her heels into the mattress, and lift her buttocks. Slide the bedpan underneath the person (if the person is holding her buttocks away from the bed by bending her knees) or place the bedpan against her buttocks and help her to roll back onto it while you press the bedpan firmly down against the mattress.

   a. A standard bedpan is positioned like a regular toilet seat.

   b. A fracture pan is positioned with the narrow end pointed toward the head of the bed.

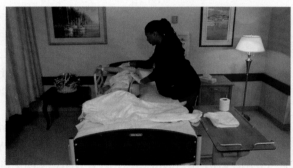

STEP 5 ■ Place the bedpan against the person's buttocks and help the person to roll back onto it.

6. Raise the head of the bed as tolerated. Draw the top linens over the person for modesty and warmth.

7. Make sure that the toilet paper and the call-light control are within reach. If the side rails are in use, return the side rails to the raised position.

8. Remove your gloves and perform hand hygiene.

9. If safety permits, leave the room and ask the person to call you when she is finished. Remember to close the door on your way out.

10. Return when the person signals. Remember to knock before entering.

11. If the side rails are in use, lower the side rail on the working side of the bed. Lower the head of the bed so that the bed is flat (as tolerated).

12. Perform hand hygiene and put on a clean pair of gloves.

13. Fanfold the top linens to the foot of the bed.

14. Ask the person to bend her knees, press her heels into the mattress, and lift her buttocks so that you can remove the bedpan and bed protector. (Or help the person to roll onto her side, facing away from you, while you hold the bedpan securely in place against the mattress to prevent the contents from spilling. Remove the bedpan and bed protector and then help the person to roll back.) If necessary, help the person to use the toilet paper.

15. Cover the bedpan with the bedpan cover or paper towels. Remove one of your gloves if you need to raise the side rails or open a door using a doorknob. Take the bedpan to the bathroom. (If the side rails are in use, raise them before leaving the bedside.)

16. Remove your gloves and dispose of them in a facility-approved waste container. Perform hand hygiene.

17. Return to the bedside. Put on a clean pair of gloves. Give the person a wet washcloth or moist hand wipes and help the person to wash her hands. Make sure that the person's perineum is clean and dry. If necessary, provide perineal care. Remove your gloves and perform hand hygiene.

18. Adjust the person's hospital gown or pajama bottoms as necessary to cover the buttocks. Help the person back into a comfortable position, straighten the bottom linens, and draw the top linens over the person. Raise the head of the bed, as the person requests. Make sure that the bed is lowered to its lowest position and that the wheels are locked.

19. Return to the bathroom. Put on a clean pair of gloves. If the person is on intake and output (I&O) status, measure the urine. Note the color, amount, and quality of the urine or feces before emptying the contents of the bedpan into the toilet. (If anything unusual is observed, do not empty the bedpan until a nurse has had a chance to look at its contents.) Clean and disinfect the bedpan according to your facility policy.

20. Gather the soiled linens and place them in the linen hamper or linen bag. Dispose of disposable items in a facility-approved waste container. Clean equipment and return it to the storage area.

21. Remove your gloves, dispose of them in a facility-approved waste container, and perform hand hygiene.

FINISHING UP

22. Complete the "Finishing Up" steps.

WHAT YOU DOCUMENT

- Date and time
- Color, amount, and quality of urine or feces
- Any abnormal observations; and if present, that a nurse was notified

PROCEDURE 25-2
Assisting a Man With Using a Urinal

Why you do it: Urinals are used for men who cannot get out of bed to urinate.

GETTING READY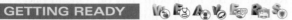

1. Complete the "Getting Ready" steps.

SUPPLIES

- gloves
- toilet paper
- urinal
- washcloth
- towel

PROCEDURE

2. Ask the man what position he prefers—lying, sitting, or standing. If necessary, raise the head of the bed as tolerated. If the man would prefer to stand, help him to sit on the edge of the bed and then to stand up.

3. Perform hand hygiene and put on the gloves.

4. Hand the man the urinal. If necessary, assist him in positioning it correctly.

5. Remove your gloves and perform hand hygiene.

6. Make sure that the toilet paper and the call-light control are within reach.

7. If safety permits, leave the room and ask the man to call you when he is finished. Remember to close the door on your way out.

8. Return when the man signals. Remember to knock before entering.

9. Perform hand hygiene and put on a clean pair of gloves. Have the man hand you the urinal, or remove it if he is unable to hand it to you. Put the lid on the urinal and hang it on the side rail while you assist the man with handwashing and perineal care as needed. Remove your gloves and perform hand hygiene. Lower the head of the bed as the man requests.

10. Put on a clean pair of gloves. Take the urinal to the bathroom. If the man is on intake and output (I&O) status, measure the urine. Note the color, amount, and quality of the urine before emptying the contents of the urinal into the toilet. (If anything unusual is observed, do not empty the urinal until a nurse has had a chance to look at its contents.) Clean and disinfect the urinal according to your facility policy.

11. Gather the soiled linens and place them in the linen hamper or linen bag. Dispose of disposable items in a facility-approved waste container. Clean equipment and return it to the storage area.

12. Remove your gloves, dispose of them in a facility-approved waste container, and perform hand hygiene.

FINISHING UP

13. Complete the "Finishing Up" steps.

WHAT YOU DOCUMENT

- Date and time
- Amount, color, and quality of urine
- Any abnormal observations; and if present, that a nurse was notified

PROCEDURE 25-3
Providing Catheter Care

Why you do it: Providing proper catheter care helps to prevent the person from getting a urinary tract infection.

GETTING READY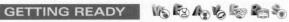

1. Complete the "Getting Ready" steps.

SUPPLIES

- gloves
- paper towels
- bed protector
- bath thermometer
- wash basin
- soap or no-rinse cleanser
- bath blanket
- washcloths
- towels
- clean clothing

PROCEDURE

2. Clean the over-bed table and cover it with paper towels.

3. Lower the head of the bed so that the bed is flat (as tolerated). Make sure that the bed is positioned at a comfortable working height (to promote good body mechanics) and that the wheels are locked.

4. Fill the wash basin with warm water (110°F [43.3°C] to 115°F [46.1°C] on the bath thermometer). Place the wash basin, soap, towels, and washcloths on the over-bed table.

5. If the side rails are in use, lower the side rail on the working side of the bed. The side rail on the opposite side of the bed should remain up.

6. Perform hand hygiene and put on the gloves.

7. Spread the bath blanket over the top linens (and the person). If the person is able, have him or her hold the bath blanket. If not, tuck the corners under the person's shoulders. Fanfold the top linens to the foot of the bed.

8. Adjust the person's hospital gown or pajama bottoms as necessary to expose the person's perineum.

9. Ask the person to open his legs and bend his knees, if possible. If the person is not able to bend his knees, help the person to spread his legs as much as possible.

10. Position the bath blanket over the person so that one corner can be wrapped under and around each leg.

11. Position a bed protector under the person's buttocks to keep the bed linens dry.

12. Lift the corner of the bath blanket that is between the person's legs upward, exposing only the perineal area.

13. Form a mitt around your hand with one of the washcloths. Wet the mitt with warm, clean water and apply soap or the no-rinse cleanser.

    a. **If the person is a woman:** Using the other hand, separate the labia. Place your washcloth-covered hand at the top of the vulva and stroke downward to the anus. Repeat, using a different part of the wash-cloth each time, until the area is clean. Rinse and dry the vulva and perineum thoroughly.

    b. **If the person is a circumcised man:** Place your washcloth-covered hand at the tip of the penis and wash in a circular motion, downward to the base of the penis. Repeat, using a different part of the washcloth each time, until the area is clean. Rinse and dry the tip and the shaft of the penis thoroughly.

    c. **If the person is an uncircumcised man:** Retract the foreskin by gently pushing the skin toward the base of the penis. Place your washcloth-covered hand at the tip of the penis and wash in a circular motion, downward to the base of the penis. Repeat, using a different part of the washcloth each time, until the area is clean. Rinse and dry the tip and the shaft of the penis thoroughly before gently pulling the foreskin back into its normal position.

(*procedure continues on page 586*)

PROCEDURE 25-3 (continued)
Providing Catheter Care

14. Using a clean washcloth, apply soap or use no-rinse cleanser and clean the catheter tubing, starting at the body and moving outward from the body about 4 inches. Hold the catheter near the opening of the urethra. This will help to prevent tugging on the catheter as you clean it.

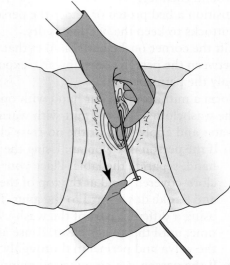

STEP 14 ▪ Clean the catheter tubing, starting at the body and moving outward.

15. Rinse the catheter tubing, if necessary, using a clean washcloth. Dry the perineal area thoroughly using a towel.

16. Check that the catheter tubing is free from kinks. Make sure that it is securely taped to the person's leg.

17. Remove your gloves and perform hand hygiene.

18. Assist the person into the supine position. Remove the bath blanket, and help the person into the clean clothing.

19. If the side rails are in use, return the side rails to the raised position. Raise the head of the bed as the person requests. Make sure that the bed is lowered to its lowest position and that the wheels are locked.

20. Put on a clean pair of gloves. Gather the soiled linens and place them in the linen hamper or linen bag. Dispose of disposable items in a facility-approved waste container. Clean the over-bed table according to facility policy. Clean equipment and return it to the storage area.

FINISHING UP

21. Complete the "Finishing Up" steps.

WHAT YOU DOCUMENT

- Date and time
- Type of care given
- Condition of skin
- Any abnormal observations; and if present, that they were reported to the nurse

PROCEDURE 25-4
Emptying a Urine Drainage Bag

Why you do it: Urine drainage bags must be emptied whenever they are full and at the end of every shift (or as ordered).

___

GETTING READY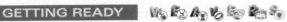

1. Complete the "Getting Ready" steps.

SUPPLIES

- gloves
- paper towels
- alcohol wipes (optional)
- graduate (each person should have his own graduate)

PROCEDURE

2. Perform hand hygiene and put on the gloves.
3. Place a paper towel on the floor, underneath the urine drainage bag. Unhook the drainage bag emptying spout from its holder on the urine drainage bag. Position the graduate on the paper towel underneath the emptying spout.
4. Unclamp the emptying spout on the urine drainage bag and allow all of the urine to drain into the graduate. Avoid touching the tip of the emptying spout with your hands or the side of the graduate.

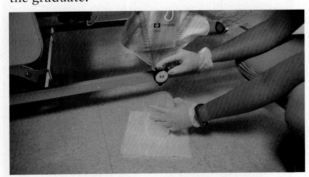

STEP 4 ▪ Unclamp the emptying spout on the urine drainage bag and allow the urine to drain into the graduate.

5. After the urine has drained into the graduate, wipe the emptying spout with an alcohol wipe (or follow facility policy). Reclamp the emptying spout and return it to its holder.
6. If the person is on intake and output (I&O) status, measure the urine. Note the color, amount, and quality of the urine before emptying the contents of the graduate into the toilet. (If anything unusual is observed, do not empty the graduate until a nurse has had a chance to look at its contents.)
7. Dispose of disposable items in a facility-approved waste container. Clean equipment and return it to the storage area.
8. Remove your gloves, dispose of them in a facility-approved waste container, and perform hand hygiene.

FINISHING UP

9. Complete the "Finishing Up" steps.

WHAT YOU DOCUMENT

- Date and time
- Amount, color, and quality of urine
- Any unusual observations

PROCEDURE 25-5
Collecting a Routine Urine Specimen

Why you do it: A routine urine specimen is often requested for urinalysis. Proper collection and handling of the urine specimen helps to ensure that the urinalysis results are accurate.

GETTING READY

1. Complete the "Getting Ready" steps.

SUPPLIES

- gloves
- paper towel
- toilet paper
- specimen container and label
- plastic transport bag (if required at your facility)
- plastic bag or waste container
- specimen collection device ("commode hat"), bedpan, or urinal

PROCEDURE

2. Complete the label with the person's name, room number, and other identifying information. Put the completed label on the specimen container. Take the specimen container to the bathroom. Place a paper towel on the counter. Open the specimen container and place the lid on the paper towel, with the inside of the lid facing up.

3. If the person will be using a regular toilet or bedside commode, fit the specimen collection device underneath the toilet or commode seat. Otherwise, provide the person with a bedpan or urinal, as applicable.

4. Assist the person with urination as necessary. Before leaving the room, remind the person not to have a bowel movement or place toilet paper into the specimen collection device, bedpan, or urinal. Provide a plastic bag or waste container for the used toilet paper.

5. Return when the person signals. Remember to knock before entering.

6. Perform hand hygiene and put on the gloves.

7. If the person used a regular toilet or bedside commode, assist the person with handwashing and perineal care as necessary and then help the person to return to bed. If the person used a bedpan or urinal, cover and remove the bedpan or urinal and assist the person with handwashing and perineal care as necessary.

8. Take the covered bedpan, urinal, or specimen collection device (if the person used a bedside commode) to the bathroom. (If the side rails are in use, raise the side rails before leaving the bedside.)

9. If the person is on intake and output (I&O) status, measure the urine. Note the color, amount, and quality of the urine.

10. Raise the toilet seat. While holding the specimen container over the toilet, carefully fill it about three-quarters full with urine from the specimen collection device, bedpan, or urinal. Discard the rest of the urine into the toilet.

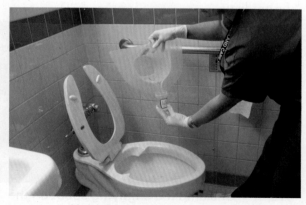

STEP 10 ■ Hold the specimen container over the toilet and fill it about three-quarters full with urine.

11. Put the lid on the specimen container. Make sure that the lid is tight. Put the specimen container on the paper towel on the counter.

12. Remove one glove and dispose of it in a facility-approved waste container. Holding the plastic transport bag in your ungloved hand, place the specimen container into the transport bag with your gloved hand. Avoid touching the outside of the transport bag with your glove.

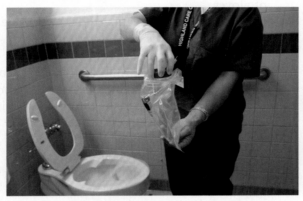

STEP 12 ■ Place the specimen container into the transport bag with your gloved hand.

13. Remove the other glove, dispose of it in a facility-approved waste container, and perform hand hygiene. Put on a clean pair of gloves.
14. Gather the soiled linens and place them in the linen hamper or linen bag. Dispose of disposable items in a facility-approved waste container. Clean equipment and return it to the storage area. Remove your gloves and perform hand hygiene.
15. Take the specimen container to the designated location.

FINISHING UP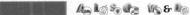

16. Complete the "Finishing Up" steps.

WHAT YOU DOCUMENT

- Date and time the specimen was collected
- Where the specimen was taken or stored for pickup

PROCEDURE 25-6
Collecting a Midstream ("Clean Catch") Urine Specimen

Why you do it: A midstream ("clean catch") urine specimen is often requested for urinalysis when the doctor suspects a urinary tract infection. Proper collection and handling of the urine specimen helps to ensure that the urinalysis results are accurate.

GETTING READY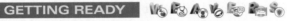

1. Complete the "Getting Ready" steps.

SUPPLIES

- gloves
- paper towel
- toilet paper
- specimen container and label
- "clean catch" kit
- plastic transport bag (if required at your facility)
- bedpan or urinal (if necessary)

PROCEDURE

2. Complete the label with the person's name, room number, and other identifying information. Put the completed label on the specimen container.

3. If the person will be using a regular toilet or bedside commode, help the person to the bathroom or bedside commode. Otherwise, provide the person with a bedpan or urinal, as applicable.
4. Perform hand hygiene and put on the gloves.
5. Place a paper towel on the counter (if the person is in the bathroom) or on the over-bed table (if the person is using a bedside commode, bedpan, or urinal). Open the specimen container and place the lid on the paper towel, with the inside of the lid facing up.
6. Open the "clean catch" kit. Have the person clean his or her perineum using the wipes in the kit. Assist as necessary:
   a. **If the person is a woman:** Use one hand to separate the labia. Hold the wipe in the

(procedure continues on page 590)

PROCEDURE 25-6 (continued)
Collecting a Midstream ("Clean Catch") Urine Specimen

other hand. Place your wipe-covered hand at the top of the vulva and stroke downward to the anus.

b. If the person is a circumcised man: Use one hand to hold the penis slightly away from the body. Hold the wipe in the other hand. Place your wipe-covered hand at the tip of the penis and wash in a circular motion, downward to the base of the penis.

c. If the person is an uncircumcised man: Retract the foreskin by gently pushing the skin toward the base of the penis. Place your wipe-covered hand at the tip of the penis and wash in a circular motion, downward to the base of the penis.

7. Assist the person with urination as necessary. Before leaving the room, remove your gloves and perform hand hygiene. Then:

a. Make sure that the toilet paper, call-light control, and specimen container are within reach.

b. Remind the person that he or she must start the stream of urine, then stop it, then restart it. The urine sample is to be collected from the restarted flow. If the person is a woman, she must hold the labia open until the specimen is collected. If the person is an uncircumcised man, he must keep the foreskin pulled back until the specimen is collected.

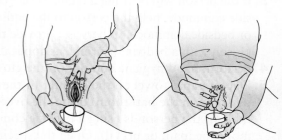

STEP 7b ■ Women must hold the labia open while voiding to prevent contamination of the urine sample. Uncircumcised men must keep the foreskin pulled back.

8. Return when the person signals. Remember to knock before entering.

9. Perform hand hygiene and put on a clean pair of gloves.

10. If the person used a regular toilet or bedside commode, assist the person with handwashing and perineal care as necessary and then help the person to return to bed. If the person used a bedpan or urinal, remove the bedpan or urinal and assist the person with handwashing and perineal care as necessary.

11. Remove your gloves and perform hand hygiene. Put on a clean pair of gloves.

12. Put the lid on the specimen container, being careful not to touch the inside of the lid or container. Make sure that the lid is tight. Put the specimen container on the paper towel on the counter or over-bed table.

13. Remove one glove and dispose of it in a facility-approved waste container. Holding the plastic transport bag in your ungloved hand, place the specimen container into the transport bag with your gloved hand. Avoid touching the outside of the transport bag with your glove.

14. Remove the other glove, dispose of it in a facility-approved waste container, and perform hand hygiene. Put on a clean pair of gloves.

15. Gather the soiled linens and place them in the linen hamper or linen bag. Dispose of disposable items in a facility-approved waste container. Clean equipment and return it to the storage area. Remove your gloves and perform hand hygiene.

16. Take the specimen container to the designated location.

FINISHING UP

17. Complete the "Finishing Up" steps.

WHAT YOU DOCUMENT

■ Date and time specimen was collected
■ Amount of assistance needed
■ Where the specimen was taken or stored for pickup

WHAT DID YOU LEARN?

Multiple Choice

Select the single best answer for each of the following questions.

1. The perineum (perineal area) is cleaned before collecting a:
   a. 24-hour urine specimen
   b. Clean-catch urine specimen
   c. Random urine specimen
   d. Stool specimen

2. The most comfortable position for using a bedpan is:
   a. Fowler's position
   b. Sims' position
   c. Prone position
   d. Supine position

3. In a person with an indwelling urinary catheter, why must the urine drainage bag be kept lower than the person's bladder?
   a. Keeping the drainage bag below bladder level will prevent a bedridden person from seeing the bag, which she might find embarrassing
   b. Keeping the drainage bag below bladder level will keep the person comfortable in bed
   c. Keeping the drainage bag below bladder level will prevent urine from returning to the bladder, where it could cause infection
   d. Keeping the drainage bag below bladder level will prevent the urine from leaking out

4. Which one of the following describes normal urine?
   a. Cloudy with a strong odor
   b. Well-formed
   c. Red-tinged
   d. Clear, light yellow, or golden with a slight odor

5. When caring for a person who is incontinent of urine, it is important to:
   a. Provide good perineal care
   b. Let the person know that his behavior is inappropriate, so it will stop
   c. Take the person to the bathroom once daily
   d. Restrict fluids to reduce the chance of an accident

6. When caring for a person with an indwelling catheter, always remember to:
   a. Leave the drainage bag above the level of the bladder while the person is in bed
   b. Tape any leaks at the connection site
   c. Wear gloves when providing daily catheter care
   d. Tape the drainage tube under the leg

Matching

Match each vocabulary word with its definition.

_____ 1. Hematuria

_____ 2. Micturition

_____ 3. Nocturia

_____ 4. Dysuria

_____ 5. Urinalysis

_____ 6. Anuria

_____ 7. Oliguria

_____ 8. Polyuria

a. Excessive urine production

b. Excessive urination at night

c. Difficulty urinating

d. No urine production

e. Urination

f. Routine urine test

g. Inadequate urine production

h. Blood in the urine

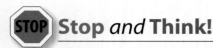 **Stop** *and* **Think!**

You are a nursing assistant in a hospital. One of your patients, Mrs. Walker, must use a bedpan because she is confined to bed, but she is having a hard time relaxing enough to urinate "in bed." What sorts of things could you do to help make using a bedpan easier for Mrs. Walker?

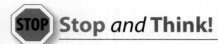 **Stop** *and* **Think!**

You are caring for Miss Smiley, who has an indwelling catheter. When you are making your end-of-shift rounds, you note that Miss Smiley's urinary drainage bag has very little urine in it. You know that the drainage bag was emptied right before you started your shift, and the output was not significant at that time. That was almost 8 hours ago. What concerns do you have regarding Miss Smiley's urine output? What would you do?

Assisting With Bowel Elimination

Bowel elimination is how the body gets rid of the waste products of digestion. In this chapter, you will learn about some common problems with bowel elimination and how the health care team assists people who are having these problems. You will also learn how to assist a patient or resident with ostomy care.

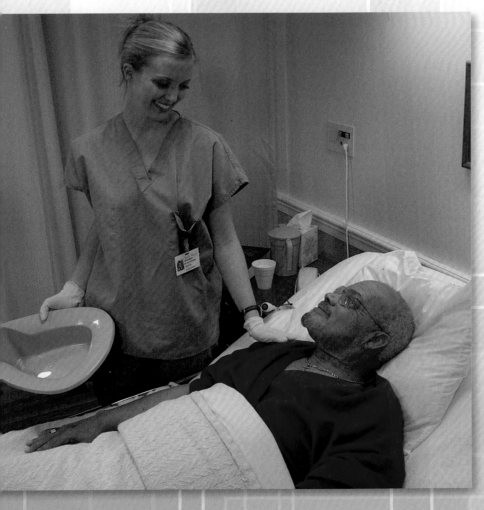

Photo: *A nursing assistant prepares to assist a resident with ostomy care.*

Introduction to Bowel Elimination

What will you learn?

When you are finished with this section, you will be able to:

1. Describe how the digestive system helps to remove waste products from the body.
2. Describe the characteristics of normal feces.
3. Discuss actions you can take to promote normal bowel elimination.
4. Define the words **chyme** and **defecate**.

The Digestive System

Chyme the liquid substance produced by the digestion of food in the stomach

The digestive tract consists of the mouth, esophagus, stomach, small intestine, large intestine, rectum, and anus (Fig. 26-1). In the stomach, the food is broken down and mixed with stomach acid and enzymes to form **chyme**. As the chyme passes through the small and large intestines (the "bowels"), nutrients and fluids

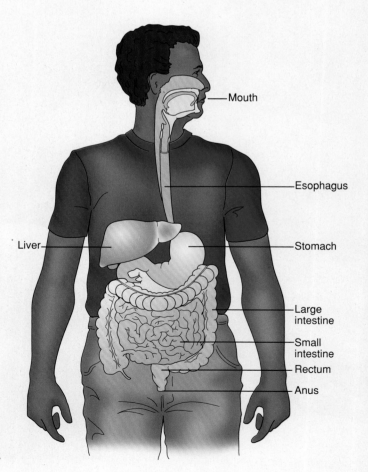

■ **FIGURE 26-1**
The digestive tract.

are absorbed into the bloodstream for use by the body's cells. By the time the chyme reaches the rectum (the last part of the large intestine), almost all of the nutrients and most of the water have been removed from it. The remaining waste material is feces.

The presence of feces in the rectum stimulates the urge to **defecate**, and the feces leave the body through the anus. The process of passing feces from the body is known by several terms, including "having a bowel movement" or "having a BM." When talking about defecation with a patient or resident, use words that the person is familiar with. This is especially important with children.

Defecate to have a bowel movement

Characteristics of Feces

In healthy people, feces are soft, brown, moist, and formed, with a distinct odor. When you are helping a patient or resident with defecation, observe the feces and report any abnormalities to the nurse. Feces with an unusual odor or appearance could be a sign of illness or infection. Certain foods and medications can also affect the odor or appearance of feces.

Defecation Habits

The frequency of a person's bowel movements and the amount of feces passed each time will differ from person to person. Many factors influence a person's defecation habits, including:

- The amount of fluid the person drinks
- The types of food the person eats
- The types of medications the person takes
- The person's age
- The person's level of activity
- The person's life-long elimination habits

For some people, one or two bowel movements a day is normal. For others, one bowel movement every 2 or 3 days is normal. You will soon become aware of the defecation habits that are normal for each person in your care. This knowledge will allow you to recognize any changes that may occur.

Promoting Normal Bowel Elimination

Being in a health care facility can change a person's normal bowel elimination habits, which can cause health problems. The most effective method of treating bowel problems is to prevent them from happening in the first place. As a nursing assistant, there are many ways you can help to promote normal bowel function for your patients or residents (Guidelines Box 26-1).

GUIDELINES BOX 26-1   Guidelines for Promoting Normal Bowel Elimination

What you do	Why you do it
Encourage drinking plenty of fluids, unless a person has a medical condition that requires fluid restriction.	*Drinking plenty of fluids helps to keep the feces soft, making bowel movements easier and preventing constipation.*
Encourage eating foods that contain fiber (such as fruits, vegetables, and whole-grain cereals and breads).	*Fiber adds bulk to the feces, causing it to hold fluid. This helps to keep the feces soft, making bowel movements easier and preventing constipation.*
Encourage regular exercise.	*Regular exercise promotes digestion and helps to prevent constipation.*
Always honor a person's request for assistance with elimination as quickly as possible.	*Holding feces for too long can lead to problems such as constipation. It is also uncomfortable to hold feces for a long time.*
Encourage your patients or residents to call when they first feel the urge to have a bowel movement.	*Holding feces for too long can lead to problems such as constipation. It is also uncomfortable to hold feces for a long time.*
Offer your patients or residents the chance to eliminate frequently, especially if they are bed-bound or require assistance.	*Some people may find it easier to accept an offer of assistance than to ask for help.*
Always provide your patients or residents with as much privacy and comfort as safety considerations will allow.	*Because of the normal odors and sounds that may accompany a bowel movement, many people have difficulty having a bowel movement if they think someone else can hear them or if someone else is in the bathroom with them.*
If a person is having difficulty moving her bowels, try having the person drink warm fluids. Also, make sure that the person does not feel rushed.	*Warm fluids, such as coffee, tea, or warm water with lemon, help stimulate the bowels to empty. Helping the person to relax can make having a bowel movement easier.*

 Putting it all together!

- The digestive system rids the body of waste products that are left over from digestion.
- Normal feces are soft, brown, moist, and formed, with a distinct odor.
- Bowel elimination habits vary from person to person.

- A change in the odor or appearance of a person's feces or in the person's bowel elimination habits could be a sign of illness or infection and should be reported immediately.
- Normal bowel elimination can be promoted by encouraging regular exercise, drinking fluids, and eating foods that contain fiber; by answering the call light promptly; and by providing for the person's privacy and comfort.

Problems With Bowel Elimination

What will you learn?

When you are finished with this section, you will be able to:

1. Discuss problems with bowel elimination that are often experienced by people in a health care setting.
2. Describe ways that the health care team assists a person who is having problems with bowel elimination.
3. State observations that you may make when assisting a person with bowel elimination that should be reported to the nurse.
4. Define the words **diarrhea**, **fecal impaction**, **flatus**, **flatulence**, and **fecal (bowel) incontinence**.

Diarrhea

If **diarrhea** is frequent or excessive, the loss of fluid from the body can quickly cause dehydration, especially in very young or elderly people. When caring for a person with diarrhea:

- Practice good infection control techniques
- Answer the call light quickly to provide access to the toilet, commode, or bedpan
- Provide gentle, thorough skin care after each bowel movement to prevent skin breakdown
- Record and report the frequency and amount of each incident of diarrhea

Diarrhea the passage of liquid, unformed feces

Constipation

Many patients or residents develop constipation (hard, dry feces that are difficult to pass). Risk factors for developing constipation include:

- Taking certain medications
- Not taking in enough dietary fiber and fluids
- Not getting enough exercise
- Delaying having a bowel movement after the urge occurs
- Lack of privacy

If a person is constipated and the regular methods of promoting normal bowel function have failed, the doctor may order a laxative, stool softener, or fiber supplement. These medications are usually given by the nurse.

- **Laxatives** are medications that chemically stimulate peristalsis (wave-like muscular movements of the intestines) so that material inside the intestines moves through at a faster pace.
- **Stool softeners** are medications that help to keep fluid in the feces, making it softer and easier to pass.
- **Fiber supplements** add bulk to the feces, causing it to hold fluid. Fiber supplements can be given in the form of tablets or as a drink additive.

If the constipation is severe, the doctor may order a rectal suppository or enema. Rectal suppositories and enemas are usually administered by the nurse, although you may be asked to assist.

- **Rectal suppositories** are small, wax-like cones or ovals that are inserted into the anus. The wax-like substance dissolves at body temperature, stimulating peristalsis or lubricating and softening the feces.
- **Enemas** are solutions that are placed in the rectum, causing the person to defecate. Enemas are discussed in more detail later in this chapter.

Fecal Impaction

Fecal impaction a condition that occurs when constipation is not relieved

In **fecal impaction**, the feces build up in the rectum, forming a mass that is impossible to pass normally. Liquid feces may seep around the mass. A person with a fecal impaction is usually very uncomfortable and may complain of abdominal or rectal pain or of liquid feces "seeping" out of the anus. The person's abdomen may be swollen.

The doctor may order a rectal suppository or an enema for a person with a fecal impaction. If the rectal suppository or enema does not remove the impaction, the nurse may need to insert a finger into the person's rectum to scoop the impacted mass out piece by piece. Many facilities require the nurse to remove an impaction, but your assistance will be necessary. If you are asked to remove an impaction, make sure that you have been adequately trained for the procedure and that it is part of your job description.

Flatulence

Flatus gas that is formed as part of the digestive process

Flatulence the presence of excessive amounts of flatus (gas) in the intestines, causing abdominal distension (swelling) and discomfort

Like feces, **flatus** is a natural by-product of digestion. **Flatulence** can result from a lack of activity or certain diagnostic and surgical procedures. Getting out of bed and walking might be all that is needed to help the person pass the gas. If walking is not allowed or possible, positioning the person on his left side may help. If the flatulence cannot be relieved by these methods, the nurse may insert a rectal tube to help the gas to escape (Fig. 26-2).

Fecal (Bowel) Incontinence

Fecal (bowel) incontinence the inability to hold one's feces, or the involuntary loss of feces from the bowel

Like urinary incontinence (see Chapter 25), **fecal (bowel) incontinence** can be temporary or permanent. Temporary fecal incontinence is a fairly common occurrence in health care facilities. The effects of medications, being in a strange place, a bout of diarrhea, reluctance to ask for help, and physical or mental disabilities can

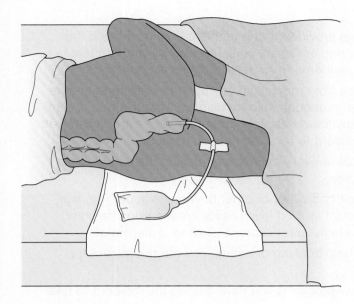

■ **FIGURE 26-2**
A rectal tube may be placed to relieve flatulence (excess gas in the intestines) if the gas cannot be passed naturally. The small bag connected to the end of the rectal tube is used to collect any liquid feces that may escape with the flatus.

all lead to accidents. Permanent fecal incontinence can be caused by many things, including:

■ Injuries or illnesses that affect the spinal cord, the brain, or the nerves that control bowel function

■ Dementia

Incontinence briefs and bed protectors may be used to help manage fecal incontinence. Because being incontinent of feces places a person at risk for developing skin problems (such as rashes and pressure ulcers), perineal care (see Chapter 21) is especially important for people who are incontinent of feces. You will be responsible for making sure that incontinence products are changed frequently and that feces are cleaned from the skin whenever a change occurs.

Bowel training is commonly used to help people who are incontinent of feces. Bowel training works to promote regular, controlled bowel movements and is very similar to bladder training (see Chapter 25). The person's care plan will note any special bowel training techniques that are being used, and the nurse will instruct you on any specific duties you will be assigned as part of that training.

Concerns for Long-Term Care

The normal effects of aging can cause the older adult to experience difficulty with bowel elimination. Slower peristalsis, inactivity, decreased food and fluid intake, certain medications, and a diet low in fiber can dramatically increase a person's risk for constipation. Aging also causes a decrease in a person's sensory perception, which decreases his or her feeling of the urge to have a bowel movement. Constipation, if not prevented and treated, can lead to fecal impaction.

Fecal impaction is considered a *sentinel event* (that is, a condition that should rarely, if ever, be seen in a resident of a long-term care facility). If a resident develops a fecal impaction, the government survey team will be observing the care that is provided to all residents to maintain regular bowel elimination. The surveyors will also check documentation to make

Tell the Nurse!

Problems with defecation

■ Diarrhea

■ Constipation

■ Blood or mucus in the feces

■ Black or dark green feces

■ Foul-smelling feces

■ Feces that are painful or difficult to pass

■ Bleeding from the anus during or after a bowel movement

■ A swollen abdomen

■ Complaints of abdominal or rectal pain

■ Liquid feces "seeping" from the anus

■ Excessive flatus (gas)

■ New fecal (bowel) incontinence

sure that proper care was provided to the resident who developed the fecal impaction. As a nursing assistant, you play a very important role in helping to prevent your residents from developing fecal impactions:

- Find out from the nurse how much fluid you need to provide to ensure that the resident takes in enough fluid to maintain effective bowel elimination and prevent dehydration. Be sure to tell the nurse immediately if you cannot get the resident to take the needed amount.
- Offer the resident fluids at every opportunity (unless the resident has orders for fluid restriction).
- If the resident does not find water or other beverages appealing, try offering snacks that count as fluid (such as ice cream, popsicles, and gelatin) or fruits with a high water content (such as watermelon).
- If the resident needs help drinking or eating, provide the necessary assistance.
- Report to the nurse any problems you have getting the resident to take fluids.
- Know what bowel habits are normal for the resident, and report changes in bowel habits to the nurse immediately. Reporting changes, such as hard stool, difficulty passing stool, or more than 2 days without a bowel movement, promptly can allow the nurse to take quick action and possibly prevent a fecal impaction from occurring.

 Putting it all together!

- Diarrhea may cause dehydration and skin breakdown. When caring for a person with diarrhea, encouraging the person to drink plenty of fluids and providing good skin care are important.
- You can help your patients or residents to avoid constipation by encouraging them to engage in regular exercise, drink plenty of fluids, and eat high-fiber foods, such as fruits and vegetables. If a person does become constipated, the doctor may order a laxative, stool softener, or fiber supplement. If the constipation is severe, the doctor may order a rectal suppository or enema.
- Prolonged constipation can lead to fecal impaction. An enema or rectal suppository may be needed to remove the mass. In some cases, the nurse may need to insert a finger into the person's rectum to break up the mass and remove it bit by bit.
- Flatulence can result from inactivity or a surgical or diagnostic procedure. Assisting the person to get out of bed and walk or positioning the person on his left side may help to pass the gas and relieve discomfort. If these methods do not work, the nurse may insert a rectal tube.
- Bowel training can help restore normal bowel function for many people with fecal (bowel) incontinence.

Obtaining a Stool Specimen

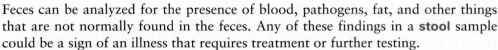

What will you learn?

When you are finished with this section, you will be able to:

1. Demonstrate proper technique for collecting a stool specimen.
2. Define the word **stool**.

Feces can be analyzed for the presence of blood, pathogens, fat, and other things that are not normally found in the feces. Any of these findings in a **stool** sample could be a sign of an illness that requires treatment or further testing.

> **Stool** a term used to refer to fecal matter after it has left the body

The nurse may ask you to collect a specimen and deliver it to the laboratory. Because people do not have bowel movements as often as they urinate, if a stool sample is needed, the person should be notified well in advance so that the specimen can be collected when it becomes available.

Stool can be collected in a bedpan, bedside commode, or collection device placed onto a regular toilet. The person must not urinate at the same time the stool sample is being collected or place toilet paper in the collection device because these actions may change the test results. When collecting a stool sample, be sure to follow the general guidelines for collecting specimens that are given in Guidelines Box 25-4 in Chapter 25.

The procedure for collecting a stool sample is given in Procedure 26-1.

Putting it all together!

- The doctor may request a stool sample to send to the laboratory for analysis. Things not normally found in feces (such as pathogens, fat, or blood) can be a sign of a disorder that requires evaluation and treatment.

- When collecting a stool specimen, it is important to remind the person not to urinate or place toilet paper in the collection device. Also, be sure to tell the person in advance that a stool sample is needed.

- Standard precautions should be taken when handling a stool specimen because contact with body fluids is likely.

Assisting With Enemas

What will you learn?

When you are finished with this section, you will be able to:

1. Describe situations when the doctor might order an enema for a person.
2. List two types of enemas.

3. Identify safety concerns related to administering an enema.
4. Demonstrate the proper technique for administering a cleansing enema.
5. Define the word **enema**.

Enema a solution that is placed into the large intestine by way of the anus for the purpose of removing feces from the rectum

An **enema** may be used to relieve constipation or a fecal impaction when other methods have not worked. An enema is also used to empty the intestine of feces before surgery or certain diagnostic tests. Sometimes enemas are used as part of a bowel training program.

An enema may come pre-packaged and ready to give or it may need to be prepared at the facility and administered using an enema bag (Fig. 26-3). The enema solution that is used varies according to the reason the enema was ordered:

- **Cleansing enemas**, sometimes called "large-volume enemas," contain from 500 to 1000 mL of solution and are primarily used to remove feces from the lower large intestine. Cleansing enemas consist of warm tap water or saline (salt water). Castile soap (a very gentle soap) may be added to the tap water or saline to create a *soapsuds enema*. The soap irritates the lining of the intestine, stimulating peristalsis. A series of cleansing enemas may be ordered prior to tests or surgery that involves the colon to totally clean out the bowel. A single cleansing enema may also be used to relieve constipation.

- **Oil retention enemas** commonly contain olive or mineral oil. The oil lubricates the inside of the rectum and any feces that are present. Oil retention enemas are useful for helping to remove fecal impactions.

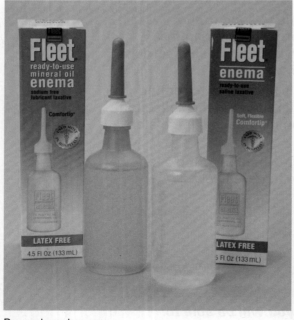

Pre-packaged enemas

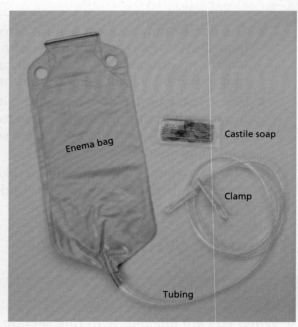

Enema bag

■ **FIGURE 26-3**

Enemas can be pre-packaged and ready to give, or they can be prepared at the facility and given using an enema bag.

■ **Commercial enemas** come pre-packaged and are used to soften the feces and irritate the lining of the rectum, stimulating defecation. Commercial enemas are useful for helping to relieve constipation and as a part of bowel training.

Enemas are ordered by a doctor and usually given by a nurse. You may be asked to assist. General guidelines for assisting with an enema are given in Guidelines Box 26-2.

Some facilities allow nursing assistants who have received the proper training to administer enemas. Make sure that you are familiar with your facility's policy and your job description. If you are permitted to give enemas, be sure to follow proper procedure and the doctor's orders closely. Procedure 26-2 describes how to administer a soapsuds enema.

GUIDELINES BOX 26-2   Guidelines for Assisting With Enemas

What you do	Why you do it
Use the correct solution and the correct amount of solution, as ordered by the doctor.	*The type of enema solution and the amount of enema solution that is given will vary according to the reason the person is receiving the enema.*
Use a bath thermometer to make sure that the enema solution is the correct temperature (usually 105°F [40.5°C]).	*If the enema solution is too cool, it may cause abdominal cramping and pain. If the enema solution is too hot, it can cause serious injury (possibly even death).*
Before beginning the procedure, make sure that a bed protector and bedpan are in place or that the path to the bathroom is clear.	*When it comes time for the person to expel the enema, she will need immediate access to toilet facilities.*
Ensure the person's privacy by closing the curtain and the door to the room and keeping the person covered with a bath blanket.	*Receiving an enema can be embarrassing. Ensuring the person's privacy and keeping the person covered help to lessen the person's embarrassment.*
Position the person on her left side in Sims' position.	*Left Sims' position allows the solution to clean a longer segment of intestine.*
After the enema has been administered, have the person hold the enema for the specified amount of time before expelling it.	*Some enema solutions require a certain amount of time to stimulate the bowels or to soften the feces.*
Cleansing enemas ordered "until clear" means that enemas are given until the enema return does not contain any feces. If you are responsible for giving cleansing enemas "until clear," ask the nurse how many enemas are allowed to be given.	*If too many enemas are given in one session, the solution can be absorbed through the intestinal walls into the bloodstream, causing a fluid imbalance in the person's body.*

Putting it all together!

- An enema is a solution that is placed in the large intestine by way of the anus to remove feces from the rectum. The doctor may order an enema to relieve constipation or a fecal impaction or to prepare the person for surgery or a diagnostic test.

- There are three main types of enemas: cleansing enemas, oil-retention enemas, and commercial enemas. The type of enema used varies according to the reason the enema was ordered.

- Some enemas are prepared by the nurse or nursing assistant and others come pre-packaged. When preparing an enema solution, make sure that it is prepared according to the nurse's instructions and that the solution is the proper temperature.

- Enemas are usually given by the nurse. If you are permitted to give enemas at your facility, always follow proper procedure and the doctor's or nurse's instructions carefully.

- Standard precautions should be taken when assisting with enemas because contact with body fluids is likely.

Assisting With Ostomy Care

What will you learn?

When you are finished with this section, you will be able to:

1. Describe the two most common types of ostomies.
2. Discuss the emotional impact that having an ostomy may have on a person.
3. Demonstrate proper technique for providing routine ostomy care.
4. Define the word **ostomy**.

Ostomy an artificial opening in the abdomen for the elimination of feces

Some of your patients or residents may have had surgery to remove part of their intestines (for example, as a result of cancer or trauma). After part of the intestine is removed, the person may not be able to eliminate feces through the anus. In this case, an artificial opening, called a *stoma*, is made in the person's abdomen, and the remaining portion of the intestine is connected to it (Fig. 26-4). The resulting **ostomy** may be temporary or permanent. The feces pass through the stoma and into a pouch (called an *ostomy appliance*) that is worn over the stoma (Fig. 26-5).

Many people who have an ostomy are able to manage their own ostomy care. Others may need help. The supplies used for ostomies vary greatly. For example, some appliances are used only once and then discarded, while others are emptied, cleaned, and used again. If providing ostomy care is within your scope of practice, make sure that you are familiar with the different types of ostomy supplies used in

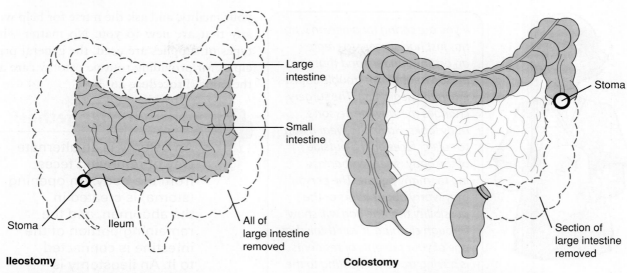

Ileostomy

- The entire large intestine is removed
- The end of the small intestine (the ileum) is attached to the abdominal wall
- Feces are very liquid and may flow continuously because the chyme does not have the chance to travel through the large intestine, where water is reabsorbed

Colostomy

- Part of the large intestine is removed
- The healthy end of the large intestine is attached to the abdominal wall
- Feces vary in consistency, depending on what portion of the intestine was removed
  - Near the beginning of the large intestine = more liquid
  - Near the end of the large intestine = more formed

■ **FIGURE 26-4**

A stoma may be located in various places on a person's abdomen, depending on what part of the intestine had to be removed.

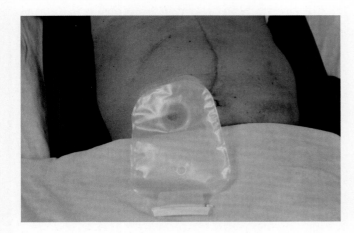

■ **FIGURE 26-5**

An ostomy appliance is worn over the stoma to collect the feces.

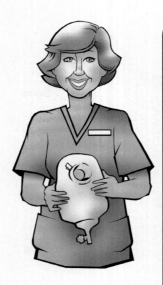

If you are caring for a person who has just had surgery to create an ostomy, understand that the person might have trouble adjusting in the beginning. The surgery changes the way the person's body looks. Having to wear a bag to collect feces on the outside of the body is very embarrassing for many people. The person may worry about odors or the possibility that the bag will show through clothing. If you think that one of your patients or residents is having trouble adjusting to the ostomy, share your concerns with the nurse.

your facility, and ask the nurse for help with any that are new to you. No matter what types of supplies are used, the general principles for providing routine ostomy care are the same (Procedure 26-3).

 Putting it all together!

- An ostomy is an alternate way of removing feces from the body. An opening (stoma) is created in the abdomen, and the remaining portion of the intestine is connected to it. An ileostomy is created if the entire large intestine must be removed. A colostomy is created when only part of the large intestine must be removed.

- For many people, having an ostomy is difficult emotionally, especially when the ostomy is new.

- Proper care of the ostomy site is necessary to keep the skin clean and healthy.

- Standard precautions should be taken when assisting with ostomy care because contact with body fluids is likely.

PROCEDURES

PROCEDURE 26-1
Collecting a Stool Specimen

Why you do it: A stool sample is often requested for analysis. Proper collection and handling of the stool sample helps to ensure that the test results are accurate.

GETTING READY
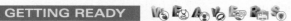

1. Complete the "Getting Ready" steps.

SUPPLIES

- gloves
- paper towel
- tongue depressor
- toilet paper
- specimen container and label
- plastic transport bag (if required at your facility)
- plastic bag or waste container
- specimen collection device ("commode hat") or bedpan

PROCEDURE

2. Complete the label with the person's name, room number, and other identifying information. Put the completed label on the specimen container. Take the specimen container to the bathroom. Place a paper towel on the counter. Open the specimen container and place the lid on the paper towel with the inside of the lid facing up.

3. Perform hand hygiene and put on gloves. If the person will be using a regular toilet or bedside commode, fit the specimen collection device underneath the toilet or commode seat. Otherwise, provide the person with a bedpan.

4. Assist the person with defecation as necessary. Before leaving the room, remind the person not to urinate or place toilet paper into the specimen collection device or bedpan. Provide a plastic bag or waste container for the used toilet paper.

5. Return when the person signals. Remember to knock before entering.

6. Perform hand hygiene and put on the gloves.

7. If the person used a regular toilet or bedside commode, assist the person with handwashing and then help the person to return to bed. Provide perineal care as necessary. If the person used a bedpan, cover and remove the bedpan and assist the person with handwashing and perineal care as necessary.

8. Take the covered bedpan or specimen collection device (if the person used a bedside commode) to the bathroom. (If the side rails are in use, raise the side rails before leaving the bedside, making sure that you remove your gloves and perform hand hygiene before touching the side rails or other items.)

9. Put on a clean pair of gloves. Note the color, amount, and quality of the feces. Using the tongue depressor, take two tablespoons of feces from the bedpan or specimen collection device and put them into the specimen container. Dispose of the tongue depressor in a facility-approved waste container. Empty the remaining contents of the bedpan or specimen collection device into the toilet.

10. Put the lid on the specimen container. Make sure that the lid is tight. Put the specimen container on the paper towel on the counter.

11. Remove one glove and dispose of it in a facility-approved waste container. Holding the plastic transport bag in your ungloved hand, place the specimen container into the transport bag with your gloved hand. Avoid touching the outside of the transport bag with your glove.

12. Remove the other glove, dispose of it in a facility-approved waste container, and perform hand hygiene.

(procedure continues on page 608)

PROCEDURE 26-1 (continued)
Collecting a Stool Specimen

13. Put on a clean pair of gloves. Gather the soiled linens and place them in the linen hamper or linen bag. Dispose of disposable items in a facility-approved waste container. Clean equipment and return it to the storage area. Remove your gloves and perform hand hygiene.
14. Take the specimen container to the designated location.

FINISHING UP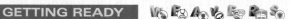

15. Complete the "Finishing Up" steps.

WHAT YOU DOCUMENT

- Date and time specimen was collected
- Color, amount, and quality of feces
- Where the specimen was taken or stored for pickup

PROCEDURE 26-2
Administering a Soapsuds (Large-Volume) Enema

Why you do it: A soapsuds enema may be ordered to remove feces from the large intestine prior to surgery or a diagnostic procedure. Proper administration of the enema is important to protect the person's safety and privacy during the procedure and to ensure that the enema is effective.

GETTING READY

1. Complete the "Getting Ready" steps.

SUPPLIES

- gloves
- paper towel
- toilet paper
- bed protector
- lubricant jelly
- 5-mL packet of castile soap
- bedpan or bedside commode
- bedpan cover (if needed)
- enema bag with tubing and clamp
- IV pole
- bath thermometer
- bath blanket
- perineal care supplies

PROCEDURE

2. Make sure that the bed is positioned at a comfortable working height (to promote good body mechanics) and that the wheels are locked.
3. Prepare the enema solution in the bathroom or utility room. Clamp the tubing and then fill the enema bag with warm water (105°F [40.5°C] on the bath thermometer) in the specified amount (usually from 500 to 1000 mL). Add the castile soap packet and mix by gently rotating the enema bag. Do not shake the solution vigorously.
4. Release the clamp on the tubing and allow a little water to run through the tubing into the sink or bedpan. This will remove all of the air from the tubing. Reclamp the tubing.
5. Hang the enema bag on the IV pole and bring it to the person's bedside. Adjust the height of the IV pole so that the enema bag is hanging no more than 18 inches above the person's anus.
6. If the side rails are in use, lower the side rail on the working side of the bed. The side rail on the opposite side of the bed should remain up. Lower the head of the bed so that the bed is flat (as tolerated).
7. Spread the bath blanket over the top linens (and the person). If the person is able, have her hold the bath blanket. If not, tuck the corners under her shoulders. Fanfold the top linens to the foot of the bed.
8. Ask the person to lie on her left side, facing away from you, in Sims' position. Help her into this position, if necessary.

9. Perform hand hygiene and put on the gloves.

10. Adjust the bath blanket and the person's hospital gown or pajama bottoms as necessary to expose the person's buttocks. Position the bed protector under the person's buttocks to keep the bed linens dry.

11. Open the lubricant package and squeeze a small amount of lubricant onto a paper towel. Lubricate the tip of the enema tubing to ease insertion.

12. Suggest that the person take a deep breath and slowly exhale as the enema tubing is inserted. With one hand, raise the person's upper buttock to expose the anus. Using your other hand, gently and carefully insert the lubricated tip of the tubing into the person's rectum (not more than 3 to 4 inches for adults). Direct the tube upward toward the umbilicus, not the bladder. Never force the tubing into the rectum. If you are unable to insert the tubing, stop and call the nurse.

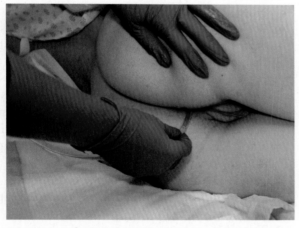

STEP 12 ■ Gently insert the top of the tubing into the person's rectum.

13. Unclamp the tubing and allow the solution to begin running slowly. Allow 5 to 10 minutes for all of the solution to be instilled. Hold the enema tubing firmly with one hand so that it does not slip out of the rectum. If the person complains of pain or cramping, slow down the rate of flow by tightening the clamp a bit. If the pain or cramping does not stop after slowing the rate of flow, stop the procedure and call the nurse.

14. When the fluid level reaches the bottom of the bag, clamp the tubing to avoid injecting air into the person's rectum.

15. Remove the tubing from the person's rectum and place it inside the enema bag. Gently place several thicknesses of toilet paper against the person's anus to absorb any fluid.

16. Ask the person to retain the enema solution for the specific amount of time.

17. Dispose of the enema bag, tubing, and other items. Remove your gloves and perform hand hygiene before touching any items that are clean, such as the side rails of the bed.

18. Perform hand hygiene and put on gloves. Assist the person with expelling the enema as necessary, using the bedpan, bedside commode, or toilet. If the person is using a regular toilet, ask her not to flush the toilet after expelling the enema.

19. If the person used a regular toilet or bedside commode, assist her with handwashing and then help her to return to bed. Provide perineal care as necessary. If the person used a bedpan, cover and remove the bedpan and assist her with handwashing and perineal care as necessary.

20. Remove your gloves and perform hand hygiene.

21. Raise the head of the bed as the person requests. Make sure that the bed is lowered to its lowest position and that the wheels are locked. (If the side rails are in use, raise the side rails before leaving the bedside.)

22. Put on gloves. Take the covered bedpan or commode bucket (if the person used a bedside commode) to the bathroom.

23. Note the color, amount, and quality of feces before emptying the contents of the bedpan or commode bucket into the toilet. (If anything unusual is observed, do not empty the bedpan or commode bucket until a nurse has had a chance to look at its contents.)

24. Gather the soiled linens and place them in the linen hamper. Dispose of disposable items in a facility-approved waste container. Clean equipment and return it to the storage area.

25. Remove your gloves, dispose of them in a facility-approved waste container, and perform hand hygiene.

(*procedure continues on page 610*)

PROCEDURE 26-2 (continued)
Administering a Soapsuds (Large-Volume) Enema

FINISHING UP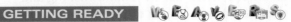

26. Complete the "Finishing Up" steps.

WHAT YOU DOCUMENT

- Date and time
- Type of enema given
- Amount of fluid instilled

- How long patient or resident "held" the enema fluid
- Complaints of pain or cramping
- Color, amount, and quality of feces and enema fluid expelled
- Any abnormal observations; and if present, that they were reported to the nurse

PROCEDURE 26-3
Providing Routine Ostomy Care

Why you do it: Because the skin around the stoma comes in contact with feces, it must be kept clean to prevent irritation.

GETTING READY

1. Complete the "Getting Ready" steps.

SUPPLIES

- gloves
- paper towels
- bed protector
- toilet paper
- 4 × 4 gauze pad
- clean ostomy appliance
- skin barrier
- bedpan
- bedpan cover (or paper towels)
- wash basin
- mild soap (or other cleansing agent, per facility policy)
- adhesive remover (optional)
- washcloths
- towel
- graduate container

PROCEDURE

2. Clean the surface of the over-bed table and cover it with paper towels. Place the ostomy supplies and clean linens on the over-bed table.
3. Make sure that the bed is positioned at a comfortable working height (to promote good body mechanics) and that the wheels are locked.
4. If the side rails are in use, lower the side rail on the working side of the bed. The side rail on the opposite side of the bed should remain up. If necessary, lower the head of the bed so that the bed is flat (as tolerated).

5. Fanfold the top linens to below the person's waist.
6. Position the bed protector on the bed alongside the person to keep the bed linens dry. Adjust the person's clothing as necessary to expose the person's stoma.
7. Perform hand hygiene and put on the gloves.
8. Remove the clamp from the end of the ostomy bag and fold the end of the pouch upward like a cuff. Empty the contents of the ostomy bag into the graduate container.
9. Wipe the lower 2 inches of the ostomy bag with toilet tissue and uncuff the pouch. Reapply the closure clip.
10. Take the graduate container to the bathroom. If you must raise the siderails on the bed or touch the door handle, remove one of your gloves.
11. Remove your gloves and perform hand hygiene.
12. Put on a clean pair of gloves. Disconnect the ostomy appliance from the ostomy belt if one is used. Remove the belt. If the ostomy belt is soiled, dispose of it in a facility-approved waste container (if it is disposable), or place it in the linen hamper or linen bag (if it is not disposable).

13. Remove the ostomy appliance by holding the skin taut and gently pushing the skin away from the appliance, starting at the top. If the adhesive is making removal difficult, use warm water or the adhesive solvent to soften the adhesive. Place the ostomy appliance in the bedpan.

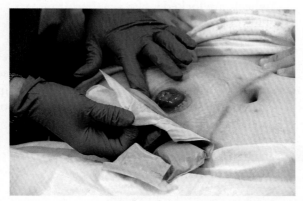

STEP 13 ■ Hold the skin taut and gently push the skin away from the appliance.

14. Gently wipe the stoma with toilet paper to remove any feces or drainage. Place the toilet paper in the bedpan. Cover the stoma with the gauze pad to absorb any drainage that may occur until the new appliance is in place.

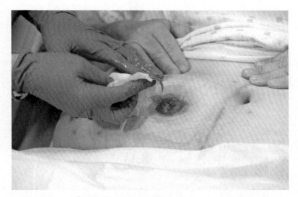

STEP 14 ■ Gently wipe the stoma with toilet tissue to remove drainage.

15. Cover the bedpan with the bedpan cover or paper towels. Take the bedpan to the bathroom. (If the side rails are in use, remove one glove and raise them before leaving the bedside.)

16. Note the color, amount, and quality of the feces before emptying the contents of the ostomy appliance and the bedpan into the toilet. (If anything unusual is observed, do not empty the ostomy appliance until a nurse has had a chance to look at its contents.)

17. Dispose of the ostomy appliance in a facility-approved waste container.

18. Remove your gloves and perform hand hygiene.

19. Fill the wash basin with warm water (110°F [43.3°C] to 115°F [46.1°C] on the bath thermometer). Return to the bedside. Place the basin on the over-bed table. If the side rails are in use, lower the side rail on the working side of the bed.

20. Perform hand hygiene and put on a clean pair of gloves.

21. Form a mitt around your hand with one of the washcloths. Wet the mitt with warm, clean water and apply mild soap (or other cleansing agent, per facility policy). Remove the gauze pad from the stoma and dispose of it in a facility-approved waste container. Clean the skin around the stoma. Rinse and dry the skin around the stoma thoroughly.

22. Apply the skin barrier if needed, according to the manufacturer's directions.

23. Put the clean ostomy belt on the person if an ostomy belt is used.

24. Make sure that the opening on the ostomy appliance is the correct size. Remove the adhesive backing on the ostomy appliance.

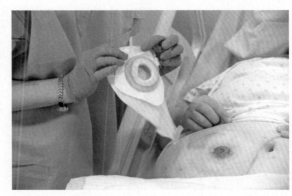

STEP 24 ■ Make sure the opening on the ostomy appliance is the correct size.

25. Center the appliance over the stoma, making sure that the drain or the end of the bag is pointed down. Gently press around the edges to seal the ostomy appliance to the skin.

(procedure continues on page 612)

PROCEDURE 26-3 (continued)
Providing Routine Ostomy Care

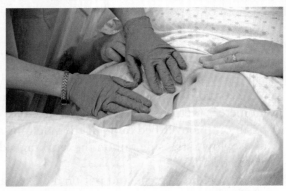

STEP 25 ▪ Gently press the edges to seal the ostomy appliance to the skin.

26. Connect the ostomy appliance to the ostomy belt, if one is used.
27. Remove the bed protector.
28. Remove your gloves and perform hand hygiene.
29. Adjust the person's clothing as necessary to cover the ostomy appliance. If the bedding is wet or soiled, change the bed linens. Help the person back into a comfortable position, straighten the bottom linens, and draw the top linens over the person. Raise the head of the bed, as the person requests.

30. If the side rails are in use, return the side rail to the raised position. Make sure that the bed is lowered to its lowest position and that the wheels are locked.
31. Put on gloves and gather the soiled linens and place them in the linen hamper or linen bag. Dispose of disposable items in a facility-approved waste container. Clean the over-bed table according to facility policy. Clean equipment and return it to the storage area. Remove your gloves and perform hand hygiene.

FINISHING UP

32. Complete the "Finishing Up" steps.

WHAT YOU DOCUMENT

- Date and time
- Type of care given
- Type of ostomy appliance used
- Condition of skin around ostomy
- Amount, color, and character of feces
- Any abnormal observations; and if present, that they were reported to the nurse

WHAT DID YOU LEARN?

Multiple Choice

Select the single best answer for each of the following questions.

1. How far is an enema tube inserted into the rectum in an adult?
   a. 3 to 4 inches
   b. 5 to 6 inches
   c. 7 to 8 inches
   d. 12 to 16 inches

2. One of your residents needs to have an enema administered. How should you position the resident in preparation for the enema?
   a. Left Sims' position
   b. Fowler's position
   c. Supine position
   d. Right Sims' position

3. A healthy person's feces will be:
   a. Black and tarry
   b. Soft, brown, formed, and moist with a distinct odor
   c. Hard and pellet-like
   d. Long and stringy

4. To help your residents or patients to maintain healthy bowel function, it is important to:
   a. Answer call lights promptly
   b. Encourage them to eat a well-balanced diet and drink plenty of fluids
   c. Assist them with exercise
   d. All of the above

5. Mr. Pak has an ileostomy, and you assist him with stoma care. What would you expect his feces to be like?
   a. Very liquid, continuously flowing
   b. Hard, dry, pellets
   c. Soft, brown, moist, and formed
   d. None of the above

6. What is the artificial opening for a colostomy called?
   a. A stoma
   b. A rectum
   c. An anus
   d. None of the above

Matching

Match each bowel disorder with its description.

_____ 1. Diarrhea

_____ 2. Fecal impaction

_____ 3. Flatulence

_____ 4. Constipation

_____ 5. Fecal (bowel) incontinence

a. Occurs when constipation is not relieved

b. The passage of liquid, unformed feces

c. Occurs when the feces remain in the intestines too long, resulting in hard, dry feces that are difficult to pass

d. Excessive amounts of gas in the intestines, causing abdominal swelling and discomfort

e. The involuntary loss of feces from the bowel

 ## Stop *and* Think!

Mr. Scott is a 42-year-old executive at an advertising agency who was recently diagnosed with colon cancer. Mr. Scott is married, with three young children. He is an avid golfer and swimmer. Following surgery to remove the cancer, Mr. Scott will have a colostomy. You are the nursing assistant who will be caring for Mr. Scott in the hospital in the days following the surgery. Describe some of the emotions Mr. Scott may be feeling after the surgery. How would you respond if Mr. Scott decided to share some of these feelings with you?

Assisting With Comfort

When we are comfortable, we feel content, without pain or distress. We are able to rest and relax. Helping patients and residents to be as comfortable as possible is an important part of providing holistic care. In this chapter, you will learn about actions nursing assistants can take to promote comfort, rest, and sleep. You will also learn about pain, which affects many patients' and residents' ability to rest and relax.

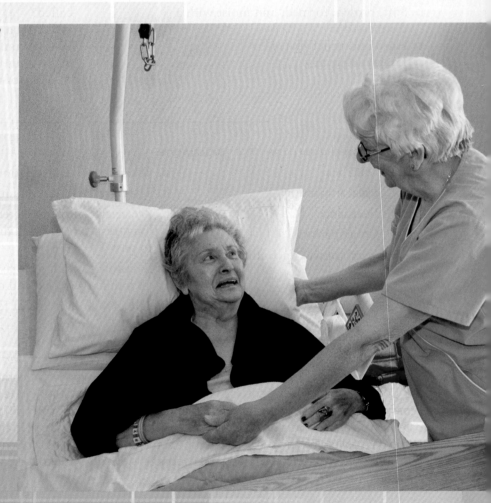

Photo: *A nursing assistant helps to position a resident comfortably.*

General Comfort Measures

What will you learn?

When you are finished with this section, you will be able to:

1. Explain why rest and sleep are important.
2. Discuss factors that may affect a person's ability to rest and sleep in a health care setting.
3. Describe ways that you can help promote rest and sleep.
4. Demonstrate proper technique for giving a back massage.

Rest and sleep are basic physical needs. Many things can affect a patient's or resident's ability to rest and sleep:

- The person may be in pain or have a chronic health condition.
- The environment may be unfamiliar. There are different sounds and smells. The bed feels different than the person's bed at home. The person may have a roommate.
- The person may be worried about his health, finances, family members, or pets that have been left at home.
- The person may have a sleep disorder that keeps him from sleeping properly.

Nursing assistants do many things to help keep their patients or residents as comfortable as possible so that they can rest and sleep (Box 27-1). Many of your daily responsibilities (such as bedmaking, assisting with elimination, and assisting with hygiene and grooming) help to keep your patients physically comfortable by helping them to meet their physical needs. You also provide emotional comfort, for example, by taking the time to sit and hold a patient's or resident's hand while the person talks.

One very common comfort measure nursing assistants use is the back massage. A back massage is relaxing for the patient or resident, and it gives you a chance to observe the person's skin for potential problems. Massaging the skin also helps to stimulate the circulation, which is important for preventing pressure ulcers. A back massage is usually given after a person's bath while rubbing lotion into the skin, after repositioning a person, or as a part of evening care to promote relaxation and sleep.

An effective back massage takes 4 to 6 minutes to complete and can be performed with the person in either the prone or the lateral position. As with any personal care procedure, always check with a nurse or read the person's nursing care plan before beginning—a person who has fractured ribs or a back injury or who has recently had back surgery should not receive a back massage. Procedure 27-1 describes how to give a back massage.

Concerns for Long-Term Care

Elderly people take longer to fall asleep and awaken more frequently during the night. As a person ages, she becomes more sensitive to noise when sleeping and will awaken more easily. This is a major concern in the long-term care setting. Because of this, an elderly person is more likely to need a regular daytime nap, which can help compensate for the loss of sleep at night and prevent daytime drowsiness.

An elderly person is also more likely to have one or more chronic health conditions that cause enough discomfort to interfere with a good night's sleep. Elderly people, especially men, wake up to urinate several times during the night and may have difficulty falling back asleep. Many people suffer from what is known as *restless leg syndrome*, an irresistible urge to move one's legs accompanied by unpleasant sensations in the legs. Many medications can cause a person to have difficulty with falling asleep or staying asleep.

Studies have shown that many residents in the long-term care setting seldom sleep for more than 1 hour at a time. A lack of sleep for elderly people can increase the risk of anxiety, delirium, and depression. Physical fatigue from the lack of sleep can also make a person more likely to fall.

BOX 27-1   Actions to Promote Rest and Sleep for Your Patients and Residents

- Encourage increased physical activity during the day. Physical activity during the day promotes better sleep at night. This is especially important for residents of a long-term care facility.

- Increase a person's exposure to daytime lighting, especially sunlight, during the day.

- Limit time for naps during the day. Although a short nap during the day can help an older person meet his sleep requirements, taking too many naps or naps that are too long can negatively affect the person's ability to sleep at night.

- Avoid giving the person beverages with caffeine (such as regular coffee, tea, or cola) in the afternoon or evening. Many people are sensitive to caffeine and find that it keeps them up at night if they have it too late in the day.

- Promote relaxation by giving the person a warm bath in the evening, or providing a massage. Finding out the person's normal bedtime routines, and following them as closely as possible, is also important for promoting relaxation and sleep.

- Offer the person a snack at bedtime.

- Assist the person with basic hygiene and elimination just before bedtime.

- Create a comfortable environment for sleeping. Straighten the bed linens and fluff the pillows. Provide a warm blanket. Make sure that items are put away and the room is neat and free of clutter. Close the blinds or draperies to darken the room, and turn off the overhead lights. (A night light may be left on for safety.) Make sure that the room temperature is not too hot or too cold.

- Position the person carefully, using good body alignment.

- Turn off the television set or radio (unless the person watches television or listens to the radio to relax before bed). Many people find soft music very relaxing at bed time. Others like to be read to from a favorite book.

- Be observant. For example, if the person seems upset or worried about something, you should report this to the nurse because stress or worry can impact the person's ability to sleep. Similarly, if the person seems to be in pain or have some other type of physical discomfort, report this to the nurse.

Putting it all together!

- Rest and sleep are basic physical needs that may be difficult to meet in a health care setting for many reasons. In order to rest and sleep, we must be comfortable, both physically and emotionally.
- Nursing assistants do many things to promote comfort and help their patients or residents to rest.
- A back massage is relaxing for the patient or resident and helps to prevent the development of pressure ulcers.

Managing Pain

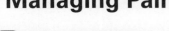 **What will you learn?**

When you are finished with this section, you will be able to:

1. Understand the different types of pain that a patient or resident may have.
2. List factors that can affect how a person responds to pain.
3. State observations that you may make that might be a sign that a person is in pain.
4. Describe how to gather information about a person's pain to report to the nurse.
5. Explain why prompt reporting of a person's pain to the nurse is important.
6. Describe medications used to control pain.
7. Describe how a nursing assistant can help a person who is in pain.
8. Define the words **acute pain** and **chronic pain**.

Pain is the body's distress signal. Pain tells us that we have been injured, that we have overworked a muscle group, that an organ is not working properly, or that we are ill. Many of the people in your care will have some type of pain. **Acute pain** occurs with an injury and lasts a short period of time. Acute pain decreases as the body's tissues repair themselves and heal. **Chronic pain** continues even after tissue healing has taken place. Chronic pain may be caused by conditions such as arthritis or cancer. Either type of pain can make it difficult for a person to rest, relax, and sleep.

It is important for the nurse to know whether a patient or resident is in pain. If the pain is new, the nurse will need to find out what is causing the pain. Even if the pain is familiar and the cause of it is known, there may still be something the nurse can do to help make the person more comfortable. As a nursing assistant, you may be the first to notice that one of your patients or residents is in pain.

Acute pain sharp, sudden pain

Chronic pain slow, diffuse, constant pain

BOX 27-2 Reporting Pain

Pain is a totally subjective experience. Only the person feeling the pain can describe what she is feeling. If a person is having pain, ask the person the following questions to get more details about her pain before reporting to the nurse:

- Where is the pain?

- How does the pain feel (for example, is it throbbing, aching, sharp, dull)?

- How long have you been feeling this pain?

- Does anything make the pain feel better (or worse)?

- How intense is the pain? (To help the person answer this question, you can ask her to rate the pain on a scale of 1 to 10, with 10 being the worst pain imaginable and 1 being slight discomfort.)

Tell the Nurse!

Nonverbal signs of pain

- Facial expressions (such as grimacing or gritting the teeth)

- The person avoids using a certain body part

- Redness and swelling of a body part

- Profuse sweating

- Changes in the person's vital signs

- Changes in the person's behavior
  - Moaning
  - Crying
  - Restlessness
  - Calling out
  - Rubbing the area of the body that is in pain

- Resisting care

Recognizing and Reporting Pain

People respond to pain in different ways. A person's culture and upbringing, past experience with pain, and sense of responsibility toward others might affect how the person responds to pain. Some people will tell you about their pain and ask for relief. Other people may try to ignore or "work through" pain. A person's body language or behavior may tell you that the person is in pain, even if the person does not actually say anything.

Report any observations that suggest that a patient or resident is in pain, or any complaints that the person may have of pain, to a nurse promptly. Providing the nurse with as much detail as possible about the person's pain is helpful (Box 27-2). Prompt and accurate reporting will help to ensure that measures are taken to make the person more comfortable, sooner.

Medications for Treating Pain

Over-the-counter medications—such as aspirin, acetaminophen (Tylenol), and ibuprofen (Advil)—can relieve mild to moderate pain. Narcotics, such as morphine or Demerol, may be needed to control severe pain. People who need narcotics to control their pain should be encouraged to ask for medication before the pain becomes too intense. Giving a small dose of a narcotic early on can help to stop the pain before it gets too bad. If left untreated, the pain will only get worse, and a higher dose of the medication will be needed to relieve it. Although giving medications is beyond the scope of practice for most nursing assistants, you will play an important role in helping the person to manage his pain by reporting requests for medication to the nurse promptly.

The Nursing Assistant's Role in Managing Pain

Although administering medications and other treatments for pain is often out of a nursing assistant's scope of practice, there are many things you can do to help a patient or resident who is in pain:

- Report complaints of pain, requests for relief from pain, and observations that suggest that a person is in pain to the nurse promptly.

- Help the person to relax using the general comfort measures described in Box 27-1. Anxiety causes the body to become tense, which increases pain.

- Some people like to be distracted from their pain by listening to music, watching television, reading, or just talking.

Remember that each person's response to pain, and the methods she is most comfortable using to find relief from it, will vary.

 ## Putting it all together!

- Pain is the body's signal that something is wrong. Acute pain lasts a short period of time and decreases as the body heals. Chronic pain is a lasting pain.

- The way a person responds to pain depends on several factors, including the person's culture and her previous experience with pain.

- A person's nonverbal communication may tell you that the person is in pain, even if he does not actually say anything to you. A patient's or resident's facial expression or a change in behavior may be the only sign that the person is having pain.

- As a nursing assistant, one of the most important things you can do for your patients or residents is notice and report pain. Prompt and accurate reporting helps to ensure that measures are taken to make the person more comfortable, sooner.

- Nursing assistants help to keep patients and residents comfortable by encouraging them to ask for pain medication when they need it and relaying these requests to the nurse.

- Simple care procedures, such as straightening the bed linens, positioning the person comfortably, giving a back massage, dimming the lights, and closing the door to the room can be very comforting to a person who is in pain.

Heat and Cold Applications

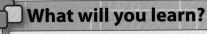 ## What will you learn?

When you are finished with this section, you will be able to:

1. Discuss the use of heat and cold applications to promote comfort.
2. Identify safety concerns related to heat and cold applications.
3. State observations that you may make when assisting with a heat or cold application that should be reported to the nurse.
4. Demonstrate proper technique for giving a moist cold application.
5. Demonstrate proper technique for giving a dry cold application.
6. Demonstrate proper technique for giving a dry heat application.

TABLE 27-1	**Effects of Heat and Cold Applications**
Heat	**Cold**
■ Widens (dilates) the blood vessels	■ Constricts (narrows) the blood vessels
■ Reduces pain and promotes circulation to speed healing	■ Reduces pain and prevents swelling
■ Relieves muscle spasms	■ Numbs sensation and controls bleeding
■ Provides warmth	■ Reduces fevers
■ Decreases muscle and joint stiffness	■ Reduces muscle spasms

The application of heat or cold can be used to reduce or prevent tissue swelling, promote healing, ease pain, and promote comfort. Heat and cold have opposite effects on the body (Table 27-1).

Heat and cold applications can be either moist or dry (Fig. 27-1):

Moist   **Dry**

Cold

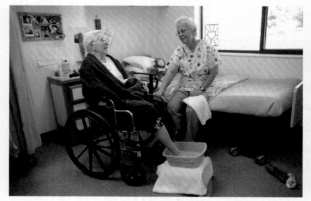

Cold compress

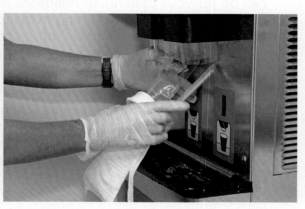

Ice bag

Heat

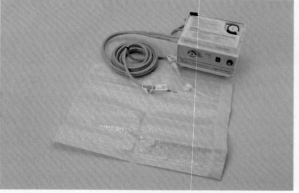

Warm soak

Aquamatic pad

■ **FIGURE 27-1**

Heat and cold applications may be either moist or dry.

- **Moist applications.** In moist applications, moisture comes in direct contact with the skin. Examples of moist applications include hot and cold compresses and warm soaks. Moist applications allow the heat or cold to penetrate the tissues more quickly and deeply.
- **Dry applications.** Dry applications prevent moisture from coming in direct contact with the skin. Examples of dry applications include ice bags, hot water bottles, and heating (Aquamatic) pads. In an Aquamatic pad, water is heated in the heating unit. The heated water passes through the tubing and into a network of tubes inside the heating pad. The hot water never comes in contact with the person's skin.

Because the application of heat or cold can be dangerous, these treatments require a doctor's order, and in some facilities, the application of heat or cold may be outside of the nursing assistant's scope of practice. Even if you are not permitted to give these treatments, you will be involved with monitoring patients or residents who are receiving them. Some people are at very high risk for injury from the application of heat or cold and must be monitored carefully:

- **Older people, very young people, and chronically ill people.** The skin of people who are very old, very young, or chronically ill can be fragile and sensitive.
- **People with fair skin.** Fair skin tends to be more sensitive to temperature changes than darker skin.
- **People with impaired sensation.** People with impaired sensation, such as those who are paralyzed or who have diabetes, are at risk for injury because they are unable to tell that an application is too hot or too cold.
- **People with impaired consciousness.** People with impaired consciousness may not be able to communicate that an application is too hot or too cold.

Guidelines for assisting with heat and cold applications are given in Guidelines Box 27-1. Procedure 27-2 describes how to give a moist cold application. Procedure 27-3 describes how to give a dry cold application. Procedure 27-4 describes how to give a dry heat application with an Aquamatic pad.

Tell the Nurse!

Heat and cold applications

- Skin that is pale and does not return to its normal color quickly after a cold application is removed
- Skin that is bright red or very pale and does not return to its normal color quickly after a heat application is removed
- Blisters
- Complaints of pain, burning, stinging, or numbness

Putting it all together!

- The use of heat and cold can help to reduce or prevent tissue swelling, promote healing, ease pain, and promote comfort.
- Heat and cold applications can cause severe injury if they are used inappropriately.
- Blistered skin, burned skin, very red skin, or very pale skin that does not return to its normal color after the application is removed should be reported to the nurse immediately.

GUIDELINES BOX 27-1 Guidelines for Assisting With Heat and Cold Applications

What you do	Why you do it
If you have questions about how to apply the heat or cold application or for how long, ask the nurse for help.	Improper application or an application that is left in place for too long can result in tissue death and skin breakdown.
Wrap dry heat or cold applications (for example, hot water bottles, ice bags) in a towel before applying them to the person's skin. Always check to make sure that the towel is in place between the application and the person's skin.	The towel is a protective layer between the person's skin and the application. If applied directly to a person's skin, dry cold or heat can cause severe burns and blisters.
Check the skin underneath both a heat and a cold application every 5 minutes.	Frequent monitoring during the procedure can help to detect problems early so that the treatment can be stopped before more damage occurs.
Never leave a heat or cold application in place for longer than 20 minutes.	Leaving a heat or cold application in place for too long can lead to burns, tissue death, and skin breakdown.
Always place a dry heat application over the treatment site, not under a body part.	Placing a dry heat application under a body part can trap too much heat between the person's body and the mattress (or other surface), resulting in a burn.
Never cover a dry heat application with the bed linens.	Covering a dry heat application with the bed linens can trap too much heat between the person's body and the bed linens, resulting in a burn.

PROCEDURES

PROCEDURE 27-1
Giving a Back Massage

Why you do it: A back message promotes comfort and relaxation. Massage also stimulates blood flow to the skin, which helps to prevent pressure ulcers.

GETTING READY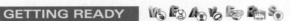

1. Complete the "Getting Ready" steps.

SUPPLIES

- gloves (if contact with broken skin is likely)
- wash basin
- lotion
- bath blanket
- towel

PROCEDURE

2. Fill the wash basin with warm water. Place the bottle of lotion in the basin of warm water to warm it.

3. Make sure that the bed is positioned at a comfortable working height (to promote good body mechanics) and that the wheels are locked.

4. Lower the head of the bed so that the bed is flat (as tolerated). If the side rails are in use, lower the side rail on the working side of the bed. The side rail on the opposite side of the bed should remain up.

5. Help the person into the prone position, or turn the person onto his side so that he is facing away from you.

6. Reposition the pillow under the person's head and adjust the bath blanket to keep the person covered, exposing only the back and buttocks.

7. Perform hand hygiene and put on the gloves if contact with broken skin is likely.

8. Pour some lotion into your cupped palm and rub your hands together to distribute the lotion onto both palms.

9. Apply the lotion to the person's back with the palms of your hands. Massage the lotion into the person's skin, using long, gliding strokes (*effleurage*), moving up the center of the back from the buttocks to the shoulders, and then back down along the outside of the back. Do not directly rub any reddened areas. Repeat four times.

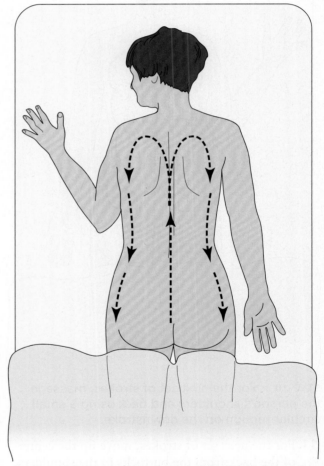

STEP 9 ■ Move up the center of the back from the buttocks to the shoulders, and then back down along the outside of the back.

(*procedure continues on page 624*)

PROCEDURE 27-1 (continued)
Giving a Back Massage

10. For the next set of strokes, move up the center of the back from the buttocks to the shoulders and then back down along the outside of the back. On the downstroke, massage the person's shoulders and back using a small circular motion. Repeat four times.

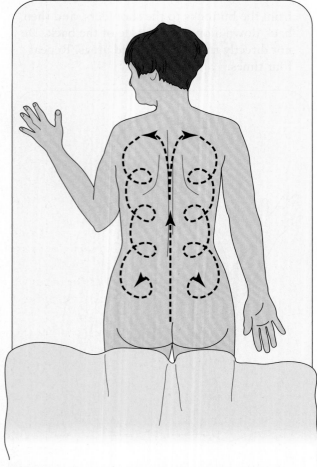

STEP 10 ■ For the next set of strokes, massage the person's shoulders and back using a small circular motion on the downstroke.

11. For the next set of strokes, move up the center of the back from the buttocks to the shoulders, and then back down along the outside of the back. On the downstroke, massage the person's shoulders, back, and buttocks using a small circular motion, paying special attention to the area at the base of the spine. Repeat four times.

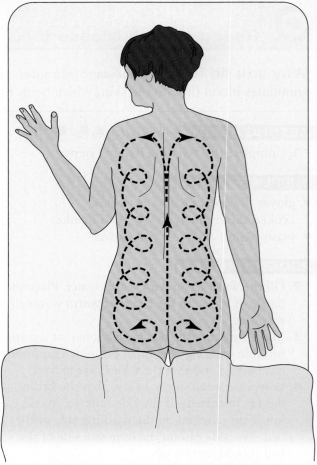

STEP 11 ■ For the final set of strokes, massage the person's shoulders, back, and buttocks using a small circular motion on the downstroke.

12. Finish with long, gliding strokes (effleurage), moving up the center of the back from the buttocks to the shoulders and then back down along the outside of the back. Repeat four times.
13. Remove your gloves, dispose of them in a facility-approved waste container, and perform hand hygiene.
14. If the back massage is being given as part of a bath, assist the person onto his back and continue with the bath. If the back massage is being given before bed or at any other time, help the person back into his pajamas, nightgown, or hospital gown.

15. If the side rails are in use, return the side rails to the raised position. Make sure that the bed is lowered to its lowest position and that the wheels are locked.

16. Gather the soiled linens and place them in the linen hamper or linen bag. Dispose of disposable items in a facility-approved waste container. Clean equipment and return it to the storage area.

FINISHING UP

17. Complete the "Finishing Up" steps.

WHAT YOU DOCUMENT

- Date and time
- Condition of the skin, especially at pressure points

PROCEDURE 27-2
Giving a Moist Cold Application

Why you do it: Cold applications reduce pain and swelling and decrease bleeding.

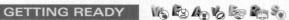

GETTING READY

1. Complete the "Getting Ready" steps.

SUPPLIES

- bed protector
- compress (for example, 4 × 4 gauze pad or washcloth)
- rolled gauze or ties (optional)
- bath basin
- ice
- bath towel

PROCEDURE

2. Put the ice in the bath basin and fill the basin with cold water at the sink.

3. Make sure that the bed is positioned at a comfortable working height (to promote good body mechanics) and that the wheels are locked.

4. Help the person to a comfortable position and expose only the area to be treated.

5. Position the bed protector as necessary to keep the bed linens dry.

6. Moisten the compress with the ice water as ordered. Wring out the compress and apply it to the treatment site.

7. Leave the compress in place for the designated amount of time, usually 15 to 20 minutes. The compress may be secured in place with ties or rolled gauze, or the patient or resident may assist by holding the compress in place.
   a. Keep the compress moistened with ice water.

b. Check the skin beneath the compress every 5 minutes. If the skin appears pale or blue or if the person complains of numbness or a burning sensation, discontinue treatment immediately and notify the nurse.

c. If you must leave the room, lower the bed to its lowest position, place the call light control within easy reach, and ask the person to signal if she experiences numbness or burning.

8. When the treatment is complete, remove the compress and carefully dry the skin.

9. Remove the bed protector. Straighten the bed linens and make sure that the person is comfortable and in good body alignment. Draw the top linens over the person.

10. Make sure that the bed is lowered to its lowest position and that the wheels are locked.

11. Gather the soiled linens and place them in the linen hamper. Dispose of disposable items in a facility-approved waste container. Clean equipment and return it to the storage area.

FINISHING UP

12. Complete the "Finishing Up" steps.

WHAT YOU DOCUMENT

- Date and time
- Type of cold application
- Body part treated
- Length of time treatment left in place
- Observation of skin after treatment
- Patient or resident comments

PROCEDURE 27-3
Giving a Dry Cold Application

Why you do it: Cold applications reduce pain and swelling and decrease bleeding.

GETTING READY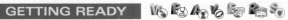

1. Complete the "Getting Ready" steps.

SUPPLIES

- rolled gauze or ties (optional)
- crushed ice
- ice bag
- towel or cloth bag cover

PROCEDURE

2. Fill the ice bag with water, close it, and turn it upside down to check for leaks. Empty the bag.

3. Fill the bag one half to two thirds full with crushed ice. Do not overfill the ice bag. Squeeze the bag to force out excess air, and close the bag.

4. Dry the outside of the bag and wrap it in the towel or place it in the bag cover.

5. Make sure that the bed is positioned at a comfortable working height (to promote good body mechanics) and that the wheels are locked.

6. Help the person to a comfortable position and expose only the area to be treated.

7. Apply the ice bag to the treatment site. Make sure that the towel is in place between the ice bag and the person's skin.

8. Leave the ice bag in place for the designated amount of time, usually 15 to 20 minutes. The ice bag may be secured in place with ties or rolled gauze, or the patient or resident may assist by holding the ice bag in place.

   a. Check the skin beneath the ice bag every 5 minutes. If the skin appears pale or blue or if the person complains of numbness or a burning sensation, discontinue treatment immediately and notify the nurse.

   b. Refill the bag with ice as necessary.

   c. If you must leave the room, lower the bed to its lowest position, place the call light control within easy reach, and ask the person to signal if he experiences numbness or burning.

9. When the treatment is complete, remove the ice bag.

10. Straighten the bed linens and make sure that the person is comfortable and in good body alignment. Draw the top linens over the person.

11. Make sure that the bed is lowered to its lowest position and that the wheels are locked.

12. Gather the soiled linens and place them in the linen hamper. Dispose of disposable items in a facility-approved waste container. Clean equipment and return it to the storage area.

FINISHING UP

13. Complete the "Finishing Up" steps.

WHAT YOU DOCUMENT

- Date and time
- Type of cold application
- Body part treated
- Length of time treatment left in place
- Observation of skin after treatment
- Patient or resident comments

PROCEDURE 27-4
Giving a Dry Heat Application With an Aquamatic Pad

Why you do it: Heat applications relax the muscles, relieve pain, and promote blood flow to the area.

GETTING READY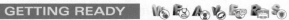

1. Complete the "Getting Ready" steps.

SUPPLIES

- aquamatic pad
- heating unit
- distilled water
- cover
- ties or tape

PROCEDURE

2. Check the pad for leaks. Make sure that the cord is not frayed and the plug is in good condition. Check the heating unit to be sure that it is filled with water. If you need to fill it, use distilled water. Tap water contains minerals that can corrode the unit.

3. Place the heating unit on a level, firm surface so that the tubing and pad are level with the heating unit at all times. Make sure that the tubing is free of kinks. Plug the cord into an outlet.

4. Allow the water to warm to the desired temperature, as specified by the nurse or the care plan (usually not to exceed 105°F to 109.4°F depending on facility policy). If the temperature is not preset, set the temperature with the key and then remove the key.

5. Place the pad in its cover.

6. Make sure that the bed is positioned at a comfortable working height (to promote good body mechanics) and that the wheels are locked.

7. Help the person to a comfortable position and expose only the area to be treated.

8. Apply the pad to the treatment site.

9. Leave the pad in place for the designated amount of time, usually 15 to 20 minutes. The pad may be secured in place with ties or tape, or the patient or resident may assist by holding the pad in place. (Do not use pins to secure the pad. Pins can puncture the pad, causing it to leak.)

   a. Check the skin beneath the pad every 5 minutes. If the skin appears red, swollen, or blistered or if the person complains of pain, numbness, or discomfort, discontinue treatment immediately and notify the nurse.

   b. Refill the heating unit if the water level drops below the fill line.

   c. If you must leave the room, lower the bed to its lowest position, place the call light control within easy reach, and ask the person to signal if she experiences numbness or burning.

10. When the treatment is complete, remove the pad.

11. Straighten the bed linens and make sure that the person is comfortable and in good body alignment. Draw the top linens over the person.

12. Make sure that the bed is lowered to its lowest position and that the wheels are locked.

13. Gather the soiled linens and place them in the linen hamper. Dispose of disposable items in a facility-approved waste container. Clean equipment and return it to the storage area.

FINISHING UP

14. Complete the "Finishing Up" steps.

WHAT YOU DOCUMENT

- Date and time
- Type of heat application
- Body part treated
- Length of time treatment left in place
- Observation of skin after treatment
- Patient or resident comments

WHAT DID YOU LEARN?

Multiple Choice

Select the single best answer for each of the following questions.

1. Which one of the following can be used to treat and control pain?
   a. Medications, such as aspirin and morphine
   b. Back massage
   c. Heat and cold applications
   d. All of the above

2. How long should a back massage last?
   a. 3 minutes
   b. 1 to 2 minutes
   c. 4 to 6 minutes
   d. 15 minutes

3. The purpose of cold applications is usually to:
   a. Prevent heat exhaustion
   b. Speed the flow of blood to an injured area
   c. Prevent swelling
   d. Prevent the formation of scar tissue

4. What is heat application used for?
   a. To relieve muscle spasms
   b. To reduce pain
   c. To promote circulation and speed healing
   d. All of the above

5. If a patient or resident is having a cold application, how often should you check the skin underneath the application?
   a. Every 15 minutes
   b. Every 10 minutes
   c. Every 5 minutes
   d. At least twice an hour

6. Heat and cold applications should not be left in place for longer than:
   a. 15 minutes
   b. 5 minutes
   c. 30 minutes
   d. 20 minutes

STOP Stop *and* Think!

Mrs. Dyatt is having a hard time getting to sleep tonight. She is restless and says that her arthritis is acting up, causing her to "ache all over." What can you do to help make Mrs. Dyatt more comfortable?

Special Care Concerns

You may be involved in caring for patients or residents who are terminally ill or dying; who have developmental disabilities, cancer, or AIDS; or who are having surgery. These patients or residents have special needs related to their condition or situation. Special care concerns are the focus of Unit 6.

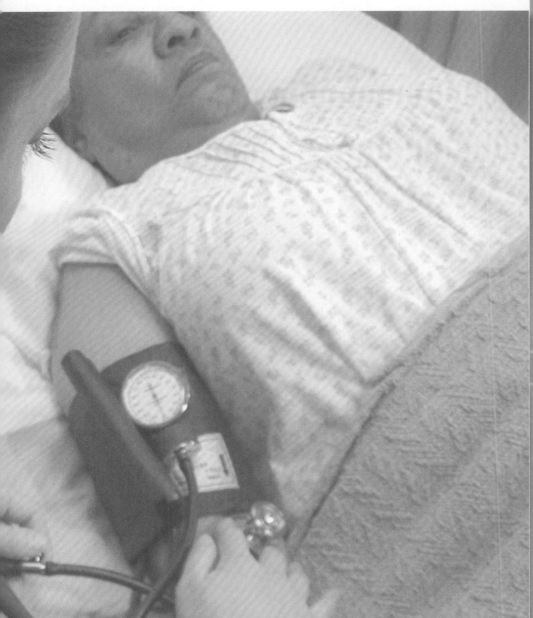

Caring for People Who Are Dying

Although everyone who lives must die, accepting the certainty of our own death or the death of someone we care about is rarely easy. As a nursing assistant, you will care for patients or residents who are dying. In this chapter, you will learn how to ensure that the time leading up to death is as comfortable and peaceful as possible for both the dying person and his or her family members.

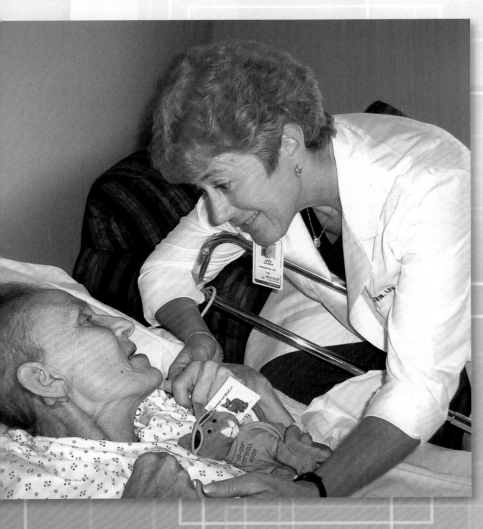

Photo: A hospice nurse cares for one of her terminally ill patients. (© Wuesthoff Brevard Hospice & Palliative Care/Brenda Spakes.)

Terminal Illness

What will you learn?

When you are finished with this section, you will be able to:

1. List the stages of grief and discuss how a person might behave during each stage.
2. Describe communication techniques that you might use to support a person during each stage of grief.
3. Discuss the role of hospice in the care of a terminally ill person.
4. Define the words **terminal illness**, **grief**, **hospice care**, **supportive care**, and **palliative care**.

Terminal illness an illness or condition from which recovery is not expected

Grief mental anguish, specifically associated with loss

Some people die suddenly of accidents or acute illnesses. Others die as a result of the natural aging process. Still others die from a **terminal illness**. Examples of terminal illnesses include some heart conditions, emphysema, dementia, and some types of cancers.

Stages of Grief

As a terminally ill person comes to terms with the knowledge that she will eventually die as a result of her disease, she will experience stages of **grief**. These stages of grief were identified by Dr. Elisabeth Kübler-Ross, a psychiatrist who worked with terminally ill people. The stages of grief that Dr. Kübler-Ross identified are denial, anger, bargaining, depression, and acceptance (Table 28-1). The terminally ill person may not pass through all of the stages of grief and may not pass through them in order.

The terminally ill person's family members will also go through the stages of grief as they prepare for their loss. Like the dying person, the family members will each pass through the stages of grief at their own order and pace. When family members are at different stages of the grieving process, emotional upset within the family can occur.

Throughout the grieving process, one emotion that usually persists is *hope*. Even the most realistic and accepting terminally ill people and their family members hold onto the hope that a cure will be found. Hope is what helps a terminally ill person to face another day or another painful treatment.

Understanding the stages of grief and how they may affect a person's behavior can help you to provide better care. Use the communication skills you learned in Chapter 4 to provide emotional support to the person. The tactics you will use will vary, depending on what stage of grief the person is in (Table 28-2).

Tell the Nurse!

Caring for a terminally ill person

- The person refuses medications or other medical treatment
- The person cries constantly, refuses food, or cannot sleep
- There is tension and disagreement within the family
- The person or a family member requests the assistance of clergy or a grief counselor
- The person expresses interest in having a will made

Hospice Care

Hospice care care provided by a health care organization for people who are dying, and their families

Terminally ill people become eligible for **hospice care** when their doctors tell them that they have approximately 6 months left to live. Hospice care is provided by a team of health care workers that includes nurses, nursing assistants, clergy, social

TABLE 28-1   **Stages of Grief**

Stage	Description	Effects on the Person's Behavior
Denial	The person refuses to accept the diagnosis or feels that a mistake has been made	■ The person may ask for a second opinion ■ The person may act as if nothing is wrong ■ The person may refuse medication or other treatments
Anger	The person realizes that she is actually going to die as a result of her illness and has feelings of rage, which may be directed toward herself or others	■ The person may become moody and withdrawn ■ The person may become uncooperative and hostile ■ The person may lose religious faith
Bargaining	The person wants to "make a deal" with someone he feels has control over his fate, such as God or a health care provider	■ The person may speak of wanting to live long enough to accomplish a goal or to witness a specific event (such as a wedding or a child's birth)
Depression	The person fully realizes that death will be the end result of the illness and experiences sadness and regret	■ The person may be sad and cry a lot ■ The person may withdraw and say little ■ The person may refuse food or have trouble falling asleep
Acceptance	The person comes to terms with the reality of his own death and is finally at peace with this knowledge	■ The person may want to complete unfinished business ■ The person may want to say goodbye to friends and loved ones ■ The person may plan his own funeral service ■ The person may want to talk about his death with others

workers, mental health providers, and others. Hospice care can be provided in a long-term care facility, in a hospital, in the person's home, or in a special hospice facility.

Although the person's illness cannot be cured, hospice workers provide **supportive care** and **palliative care** to keep the person as comfortable as possible as death approaches. Hospice workers also provide emotional support to both the terminally ill person and the family. After the person dies, hospice workers continue to support the family by providing grief counseling and other types of assistance.

Supportive care treatments that will not prolong life, but will make a person more comfortable, such as oxygen therapy, nutritional supplementation, pain medication, range-of-motion exercises, grooming and hygiene, and positioning assistance

Palliative care care that focuses on relieving uncomfortable symptoms, not on curing the problem that is causing the symptoms; examples include pain medication, chemotherapy or radiation to shrink a tumor, oxygen to make breathing easier, and some surgical procedures

	TABLE 28-2	**Communication Throughout the Grieving Process**	

Stage	Sample Dialogue	Appropriate Response From Nursing Assistant
Denial	**Person:** "They don't know what they're talking about. I can't possibly have cancer." **Nursing assistant:** "I'm sorry; it must have been very hard for you to hear the test results."	■ Acknowledges what the person is saying by responding in an honest, yet neutral way
Anger	**Person:** "If you weren't so incompetent, I wouldn't be so sick!" **Nursing assistant:** "Mr. Smith, you seem so angry."	■ Acknowledges the person's anger and allows him to talk about it ■ Avoids feeling defensive or taking the person's anger personally
Bargaining	**Person:** "If I could just hang on until my sister arrives. . . ." **Nursing assistant:** "We'll do all we can to help you do that. But until then, I'll be with you."	■ Offers support that she can realistically provide and reassures the person that she will be cared for
Depression	**Person:** "I don't want to die. . . . I'm so sad." **Nursing assistant** (sitting quietly and holding the person's hand): "I'm here for you."	■ Offers comfort in the form of touch and silence ■ Does not attempt to "cheer the person up"
Acceptance	**Person:** "It won't be long until I'm going on to my reward." **Nursing assistant:** "You're going on to your reward?"	■ Uses communication techniques that encourage the person to talk, such as rephrasing the person's statement as an open-ended question

Putting it all together!

■ A terminally ill person will eventually die as a result of his disease. The health care team's primary goal is to help the terminally ill person to continue to live, and eventually to die, in comfort and with dignity.

■ The five stages of grief identified by Dr. Elisabeth Kübler-Ross are denial, anger, bargaining, depression, and acceptance. Being able to recognize the stages of grief will help you to provide better care for a terminally ill person and his family members.

■ Hospice care focuses on supportive and palliative care measures to ensure that a terminally ill person faces the end of life with comfort and dignity.

Advance Directives and Wills

What will you learn?

When you are finished with this section, you will be able to:

1. Describe ways that a person can specify her wishes for end-of-life care in advance.
2. Describe how a person can specify his wishes for the management of his affairs after death.
3. Define the words **do not resuscitate (DNR) order** and **will**.

Advance Directives

In Chapter 2, you learned that advance directives are documents that allow a person to make her wishes regarding health care known to family members and health care workers, in case the time comes when she is no longer able to make those wishes known herself. The person's advance directive could include a living will, the naming of a durable power of attorney for health care (also known as a health care agent), or both. The person may specify that only supportive care is to be provided as the time of death approaches. If this is the case, the doctor will place a **do not resuscitate (DNR) order** in the person's medical record. All members of the health care team who provide direct care to the person should be aware of this order to ensure that the person's wishes for end-of-life care are carried out.

Do not resuscitate (DNR) order an order written on a person's chart specifying the person's wishes that the usual efforts to save his life will not be made; also called a *no-code order*

Wills

Many people want to leave instructions about how their affairs and belongings are to be managed after they die. These instructions are called a **will**. A patient's or resident's request for help in making a will should be relayed to the nurse promptly. Many health care facilities have people on site who are able to provide assistance when people wish to make or update a will.

Will a legal statement that expresses a person's wishes for the management of his or her affairs after death

Putting it all together!

- Advance directives help to ensure that a person's wishes regarding end-of-life care are honored, even if the person is no longer able to express those wishes verbally. Advance directives preserve the person's right to die in as peaceful and dignified a manner as possible.
- A person may only wish for supportive care at the end of life. In this case, a DNR order is placed in the person's chart and must be respected.
- A will contains instructions about how the person's affairs and belongings are to be managed after she dies.

Attitudes Toward Death and Dying

What will you learn?

When you are finished with this section, you will be able to:

1. Discuss factors that can affect how a person views death.
2. Explain why it is important for health care workers to examine their own feelings about death.
3. Define the words **afterlife** and **reincarnation**.

Some people have many fears regarding death. People may fear the unknown. They may worry about losing control over their own bodies. They may be afraid of dying alone or dying in pain. Other people accept death with calmness, serenity, and possibly even anticipation.

Many factors influence a person's attitude toward death, including:

- The person's cultural beliefs
- The person's religious or spiritual beliefs
- The person's previous experience with death (for example, the death of a friend or loved one)
- The person's sense of having accomplished everything she wanted to do in life

When faced with their own death or that of a loved one, many people find comfort in their cultural and religious or spiritual beliefs. People may want to visit with clergy members; surround themselves with religious items; or spend time alone praying, meditating, or reading religious texts. When cultural and religious or spiritual beliefs provide an explanation for what happens to a person after death, they can be a source of comfort for the dying person and her family members. Many people believe in an **afterlife**. Others believe in **reincarnation**. It is important for you to respect the person's cultural and religious or spiritual beliefs, even if they are different from your own. Some examples of death rituals associated with specific cultural groups are shown in Box 28-1.

Afterlife a state of being where the dead meet again with loved ones who have passed on before them

Reincarnation the idea that a person's spirit or soul will live again on Earth in the form of an animal or human being yet to be born

BOX 28-1   Common Death Rituals of Specific Cultural Groups

Group	Death Ritual	Intervention
African Americans	May respond to news of death of a loved one by *falling out* (that is, sudden collapse, paralysis, and inability to see or speak).	Recognize that this is a culturally based response and not an emergency medical condition; provide support.
Amish Appalachians	Provide a wake-like "sitting up" during the night for seriously ill and dying family members.	Arrange for privacy and accommodate family members staying overnight.
Cubans, Filipinos, Mexicans	A large gathering of relatives and friends may attend the dying person and place religious artifacts around the person; candles are lit after death to illuminate the path of the spirit to the afterlife.	Arrange for a gathering place close to the dying person; find electric candles if open flames are not allowed; summon clergy for religious rituals; do not move religious items.

Group	Death Ritual	Intervention
Europeans	Believe that the dying person should not be left alone.	Make accommodations for family members to be present at all times.
Haitians	Family members gather and pray when death is imminent and may cry uncontrollably; all family members try to be at the person's bedside at the time of death.	Make accommodations for privacy, encourage family to bring in religious objects, allow families to participate in postmortem care if they desire to do so.
Hindus, Indians	Priest and the eldest son may perform death rites, with all male relatives assisting; women may respond with loud wailing.	Provide a supportive and private environment; offer understanding of death rituals and grief behaviors.
Japanese	Family members gather at the bedside at the time of death, with the eldest son having particular responsibilities at the time.	Notify the eldest son of pending death, identify lines of communication if the eldest son is not available.
Jews	Dying person should not be left alone; death rituals vary and some are not performed on the Sabbath or holy days.	Ask the closest relative specifically about postmortem practices.
Koreans	Family members are expected to stay with the person who is dying and assist with care.	Support family in caring for the person.
Mexicans	Some, especially women, may have an *ataque de nervios* (that is, the person exhibits hyperkinetic and seizure-like activity to release strong emotions) on hearing of the death of a loved one.	Recognize that this is a culture-bound syndrome and treatment is usually not necessary; remain with the person, provide support, and involve family with assistance, if possible.
Muslim groups	The bed should be turned to face the holy city of Mecca; family recites prayers from the Qur'an.	Facilitate positioning of the bed whenever possible, provide privacy for prayers.
Navajo Indians	It is taboo to talk about a fatal disease or dying; the issue needs to be discussed in the third person, as if it is occurring in someone else.	Avoid suggesting that someone is dying because this may be interpreted as a wish that the person be dead.
Puerto Ricans	Death is perceived as a time of crisis; the head of the family (that is, usually the oldest daughter or son) is responsible for receiving the news of death.	Allow time for the family to view, touch, and stay with the body before it is removed; ask if the family wants a clergy member called.
Vietnamese	Flowers are avoided during illness because they are usually reserved for rites of the dead.	Ask permission from the patient or family before placing flowers in a room.

Source: Purnell, L. D. (2009). *Culturally competent health care.* Philadelphia, PA: F. A. Davis.

It is important for you to be aware of your own feelings and beliefs about death. Many nursing assistants (especially new nursing assistants) compromise the care they give a dying patient or resident without being fully aware that they are doing so. For example, a nursing assistant might not check in on the dying person as often as he checks on other patients or residents. He might provide only the necessary care and then leave the person's room quickly because of the fear that if he stays, the person will want to talk about death. Or he may be overly cheerful around the person. These are called *avoidance behaviors*, and they usually occur because the nursing assistant has not yet explored his own feelings about death. Talking to your supervisor, a clergy member, or a mental health counselor about questions and fears you have about death can help you to clarify your feelings about death and dying.

> **Concerns for Long-Term Care**
>
> In older adults, death is usually associated with a combination of chronic illnesses and the aging process. Society, as a whole, tends to view the death of an elderly person as "just a part of life." Interestingly, the American Geriatrics Society (AGS) states that "birth and death give definition to life as the period in between." For many older adults, having a "good death" is just a part of the process of living and is strongly influenced by that person's cultural and spiritual beliefs.
>
> Facing the death of a resident never gets any easier. You will become very attached to your residents. Although the relationship you have with the resident can make providing end-of-life care very emotionally difficult for you, it is this relationship that will allow you to provide the holistic care that the dying person needs so much.

 ## Putting it all together!

- A person's culture and religious or spiritual beliefs often influence how the person feels about death and prepares for it.
- Talking to your supervisor, a clergy member, or a mental health counselor can help you to come to terms with your own feelings and beliefs about death. Being aware of your own feelings about death and dying helps you to provide the best care possible to a dying patient or resident.

Care and Support of the Dying Person and the Family

 ## What will you learn?

When you are finished with this section, you will be able to:

1. Discuss the physical changes that occur as death nears.
2. Describe how you can help to keep a dying person physically comfortable.
3. Describe how you can help to support a dying person emotionally.
4. Discuss ways that you can help the family of a dying person.

BOX 28-2 The Dying Person's Bill of Rights

I have the right to be treated as a living human being until I die.

I have the right to maintain a sense of hopefulness, however changing its focus may be.

I have the right to be cared for by those who can maintain a sense of hopefulness, however changing this might be.

I have the right to express my feelings and emotions about my approaching death in my own way.

I have the right to participate in decisions concerning my care.

I have the right to expect continuing medical and nursing attention even though "cure" goals must be changed to "comfort" goals.

I have the right not to die alone.

I have the right to be free from pain.

I have the right to have my questions answered honestly.

I have the right not to be deceived.

I have the right to have help from and for my family in accepting my death.

I have the right to die in peace and dignity.

I have a right to retain my individuality and not be judged for my decisions, which may be contrary to beliefs of others.

I have the right to discuss and enlarge my religious and/or spiritual experiences, whatever these may mean to others.

I have the right to expect that the sanctity of the human body will be respected after death.

I have the right to be cared for by caring, sensitive, knowledgeable people who will attempt to understand my needs and will be able to gain some satisfaction in helping me face my death.

Created at the workshop *The Terminally Ill Patient and the Helping Person*, Lansing, Michigan, sponsored by the Southwestern Michigan Inservice Education Council and conducted by Amelia J. Barbus, Associate Professor of Nursing, Wayne State University, Detroit.

Every person has the right to die in peace and with dignity (Box 28-2). As a nursing assistant, it is your job to do everything you can to ensure that this right is honored. A holistic, humanistic approach to care is taken with a dying person, just as with any other person.

Meeting the Dying Person's Physical Needs

As death draws near, the person may show certain physical signs, caused as the body begins to "shut down." These signs may appear over the course of a few hours or a few days, or even within the space of a few minutes. Some people may not show these signs. However, recognizing these physical signs and understanding why they occur will help you to know what type of care to give the dying person (Table 28-3). As you are providing care for a person who is dying, take note of any physical changes that you observe. Report these changes to the nurse and record them in the person's medical chart, per facility policy.

Promote general comfort by keeping the person's room well lit. Control odors by keeping the room well ventilated, removing odorous items such as soiled linens, and using an

Although the relationship you have with your patient or resident can make providing end-of-life care very emotionally difficult for you, it is this relationship that will allow you to provide the holistic, humanistic care that the dying person needs so much. Helping to meet the person's physical and emotional needs helps to ensure that the person dies peacefully and with dignity.

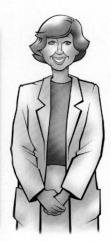

TABLE 28-3 **Physical Changes That Occur as Death Approaches and Corresponding Care Measures**

Organ System	Physical Change	Care Measures
Circulatory system	■ As the circulation fails, the blood pressure drops and the pulse becomes rapid and weak. The body temperature rises, but the skin feels cool and clammy. The person may perspire heavily, and the skin may look pale, gray, or bluish.	■ Cover the person with light bed linens. Provide frequent skin care and linen changes to prevent skin breakdown and promote comfort.
Respiratory system	■ The respiratory pattern changes to very irregular, shallow breathing or an alternating fast–slow pattern. Fluid or mucus may collect in the air passages causing the noisy, rattling breathing that is often known as the "death rattle."	■ Report observations of labored breathing to the nurse. The nurse may be able to provide suctioning (to clear secretions) and oxygen therapy. For some people, elevating the head of the bed makes breathing less of an effort. Oxygen cannulas may cause irritation and crusting around the nostrils. Clean the area gently with a clean, moist washcloth and apply a lubricant.
Digestive system	■ The digestive system slows down. The person may experience nausea, vomiting, abdominal swelling, fecal impaction, or bowel incontinence. The person may not want food or water.	■ Offer ice chips and provide frequent oral care to keep the mouth moist and promote comfort. Enemas may be necessary to assist with bowel elimination.
Urinary system	■ Urine output decreases as the kidneys respond to the lack of blood flow. The person may become incontinent of urine.	■ Check the person regularly for incontinence. Clean the skin gently and change soiled or wet clothing and bed linens. Bed protectors or indwelling urinary catheters may be needed.
Musculoskeletal system	■ The muscles relax and the person may be too weak to reposition himself.	■ Provide frequent, regular position changes to prevent pressure ulcers and promote comfort.
Nervous system	■ Some people lose the ability to speak. ■ Vision may become blurred. ■ Pain is usually diminished. ■ Hearing usually remains sharp. ■ Consciousness may be altered.	■ Ask the person questions that can be answered by a nod or shake of the head. ■ Keep the room well lit and make sure that you introduce yourself when entering the room. Explain procedures. ■ Observe the person for pain and report findings to the nurse so that the person can receive medication to remain comfortable. ■ Always talk to the person as if he is able to hear you, even if he cannot respond. Encourage family members to talk to the dying person also.

air freshener as needed. Giving the person a back massage, playing soft music, or reading aloud to the person are also activities that promote rest and comfort.

Meeting the Dying Person's Emotional Needs

Listening and Touch

A nursing assistant can help meet a dying person's emotional needs by being a good listener. A dying person may want to talk about his fears related to dying or what he expects the afterlife to be like. Or the person may just want to share memories with you. Use the communication skills that you learned in Chapter 4 to encourage the person and let him know that you are there to listen. In many instances, you do not need to say anything—you just need to listen to what the person wants to tell you.

Other dying people will not want to talk. A person who does not want to talk still needs to know that you are close by and available if she needs you. Check on the person frequently. Many dying people appreciate it when someone takes the time to sit near them quietly. Touch is also an effective way to let the person know that you care. Gently hold the person's hand or touch her shoulder when you are speaking to her.

Assisting With Requests for Clergy

As part of preparing for death, the person may want to confess or receive a religious blessing. If a patient or resident requests that you call a clergy member, you should notify the nurse immediately. When the clergy member arrives, make sure that there is a place for the clergy member to sit, and ensure privacy.

Supporting the Family

There are many simple things you can do to comfort the family of a dying person:

- **Ensure good communication between the family members and the health care team.** Answer any questions about the patient's or resident's care that you are qualified to answer. Relay any questions that you are not able to answer to the nurse promptly.

- **Allow family members to stay with the dying person.** Visiting hours are usually relaxed, allowing family members to stay with the dying person as long as they like. Just be sure to ensure the person's privacy when you are providing physical care by asking the family members to step outside until the procedure is completed.

- **Allow family members to participate in the person's care if they want to.** Some family members may ask to help provide physical care for the dying person. Participating in the care of a dying loved one can help a family member to feel better about the situation (Fig. 28-1).

- **Ensure that the family members' basic needs are met.** Make sure that there are enough chairs in the room. Encourage family members to rest and take meals as necessary. Show them how to find the restrooms, public telephones, vending machines, and cafeteria.

- **Be readily available to provide needed care to the patient or resident without being intrusive of the family's privacy.** It can be comforting to family members to know that you are nearby and available to help as needed.

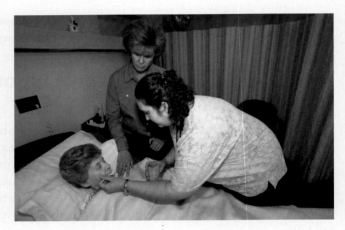

■ **FIGURE 28-1**

If a family member wants to help care for the dying person, suggest simple care measures that the family member can perform. Here, a nursing assistant is showing a family member how to ease the person's thirst by giving ice chips.

 Putting it all together!

- A dying person becomes dependent on others for physical care as death approaches. Basic care measures include skin care, oral care, and assistance with positioning.
- Providing holistic, humanistic care means helping a dying person to meet his emotional needs as well as physical ones. Listening and touch let the person know that he is cared for and not alone.
- Family members of a dying person require support as well. Being respectful, thoughtful, and kind can do much to make family members feel better.

Postmortem Care

What will you learn?

When you are finished with this section, you will be able to:

1. Discuss the responsibilities you may have following the death of a patient or resident.
2. Demonstrate proper technique for providing postmortem care.
3. Define the words **postmortem care**, **rigor mortis**, **shroud**, and **autopsy**.

Postmortem care the care of a person's body after the person's death

If you are present when one of your patients or residents dies, notify the nurse that the person has died, and note the time. You may need to document the absence of vital signs. The doctor will legally pronounce the person dead. The time of death is recorded on the person's death certificate. After the doctor has pronounced the person dead, you may be required to assist the nurse in giving **postmortem care**. Be aware that cultural and religious beliefs often dictate how the body is to be cared for after death (and by whom). Family members may want to help clean and prepare the body in accordance with cultural and religious traditions.

Postmortem care is necessary to keep the body in proper alignment and to prevent skin damage and discoloration. During postmortem care:

- The skin is cleaned of any mucus, urine, feces, or other fluids. Standard precautions are followed when performing postmortem care because body fluids are still potentially infectious, even after death.

- The body is placed in proper alignment before **rigor mortis** occurs. Be aware that during repositioning, trapped air may escape from the lungs or digestive tract, making a sound like a sigh or a moan. Although these sounds may startle you, they are normal.

- A **shroud** may be applied (Fig. 28-2).

Rigor mortis the stiffening of the muscles that usually develops within 2 to 4 hours of death

Shroud a covering used to wrap the body of a person who has died

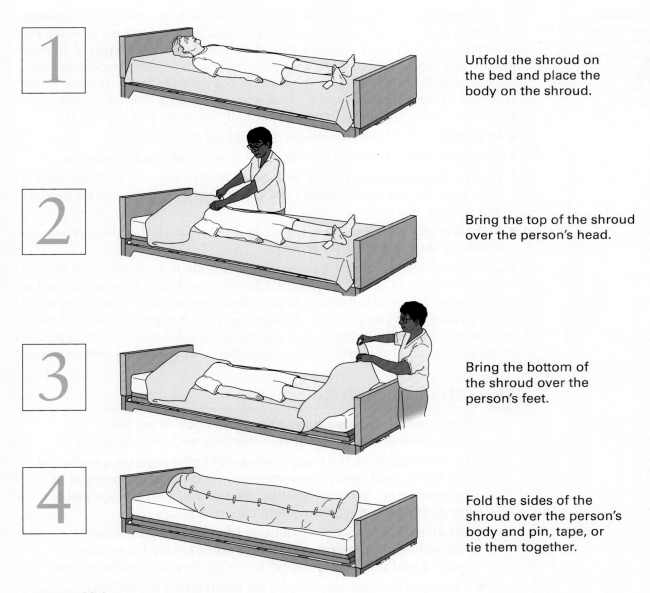

1. Unfold the shroud on the bed and place the body on the shroud.

2. Bring the top of the shroud over the person's head.

3. Bring the bottom of the shroud over the person's feet.

4. Fold the sides of the shroud over the person's body and pin, tape, or tie them together.

■ **FIGURE 28-2**

How to wrap the body in a shroud.

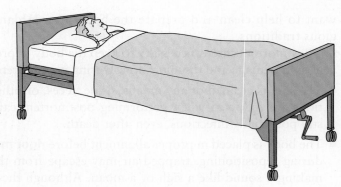

■ **FIGURE 28-3**

The body is placed in the supine position for viewing by the family. A pillow is placed under the person's head and shoulders.

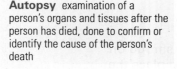

Autopsy examination of a person's organs and tissues after the person has died, done to confirm or identify the cause of the person's death

■ The person's personal belongings are collected and packed up to send with the family.

If an **autopsy** is to be performed, medical devices such as tubes, drains, catheters, and intravenous (IV) lines are not removed as part of postmortem care. If an autopsy is not necessary, the nurse will usually remove these medical devices as part of the postmortem care procedure. Procedure 28-1 describes how to provide postmortem care.

Many facilities only prepare the person's body for the family to view before sending it to the morgue or funeral home, where the funeral director completes the postmortem care procedure. To prepare the body for viewing by the family:

■ Straighten the bed linens (or change them, if they are soiled).

■ Wash the person's body and dress the person in a clean gown or pajamas.

■ Position the person in a natural position on the bed (Fig. 28-3). Draw the top sheet up to the person's shoulders and cuff it neatly. Do not cover the person's face with the sheet.

■ Make sure that the room is neat and adjust the lights so that they are not too bright. As always, provide for privacy.

Providing postmortem care can be emotionally difficult. It is normal to feel sad and cry at the passing of a patient or resident. Allow yourself to be a human being and to feel emotions. Talking about your feelings with a co-worker, supervisor, clergy member, or counselor can help you work through your grief. It might also help to think of providing postmortem care as a way of paying your last respects to the dead person. In this way, the ritual of providing this care becomes a way of coping with your grief.

Putting it all together!

■ Postmortem care is done to keep the body in proper alignment and to prevent skin damage and discoloration.

■ In some facilities, the body is prepared for immediate viewing by the family, and then postmortem care is done at the morgue or funeral home. In other facilities, the nursing staff is responsible for completing the postmortem care procedure.

■ When caring for a person's body after death, you show respect for the person and the person's family by working quietly and protecting the person's privacy, even after death.

■ Standard precautions should be taken when providing postmortem care because contact with body fluids is likely.

CHAPTER 28 PROCEDURES

PROCEDURE 28-1
Providing Postmortem Care

Why you do it: Postmortem care keeps the body in proper alignment and prevents skin damage and discoloration.

GETTING READY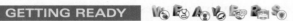

1. Complete the "Getting Ready" steps.

SUPPLIES

- gloves
- paper towels
- cotton balls
- bed protector
- postmortem kit*
- wash basin
- soap or no-rinse cleanser
- comb
- bath blanket
- washcloth
- towel
- clean gown
- clean linens (if necessary)

PROCEDURE

2. Cover the over-bed table with paper towels. Place your supplies on the over-bed table.
3. Make sure that the bed is positioned at a comfortable working height (to promote good body mechanics) and that the wheels are locked. Lower the head of the bed so that the bed is flat. Fanfold the top linens to the foot of the bed.
4. Put on the gloves.
5. If instructed to by the nurse, remove or turn off any medical equipment.
6. Place the body in the supine position. Position the pillow under the person's head and shoulders. Undress the body and cover it with the bath blanket.

*The contents of the postmortem kit vary, but most contain a shroud, something for securing the shroud, ties, gauze pads, a chin strap, identification tags, and a plastic bag or envelope for the person's belongings.

7. Close the eyes. Put a moistened cotton ball on each eyelid if the eyes do not stay closed. If the person has an artificial eye, this should be in place, unless you are instructed otherwise.
8. Replace the person's dentures, unless you are instructed otherwise. Close the mouth and, if necessary, gently support the jaw with the chin strap, a light bandage, or a rolled hand towel.
9. Remove any jewelry and place it in a plastic bag or envelope for the family. List each piece of jewelry as you remove it. Do not remove engagement or wedding rings, unless it is your facility's policy to do so.
10. Fill the wash basin with warm water. Place the basin on the over-bed table. Wash the body and comb the hair.
11. If the family is to view the body, dress the body in a clean gown. If the bedding is wet or soiled, change the bed linens. Draw the top linens over the person, forming a cuff at the shoulders. (Do not cover the person's face.) Straighten the room, lower the lights, and provide for the family's privacy.
12. After the family leaves, collect all of the person's belongings, noting each item on your list.
13. Fill out three identification tags:
    a. Attach one to the right great toe or the right ankle.
    b. Attach one to the person's belongings.
    c. Save the last to be attached to the outside of the shroud (if used).
14. If a shroud is to be used, put on a clean pair of gloves, apply it now, and attach the third identification tag to the outside of the shroud.

(procedure continues on page 646)

PROCEDURE 28-1 (continued)
Providing Postmortem Care

15. Gather the soiled linens and place them in the linen hamper. Dispose of disposable items in a facility-approved waste container. Clean equipment and return it to the storage area.

16. Remove your gloves, dispose of them in a facility-approved waste container, and perform hand hygiene.

17. Transfer the body from the bed to a stretcher for transport to the morgue, if appropriate. If the family has made funeral arrangements, leave the body in the room with the door or curtain closed.

18. Report the time the body was transported and the location of the person's belongings to the nurse.

FINISHING UP

19. Complete the "Finishing Up" steps.

WHAT YOU DOCUMENT

- Date and time
- Care given
- Description of items removed from the body, for example, jewelry, dentures
- Who received the removed items and other personal belongings
- Time the body is taken to morgue or funeral home

WHAT DID YOU LEARN?

Multiple Choice

Select the single best answer for each of the following questions.

1. Denial is:
   a. The stage of the grieving process in which the person becomes very depressed
   b. A form of bargaining with God for more time
   c. The final step of the grieving process
   d. The time during the grieving process when the person believes the diagnosis is incorrect

2. An agency that cares only for people who are dying is a:
   a. Skilled facility
   b. Sub-acute care unit
   c. Long-term care facility
   d. Hospice organization

3. The stage of grief when a person begins to say goodbye and make arrangements for his or her death is the:
   a. Bargaining stage
   b. Anger stage
   c. Denial stage
   d. Acceptance stage

4. Hospice care is designed to:
   a. Keep the person comfortable
   b. Prolong the person's life
   c. Treat the person aggressively
   d. All of the above

5. A patient with terminal cancer says he plans to live long enough to go to his daughter's wedding. This is an example of:
   a. Acceptance
   b. Depression
   c. Bargaining
   d. Denial

6. A legal document that expresses a person's wishes for the management of her affairs after death is a/an:
   a. Advance directive
   b. Living will
   c. Durable power of attorney
   d. Will

7. When caring for a person who is dying, you should:
   a. Keep family members away from the dying person
   b. Keep the room dark
   c. Provide for the person's physical and emotional needs
   d. Change the subject if the person starts to talk about death or dying

8. A common sign of approaching death is:
   a. Severe pain that gets worse
   b. Normal or increased vital signs
   c. Cool, moist skin
   d. Increased appetite

9. Postmortem care is done:
   a. Right before the person dies
   b. After the doctor pronounces the person dead
   c. After rigor mortis sets in
   d. If there is time

10. As death approaches, the last sense to be lost is:
    a. Sight
    b. Hearing
    c. Smell
    d. Taste

11. Which one of the following is a true statement about providing postmortem care?
    a. Standard precautions are used because the body may be infectious
    b. Dentures are removed from the mouth and given to the family to take home
    c. There is no need for privacy because the person is dead
    d. All of the above

12. In caring for the dying person, the nursing assistant also needs to care for the family. Which of the following can the nursing assistant do to support the family?
    a. Allow family members to stay with the dying person
    b. Be respectful of the family
    c. Provide the family with privacy
    d. All of the above

Matching

Match each vocabulary word with its definition.

_____ **1.** Reincarnation

_____ **2.** Rigor mortis

_____ **3.** Postmortem care

_____ **4.** Autopsy

a. Examination of a person's tissues and organs after death

b. Stiffening of the muscles that occurs 2 to 4 hours after death

c. Care of a body after death

d. The belief that the soul of a dead person returns to Earth in the form of another human being or animal yet to be born

 Stop *and* **Think!**

Wendy has been caring for Mr. Cole, who is dying. Now it appears that the time of death is rapidly approaching. Even though Mr. Cole is having trouble talking, he does manage to say to her, "I don't want to die alone." What can Wendy do to help Mr. Cole?

 Stop *and* **Think!**

Mrs. Brown has a history of depression, and years ago, she attempted suicide. Mrs. Brown's husband has been told that his wife has terminal cancer. He does not want her to know her diagnosis because he thinks she will become depressed and attempt suicide again. When you are giving Mrs. Brown a bed bath, she asks you if she is dying. How would you respond?

Caring for People With Developmental Disabilities

Developmental disabilities affect a person's physical or intellectual development or both. In this chapter, you will learn about some common developmental disabilities and the special needs of patients and residents with these conditions.

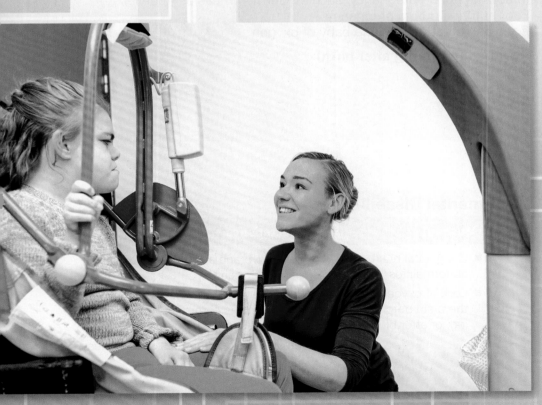

Photo: *Good communication skills are especially important when working with people with developmental disabilities.*

Introduction to Developmental Disabilities

What will you learn?

When you are finished with this section, you will be able to:

1. Discuss causes of developmental disabilities.
2. Discuss eight common types of developmental disabilities.
3. Define the word **developmental disability**.

Developmental disability
a permanent disability that affects a person before he or she reaches adulthood (that is, before 19 to 22 years of age) and interferes with the person's ability to achieve developmental milestones

A **developmental disability** may be congenital (something a child is born with) or acquired (occurring after birth, as a result of trauma or illness) (Box 29-1). The same developmental disability can be severe in one person and mild in another. Table 29-1 reviews common types of developmental disabilities.

BOX 29-1 **Common Causes of Developmental Disabilities**

Congenital (present at birth):
Genetic (inherited) disorders
Consumption of alcohol, drugs, or other toxic substances during pregnancy
Infections during pregnancy, such as German measles (rubella)
Poor nutrition during pregnancy
Conditions that deprive the baby of oxygen

Acquired (occurring after birth):
Birth trauma
Head injury
Near-drowning
Poisoning

TABLE 29-1 **Common Developmental Disabilities**

Developmental Disability	Causes	Characteristics
Intellectual disability (known as mental retardation in the past)	■ Congenital brain abnormalities ■ Lack of oxygen to the brain before, during, or after birth	■ Below-average ability to reason, think, and understand ■ Problems with skills needed to live and work, such as communication skills, social skills, and self-care skills ■ Intelligence quotient (IQ) score of less than 70 ■ Loving and trusting demeanor

Developmental Disability	Causes	Characteristics
Down syndrome	■ Genetic disorder	■ Some degree of intellectual disability ■ Some degree of muscle weakness ■ Commonly, heart defects and respiratory tract infections ■ Almond-shaped eyes ■ Large tongue in a small mouth ■ Square hands with short fingers ■ Small, wide nose and small ears ■ Short stature and wide, short neck ■ Loving and trusting demeanor
Autism	■ Unknown, possibly a genetic disorder	■ Extreme difficulty communicating with, and relating to, other people and surroundings ■ Average or above-average intelligence or some degree of intellectual disability ■ May have seizures
Cerebral palsy	■ Congenital brain abnormalities ■ Lack of oxygen to the brain before, during, or after birth ■ Early childhood accidents that cause brain injury or deprive the brain of oxygen	■ Difficulty controlling movement ■ Spasms and shortening of the muscles, possibly contractures ■ Possibly some degree of intellectual disability
Fragile X syndrome	■ Genetic disorder	■ Some degree of intellectual disability ■ Behavioral problems ■ Delayed speech and communication skills ■ Large, cupped ears ■ Slim build ■ Wide-set eyes ■ Velvet-like skin

(*table continues on page 652*)

TABLE 29-1 Common Developmental Disabilities (continued)

Developmental Disability	Causes	Characteristics
Fetal alcohol syndrome 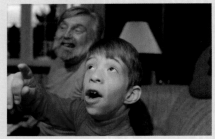 (©David H. Wells/CORBIS)	■ Consumption of alcohol by mother during pregnancy	■ Smaller-than-normal size ■ Some degree of intellectual disability ■ Behavioral problems ■ Learning difficulties ■ Facial deformities
Spina bifida 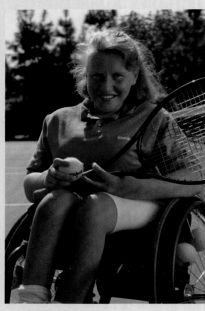 (©Jim Sugar/CORBIS)	■ Congenital spinal column abnormality	■ Weakness or paralysis from the waist down, depending on the severity of the defect ■ Commonly, problems with bowel and bladder control ■ Possibly some degree of intellectual disability
Hydrocephalus 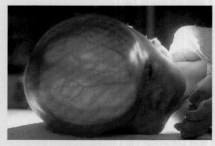 (© Southern Illinois University/Science Source)	■ Congenital brain or spinal column abnormalities that lead to a build-up of cerebrospinal fluid (CSF) ■ Tumor ■ Head trauma ■ Infection	■ Enlarged head (when condition occurs in a child younger than 2 years) ■ Some degree of intellectual disability (if pressure on brain is not relieved) ■ Possibly some motor disability (if pressure on brain is not relieved)

Putting it all together!

- A developmental disability is a permanent disability that affects a person before he reaches adulthood. A developmental disability may be congenital or acquired.

- A developmental disability can affect a person's intellectual function, physical function, or both. The severity of the disability varies from person to person, even among people with the same condition.

- Common developmental disabilities include intellectual disability, Down syndrome, autism, cerebral palsy, fragile X syndrome, fetal alcohol syndrome, spina bifida, and hydrocephalus.

Education and Protection of Rights

What will you learn?

When you are finished with this section, you will be able to:

1. Describe special education programs that can help a person with developmental disabilities to become less reliant on others for care.
2. Describe laws and organizations that have been established to protect the rights of people who have developmental disabilities.

Special Education

Special educational programs are focused on the individual's needs and may cover a wide range of topics:

- **Self-care skills** (for example, eating and dressing)
- **Life skills** (for example, counting money)
- **Social skills** (for example, understanding appropriate behavior and "limits")

Vocational training focuses on teaching work skills that help people with disabilities to become less dependent on others for their care (Fig. 29-1).

Protection of Rights

The Americans with Disabilities Act (ADA) ensures that people who have disabilities are treated the same as those without disabilities. The ADA guarantees people with disabilities access to public education, employment, and public places such as parks, restaurants, and transportation. The Arc of the United States is an organization that helps to protect the rights of people with intellectual disabilities, very similar to how the Omnibus Budget Reconciliation Act (OBRA) helps to protect the rights of the elderly people.

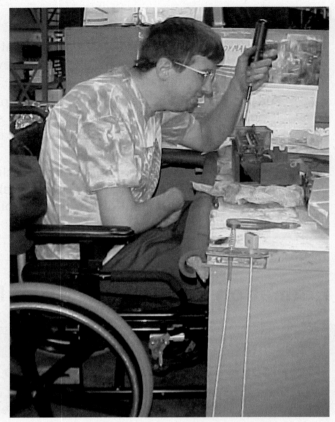

■ **FIGURE 29-1**

Vocational training helps
to prepare people with
developmental disabili-
ties for the work force.
(Courtesy of the Wood County
Board of Mental Retardation
and Developmental Disabilities,
Bowling Green, OH.)

Putting it all together!

- A person with developmental disabilities may attend a special
  education program to learn self-care skills, life skills, or social
  skills. Vocational training teaches work skills that will enable the
  person to get a job.
- Legislation (such as the Americans with Disabilities Act) and
  organizations (such as the Arc of the United States) help to
  protect the rights of people with disabilities.

Caring for People With
Developmental Disabilities

What will you learn?

When you are finished with this section, you will be able to:

1. Describe special considerations that you should keep in mind
   while helping a person with developmental disabilities with
   activities of daily living (ADLs).

2. Explain methods used to help people with developmental disabilities maximize their abilities and become less dependent on others.

3. State observations that you may make when caring for a person with developmental disabilities that should be reported to the nurse.

Meeting the Physical Needs of a Person With Developmental Disabilities

Developmental disabilities can cause mild or severe impairment. When you are caring for a person with developmental disabilities, focus on the individual. Do not expect the person to have the same abilities or disabilities as another person with the same condition.

Encourage and allow the person to do as much as possible on her own to help promote independence. Many people with developmental disabilities are able to manage their activities of daily living (ADLs) quite independently by using assistive devices. A person with intellectual disabilities may simply need to be reminded of what to do next to accomplish self-care tasks.

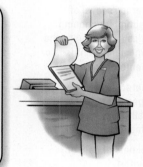

When caring for a person with a developmental disability, make sure to learn as much as you can about that person. Focusing on the person's abilities instead of disabilities will help you to provide the standard of care that each of your patients or residents needs from you.

Physical rehabilitation may be used to maximize the person's independence and maintain levels of function. You may be responsible for helping the person with physical rehabilitation (for example, by assisting the person with range-of-motion exercises).

Communicating With a Person With Developmental Disabilities

Many people with developmental disabilities have difficulty communicating. Some people are physically unable to form words to speak. Others lack the intellectual ability to use or understand language. Many people with developmental disabilities also have vision or hearing problems. When caring for a person with developmental disabilities:

- Ask family members what communication techniques work best with the person.
- Pay attention to the person's nonverbal communication (facial expressions, body language).
- If the person has an intellectual disability, use simple words and short phrases.
- Remember that a touch, a smile, and a kind word communicate care and compassion.

Because many people with severe developmental disabilities have difficulty communicating, they may be unable to tell you if they are experiencing pain or discomfort. Watch for small changes in a person's behavior, eating habits, or sleeping habits. Changes like these may be a sign that the person is ill.

Tell the Nurse!

Caring for a person with a developmental disability

- The person's vital signs change (especially body temperature or pulse rhythm)

- The person's appetite changes

- The person's level of activity changes

- The person's physical ability changes (for example, a person who usually has no trouble walking starts having falls)

- The person's level of intellectual functioning changes (for example, the person seems confused or disoriented)

- The person's behavior changes (for example, a normally gentle person becomes aggressive)

- Complaints of pain or discomfort

- Red or swollen areas

- Signs of physical or emotional abuse

Concerns for Long-Term Care

Today, because of improvements in medical care and nutrition, people who have developmental disabilities are living much longer than they used to. People with developmental disabilities experience the same changes that occur as a result of aging as everyone else. However, they usually experience these changes earlier, in middle age. In addition, many people with developmental disabilities are at risk for developing certain other health conditions as they age. As a result of these changes, a person with a developmental disability may require more care and assistance as he ages. The aging parents of an adult child with a developmental disability may find it difficult to provide that care for their son or daughter, due to their own frailty or disability.

Moving to a long-term care facility can be difficult for the person, as well as his family members. Having to leave home—where the person felt comfortable and safe—and move into a long-term care facility can be incredibly traumatic for a person with a developmental disability, just as it can be for any other resident. The person may feel angry, deserted, or alone, and will need your compassion and understanding to help become comfortable in his new surroundings.

Family members may have difficulty adjusting as well. A parent may have difficulty trusting the care of his or her child to someone else. In many cases, the parent has been the child's primary caregiver for the child's entire life. You can imagine how hard it would be to give up that role after 30, 40, or even 50 years! The parents may worry about how to afford their own care, as well as that of their child. In addition, they may worry about paying for the continued care that their child will need after their death.

Putting it all together!

- A person with developmental disabilities may require a lot of assistance with activities of daily living (ADLs) or very little. Assistive devices and rehabilitation can help a person with a developmental disability to maximize his abilities and maintain independence.

- As a nursing assistant, you may be involved in assisting people with developmental disabilities with tasks related to rehabilitation.

- Because people with developmental disabilities may have difficulty communicating, you may need to rely on your observation skills to tell when something is wrong. Be alert to changes in the person's vital signs, sleeping or eating habits, or behavior.

WHAT DID YOU LEARN?

Multiple Choice

Select the single best answer for each of the following questions.

1. Which one of the following statements about intellectual disabilities is correct?
   a. It affects the motor region of the brain
   b. It can occur before, during, or after birth
   c. It is always severe
   d. None of the above

2. What physical characteristics does a person with Down syndrome have?
   a. Large, cupped ears; a slim build; wide-set, somewhat squinting eyes; and velvet-like skin
   b. Almond-shaped eyes, square hands with short fingers, large tongue in a small mouth
   c. A large head
   d. Facial deformities and small stature

3. What do scientists think is a cause of autism?
   a. Genetics
   b. Oxygen deprivation at birth
   c. Drugs
   d. Trauma at birth

4. Cerebral palsy can be caused by:
   a. Alcohol intake during pregnancy
   b. A lack of oxygen to the brain
   c. An extra chromosome
   d. A bad cold

5. A person with autism has:
   a. An enlarged head
   b. Hearing and vision problems
   c. Problems relating to others
   d. Muscle weakness

6. A person with Down syndrome always has some degree of:
   a. Intellectual disability
   b. Spastic movements
   c. Cerebral palsy
   d. Autism

7. Which one of the following statements about fetal alcohol syndrome is correct?
   a. It occurs when a woman smokes during pregnancy
   b. A newborn with fetal alcohol syndrome is larger than normal
   c. It occurs when a woman drinks alcohol during pregnancy
   d. It is caused by oxygen deprivation at birth

8. What is spina bifida?
   a. A seizure disorder
   b. A defect of the spinal canal
   c. A shunt
   d. Another name for fragile X syndrome

9. What is common in a person with spina bifida?
   a. Autism
   b. Bowel and bladder incontinence
   c. Drooling
   d. Seizures

10. Hydrocephalus occurs when:
    a. Cerebrospinal fluid (CSF) builds up
    b. The person has a seizure
    c. A person is born with an extra chromosome
    d. A person has nerve damage

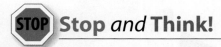 Stop *and* Think!

Today a new resident has been admitted to the long-term care facility where you work. Mr. Theodore has severe cerebral palsy. He is an only child. His parents, who are in their 80s, are no longer able to provide the physical care that Mr. Theodore needs. Mr. Theodore is very upset. He is crying, and he keeps asking why his family doesn't want him anymore. What can you do in the coming days and weeks to help Mr. Theodore make the adjustment to his new home?

Caring for People With Cancer

Any organ system can be affected by cancer. In fact, it is estimated that 200 different types of cancer can affect the human body. In this chapter, you will learn about how cancer is diagnosed and treated. You will also learn about the special physical and emotional needs of people with cancer.

Photo: *A nursing assistant talks with a patient who is receiving chemotherapy to treat cancer. A common side effect of chemotherapy is hair loss. (© Colin Cuthbert/Science Source.)*

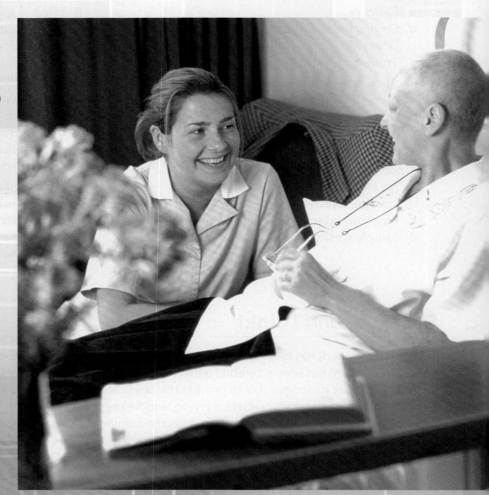

Introduction to Cancer

What will you learn?

When you are finished with this section, you will be able to:

1. Describe the difference between benign and malignant tumors.
2. List risk factors for cancer.
3. Define the words **tumor**, **benign**, **malignant**, and **metastasis**.

A **tumor** is either **benign** or **malignant**. We often refer to malignant tumors as "cancer." Malignant tumors grow rapidly and invade nearby healthy tissue. Cells from malignant tumors can also travel through the bloodstream to other parts of the body, where they "take root" and start a new cancerous tumor. This process is called **metastasis**.

The exact cause of cancer is unknown. Risk factors for developing cancer may include:

- A family history of cancer
- Environmental factors, such as exposure to pollution, tobacco smoke, radiation, or chemicals
- A high-fat diet
- A sedentary lifestyle

According to the National Cancer Institute, age is the single most important risk factor for cancer. Most new cancer cases are diagnosed in older adults and cancer is the second leading cause of death in people who are 65 years old and older.

Tumor an abnormal growth of tissue; the cells that form the tumor may be benign or malignant

Benign "good" or "kind"; adjective used to describe a non-cancerous tumor (that is, one that grows slowly and does not spread)

Malignant "evil"; adjective used to describe a cancerous tumor (that is, one that grows rapidly and spreads)

Metastasis the process by which cancer cells spread from their original location in the body to a new location, which may be quite distant from the first

Putting it all together!

- A tumor, or mass of abnormal cells, may be malignant (cancerous) or benign (not cancerous). The cells that make up malignant tumors divide rapidly and spread into nearby tissues. They can also enter the bloodstream and spread to distant organs, a process called metastasis.
- Risk factors for cancer include a family history of cancer, environmental factors, a high-fat diet, a sedentary lifestyle, and age. Eating a healthy diet, exercising, and avoiding smoking and job-related carcinogens are important steps that people can take to lower their risk of developing cancer.

Detecting and Treating Cancer

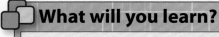

What will you learn?

When you are finished with this section, you will be able to:

1. Describe observations that could be early warning signs of cancer.

2. Explain why early detection of cancer is important.
3. Describe methods used to diagnose cancer.
4. Describe methods used to treat cancer.
5. Define the words **biopsy** and **prognosis**.

Detecting Cancer

Early detection of cancer can lead to early treatment, which greatly improves a person's chances of surviving the disease. Many cancers are caught in their early stages when a person notices a change and reports it to the doctor promptly (Box 30-1). Other cancers are caught in their early stages through routine physical check-ups and screening tests.

If a person is thought to have cancer, the doctor may order additional tests to diagnose the cancer, determine what type it is, and determine how far it has spread.

- **Imaging studies,** such as x-rays, computed tomography (CT) scans, and magnetic resonance imaging (MRI) scans, allow the doctor to see the tumor without actually entering the body.
- **Endoscopic examinations** involve using a lighted instrument to look inside the body and obtain tissue or fluids for analysis.
- **Biopsy** can be performed by surgically removing all or part of the tumor or by using a needle to obtain tissue or fluids for analysis.

Biopsy a diagnostic procedure that involves obtaining a cell or tissue sample for examination under a microscope

---

BOX 30-1 CAUTIONS: Warning Signs of Cancer

Change in bowel or bladder habits. A person with colon cancer may have diarrhea or constipation or may notice that the stool has become smaller in diameter. A person with bladder or kidney cancer may have urinary frequency and urgency.

A sore that does not heal. Small, scaly patches on the skin that bleed or do not heal may be a sign of skin cancer. A sore in the mouth that does not heal can indicate oral cancer.

Unusual bleeding or discharge. Blood in the stool is often the first sign of colon cancer. Similarly, blood in the urine is usually the first sign of bladder or kidney cancer. Postmenopausal bleeding (bleeding after menopause) may be a sign of uterine cancer.

Thickenings or lumps. Enlargement of the lymph nodes or glands (such as the thyroid gland) can be an early sign of cancer. Breast and testicular cancers may also present as a lump.

Indigestion or difficulty in swallowing. Cancers of the digestive system may cause indigestion, heartburn, or difficulty swallowing.

Obvious change in a wart or mole. Moles or other skin lesions that change in shape, size, or color should be reported.

Nagging or persistent cough or hoarseness. Cancers of the respiratory tract, including lung cancer and laryngeal cancer, may cause a cough that does not go away or a hoarse (rough) voice.

Sudden, unexplained weight loss. Loss of a significant amount of weight (for example, about 10 pounds) without trying may be the first sign of cancer, especially cancer of the pancreas, stomach, esophagus, or lung.

You may need to help prepare a patient or resident for a diagnostic test. Be aware that a person awaiting test results is likely to be anxious about his **prognosis**. Use the communication skills you learned in Chapter 4 to encourage the person to talk about his fears and to ask any questions he may have. Report questions to the nurse so that they can be answered promptly.

> **Prognosis** a doctor's prediction of the course of a person's disease, and his or her estimation of the person's chances for recovery

Treating Cancer

Many types of cancer can be successfully treated. There are three main approaches to treating cancer (Fig. 30-1). The approach used depends on the type of cancer and the extent to which the cancer has spread to other tissues and organs. Treatment methods may be used alone or in combination with each other, depending on the type and extent of the cancer.

In addition to the three conventional types of cancer treatment, some people choose to add other therapies. *Biologic therapy* involves the use of living organisms (such as bacteria), substances produced by living organisms or similar substances that can be produced in the laboratory (such as vaccines or antibodies). Biologic therapy can be used to either boost a person's immune system to act against cancer cells or to prevent infections from other organisms. *Complementary and alternative medicine therapies (CAM)* may be used in addition to chemotherapy

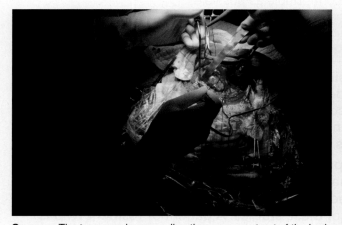

Surgery: The tumor and surrounding tissues are cut out of the body.

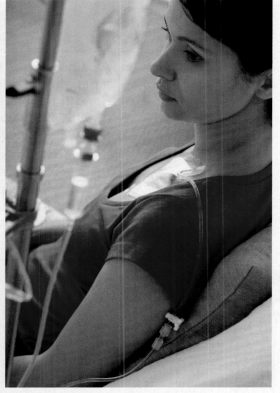

Chemotherapy: Medications destroy the cancer cells.

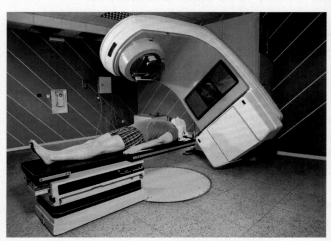

Radiation: Powerful x-ray beams destroy the cancer cells.

■ **FIGURE 30-1**

The three main approaches to treating cancer.

and radiation. CAM includes techniques such as special diets, massage, acupuncture, special herbs, and meditation.

In some cases, a person's cancer cannot be cured. The person may still be treated with surgery, chemotherapy, radiation, or a combination of the three. However, in this case, the goal of treatment is to help make the person more comfortable, not to get rid of the cancer.

> **Concerns for Long-Term Care**
>
> Many of your older residents with cancer will receive palliative treatment, or no treatment at all. Because of advanced age, a chronic health condition, or both, the person may be too frail to tolerate aggressive treatment of the cancer. For example, a resident with heart disease may not be able to tolerate the recommended chemotherapy because the medications are potentially toxic to the heart. Another resident may not be able to have surgery because his chronic respiratory disorder makes anesthesia too risky. A resident with dementia may not be able to be still through radiation treatments. In cases like this, the treatment may be harder on the person than the cancer itself. As a result, the person (or his health care agent) and the doctor may agree not to screen for common cancers (or not to do further testing for cancer even if the person has symptoms that suggest cancer). Instead, palliative care is provided to minimize symptoms and keep the person as comfortable as possible.

 ## Putting it all together!

- As a nursing assistant, you may be the first to notice that a patient or resident has an early warning sign of cancer. Reporting your concerns to the nurse immediately can lead to early detection and treatment, which greatly improves the person's chances of surviving the disease.

- If the doctor suspects cancer, he or she might order follow-up tests (such as imaging studies, endoscopic studies, or biopsy). You may be responsible for helping to prepare a patient or resident for one of these studies. A patient or resident who is awaiting test results is likely to be upset and anxious.

- The three main approaches to treating cancer are surgery, chemotherapy, and radiation. These approaches may be used alone or in combination, depending on the type of cancer and whether it has spread. Many people also choose to add biologic therapy or complementary and alternative medicine to their conventional cancer treatment. These methods may be used to cure the cancer or, if the cancer cannot be cured, to help make the person more comfortable.

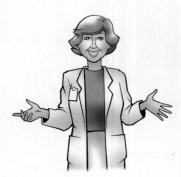

A person with cancer often faces many treatment choices, including the choice of not having treatment at all. It is important to respect the person's choice, even if you do not agree with it. When you respect the decisions of the people you provide care for and support them emotionally, you demonstrate true compassion and caring.

Caring for a Person With Cancer

What will you learn?

When you are finished with this section, you will be able to:

1. Describe some of the side effects of cancer treatment.
2. Discuss how you can help a person who is experiencing side effects of cancer treatment feel more comfortable.
3. Discuss how cancer affects a person emotionally.
4. Define the words **alopecia** and **stomatitis**.

Meeting the Physical Needs of a Person With Cancer

Managing Pain

Cancer can be very painful. The pain may be temporary, related to surgery or radiation treatment, or it may be chronic, related to the cancer itself. Chapter 27 describes how you can help a person who is in pain.

Managing Side Effects of Treatment

The treatments used for cancer, especially chemotherapy and radiation therapy, may have severe side effects:

- **Nausea, vomiting, diarrhea,** and **loss of appetite (anorexia)** are common with chemotherapy and radiation treatments. Provide frequent mouth care and offer small, frequent meals. If the person has an appetite for a particular food or beverage, try to accommodate the person's request.
- **Constipation** is often a side effect of pain medication. Chapter 26 describes methods of preventing and treating constipation.
- **Skin irritation** can result from radiation treatment. Prevent skin breakdown by providing gentle, thorough skin care.
- **Alopecia** can result from chemotherapy. A hat or scarf can be used to keep the head warm.
- **Stomatitis** can result from chemotherapy. Stomatitis is painful and may affect the person's ability to eat. Provide frequent, gentle oral care to prevent infection. Offer the person drinks that are blended with ice, ice cream, yogurt, or fruit to soothe the mouth and provide nutrition.
- **Fatigue.** People who are being treated for cancer may be very tired all of the time. Assist the person with mild exercise combined with periods of rest to maintain muscle strength.
- **Increased risk for infection.** Cancer treatments can temporarily interfere with the body's ability to fight off infections. Prevent the person from being exposed to pathogens by practicing good infection control at all times and asking people with contagious illnesses to delay visiting.

Alopecia baldness, loss of hair

Stomatitis inflammation of the mouth, often seen in people who are receiving chemotherapy

Tell the Nurse!

Caring for a person with cancer

- Severe nausea, vomiting, or both

- Pain or sores in the mouth

- Red or irritated skin

- Unusual discharge or bleeding from the vagina, urethra, or rectum

- Pain

- Diarrhea or constipation

- Redness, swelling, or pain around an intravenous (IV) or venous access site

- Fever or other signs of infection

Meeting the Emotional Needs of a Person With Cancer

A person who has cancer may have many concerns. For example, the person may fear the side effects of treatment or worry about having a great deal of pain. The person may worry about how the cancer, its treatment, or both will affect her appearance. The person may worry that even if the cancer is treated successfully now, it may return later in life. Be a good listener and allow the person to verbalize her fears and feelings.

Many people are uncomfortable with the subject of cancer, and as a result may avoid a person with cancer without even being aware that they are doing so. If one of your patients or residents has been diagnosed with cancer, be sure to check in on the person as often as you check in on your other patients or residents. Spend time with the person and offer as many physical comforts as possible. Remember the value of a comforting touch.

Many people with cancer find comfort in their spiritual beliefs and practices. As always, report requests for clergy to the nurse promptly and provide privacy for time spent with clergy or in prayer or meditation.

Putting it all together!

- A person with cancer has many physical needs that are directly related to the cancer or to its treatment. You will play an important role in helping your patients or residents who have cancer to manage their pain and deal with the unpleasant side effects of treatment.

- A person with cancer will need assistance to meet emotional and spiritual needs as well. Often, the best thing you can do is listen if the person wants to talk or spend quiet time with the person if he does not want to talk.

WHAT DID YOU LEARN?

Multiple Choice

Select the single best answer for each of the following questions.

1. Which one of the following statements best describes a malignant (cancerous) tumor?
   a. It consists of abnormal cells that divide rapidly and are capable of spreading to nearby tissues and distant organs.
   b. It consists of abnormal cells that divide slowly and tend to stay together.
   c. All tumors are malignant.
   d. All malignant tumors are fatal.

2. Which one of the following factors plays a role in whether or not a person develops cancer?
   a. Inheritance (genes)
   b. Lifestyle choices, such as diet and exercise
   c. Environment
   d. All of the above

3. Mrs. Worthington is receiving chemotherapy following surgery to remove a malignant tumor. Following each treatment, she is very nauseated, and often she vomits. What could you do to help Mrs. Worthington feel better?
   a. Offer her strong pain medications
   b. Offer her ice chips and sit with her and hold her hand
   c. Enter her room only when necessary to avoid disturbing her
   d. Serve her meal tray as usual, in hopes that the smell of the food will increase her appetite

Matching

Match each vocabulary word with its definition.

_____ 1. Stomatitis

_____ 2. Biopsy

_____ 3. Metastasis

_____ 4. Tumor

_____ 5. Prognosis

a. A diagnostic procedure that involves obtaining a cell or tissue sample for examination under a microscope

b. The doctor's prediction of the course of a person's disease and the person's chance of recovering from it

c. Inflammation of the mouth

d. The spread of malignant cells to other parts of the body

e. Abnormal growth of tissue

Stop *and* Think!

You are caring for Mr. Lukens, a resident who was recently diagnosed with cancer. The doctors have presented Mr. Lukens and his family with a number of different treatment options, and for the last few days, Mr. Lukens has been weighing the pros and cons of each. In addition, he is still trying to adjust to the diagnosis he has just been given and what it means for his future. One morning, while you are making Mr. Lukens' bed, he starts to talk to you about his father, who died of cancer after going through several months of agonizing treatments. He tells you that he is scared that he, too, will go through the treatments and that in the end, all of his suffering might be for nothing. "Maybe it would just be easier to give up now and die peacefully," he says. How would you react to what Mr. Lukens is telling you? Is there anything you can do or say that might help Mr. Lukens with the difficult choices he needs to make?

Caring for People With HIV/AIDS

More than 1.1 million people in the United States are infected with HIV, the virus that causes AIDS. HIV/AIDS is a global health crisis. The rate of infection continues to increase around the world, and there is no cure for this devastating disease. In this chapter, you will learn more about HIV/AIDS and how it affects the people who have it, physically and emotionally.

Photo: Seniors attend an HIV/AIDS educational presentation and screening held by the New York City Department of Aging. Although many people think of HIV/AIDS as a disease that affects young people, older people are at risk too. (AP Photo/Bebeto Matthews.)

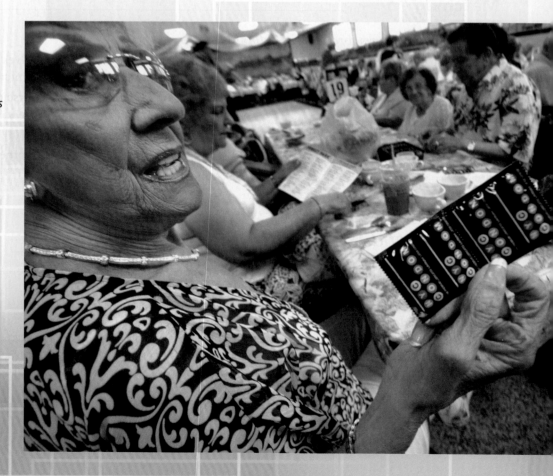

Introduction to HIV/AIDS

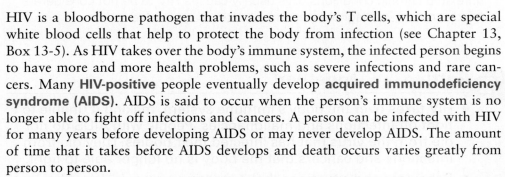

What will you learn?

When you are finished with this section, you will be able to:

1. Describe how HIV infection affects the body.
2. Describe situations and behaviors that increase a person's risk of becoming infected with HIV.
3. Define the words **HIV-positive, acquired immunodeficiency syndrome (AIDS), homosexual,** and **heterosexual**.

HIV is a bloodborne pathogen that invades the body's T cells, which are special white blood cells that help to protect the body from infection (see Chapter 13, Box 13-5). As HIV takes over the body's immune system, the infected person begins to have more and more health problems, such as severe infections and rare cancers. Many **HIV-positive** people eventually develop **acquired immunodeficiency syndrome (AIDS)**. AIDS is said to occur when the person's immune system is no longer able to fight off infections and cancers. A person can be infected with HIV for many years before developing AIDS or may never develop AIDS. The amount of time that it takes before AIDS develops and death occurs varies greatly from person to person.

Anyone can be infected with HIV and get AIDS—young, old, **homosexual, heterosexual,** male, or female. Behaviors and situations that increase a person's risk for becoming infected with HIV include the following:

- **Having unprotected sex.** Unprotected sexual intercourse, both homosexual and heterosexual, is the most common method of HIV transmission.
- **Sharing needles.** Sharing of needles among people who abuse intravenous drugs is the second most common method of transmission.
- **Receiving tissue transplants or transfusions of blood or blood products.** This method of transmission is less common now in the United States because donated blood and tissue are screened for the virus.
- **Having an HIV-positive mother.** HIV can be transmitted from mother to baby before or during birth or through breast milk.

To date, there is no cure or vaccine for HIV/AIDS. However, early diagnosis of HIV infection and early treatment with antiretroviral therapy (ART) can help delay or prevent the onset of HIV and reduce the risk of transmission of the virus to other people. These medications can cost more than $10,000 per year and are not always successful. In addition, they often cause side effects, such as headache, dizziness, nausea, diarrhea, fever, skin rash, severe anemia, and extreme fatigue. The number of people becoming infected with HIV/AIDS in the United States and many European countries has decreased due to new medications and AIDS awareness education. However, in many developing nations, the rate of HIV infection is increasing, and the number of people dying from AIDS is doubling and even tripling due to a lack of medical services and HIV/AIDS education.

HIV-positive the state of being infected with human immunodeficiency virus (HIV)

Acquired immunodeficiency syndrome (AIDS) a disease caused by human immunodeficiency virus (HIV), a bloodborne virus that attacks the body's immune system; death usually results when the body becomes unable to recognize and fight off infections

Homosexual a person who is sexually attracted to members of the same sex

Heterosexual a person who is sexually attracted to members of the opposite sex

> ### Concerns for Long-Term Care
>
> Although many people do not consider the elderly population to be at risk for becoming infected with HIV, the Centers for Disease Control and Prevention (CDC) reports that the number of people diagnosed with HIV has increased more than twice as quickly in people over age 50 than in younger adults. People aged 50 years and above make up approximately 30% of the total number of HIV/AIDS cases nationwide.
>
> AIDS awareness programs, which teach people about AIDS and how to lower their risk of becoming infected with HIV, have traditionally been aimed at younger people, rather than older people. Many older people are not aware of how HIV is transmitted or behaviors that put them at risk for getting HIV. As a result, sexually active older adults may engage in unprotected sex, which puts them at risk for HIV infection.
>
> AIDS-related symptoms may be attributed to growing older or other unrelated chronic conditions. This usually causes HIV to be not considered, misdiagnosed, or diagnosed at a much later stage in older adults.

Putting it all together!

- HIV takes over the body's immune system, making it unable to fight off infections and malignancies. People with AIDS do not die from the virus that has infected their bodies. They die from infections and cancers that the body is no longer able to fight.
- Behaviors and situations that increase a person's risk of being infected with HIV include having unprotected sex, sharing needles, receiving contaminated tissue transplants or blood transfusions, and being born to an HIV-positive mother.
- Anyone—young, old, male, female, heterosexual, or homosexual—can become infected with HIV!

Attitudes Toward People With HIV/AIDS

What will you learn?

When you are finished with this section, you will be able to:

1. Discuss why people with HIV/AIDS are at risk for discrimination and poor treatment.
2. Discuss some of the rights of people with HIV/AIDS that are protected by law.
3. Discuss measures you can take to help protect a person with HIV/AIDS from discrimination and poor treatment.

In many cultures, being HIV-positive or having AIDS is considered shameful. As a result, a person with HIV/AIDS may experience discrimination and poor treatment by others. There are many factors that contribute to the negative attitude many people have toward those who are HIV-positive or have AIDS:

- Because HIV infection is associated with many behaviors that people can control (such as whether or not they practice safe sex), some people may feel that the person with HIV/AIDS "has only herself to blame."

- Many of the behaviors associated with HIV infection are behaviors that many people do not approve of for moral or religious reasons (such as abusing street drugs or being homosexual).

- Many people lack information about how HIV is transmitted and, as a result, fear becoming infected with HIV through casual contact with an infected person.

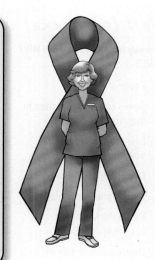

Remember that it does not really matter how a person became infected with HIV. Even if you do not approve of the person's lifestyle, you must not let your personal beliefs affect the care that you give the person. Instead of focusing on how the person got HIV, focus on who the person is. Your ability to provide supportive and compassionate care to your patients or residents with HIV/AIDS will make a significant difference in their quality of life.

Because a person with HIV/AIDS is at risk for discrimination, many states have laws designed specifically to protect the rights of people with HIV/AIDS. These laws ensure the person's right to employment, education, privacy, and health care. In most states, people with AIDS are protected under the Americans with Disabilities Act (ADA).

As with all of your patients or residents, protecting the person's privacy and right to confidentiality is very important. This is especially true when a person has a condition, such as HIV/AIDS, that could cause him to experience discrimination. For example, if a person is known to be HIV-positive, he may have trouble getting a job, obtaining health insurance, or renting an apartment. Although laws are in place to protect the person from discrimination, discrimination can still occur. Know your facility's or agency's policies related to keeping health information private and follow these policies carefully at all times with all patients and residents.

 Putting it all together!

- A person with HIV/AIDS is at risk for discrimination because of negative attitudes that many people have toward this disease.

- Many states have passed laws to help ensure the right to employment, education, privacy, and health care for people with HIV/AIDS.

- You need to know the HIV status of a person to whom you are providing care. However, no one else needs to know. You must keep information about a person's HIV status or any other medical condition private and confidential.

Caring for a Person With HIV/AIDS

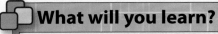 **What will you learn?**

When you are finished this section, you will be able to:

1. Describe special considerations you should keep in mind when providing physical care for a person with HIV/AIDS.
2. Discuss how HIV/AIDS affects a person emotionally.

A person with HIV/AIDS may receive care from many different health care organizations. Throughout the course of the illness, people with HIV/AIDS require hospitalization for the treatment of severe infections and other problems. Toward the end of their lives, most people with AIDS require almost complete assistance with activities of daily living (ADLs). As a result, many seek care from home health care agencies or move to long-term care facilities. Most people with AIDS also eventually require hospice care.

Meeting the Physical Needs of a Person With HIV/AIDS

As HIV infection progresses, the person is likely to develop many health problems, including:

- Loss of appetite (anorexia), nausea, vomiting, or diarrhea
- Weight loss
- Fever (with or without night sweats)
- Pain or difficulty swallowing (dysphagia)
- Fatigue
- Swollen lymph nodes in the neck, armpits, and groin
- A cough or recurrent episodes of pneumonia
- Sores or white patches in the mouth
- Bruises or dark bumps on the skin that do not heal (Fig. 31-1)
- Forgetfulness and confusion
- Dementia

Table 31-1 describes some of the care measures nursing assistants use to help meet the physical needs of people with HIV/AIDS. You may find it frightening to provide physical care for a person who is known to have a communicable, potentially deadly illness. Know that with the proper and consistent use of standard precautions, your risk of exposure to HIV and other bloodborne pathogens in the workplace is actually quite low.

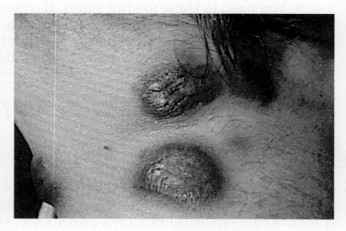

■ **FIGURE 31-1**

Kaposi's sarcoma, a type of cancer, may be seen on the skin and mucous membranes of people with advanced HIV infection (AIDS). Courtesy of Goodheart, H.P. [2003]. *Goodheart's photoguide of common skin disorders: Diagnosis and management* [p. 374]. Philadelphia: Lippincott Williams & Wilkins.

TABLE 31-1 **Physical Problems Related to HIV/AIDS and Corresponding Care**

Physical Problem	Cause	Care Measures
Poor nutrition	■ Painful sores in the mouth can make eating difficult. Nausea can cause anorexia.	■ Provide frequent oral care. ■ Use a special numbing spray or mouthwash as ordered to ease the pain of mouth sores. ■ Offer nutritious drinks made from yogurt or ice cream combined with fruit. ■ Serve nutritional supplements as ordered.
Fluid imbalance	■ Chronic diarrhea and vomiting can cause dehydration.	■ Measure and record intake and output as ordered.
Rashes and skin infections	■ Rashes and skin infections can develop as a result of both the disease and the medications used to treat it.	■ Use special cleansing agents, special bathing techniques, or both as ordered. ■ Keep the skin clean and dry and change clothing and linens as needed.
Weakened immune system	■ HIV destroys the cells that help the body to fight off infections.	■ Ask visitors with colds or other contagious illnesses to delay visiting. ■ Ensure that foods are cooked thoroughly. ■ Practice proper infection control measures, especially good hand hygiene.
Pain, weakness, and fatigue	■ Pain, weakness, and fatigue occur as a result of both the disease and the medications used to treat it.	■ Assist the person with ADLs as needed, being sure to let the person do as much for herself as possible for as long as possible. ■ Assist the person with mild exercise combined with periods of rest to maintain muscle strength. ■ Position the person for comfort using pillows and other supportive devices. ■ Provide back massages and a quiet room to promote rest and relaxation.

Meeting the Emotional Needs of a Person With HIV/AIDS

People with HIV/AIDS have a great deal of emotional stress.

■ Many HIV-positive people are abandoned by friends and family members due to fear, shame, or disapproval.

■ The person may have worries about money. The person may lose a job (and health care benefits) because of the disease. Health care and the medications used to slow the progression of the disease are very expensive.

- The person may suffer from guilt, especially if risky behavior led to the infection.
- The person may have many fears related to failing health, disability, pain, or death.

Clinical depression and suicide are common among people with HIV/AIDS. When caring for a person with HIV/AIDS, pay attention to changes in the person's behaviors or moods that may be signs of clinical depression (see Chapter 8). Also, if the person talks of suicide, report this to the nurse immediately.

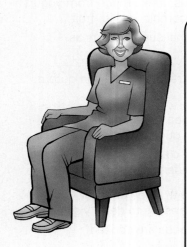

How would you feel if people were afraid to touch you? Would you feel dirty, unloved, and alone? Sometimes, the only human touch a person with HIV/AIDS will experience will come from caregivers. When caring for a person with HIV/AIDS, you can use touch to comfort the person, spend time listening and talking with the person, or hug the person. None of these activities will transmit the virus to you, and these simple actions can help the person with HIV/AIDS feel much better.

Putting it all together!

- People with HIV/AIDS require the services of many different types of health care organizations throughout the course of their illness.
- HIV infection and the medications used to slow its progression can cause many physical problems, including poor nutrition; fluid imbalance; rashes and other skin disorders; a high risk for infection; and pain, weakness, and fatigue. There are many things you can do to help keep the person physically comfortable and relieve or prevent some of these problems.
- In addition to providing physical care, you will play an important role in providing emotional care to the person with HIV/AIDS. You cannot get HIV from holding a person's hand or giving a person a hug.
- With the proper and consistent use of standard precautions, your risk of exposure to HIV in the workplace is quite low.

WHAT DID YOU LEARN?

Multiple Choice

Select the single best answer for each of the following questions.

1. When are standard precautions used?
   a. When a person who is HIV-positive develops AIDS
   b. When a person is HIV-positive or has AIDS
   c. When caring for a patient or resident who is homosexual
   d. When caring for any patient or resident and contact with blood or body fluids is possible

2. Which one of the following statements about HIV infection and AIDS is true?
   a. Anyone can become infected with HIV, regardless of age, gender, sexual orientation, or race.
   b. People who become infected with HIV and get AIDS are only drug abusers or homosexuals.
   c. HIV infection and AIDS are not a problem among the elderly people.
   d. AIDS usually develops soon after a person is first exposed to HIV.

3. When caring for a person who is HIV-positive, which one of the following observations should be reported to the nurse?
   a. The person has diarrhea
   b. The person seems depressed
   c. The person seems disoriented
   d. All of the above

4. Why is it especially important for nursing assistants to keep information about a person's HIV status private and confidential?
   a. AIDS is a shameful disease and should not be discussed in public.
   b. A person with HIV/AIDS can face discrimination because of the stigma of the disease.
   c. Nursing assistants have a responsibility to make sure that everyone who might come in contact with the person knows the person's HIV status so that others can protect themselves.
   d. AIDS is a global health crisis.

5. Which one of the following physical problems is a person with AIDS at risk for?
   a. Hair loss due to the medications used to slow the progression of HIV to AIDS
   b. Dehydration due to chronic diarrhea
   c. Blindness due to nerve damage as a result of HIV infection
   d. Heart failure due to myocardial infarction

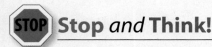 **Stop** *and* **Think!**

You work in a hospital. One of the patients you will be caring for today, Camilla, is a 34-year-old woman who has been admitted for the treatment of AIDS-related pneumonia. You have never cared for a patient with AIDS. Frankly, you are a little bit nervous about meeting Camilla and about providing hands-on physical care to a person who is known to be HIV-positive. What will be your approach to Camilla and to your responsibilities as a nursing assistant?

Caring for People Who Are Having Surgery

Surgery is a branch of medicine that involves treating disorders by entering the body and physically removing or repairing damaged organs or tissues. As a nursing assistant, you will help to prepare people for surgery and care for them afterward. This chapter discusses the special types of care that you will give to people both before and after surgery.

Photo: *A surgical team performs an operation.*

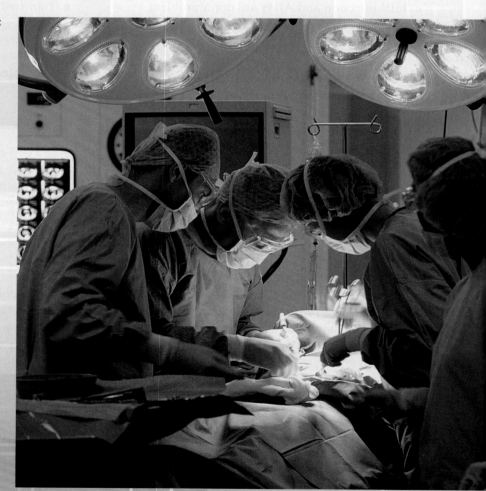

Introduction to Surgery

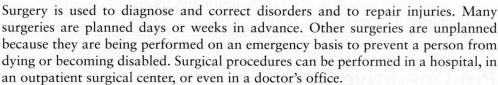

What will you learn?

When you are finished with this section, you will be able to:

1. Explain why a person might need surgery.
2. Define the words **peri-operative period**, **pre-operative phase**, **intra-operative phase**, and **post-operative phase**.

Surgery is used to diagnose and correct disorders and to repair injuries. Many surgeries are planned days or weeks in advance. Other surgeries are unplanned because they are being performed on an emergency basis to prevent a person from dying or becoming disabled. Surgical procedures can be performed in a hospital, in an outpatient surgical center, or even in a doctor's office.

In the past, people who were having a planned surgical procedure were admitted to the hospital a day or so before surgery. Now, changes in how we pay for health care have led to shorter hospital stays. Most people are admitted to the hospital or surgical center an hour or two before the surgery is scheduled. After the surgery, the person is often discharged within a few hours to recover at home, in an extended care facility, or in a long-term care facility. These changes mean that as a nursing assistant, you can expect to care for people who are either preparing for surgery or recovering from it, no matter where you work.

The **peri-operative period** has three phases: the **pre-operative phase**, the **intra-operative phase**, and the **post-operative phase** (Fig. 32-1).

Peri-operative period the term used to describe all three phases of the surgical process as a whole—the pre-operative, intra-operative, and post-operative phases

Pre-operative phase the phase before the surgery is actually performed

Intra-operative phase the phase during which the surgery is actually performed

Post-operative phase the phase after the surgery is actually performed

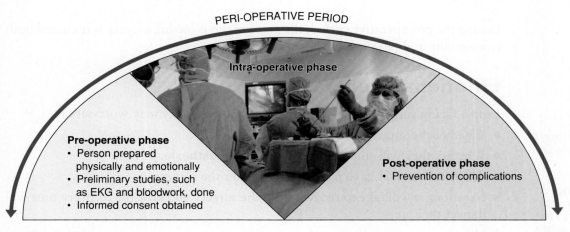

PERI-OPERATIVE PERIOD

Intra-operative phase

Pre-operative phase
- Person prepared physically and emotionally
- Preliminary studies, such as EKG and bloodwork, done
- Informed consent obtained

Post-operative phase
- Prevention of complications

■ **FIGURE 32-1**

The three phases of care for a person having surgery.

Putting it all together!

- Surgery is a branch of medicine that involves treating disorders by removing or repairing damaged tissues or organs. Some surgeries are planned in advance. Others are done on an emergency basis.

- Because many surgeries are now done on an outpatient basis, you may be responsible for helping a person to prepare for and recover from surgery even if you do not work in a hospital.

- The three phases of the surgical process are the pre-operative, intra-operative, and post-operative phases. The term *peri-operative period* is used to describe the three phases of the surgical process as a whole.

Pre-Operative Care

What will you learn?

When you are finished with this section, you will be able to:

1. Understand the concerns that a person who is about to have surgery may have and describe actions you can take to help relieve some of these worries.
2. Describe what needs to be done to physically prepare a person for surgery and explain your role in these preparations.
3. Explain the purpose of the pre-operative checklist.
4. Define the words **anesthesia** and **pre-operative teaching**.

During the pre-operative period, the person who is having surgery is prepared both emotionally and physically for the procedure.

Emotional Preparation

People facing surgery usually have many concerns. They may worry about:

- Whether the surgery will be successful
- Whether they will survive the surgery, the **anesthesia**, or both
- Whether they will have pain during or after the surgery
- How long it will take to recover from the surgery and how the recovery time will impact their lives
- How the surgery will affect their appearance

    To help reduce a person's anxiety about the upcoming surgery, the health care team talks with the person and his family members about the procedure, its benefits and possible risks, and what can be expected during the post-operative recovery period. You will assist the nurse and the doctor with this **pre-operative teaching**

Anesthesia loss of the ability to feel pain, caused by administration of a medication

Pre-operative teaching teaching done by members of the health care team to prepare a person and his or her family members for surgery; during pre-operative teaching, the person learns about the surgical procedure, its benefits and possible risks, and what can be expected during the post-operative recovery period

by reinforcing what the nurse has told the person and by keeping the nurse and doctor informed of any questions the person may ask you about the procedure. If the person seems very anxious or upset, be sure to report this observation to the nurse as well.

Physical Preparation

Several things are done to physically prepare the person for surgery:

- Several days before the surgery, the doctor may order laboratory studies (such as blood work, urine tests, and X-rays) to assess the person's level of health.

- The person may be placed on NPO (nothing by mouth) status for 6 to 8 hours before surgery. An empty stomach at the time of surgery helps to prevent vomiting, a common occurrence with some types of anesthesia. Frequent mouth care helps to keep the person on NPO status comfortable.

- A bowel prep and/or a cleansing enema may be ordered to empty the bowel before some types of abdominal or rectal surgery.

- The skin and hair are washed. Special antimicrobial soaps may be ordered. Removal of body hair (if ordered) and final skin preparations are usually performed in the operating room immediately before the procedure.

- Make-up and nail polish are usually not permitted. Prosthetic devices, glasses, contact lenses, hearing aids, dentures, wigs, jewelry, and hair ornaments may also be removed prior to surgery.

- The person is brought to a preparation area next to the operating room. The person is dressed in a clean hospital gown and surgical cap, and sedatives (to relieve anxiety) may be given. After these medications have been given, the person must remain in bed with the side rails up to reduce the risk of falling.

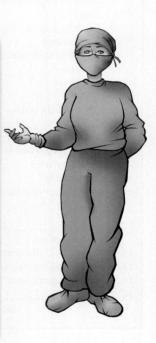

It is easy to tell a person that a surgical procedure is "minor" or "routine." Indeed, to health care workers who see similar surgeries every day, these procedures might be very routine! But no matter how simple or low-risk a surgical procedure is, there is nothing minor or routine about it to the person who is having it. Recognizing the person's fears, listening to the person's questions and concerns, and taking action to get those questions or concerns addressed are all very important things that you can do to help a person prepare emotionally for the upcoming surgery.

Documentation

After all other preparations have been made for surgery, a pre-operative checklist is completed (Fig. 32-2). The checklist is used to confirm that all pre-operative tests and procedures have been completed and that informed consent (see Chapter 2) has been obtained. Nursing assistants are often responsible for completing and recording many of the tasks on the checklist.

1. Patient's name: _____ Date: _____ Height: _____ Weight: _____
   Identification band present: _____
2. Informed consent signed: _____ Special permits signed: _____
3. Surgical site: _____ (Ex: Sterilization)
4. History & physical examination report present: _____ Date: _____
5. Laboratory records present: _____
   CBC: _____ Hgb: _____ Urinalysis: _____ Hct: _____

6. Item	Present	Removed
a. Natural teeth		
Dentures; upper, lower, partial	_____	_____
Bridge, fixed; crown	_____	_____
b. Contact lenses	_____	_____
c. Other prostheses—type: _____	_____	_____
d. Jewelry:		
Wedding band (taped/tied)	_____	_____
Rings	_____	_____
Earrings: pierced, clip-on	_____	_____
Neck chains	_____	_____
Any other body piercings	_____	_____
e. Make-up	_____	_____
Nail polish	_____	_____
7. Clothing		
a. Clean patient gown	_____	_____
b. Cap	_____	_____
c. Sanitary pad, etc.	_____	_____

8. Family instructed where to wait? _____
9. Valuables secured? _____
10. Blood available? _____ Ordered? _____ Where? _____
11. Preanesthetic medication given: _____
    Type: _____ Time: _____

12. Voided: _____ Amount: _____ Time: _____ Catheter: _____
    Mouth care given: _____
13. Vital signs: Temperature: _____ Pulse: _____ Resp: _____ Blood Pressure: _____
14. Special problems/precautions: (Allergies, deafness, *etc.*): _____
15. Area of skin preparation: _____
16. _____ Date: _____ Time: _____
    Signature: Nurse releasing patient

■ **FIGURE 32-2**

A pre-operative checklist documents that all of the tasks that must be completed during the pre-operative period have been completed. The pre-operative checklist goes in the person's medical record and must be completed before the person goes into surgery.

Putting it all together!

- During the pre-operative phase, the person is prepared both emotionally and physically for the surgery.
- People who are about to have surgery often have many concerns. Pre-operative teaching helps to relieve some of the person's concerns. By listening to the person and promptly relaying any questions she may have to the nurse, you can make an important contribution to the pre-operative teaching process.

- Tasks related to physically preparing the person for surgery that you may be responsible for include maintaining NPO status, assisting with the administration of a bowel prep and/or a cleansing enema, assisting with skin preparation, assisting the person to dress, and helping to keep the person safe.
- A pre-operative checklist is completed to verify that the tasks needed to prepare the person physically for surgery have been accomplished and that informed consent has been obtained.

Intra-Operative Care

What will you learn?

When you are finished with this section, you will be able to:
1. Explain how the person's room is prepared for the person to return to after surgery.
2. List items you may need to gather and place in the person's room.

While the person is in surgery, you may be responsible for preparing the person's room for the person's arrival post-operatively. To ready the room, you will:

- Change the bed linens and make a surgical bed (see Chapter 19)
- Raise the bed so that it will be level with the stretcher to make it easier to transfer the person from the stretcher to the bed (see Chapter 17, Procedure 17-11)
- Clear furniture to provide a pathway for the stretcher
- Gather items that may be needed at the time of the person's arrival (Box 32-1) and place them in the room

BOX 32-1 Equipment for Post-Operative Care

- Equipment for taking vital signs and a flow sheet for recording the vital signs
- An intravenous (IV) pole
- A towel and washcloth
- An emesis basin
- A bed protector
- Suction to connect to drainage devices
- Supplemental oxygen
- Pillows or other positioning aids to elevate the arms or legs
- Warmed blankets

Putting it all together!

- Preparing the person's room while the person is in surgery helps to promote comfort and efficiency.
- To prepare the room, the linens are changed and a surgical bed is made, furniture is moved out of the way to make room for the stretcher, and equipment that will be needed during the post-operative phase is gathered and placed in the room.

Post-Operative Care

What will you learn?

When you have finished with this section, you will be able to:

1. Describe potential complications that may occur as the result of surgery and the measures taken to prevent them.
2. State observations that you may make when caring for a person who has just had surgery that should be reported to the nurse.
3. Demonstrate proper technique for applying anti-embolism (TED) stockings.
4. Define the word **post-anesthesia care unit (PACU)**.

Post-anesthesia care unit (PACU) the recovery room where patients are taken following surgery so that they can be closely monitored by the health care team to make sure that they are recovering without complications from the surgery or the anesthesia

Immediately after surgery, the person is taken to the **post-anesthesia care unit (PACU)**. Once the person is awake, breathing normally, and has stable vital signs, she is moved from the PACU to a hospital room or designated area in the surgical center until ready to be discharged home. This period of recovery before the person is ready to go home could last from a few hours up to a few days, depending on the surgery.

When the person is returned to her room, you will assist in transferring the person from the stretcher to the bed. The person may need to be positioned in a particular way post-operatively. Make sure to ask the nurse for any special instructions. If the person had surgery on an arm or leg, the arm or leg is usually elevated on a pillow or folded blanket to prevent swelling and pain. Vital signs are taken as ordered and recorded on the flow sheet (Fig. 32-3).

Preventing Complications

In the hours and days that follow surgery, the health care team focuses on preventing complications.

Respiratory Complications

Drowsiness from anesthesia and pain medications, as well as post-operative pain, can make it difficult for the person to clear the lungs and airways of fluid and mucus. As a result, the tiny air sacs in the lungs may fill with fluid (pneumonia) or collapse (atelectasis). Both of these conditions make it difficult for oxygen to pass

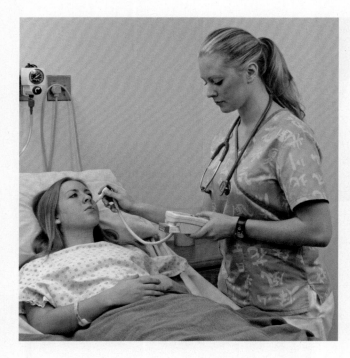

■ **FIGURE 32-3**
Vital signs are taken frequently during the immediate post-operative period because a change in vital signs could signal a complication of the surgery or the anesthesia.

into the blood and carbon dioxide to pass out of it. To prevent fluid and mucus from collecting the lungs, you may need to assist the person with frequent repositioning and with performing respiratory exercises (Fig. 32-4).

Cardiovascular Complications

Anesthetic agents, pain medications, and immobility after surgery cause the body's circulation to slow down. This increases the person's risk of forming blood clots, especially in the lower legs. These blood clots can break loose and move to the lungs, heart, or brain. If this occurs, the person may die. To prevent clots from forming, the doctor may order the use of a sequential compression device (SCD),

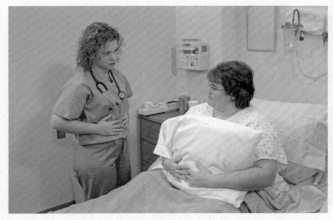

Coughing and deep breathing exercises: The person takes a few deep breaths and then coughs forcefully. Supporting the incision site with a pillow helps to minimize pain.

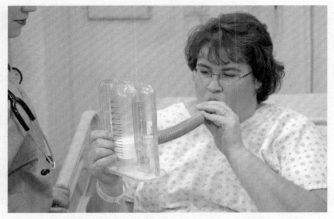

Incentive spirometry: The person inhales through the incentive spirometer. The goal is to raise the balls in the chamber.

■ **FIGURE 32-4**
Respiratory exercises used to prevent respiratory complications.

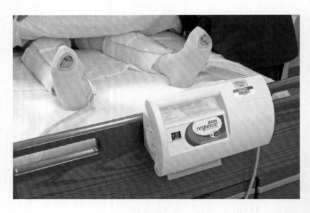

Sequential compression device (SCD): Plastic sleeves wrapped around the person's lower legs inflate and deflate in a regular cycle to promote circulation.

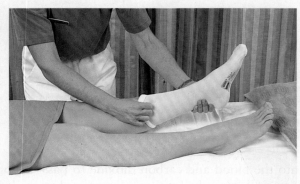

Anti-embolism (TED) stockings: Tight-fitting elastic fabric applies pressure to the lower legs and helps blood return to the heart.

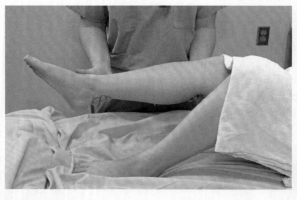

Leg exercises: The person rotates the ankle, flexes and points the foot, flexes and extends the knee, raises the leg off the bed, and then lowers it. This sequence is repeated five times, every 1 to 2 hours, to promote circulation.

■ **FIGURE 32-5**

Methods of preventing cardiovascular complications.

anti-embolism (TED) stockings, or leg exercises (Fig. 32-5). Procedure 32-1 describes how to apply anti-embolism stockings.

Assisting With Activities of Daily Living (ADLs)

During the post-operative period, the person will need assistance with ADLs:

- **Repositioning:** Pain and weakness may make assistance with repositioning necessary. Assisting the person with repositioning at least every 1 to 2 hours (or as ordered) promotes comfort and helps to prevent complications of immobility.
- **Nutrition:** Once the person is able to take fluids orally and is no longer nauseated, he will usually be started on a clear liquid diet. The diet is progressed as the person's condition improves. Good hydration and a proper diet help with the healing process.

- **Elimination:** You will be responsible for recording the person's first voiding after surgery and measuring and recording intake and output (I&O) as ordered. You may need to assist the person with a bedpan or urinal or provide catheter care.
- **Hygiene:** Providing frequent oral care, changing soiled gowns and linens, and assisting with bathing help to promote comfort.
- **Ambulation:** Early and frequent ambulation is helpful in preventing many of the complications that can result from surgery. The person may be weak and unsteady. Allow the person time to dangle before getting out of bed. At first, you will take short walks. As the person's strength returns, you can go for longer walks.

Concerns for Long-Term Care

Many elderly people who are residents in a long-term care facility will need surgery at some point. If you work in this type of health care setting, you will have many responsibilities related to preparing your residents for their surgical procedures and then caring for them after they return to the facility after surgery. Many people, especially elderly people, may need to go to a long-term care facility for a short period of time after having surgery. There they can continue to recover and receive any necessary therapy until they are strong enough to return to their own homes.

An elderly person is more likely to suffer complications related to surgery than is a younger person. Many elderly people have other chronic health conditions, not directly related to the reason they are having surgery. It takes an elderly person longer to wake up completely from sedation or general anesthesia. As a result, you will need to monitor their respirations and level of consciousness closely. An elderly person is more likely to become dizzy and fall when trying to get out of bed and walk after surgery. The use of side rails to help prevent falling out of bed and reminding the person to call for assistance may be necessary for a while.

Respiratory complications are more likely to occur in an older person after surgery. Confusion and restlessness may be an indication of decreased oxygenation and not pain. Some types of sedation and pain medication can cause temporary delirium in older people. Make sure that you observe your residents closely as they recover from surgery and report anything that does not seem quite normal to the nurse immediately.

Tell the Nurse!

Post-operative care

- An increased amount of bright red drainage (blood) on the person's wound dressing or in the drainage collection device
- A significant change in the person's vital signs (blood pressure, pulse, respirations, temperature)
- Trouble breathing, or wheezing or gurgling sounds
- Restlessness, confusion, or disorientation
- Very pale or bluish lips or nailbeds
- Cool, clammy skin
- Increased pain, tingling, or numbness in an arm or leg with a cast or bandage
- Pain or swelling at the IV site, or the IV is not dripping
- Abdominal pain, nausea, or vomiting

Putting it all together!

- People who have had surgery are at risk for developing complications, especially those related to breathing and circulation. Frequent repositioning, respiratory exercises, and the use of devices that increase circulation in the lower legs help prevent these complications.
- You may be the first to notice that a person is developing complications from surgery. Reporting your observations to the nurse promptly helps to ensure that action will be taken quickly to prevent the person's condition from getting worse.
- In addition to performing tasks related to preventing complications, you may need to assist your surgical patients with their ADLs during the post-operative period.

Oxygen Therapy

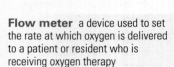

Flow meter a device used to set the rate at which oxygen is delivered to a patient or resident who is receiving oxygen therapy

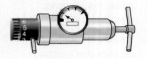

What will you learn?

When you are finished with this section, you will be able to:

1. Explain why a person may need oxygen therapy.
2. List four sources of oxygen for oxygen therapy.
3. Describe two methods of delivering oxygen to the person.
4. State observations you may make when caring for a person who is receiving oxygen therapy that should be reported to the nurse.
5. Describe safety guidelines that you should follow when caring for people receiving oxygen therapy.
6. Define the word **flow meter**.

Tell the Nurse!

Oxygen therapy

- A reading below 90% on the pulse oximeter
- The flow rate on the flow meter does not match the ordered flow rate
- Low pressure reading on the dial of a pressurized oxygen tank
- Difficult or labored breathing
- Increase or decrease in respiratory rate
- Lips, nailbeds, or face are bluish or gray
- A sudden onset of chest pain or difficulty breathing
- Noisy breathing (for example, wheezing, "barking," or "crowing"
- Fluid-like, gurgling sounds (especially if the person is very weak or comatose)
- Coughing up sputum that is discolored
- Respirations that become very slow and shallow, or they stop

Room air contains only about 20% oxygen. People who have just had surgery or who have lung disorders may have trouble getting the oxygen their bodies need from inhaled air alone. For these people, the doctor might order extra (supplemental) oxygen to increase the amount of oxygen they take in with each breath. Sources of oxygen for oxygen therapy include wall-mounted delivery systems, pressurized tanks, oxygen concentrators, and small portable tanks containing liquid oxygen (Fig. 32-6). Because oxygen therapy can be very drying to a person's mouth or nose, moisture is often added to the oxygen using a humidifier bottle.

Oxygen is considered a medication and requires a doctor's order to be used. The doctor determines the flow rate (the rate at which the oxygen should be delivered). The flow rate is set using a device called a **flow meter**. The doctor also specifies how the oxygen should be given. The device used to deliver oxygen to the person depends on several factors, including the amount of oxygen ordered, the condition being treated, and the person's overall physical condition (Fig. 32-7). A nurse or respiratory therapist is responsible for setting up and adjusting the oxygen therapy.

People who are receiving oxygen therapy are often monitored to make sure that the supplemental oxygen is meeting the body's demand for oxygen. A device called a *pulse oximeter* is clipped to the person's fingertip or earlobe to monitor oxygen levels in the bloodstream (Fig. 32-8). A normal reading is between 95% and 100%. Readings below 90% indicate that the person's tissues are not receiving enough oxygen, and you should report this to the nurse immediately.

General guidelines for the safe use of oxygen therapy are given in Guidelines Box 32-1.

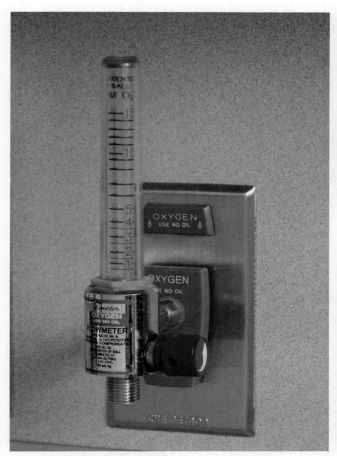

A. Wall-mounted delivery system

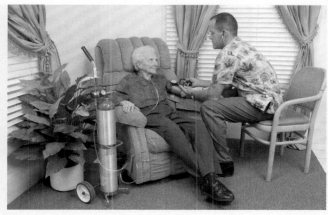

B. Pressurized tank

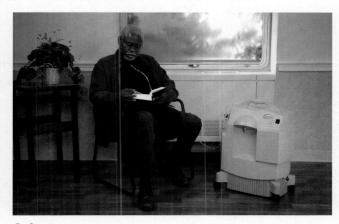

C. Oxygen concentrator

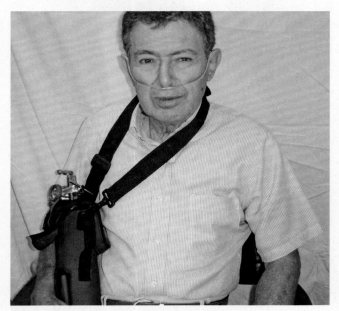

D. Liquid oxygen tank

■ **FIGURE 32-6**

Supplemental oxygen can be supplied in various ways. **(A)** With a wall-mounted delivery system, the oxygen is piped into the person's room from a central location. A valve and flow meter device is inserted into the wall outlet to access the oxygen. **(B)** A pressurized tank of oxygen can go where the person goes. **(C)** An oxygen concentrator is often used in the home and long-term care settings, especially when the person only needs to use oxygen on an as-needed basis. Oxygen concentrators produce 100% oxygen by filtering the nitrogen out of room air. **(D)** Small portable liquid oxygen tanks are lightweight and allow a person more freedom of movement.

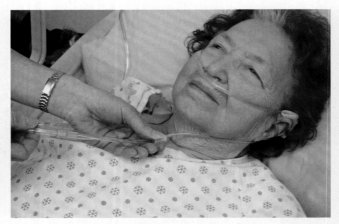

Nasal cannula: a two-pronged device that is inserted into the nostrils

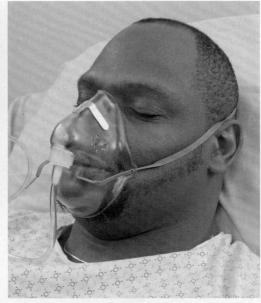

Facemask: fits over the person's nose and mouth

■ **FIGURE 32-7**

Devices used for oxygen delivery.

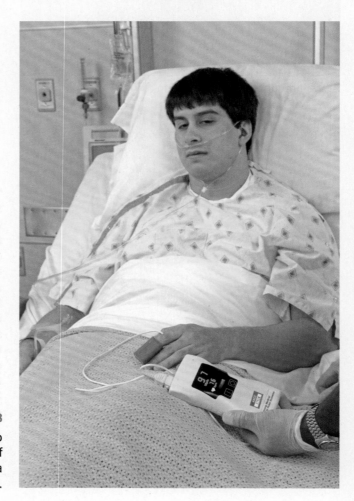

■ **FIGURE 32-8**

Pulse oximetry is used to monitor the amount of oxygen that is reaching a person's tissues.

GUIDELINES BOX 32-1   Guidelines for Oxygen Therapy

What you do	Why you do it
Avoid lighting matches or cigarette lighters in the person's room. Post a "No Smoking" sign and remind the patient or resident and any visitors not to smoke when oxygen is in use.	*Use of oxygen therapy can increase the oxygen content of linens and clothing in the immediate area. Fires are more likely to start and will burn much faster as a result of the added oxygen.*
Make sure that any electrical equipment is in good working order and that cords are not frayed. Use a battery-operated razor or a blade razor when shaving a person who is receiving supplemental oxygen.	*Electrical equipment that is not properly maintained can be the source of a spark, which could start a fire.*
Make sure that the tubing through which the oxygen is delivered is free of kinks and that the person is not lying on it.	*If the tubing is obstructed in any way, oxygen flow will be impaired and the person will not receive the correct amount.*
Do not adjust the flow rate of oxygen.	*Adjusting the flow rate of oxygen is out of the nursing assistant's scope of practice. Receiving too much oxygen can be as harmful to the patient or resident as receiving too little oxygen. The doctor decides how much oxygen the patient or resident should receive.*
When you are caring for a person who is receiving supplemental oxygen, be aware of the ordered flow rate and tell the nurse if the flow rate on the flow meter does not match the ordered flow rate.	*The setting on the flow meter may get changed accidentally. Checking frequently to make sure that the ordered flow rate matches the flow rate on the person's medical chart helps to keep your patient or resident safe. Receiving too much oxygen can be as harmful to the patient or resident as receiving too little oxygen.*
When providing personal care, do not remove a person's facemask or nasal cannula, unless you are specifically told to do so by the nurse.	*Removing the facemask or nasal cannula will deprive the person of the supplemental oxygen. Some people may not be able to tolerate a decrease in the amount of oxygen they are receiving, even for just a few minutes.*
Check the humidifier bottle frequently for bubbles.	*Bubbles indicate that the oxygen is flowing freely.*
Make sure that the water level in the humidifier bottle does not get too low.	*Oxygen that is not humidified prior to delivery can be very drying to the mucous membrane lining of the person's nasal cavity and mouth. This dryness can be uncomfortable for the patient or resident.*
Provide oral care frequently, as directed by the nurse.	*Frequent oral care helps to relieve some of the dryness of the nose and mouth that occurs with supplemental oxygen therapy.*
Watch for signs of skin irritation behind the person's ears, over his cheeks, or under his nose.	*The pressure and friction from the tubing that holds the facemask or nasal cannula in place can cause skin breakdown.*

Putting it all together!

- Oxygen therapy is the administration of supplemental oxygen. A person who is recovering from surgery or who has a lung disorder may need supplemental oxygen.
- Oxygen is a medication and requires a doctor's order to be used. Oxygen therapy is administered by a respiratory therapist or nurse.
- Oxygen may be supplied by way of a wall-mounted system, a pressurized tank, an oxygen concentrator, or a portable liquid oxygen tank.
- Oxygen can be administered through a nasal cannula or a facemask.
- Observing safety precautions when oxygen therapy is in use is important to prevent fires and injury to the patient or resident.

PROCEDURES

PROCEDURE 32-1
Applying Anti-Embolism (TED) Stockings

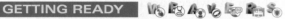

Why you do it: Use of anti-embolism (TED) stockings as ordered helps to prevent the formation of blood clots in the lower legs.

GETTING READY

1. Complete the "Getting Ready" steps.

SUPPLIES

- anti-embolism (TED) stockings in the correct size

PROCEDURE

2. Make sure that the bed is positioned at a comfortable working height (to promote good body mechanics) and that the wheels are locked. If the side rails are in use, lower the side rail on the working side of the bed. The side rail on the opposite side of the bed should remain up.
3. Help the person into the supine position.
4. Fanfold the top linens to the foot of the bed. Adjust the person's hospital gown or pajama bottoms as necessary to expose one leg at a time.
5. Turn the stocking inside out down to the heel.

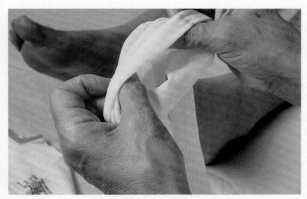

STEP 5 ■ Turn the stocking inside out down to the heel.

6. Slip the foot of the stocking over the person's toes, foot, and heel. The stocking has an opening in the toe area, which allows the health care team to assess the person's toes to make sure they are receiving enough blood. Depending on the manufacturer, this opening may be on the top or on the bottom of the stocking.

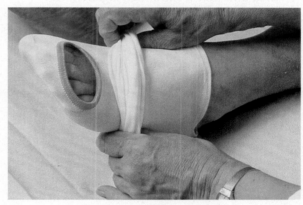

STEP 6 ■ Slip the foot of the stocking over the person's toes, foot, and heel.

7. Grasp the top of the stocking and pull it up the person's leg. The stocking will turn itself right-side out as you pull it up the person's leg.

(*procedure continues on page 690*)

PROCEDURE 32-1 (continued)
Applying Anti-Embolism (TED) Stockings

■

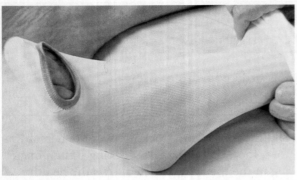

STEP 7 ■ Grasp the top of the stocking and pull it up the person's leg.

8. Check to make sure that the stocking is not twisted and that it fits snugly against the person's leg, with no wrinkles. Also make sure that the stocking fits smoothly over the heel and that the opening in the toe area is correctly located in the toe region.

9. Cover that leg, expose the other leg, and repeat steps 5 through 8.

10. Help the person back into a comfortable position, straighten the bottom linens, and draw the top linens over the person. Raise the head of the bed as the person requests. Make sure that the bed is lowered to its lowest position and that the wheels are locked.

FINISHING UP

11. Complete the "Finishing Up" steps.

WHAT YOU DOCUMENT

■ Date and time
■ Condition of person's skin on legs and feet (Be especially observant of reddened, warm, or painful areas on the calves.)

WHAT DID YOU LEARN?

Multiple Choice

Select the single best answer for each of the following questions.

1. Mrs. Jones is recovering from surgery. How often will she need assistance with repositioning?
   a. Every shift
   b. Every 1 to 2 hours
   c. Every 3 to 4 hours
   d. Every 15 minutes

2. The nurse asks you to help Mr. Huang in Room 340 with coughing and deep breathing exercises. What is the purpose of these exercises?
   a. To help Mr. Huang build up his strength following the surgery
   b. To lower Mr. Huang's risk of pulmonary embolism
   c. To lower Mr. Huang's risk of pneumonia or atelectasis
   d. All of the above

3. Which one of the following activities takes place before surgery?
   a. Frequent ambulation
   b. Completion of the pre-operative checklist
   c. Performance of coughing and deep breathing exercises
   d. Careful monitoring in the post-anesthesia care unit (PACU)

4. Why must a person who is having surgery avoid taking food or fluids by mouth for 6 to 8 hours before the surgery?
   a. An empty stomach helps to prevent vomiting during or after surgery
   b. An empty stomach is necessary to prevent infection of the abdominal cavity
   c. The anesthesia is more effective if the person's stomach is empty
   d. An empty stomach helps to prevent problems with elimination after the surgery

5. Who has to write the order for oxygen to be used?
   a. The nurse
   b. The respiratory therapist
   c. The doctor
   d. No order is necessary; if someone needs oxygen, it must be given immediately.

6. One of your responsibilities is to assist Mr. Tang with shaving. Mr. Tang is receiving continuous oxygen via a nasal cannula. What should you do when helping Mr. Tang to shave?
   a. Remove the nasal cannula before you begin the procedure.
   b. Use a battery-operated razor or a blade razor instead of an electrical razor.
   c. Increase the flow of oxygen during the procedure.
   d. Decrease the flow of oxygen during the procedure.

 Stop *and* Think!

You are a nursing assistant in an assisted-living facility. One of your residents, Mrs. Wight, is scheduled to have an outpatient surgical procedure done at a local hospital. Mrs. Wight is a very stylish woman who takes a lot of pride in her appearance. She knows that she is not permitted to wear make-up during surgery, but when you arrive in her room to help her get ready the day of the surgery, you find that she is looking like her usual self—nails done, jewelry on, lipstick applied. What would you do, and why?

(STOP) Stop *and* Think!

You work as a nursing assistant in a hospital. One of your patients, Mr. Newman, is scheduled for exploratory surgery to determine whether a tumor in his brain is cancerous. Mr. Newman is married and has three children ranging in age from 8 to 14 years. He has a very large extended family, many of whom have been staying at the hospital day and night since Mr. Newman was admitted. How might Mr. Newman and his family members be feeling right now? Is there anything you could do to help them?

Caring for People in the Home Environment

Home health care is skilled nursing care that is given to a person in his or her home. People who have been injured or ill and have been receiving care in a hospital or other acute care setting are being sent home sooner and sicker than ever before and may still need some type of nursing care.

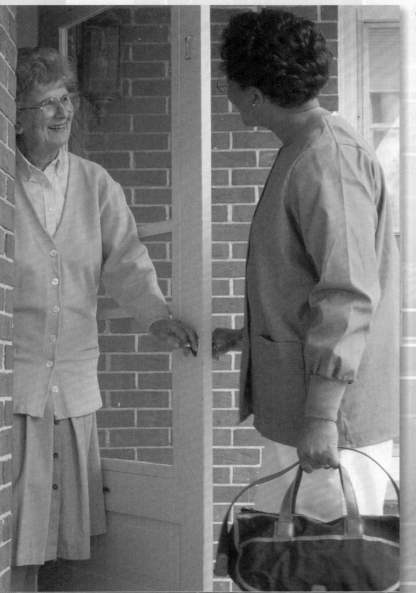

Photo: *Home health aides care for clients in their homes.*

Introduction to Home Health Care

What will you learn?

When you are finished with this section, you will be able to:

1. Describe why a person might need home health care.
2. List some of the members of the home health care team.
3. Describe some of the types of treatment a person may receive in his or her home.
4. Define the words **respite care** and **homebound**.

Given a choice, most people would prefer to stay in the comfort of their own homes when they are sick or recovering from an injury or surgery. Home health care, also known as *home care*, makes it possible for people who are not critically ill to receive health care in the comfort of their own homes. A person who is receiving the services of a home health care agency is called a *client*, instead of a "patient" or a "resident." There are many reasons why a person might become a client of a home health care agency:

- **The person may have just been released from the hospital following an acute illness or injury.** Many of these clients will continue to need intravenous (IV) antibiotics or other medications, wound care, or physical therapy before they fully recover.

- **The person may have a chronic illness or disability that makes it hard for him or her to manage some tasks independently.** For example, a person who is paralyzed might need assistance in order to get out of bed and ready for work each morning.

- **The person may have a condition, such as dementia, that makes it dangerous for the person to be left alone in the house.** Home health care agencies offer **respite care** services that allow a primary caregiver a chance to "take a break" or leave the house to go to his or her own appointments or run errands.

- **The person may be terminally ill.** Hospice care is often provided in the person's home.

Home health care services are usually divided into two different categories. *Skilled home care* services are meant to be short-term and are usually paid for by Medicare and some other health insurance programs. In order to qualify for skilled home care, a client must meet all of the following criteria:

- The person must be **homebound**
- The services must be ordered by the person's primary care doctor
- There must be a need for skilled nursing or rehabilitative care
- The person must require intermittent (several times a day), but not full-time, care

After meeting the criteria, Medicare will pay for home health services for a period of 60 days. The goal of skilled home care services is to help the client return to his or her most optimal health. At the end of the 60-day period, the client's condition is reevaluated and if necessary, the services can be extended for an additional 60 days.

Long-term home care services (also referred to as home health sitting services) are available for many elderly people who need home care but do not meet the

Respite care home care that gives the primary caregiver an opportunity to rest or leave the home for a short period of time

Homebound the person is unable to leave the house without a lot of help from another person

criteria for skilled home care. Long-term care services are usually made up of non-skilled duties, such as meal preparation, light housekeeping, assistance with personal care, grocery shopping, and other errands. This type of home care service is usually paid for by the individual or his or her family members. Some services may be offered as part of a community's outreach project.

BOX 33-1	**Members of the Home Health Care Team**
Doctor	The doctor usually initiates the order for the client to receive home health care services. The doctor is responsible for writing orders for the treatment, therapy, special diets, and medications that the client will receive.
Case Manager	The clinical case manager, usually a registered nurse (RN), is responsible for overseeing all of the client's care, from admission to discharge. The case manager assesses the client and works with the client and his or her family members to create the care plan. He or she will also coordinate the client's care and make assignments to the home health care aide and other members of the care team. The case manager receives input from other team members and is responsible for reevaluating the client's care needs should their condition decline or improve.
Registered Nurse (RN) and Licensed Practical Nurse (LPN)	RNs and LPNs visit the client and provide skilled nursing care that may be needed. For example, the nurses will provide wound care, IV medications, specialized procedures, and client/family teaching about the client's condition or care measures.
Home Health Aide	The home health aide follows the care plan set up by the case manager and provides personal care for the client. Home health aides assist clients with hygiene and grooming needs, toileting, positioning and transferring, monitoring vital signs, observing and reporting any changes in the client's condition, and other duties required to ensure the client's safety and comfort. The home health aide may visit a client two times a week or up to twice a day, each day of the week, depending on the client's needs and the care plan.
Physical Therapist	Physical therapists provide exercises geared toward helping clients gain strength, balance, mobility, movement, and gait.
Occupational Therapist	Occupational therapy assists clients to relearn and gain the ability to perform ADLs. The occupational therapist makes recommendations for home safety modifications or adaptive equipment that will improve the client's level of independence.
Speech Therapist	Speech therapy helps clients improve their ability to speak and communicate more clearly, especially after an accident or stroke that causes aphasia. Speech therapists also assist clients who have eating and swallowing difficulties.
Registered Dietician	Registered dieticians provide consultation and teaching on diet and nutrition choices and concerns, especially for those with a medically prescribed diet.
Social Services/ Social Worker	Social workers provide assistance to clients and their families with needs such as financial issues, meal assistance, or obtaining medical or assistive devices (for example, hospital beds, bedside commodes, ambulation devices). Some social workers provide counseling services, advance directives, and ongoing support in the home, such as respite care.

Members of the Home Health Care Team

Just as in other health care settings, health care that is provided in the home is provided by a health care team. Box 33-1 lists the members of the home health care team and gives a brief description of each member's primary role.

Putting it all together!

- Home health care makes it possible for people who are not critically ill to receive health care in the comfort of their own home.
- There are many reasons a person may need home health care.
- In order to be eligible to receive skilled home health care, a client must be homebound and meet other established criteria.
- Home health care is provided by an entire team of health care workers.

The Home Health Aide

What will you learn?

When you are finished with this section, you will be able to:
1. Describe the primary duties of a home health aide.
2. List personal qualities that a home health aide must have to be successful.
3. Define the word **abandonment**.

Responsibilities of the Home Health Aide

The home health aide is a very important member of the home health care team. The home health aide usually assists clients with tasks related to personal care. Many of your responsibilities will be related to helping your clients with activities, such as bathing, eating, getting dressed, exercising, toileting, repositioning, and transferring (Fig. 33-1). As always, the amount of help you will need to provide will vary from client to client, and you should encourage the client to do as much as possible for himself or herself.

If a client starts to decline your assistance with ordered tasks that are listed on the person's care plan, it may indicate the need to reevaluate the care plan or the need for continuing care. Make sure that you report this to your case manager.

Depending on the client's needs, the home health aide may also be assigned light housekeeping duties, such as cleaning, preparing meals, and doing laundry. The home health aide's responsibilities will be clearly outlined in the client's care plan. You must follow the care plan exactly. Any changes to the care plan must first be approved by the case manager.

As in other health care settings, the home health aide is usually the person who spends the most one-on-one time with a client. Because you will most likely be the one providing "personal care" to the client, you will also be in the best position to make

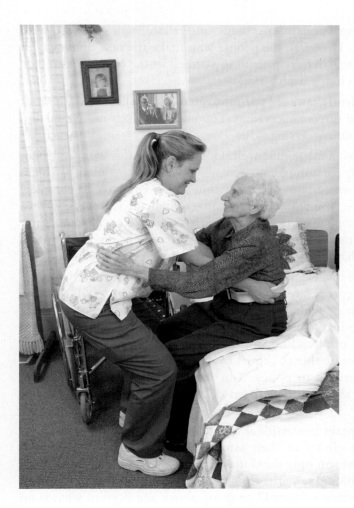

■ **FIGURE 33-1**

Home health aides assist with all types of personal care. Here, a home health aide helps a client to transfer out of bed.

important observations about changes in the client's well-being. By communicating his or her observations to the rest of the health care team, the home health aide becomes the "eyes and ears" of the members of the team who do not see the client as frequently. For this reason, communicating with the case manager and other members of the health care team is an essential part of the home health aide's responsibilities.

Sharing information with other health care team members about a person's care in most health care settings usually involves face-to-face communication. However, in the home health care setting, team members may rarely see each other. As a result, most communication among team members takes place through documentation. The documentation may be entered on an electronic device or handwritten on paper. As always, you must accurately document the care you provide using the method approved by your agency, including the date, time, and duration of the visit. Proper documentation is necessary to ensure that all members of the home health care team are kept "in-the-know." The proper documentation is also an essential requirement to ensure that payment is received for the care from Medicare, Medicaid, and other insurance agencies.

Qualities of the Successful Home Health Aide

So maybe you are thinking that you would like to work in the home health setting. Of course, just as in any health care setting, a strong work ethic is important. For

Tell the Nurse!

As a home health aide, you will play an important role in reporting changes in a client's medical condition that could indicate a serious problem. Your agency will have written guidelines about observations that should be reported. Make sure that you are familiar with these guidelines, and if you are ever in doubt about whether an observation should be immediately reported to the case manager, choose to err on the side of safety and report it. Make sure that you report any of the following observations to the case manager immediately:

■ One or more of the client's vital signs are above or below the standards set by the agency.

■ The client has a fever or other signs of infection.

■ There is a change in the client's mental alertness or orientation.

■ The client has signs of skin breakdown or pressure sores.

■ The client has signs or symptoms that could indicate a medical emergency.

■ You suspect that the client is being abused (physically, sexually, or psychologically).

■ There are unsafe or unsanitary conditions in the home.

example, being honest, compassionate, courteous, and reliable will serve you well, no matter where you work. However, the people who make the best home health aides also have other qualities that help them to succeed in the home health care setting. The most successful home health aides:

- **Enjoy working independently and are self-motivated.** Home health aides work in a client's home without direct supervision. You need to be self-motivated and very comfortable with your caregiving skills.

- **Are organized and able to manage time well.** Home health aides work independently and are responsible for completing assigned duties as scheduled. Each client you visit will have a set amount of time within which you have to complete that person's ordered care. You will need to be able to manage your time well so that you have time to complete all the assigned care duties for each client. Since you will be traveling from client to client, you must plan your day so that you visit clients in an order that allows for the most efficient use of travel time.

- **Are reliable.** Clients who receive home care depend on the home health aide to arrive and provide the appropriate care. A home health aide who fails to show up at a client's home to provide scheduled care is guilty of **abandonment**. A home health aide who leaves a client's home without completing scheduled tasks may also be guilty of abandonment. If you are unable to arrive at a client's home on time or are unable to report to work at all, make sure that you notify your agency according to policy. You should also contact your client to let him or her know that you have been delayed and when you expect to arrive.

- **Are able to set and maintain professional boundaries.** Professional boundaries are necessary to prevent clients or their family members from taking advantage of you. You may perform only the duties that are listed on the client's care plan and report any additional requests for care to your supervisor for approval before doing them. Becoming a "friend" or going above and beyond what is on the plan of care can set the client, and possibly his or her family, up to become more dependent on the agency than is necessary or appropriate. Make sure that you follow agency policies regarding personal relationships between health care professionals and clients, and the acceptance of gifts.

- **Have good communication skills.** Clear communication with the other members of the home health care team has already been discussed. You also need to remember the communication skills you learned in Chapter 4 when working with your clients and their family members.

- **Look and act professional.** Dress and personal hygiene are very important. Dress according to your agency's policy and always wear the proper identification. Since mishaps can occur, either while providing care in a client's home or while traveling between visits, that can cause your clothing to become soiled, it is a good idea to carry an additional set of clothing. That way, you can always look clean and neat for every client.

Abandonment the term abandonment means to withdraw one's support or help from another person, in spite of duty or responsibility

Putting it all together!

- The home health aide is usually responsible for assisting clients with personal care.

- The home health aide's responsibilities will be clearly outlined in the client's care plan. You must follow the care plan exactly.

- The home health aide becomes the "eyes and ears" of the members of the health care team who do not see the client as frequently.
- Documentation is a very important communication tool in the home health care setting.
- To succeed as a home health aide, a person must have several distinct qualities.

The Home Health Care Environment

What will you learn?

When you are finished with this section, you will be able to:

1. Describe how the home health care environment is different from other health care settings.
2. List safety concerns that are unique to the home health care environment.
3. Discuss the responsibilities of the home health aide in an emergency situation.
4. Describe measures that the home health aide should take to help ensure his or her own personal safety.

Health care facilities are able to provide care to patients and residents under very controlled conditions. Facilities are required to meet guidelines and regulations that help to maintain cleanliness, provide privacy, and remain safe for all the people who receive care there. Other members of the health care team who do not provide direct personal care are responsible for cleaning, preparing meals, and making sure that equipment works properly. The home health care setting is a very different type of environment.

You will most likely provide care for many clients who live in very different types of homes. A client may live in a single-family house in a quiet neighborhood. Another client may live in an inner-city apartment building. Some clients may be wealthy and have beautiful homes with modern accommodations. Others may live on very limited funds and have a house or apartment that is old and in need of repair. Some clients may not even have modern plumbing and no bathtub or shower. Regardless of the setting, you are responsible for providing the same quality of care for each of your clients.

> *No matter what type of home environment your client lives in, you must always remember that he or she is a unique individual in need of health care and that you are responsible for providing that care to the best of your ability. Do not make judgments about a person based on the type of home he or she lives in.*

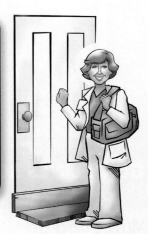

Safety Concerns in the Home Health Setting

Many of us consider our homes places of safety and security. However, the home environment can actually be quite dangerous. As a home health aide, you need to be aware of conditions in the home that put the client at risk. You also need to know how to react in the event of an emergency.

Falls

Chapter 15 taught you that falling is the most common type of accident that occurs in the health care setting and the number one cause of accidental death among elderly people. Many factors in the home can also put a person at risk for falling, especially if the person has limited mobility or poor eyesight:

- Many homes are old, with worn carpets or uneven floors.
- Hallways, rooms, and staircases might be dimly lit, or not lit at all.
- The bathroom may be small, or not located in a place that is easy for a person with poor mobility to reach.
- The bathroom may not be equipped with handrails to assist a person with poor mobility to get on and off the toilet or in and out of the bathtub.
- The home may be filled with a lifetime of collected objects and furniture, which can lead to crowding and clutter.
- Many people have pets, which can run underfoot.

Fire

Fire danger is also a concern in the home:

- The wiring in the house may be old.
- Outlets may be overloaded. Overload can be caused by plugging too many cords into a single outlet, or by using extension cords.
- Electrical cords may be covered by carpet. This is a fire hazard as well as a tripping hazard.
- The family may rely on space heaters, wood-burning stoves, or fireplaces to provide heat.
- Many people do not have functioning smoke detectors in their homes.

Guidelines for helping to maintain a safe home environment are given in Guidelines Box 33-1.

GUIDELINES BOX 33-1   Guidelines for Maintaining a Safe Home Environment

What you do	Why you do it
Make sure that the furniture is arranged to allow for wide walkways. Chairs and small tables should be placed around the edges of the room, rather than in the center.	*A cluttered, narrow walkway increases a person's risk of tripping and falling.*
Remove any clutter or obstacles from indoor and outdoor walkways and steps. Provide adequate lighting.	*Proper lighting enhances the ability to see, which helps to prevent falls. Removing obstacles and clutter that a person could trip over helps to prevent falls as well.*

What you do (continued)	**Why you do it** (continued)
Place a small lamp and a telephone on the person's bedside table.	*Having these items close at hand can help to prevent falls. If the phone rings, the person can answer it without getting out of bed. If the person needs to get out of the bed in the middle of the night, he or she can turn on the light first. The ability to see helps to prevent falls.*
Install night-lights as needed.	*Some people may hesitate to turn on the light when they get up in the middle of the night. Night-lights can help the person to see the route to the bathroom or kitchen without turning on the lights in the room or hallway. The ability to see helps to prevent falls.*
Avoid running cords across walkways. Instead, move the furniture so that the electrical cords for lamps and other appliances are close to the outlet.	*A person could trip over a cord that is stretched across a room or walkway.*
In wintry climates, make arrangements for snow and ice to be removed from outdoor walkways and steps.	*A person could easily slip and fall on icy or snowy walk-ways and steps.*
Clean up spills on the bathroom or kitchen floor promptly.	*Tile or linoleum floors become very slippery when wet, increasing the person's risk of falling.*
Use a no-slip rubber bath mat on the floor of the bathtub.	*A no-slip rubber bath mat helps to provide traction, reducing the person's risk of falling while getting into or out of the bathtub.*
Provide a bath bench or a shower chair for the person to use while showering.	*An unsteady person will be more stable and at less risk for falling if he or she can sit down during the shower.*
Be aware of potential fire hazards (for example, frayed wires and overloaded outlets) and report these immediately.	*A house fire can have tragic consequences, especially when the people who live in the home are relatively unable to help themselves should a fire break out.*
Keep chemicals, cleaning solutions, and other poisonous substances in a locked storage area.	*Poor eyesight, confusion, or a decreased sense of taste or smell can cause an elderly person to eat or drink something that will cause harm. Children are also at risk for accidental poisonings because they are curious.*
Program emergency telephone numbers into the telephone (for example, for the person's doctor, a family member, and emergency services), or keep a written list next to the telephone.	*Having emergency phone numbers handy will make it easier for the person to call for help in the event of an emergency.*

It is not your responsibility to change the client's home to ensure safe conditions. However, your observations about the overall safety of the home are important and should be reported to the case manager. The case manager will arrange for the necessary modifications and equipment. Your job is to make the case manager aware of the client's needs.

Emergency Situations

It is quite possible that despite your efforts to maintain a safe home environment, an accident, fire, or medical emergency will occur. You may arrive at the home of a client and find that the person has fallen and hurt himself or herself. You may smell smoke or gas when you enter the client's home. The client may have a medical emergency, such as a heart attack or stroke, while you are there. Remember what you learned in Chapters 14 and 16 about reacting to fire and medical emergencies. Remain calm, and use good judgment. Activate the emergency medical services (EMS) system by calling "911" or the emergency telephone number specified by your agency. Then provide appropriate care until help arrives. After the situation has been resolved, you will need to report and record according to your agency's policy.

Abusive Situations

In Chapter 2, you learned about abuse. Abuse can be physical, emotional, or sexual. Anyone can be a target for abuse. Families are complex, and many things go on in the privacy of a person's home "behind closed doors." As a home health aide, you may witness some of these things. A disabled or elderly person is more likely to be abused in the privacy of his or her own home because the abuser may feel that the abuse will go undiscovered.

As a home health aide, you may find yourself in a situation where you suspect that one of your clients is being abused. Laws require that any health care worker who suspects the abuse of a child or a vulnerable adult must report his or her suspicions to the proper authorities. Your agency will have specific policies about how you are to report any suspected abuse.

If a family situation turns violent while you are in the client's home, and you feel unsafe, you should leave the home after doing your best to make sure that the client is also safe. Please do not try to intervene if the situation is turning violent or you may become a victim yourself. Activate the EMS system by calling "911" or the emergency telephone number specified by your agency if you feel that someone in the house is in immediate danger, and then report the situation to the case manager.

Other Safety Concerns

The home health care setting presents some safety concerns that are unique to that environment. Many of your clients may have pets in the home. Dogs, either large or small, that are normally friendly may become protective of an owner who is ill. A dog may think you are a threat to its owner, especially when you are touching or moving a client while providing personal care. The dog may become nervous and protective, resulting in bites or scratches to the home health aide. It is a good idea to call the client before entering the home and request that the dog be confined to another room or area while you are providing care.

Many people have multiple pets in their homes. If a client or family members are unable to care for multiple pets, you may notice unsanitary conditions involving pet waste, food, or other issues. You may also notice conditions in which there are insect, mouse, or rat infestations in a client's home. Any of these situations can create a health concern and should be reported to the case manager.

Depending on where you live, inclement weather can also create safety concerns both for the client and for the home health aide. Snow and ice can make steps and sidewalks treacherous and lead to falls. Heavy rains that can lead to flooding and storms can cause structural damage to a person's home. Weather conditions can make it difficult for you to even reach a client's home.

Personal Safety

As a home health aide, you will use standard methods to keep yourself safe on the job. For example, you will use proper body mechanics to minimize your risk of physical injury when lifting or transferring clients, and you will use standard precautions to protect yourself from infection. But some aspects of the home health aide's job pose unique safety risks. Instead of working in one building, you will be required to travel from one client's home to another. This puts you at an increased risk for traffic accidents, flat tires, and other hazards of driving. In addition, some of your clients may live in unsafe neighborhoods, which could put you at risk for being attacked. Protecting yourself while traveling to and from your clients' homes is a top priority. Box 33-2 describes some things you can do to keep yourself safe while traveling between clients' homes.

BOX 33-2   Personal Safety Suggestions

- Keep your car in good repair, and always start out with a full tank of fuel.

- Choose the safest route of travel. Avoid driving or walking through unknown areas and alleys.

- Take a defensive driving course.

- Keep an emergency kit in the trunk of your car specific for your type of weather conditions. Include flares, a blanket, a shovel, food, drinking water, a flashlight and batteries, jumper cables, and a tire jack.

- Be aware of the dangers of driving in ice and snow. When the weather is bad, be prepared with snow tires, a bag of sand or kitty litter (for weight and traction), antifreeze, and windshield washer fluid.

- Always keep your car doors locked and stay alert for strangers who may wish to cause you harm.

- Leave excessive amounts of cash and expensive personal items (such as jewelry or electronics) at home. Do not leave items in plain view on the car seat. Instead, take them with you or put them in the trunk or under the seat before leaving the car. Always lock your car.

- Visit clients who live in unsafe neighborhoods during the day, preferably during the morning hours. Or, speak with the case manager about arranging an escort to help ensure your safety.

- Park your car in a safe, well-lighted area as close to the client's home as possible.

- Choose the safest walking route to reach the home. When walking from your car to the client's home and back, be aware of other people, strange animals, and your surroundings in general.

- Wear a name badge identifying yourself as a home health care provider according to your agency policy. If you are attacked, let the attacker know that you do not carry syringes, needles, or medication.

- Consider taking a self-defense course. If you are attacked, use your bag, arms, and hands to protect your face, neck, and throat. Kick the attacker with your legs. Use your car keys to slash the attacker's face. Scream or yell loudly to attract attention.

- Make sure that someone else (your case manager, a friend, or family member) knows your planned schedule. Follow your schedule and check in with the office frequently.

- Carry a fully charged cell phone with you at all times.

Putting it all together!

- Home health aides are responsible for protecting themselves and those in their care from physical harm.
- The home environment poses many safety risks. Home health aides are responsible for noting dangerous situations in the home and reporting their observations to the case manager and for knowing how to react should an emergency occur.
- Home health aides must be concerned with keeping themselves safe while traveling between clients' houses.

Infection Control

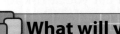

What will you learn?

When you are finished with this section, you will be able to:

1. Describe ways that home health aides can spread infection.
2. Identify ways to reduce the spread of infection within the home.
3. Discuss how standard precautions are used in the home environment.
4. Describe how to properly prepare and store food.
5. Define the word **bag technique**.

Just as in any other health care setting, infection control in the home is very important. Many of your clients will have risk factors for infection. Your clients will be sick, recovering from surgery, elderly, or have a chronic illness or condition that will increase their risk of getting an infection. One of your most important responsibilities is to protect the people you care for from infection.

As a home health aide, you will visit several clients' homes each day. Improper or careless use of infection control methods can result in pathogens being carried from the home of one client to the home of another one. You can transmit pathogens on your hands, clothes, or equipment. By maintaining a sanitary environment and using standard precautions, you can protect your clients and yourself from communicable disease.

Maintaining a Sanitary Environment

No matter where you work, you will do many things to help maintain a sanitary work environment (see Chapter 13, Guidelines Box 13-1). When working in a client's home, you will have additional responsibilities related to maintaining a sanitary environment and preventing the spread of infection.

Using Proper Bag Technique

Many items that you will use to provide personal care for your clients may be stored in the client's home in a designated place (Fig. 33-2). Other needed supplies may need to be taken to the client's home each time you visit. Supplies specific

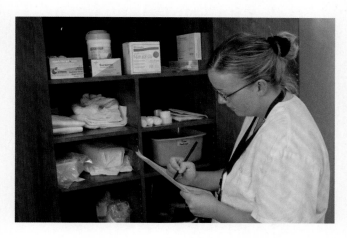

■ **FIGURE 33-2**
Some of the supplies and equipment you will need to care for your client will be kept in a special place in the client's home. Here, a home health aide is checking to see if any of the supplies are getting low.

for each client are usually filled by your agency from a central area and placed in delivery bags. This helps to ensure that you have the necessary supplies available for each of your clients. It not only helps to prevent the transmission of infection because you are not taking container bags from one client's house to another but also helps control cost.

Only supplies specific to that client are taken into the house. Unused supplies are not to be returned to the agency after being taken into the home. This practice is for infection control, in addition to cost management.

Equipment that is used with each client, such as equipment for measuring vital signs, is carried in a small tote bag. Other things that you may carry in your tote bag include:

- Forms needed for documentation and a pen
- Personal protective equipment (PPE)
- Supplies for cleaning your equipment
- Alcohol-based hand rub
- Storage bags to enclose any specimens or small equipment that is to be returned to the agency
- Barrier to place tote bag on (disposable water-proof sheets of paper)

Bag technique is used to help prevent the transmission of microbes from one client's home to another client's home, or to your car. To practice proper bag technique:

1. When you arrive at the client's home, place your tote bag on a clean surface, such as the kitchen table, after laying down a clean barrier. Placing a barrier between your tote bag and the surface helps to prevent contamination of the bag.

2. After performing proper hand hygiene, remove the equipment you will need from your tote bag.

3. After you use the equipment, clean it and disinfect it according to agency policy and return it to your tote bag (Fig. 33-3).

4. Some items that are used for a client's care may need to be returned to the agency for proper cleaning and disinfection before they are used again. Any dirty equipment should be contained in a sealed plastic bag for transport back to the agency. When placing the dirty bag into your car, do not place it near clean supply bags that are to be used for other clients. Have a separate area to keep those supplies.

Bag technique an infection control procedure used in the home health care setting to keep the home health aide's tote bag free from contamination

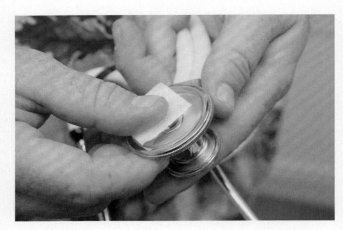

■ **FIGURE 33-3**
Equipment that is used for each client, such as equipment for measuring vital signs, is cleaned after each use and before placing it back in your tote bag.

Cleaning Equipment and Household Surfaces

You will use many pieces of equipment as you care for your clients. Bedside commodes, equipment used for bathing and grooming, and many other things will need to be properly cleaned and disinfected after each use. A commercial disinfectant solution or a solution of bleach and water mixed 1:10 (1 cup of bleach to 10 cups of water) may be used, according to your agency's policy. Make sure that you wear gloves when cleaning any equipment.

Many of your duties as a home health care nurse may include keeping areas where food is prepared and personal care is given clean. A disinfectant solution is used to clean floors, kitchen counters, bathroom fixtures (including the toilet, bathtub, sink, and counters), and surfaces that are frequently touched by many people (such as doorknobs, telephone receivers, and refrigerator handles).

Assisting Clients With Personal Hygiene

Helping your clients to maintain good personal hygiene is essential to maintaining a sanitary environment. Bathing, washing hair, brushing teeth, and wearing clean clothing are all practices that help prevent the spread of infection. Change the client's bed linens frequently and encourage the client to wear clean clothing each day. (As always, soiled bed linens and clothing should be changed immediately.)

If light housekeeping duties are part of the person's care plan, you may need to assist with some laundry items.

■ Wash soiled bed linens and clothing in the washing machine, using the warmest water temperature available.

■ Use a lengthy wash cycle and laundry detergent.

■ Add bleach if fabrics are colorfast.

■ Make sure to follow laundering directions found on a garment's tag so that you do not damage it.

■ Dry the laundry on the appropriate heat setting in the dryer. If a dryer is unavailable, hang laundry in the sun to dry.

Using Standard Precautions

Maintaining a sanitary workplace is one important way to limit the spread of infection. In addition, you must always use standard precautions when providing client care. Standard precautions, covered in detail in Chapter 13, are used to reduce your risk of getting a communicable disease from a client. Proper use of standard precautions also helps to prevent the transmission of an infection to family members or clients.

Hand Hygiene

Proper hand hygiene is the single most important method of preventing the spread of infection in any type of health care setting (see Chapter 13). Always perform proper hand hygiene:

- When you first arrive at a client's home
- Whenever your hands become visibly soiled with blood or other body fluids or substances
- Whenever you remove your gloves
- After each task or procedure you perform
- Before you leave the client's home

Wash your hands with soap and warm water, using the technique you learned in Chapter 13. If paper towels are not available, use a *clean* cloth towel to dry your hands.

If handwashing facilities are not available or are inadequate, and your hands are not visibly soiled with dirt, blood, or other bodily fluids or substances, you can use an alcohol-based hand rub to decontaminate your hands (Fig. 33-4). If your hands are visibly soiled, then you should seek proper handwashing facilities as soon as possible.

Using Personal Protective Equipment (PPE)

As in other health care settings, gloves, gowns, masks, and goggles are worn as necessary to control the spread of pathogens. Your agency is required by the Occupational Safety and Health Administration (OSHA) to provide you with

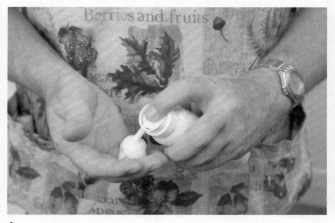
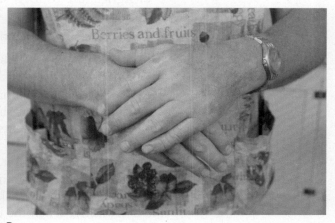

A   **B**

■ **FIGURE 33-4**

An alcohol-based hand rub can be used for routine hand hygiene. Alcohol-based hand rubs are easy to use. **A.** Apply the recommended amount of product to one of your palms. **B.** Rub your hands together, covering your hands and fingers (front and back) with the product. Keep rubbing your hands together until your skin is dry.

adequate PPE. You may carry PPE in your tote bag, or it may be included in the client's supply bag or stored in the home. It is your responsibility to make sure that you have the PPE that you need before you leave for work and to use the PPE consistently, conscientiously, and correctly (see Chapter 13). Eye protection that is not disposable must be cleaned and disinfected after each use.

Disposing of Sharps

Many clients will use needles, lancets, or other sharp items on a routine basis due to a medical condition. Clients who routinely use needles and lancets will be taught by the nurse how to properly dispose of these items safely. You may use disposable razors when providing care to your clients. These razors should also be disposed of safely. Clients may be provided with an OSHA-approved sharps disposal container by the home health agency. One of your duties may be to close and dispose of the sharps containers as they become full. Follow your agency's policy on proper sharps disposal measures.

Handling Food Properly

Depending on a client's care plan, you may be responsible for preparing simple meals or snacks. Before preparing any food, always perform hand hygiene using proper handwashing technique, and make sure that the surface where you will be preparing the food is clean. When preparing foods, remember to:

- Take note of expiration dates on packaged foods
- Avoid using eggs that are cracked
- Thoroughly wash and dry fresh fruits and vegetables before serving them
- Wash your hands after handling raw meat or poultry, and before touching anything else
- Wash cutting boards, utensils, and dishes used to prepare raw meat or poultry in hot, soapy water immediately after use
- Cook meat and poultry thoroughly, according to the United States Department of Agriculture (USDA) safe food handling labels that are attached to all supermarket meat packages
- Use a clean spoon each time if you must taste the food to check for seasonings
- Prepare food according to the client's dietary orders (see Special Diets in Chapter 24)

Raw or cooked food that is not stored properly can easily spoil and cause foodborne illnesses. Leftovers should be placed in appropriate sealed containers, labeled with the date and contents, and refrigerated. Food in the refrigerator should be inspected and disposed of before it is outdated or spoiled. The refrigerator itself should be cleaned with hot, soapy water periodically.

After each use, clean kitchen counters and stovetops with a disinfectant solution. If the house has a dishwasher, rinse the dishes and utensils and place them in the dishwasher. When the dishwasher is full, run it using the hot water cycle and dishwasher detergent. Items that are not "dishwasher safe" should be washed by hand using hot, soapy water. If possible, allow these items to air dry in a rack. Otherwise, use a clean dish towel or paper towels to dry them. If no dishwasher is available, the dishes and utensils will need to be washed by hand and dried. Be sure to wear gloves when washing dishes.

Putting it all together!

- Infection control is a priority in the home health care setting, just as it is in any other health care setting. The home health aide helps to prevent the spread of infection by maintaining a sanitary environment and using standard precautions.

- Using proper bag technique helps to prevent the spread of microbes from one client's home to another client's home.

- Disinfecting household surfaces, especially those where food is prepared or personal care is given, is essential to maintaining a sanitary environment.

- Practicing good personal hygiene, and helping clients do the same, is an important part of infection control.

- Standard precautions are used in the home setting just as they are in any other health care setting. Standard precautions are used to reduce your risk of acquiring a communicable disease from your clients and to help prevent their spread to family members or other clients.

- Handling and storing food properly is important for preventing food-borne illnesses.

WHAT DID YOU LEARN?

Multiple Choice

Select the single best answer for each of the following questions.

1. Which one of the following is a routine responsibility of a home health aide?
   a. Providing personal care for a client who is recovering from a stroke
   b. Grocery shopping for the client's family
   c. Administering medications to the client
   d. Washing windows and walking the dog

2. You are scheduled to work today, but the weather is beautiful and your best friend is begging you to take the day off and go to the beach with her. What should you do?
   a. Rush through the clients on your list so that you can leave work early and go to the beach.
   b. Call the case manager on the way to the beach and tell him or her you will not be able to visit your clients today.
   c. Tell your friend that you are sorry that you cannot go to the beach today.
   d. Call each of your scheduled clients and ask them if it would be okay if you came tomorrow instead.

3. Why is documentation a very important responsibility of the home health aide?
   a. Documentation is the main way that the members of the home health care team communicate with each other about the care given to the client and the client's condition.
   b. Documentation provides information that is used to determine if a client is recovering or getting worse.
   c. Documentation of all care provided is needed to justify continued payment for home care services.
   d. All of the above

4. You have just entered a client's home and are preparing to wash your hands at the kitchen sink when you notice that there is no soap. How else could you accomplish the task of decontaminating your hands?
   a. Wipe your hands with a moisturizing hand lotion and a tissue.
   b. Use an alcohol-based hand rub.
   c. Run your hands under hot water and dry them with a dish towel.
   d. Skip washing your hands at this time because you have just arrived at the home, and you have not done anything yet.

5. You are caring for Mrs. DiTomo, who has advanced emphysema. Mr. DiTomo, who also has health problems, complains of chest pain and slumps to the floor. What should you do first?
   a. Call the case manager.
   b. Dial "911" to activate the emergency medical services (EMS) system.
   c. Call the DiTomo's daughter and ask her to come over right away.
   d. Leave for your next assignment. You owe it to your next client to be on time, and caring for Mr. DiTomo is not your responsibility.

6. You arrive at a client's home and find the client tied down in bed. The client's daughter tells you that her mother keeps getting out of bed, so she has tied her down to the bed because she does not have time to keep checking on her. What should you do about this situation?
   a. Ignore it. The client's daughter obviously knows what is best for her mother.
   b. Report your observations to the case manager immediately.
   c. Call the police.
   d. Untie the client and tell the daughter that she is guilty of abusing her mother.

7. Which of the following observations about a client's home should be reported to the client's case manager?
   a. The client has the most modern kitchen appliances.
   b. The client has newspapers stacked everywhere and you saw three mice in the home today.
   c. The client has a large collection of dishes.
   d. The client has very poor taste in decorating.

Matching

Match each numbered item with its appropriate lettered description.

_____ **1.** Case manager

_____ **2.** Care plan

_____ **3.** Respite care

_____ **4.** Hospice care

_____ **5.** Bag technique

a. End-of-life care provided to a person who is terminally ill

b. An infection control procedure used in the home health care setting to keep the home health aide's tote bag free from contamination

c. Member of the health care team responsible for overseeing a client's care, from admission through discharge

d. A set of instructions for the client's care

e. Care that allows the primary caregiver to rest or leave the house for a short period of time

STOP Stop *and* Think!

You have been assigned to provide home health care for Mr. Adams, a new client at your agency. Mr. Adams recently had a stroke, which left him partially paralyzed on his left side and he just returned home from the hospital this week. Mr. Adams' wife has said that she is very anxious about how she will care for him properly in the home. Today, you arrive at 10 AM to assist Mr. Adams with his shower and other grooming needs. After his shower, you dress him and assist him into the living room so that he can watch TV for a while. After you change his bed linens and clean up your supplies in the bathroom, Mrs. Adams asks you if you mind doing the vacuuming so that she can just rest with her husband. You note that you have accomplished all of the assigned duties listed on Mr. Adams' care plan and it is now time for you to leave and move on to your next client. What should you do?

Answers to the **What Did You Learn?** *Exercises*

Chapter 1: The Health Care System
Multiple choice: 1-d, 2-c, 3-b
Matching set 1: 1-a, 2-c, 3-d, 4-b, 5-e
Matching set 2: 1-c, 2-e, 3-a, 4-d, 5-b

Chapter 2: The Nursing Assistant's Job
Multiple choice: 1-c, 2-b, 3-c, 4-b, 5-b, 6-b, 7-d, 8-b, 9-a, 10-b, 11-d, 12-d, 13-c, 14-a, 15-b, 16-a, 17-d

Chapter 3: Professionalism and Job-Seeking Skills
Multiple choice: 1-b, 2-d, 3-d, 4-b, 5-c, 6-c, 7-d, 8-a, 9-b, 10-c, 11-c

Chapter 4: Communication Skills
Multiple choice: 1-b, 2-a, 3-d, 4-b, 5-c, 6-a, 7-b, 8-c, 9-b, 10-b, 11-a
Matching: 1-e, 2-a, 3-d, 4-c, 5-b

Chapter 5: Those We Care For
Multiple choice: 1-d, 2-a, 3-b, 4-b, 5-d, 6-d
Matching: 1-e, 2-f, 3-b, 4-a, 5-g, 6-c, 7-d

Chapter 6: The Patient's or Resident's Environment
Multiple choice: 1-c, 2-d, 3-b, 4-a, 5-d

Chapter 7: Basic Body Structure and Function
Multiple choice: 1-c, 2-b, 3-d, 4-c, 5-b, 6-a, 7-d, 8-b, 9-d, 10-a, 11-c, 12-c, 13-a, 14-b, 15-d, 16-a, 17-d, 18-b, 19-a, 20-a, 21-c, 22-a, 23-d, 24-d, 25-c
Matching: 1-b, 2-j, 3-g, 4-a, 5-h, 6-c, 7-e, 8-i, 9-f, 10-d

Chapter 8: Common Disorders
Multiple choice: 1-d, 2-c, 3-a, 4-b, 5-c, 6-d, 7-a, 8-d, 9-c, 10-b, 11-a, 12-b, 13-c, 14-b, 15-a, 16-a, 17-d
Matching: 1-c, 2-h, 3-f, 4-i, 5-g, 6-e, 7-b, 8-d, 9-a, 10-j

Chapter 9: Rehabilitation and Restorative Care
Multiple choice: 1-d, 2-d, 3-c, 4-b
Matching: 1-b, 2-c, 3-a

Chapter 10: Overview of Long-Term Care
Multiple choice: 1-a, 2-c, 3-b, 4-c
Matching: 1-e, 2-a, 3-d, 4-c, 5-b

Chapter 11: The Long-Term Care Resident
Multiple choice: 1-b, 2-d, 3-a, 4-d, 5-d
Matching: 1-g, 2-e, 3-b, 4-c, 5-f, 6-d, 7-a

Chapter 12: Caring for People With Dementia
Multiple choice: 1-d, 2-a, 3-b, 4-c, 5-d, 6-a, 7-b, 8-a, 9-d

Chapter 13: Infection Control
Multiple choice: 1-d, 2-b, 3-b, 4-d, 5-c, 6-d, 7-d, 8-c, 9-d, 10-b, 11-d, 12-d, 13-b, 14-b, 15-c
Matching: 1-b, 2-c, 3-d, 4-e, 5-a

Chapter 14: Workplace Safety
Multiple choice: 1-a, 2-b, 3-c, 4-c, 5-a, 6-a, 7-c, 8-b, 9-b, 10-b

Chapter 15: Patient and Resident Safety
Multiple choice: 1-d, 2-b, 3-c, 4-a, 5-b, 6-c, 7-c, 8-b

Chapter 16: Basic First Aid and Emergency Care
Multiple choice: 1-d, 2-c, 3-b, 4-d, 5-d, 6-d, 7-d
Matching: 1-g, 2-h, 3-b, 4-c, 5-a, 6-f, 7-d, 8-e

Chapter 17: Assisting With Repositioning and Transferring
Multiple choice: 1-a, 2-a, 3-d, 4-c, 5-d, 6-d, 7-c, 8-b, 9-c, 10-d, 11-b, 12-d, 13-d, 14-a, 15-c

Chapter 18: Assisting With Exercise
Multiple choice: 1-d, 2-c, 3-c, 4-a
Matching: 1-f, 2-c, 3-d, 4-e, 5-b, 6-a

Chapter 19: Bedmaking
Multiple choice: 1-b, 2-d, 3-c, 4-a, 5-d, 6-c

Chapter 20: Measuring and Recording Vital Signs, Height, and Weight
Multiple choice: 1-c, 2-a, 3-b, 4-c, 5-d, 6-d, 7-a, 8-d, 9-d, 10-b, 11-c

Chapter 21: Assisting With Hygiene

Multiple choice: 1-a, 2-c, 3-d, 4-d, 5-c, 6-d, 7-b, 8-a, 9-d, 10-d, 11-d
Matching: 1-f, 2-e, 3-c, 4-d, 5-a, 6-b

Chapter 22: Preventing Pressure Ulcers and Assisting With Wound Care

Multiple choice: 1-d, 2-c, 3-a, 4-d, 5-b, 6-d, 7-c, 8-a

Chapter 23: Assisting With Grooming

Multiple choice: 1-c, 2-a, 3-a, 4-c, 5-b, 6-d, 7-d, 8-c, 9-c, 10-a, 11-d

Chapter 24: Assisting With Nutrition

Multiple choice: 1-c, 2-b, 3-c, 4-b, 5-b, 6-a, 7-c, 8-b, 9-b, 10-d
Matching: 1-c, 2-f, 3-a, 4-e, 5-d, 6-b

Chapter 25: Assisting With Urinary Elimination

Multiple choice: 1-b, 2-a, 3-c, 4-d, 5-a, 6-c
Matching: 1-h, 2-e, 3-b, 4-c, 5-f, 6-d, 7-g, 8-a

Chapter 26: Assisting With Bowel Elimination

Multiple choice: 1-a, 2-a, 3-b, 4-d, 5-a, 6-a
Matching: 1-b, 2-a, 3-d, 4-c, 5-e

Chapter 27: Assisting With Comfort

Multiple choice: 1-d, 2-c, 3-c, 4-d, 5-c, 6-d

Chapter 28: Caring for People Who Are Dying

Multiple choice: 1-d, 2-d, 3-d, 4-a, 5-c, 6-d, 7-c, 8-c, 9-b, 10-b, 11-a, 12-d
Matching: 1-d, 2-b, 3-c, 4-a

Chapter 29: Caring for People With Developmental Disabilities

Multiple choice: 1-b, 2-b, 3-a, 4-b, 5-c, 6-a, 7-c, 8-b, 9-b, 10-a

Chapter 30: Caring for People With Cancer

Multiple choice: 1-a, 2-d, 3-b
Matching: 1-c, 2-a, 3-d, 4-e, 5-b

Chapter 31: Caring for People With HIV/AIDS

Multiple choice: 1-d, 2-a, 3-d, 4-b, 5-b

Chapter 32: Caring for People Who Are Having Surgery

Multiple choice: 1-b, 2-c, 3-b, 4-a, 5-c, 6-b

Chapter 33: Caring for People in the Home Environment

Multiple choice: 1-a, 2-c, 3-d, 4-b, 5-b, 6-b, 7-b
Matching: 1-c, 2-d, 3-e, 4-a, 5-b

Introduction to the Language of Health Care

All professions have their own sets of words and abbreviations that are used to describe objects and situations that are specific to that particular profession. Understanding the words and abbreviations that are unique to the health care profession is essential if you expect to be able to communicate effectively with the other members of the health care team. Not knowing these words and abbreviations will make it difficult for you to read and follow orders for patient or resident care. In addition, you will need to know these words and abbreviations to accurately record and report.

In this appendix, you will learn some tricks that will allow you to figure out the meaning of many unfamiliar words you may hear or read. We will also introduce you to some commonly used medical words and abbreviations. Finally, you should always make it a point to look up new words or abbreviations in a medical dictionary as soon as you hear or read them. Alternatively, you can ask the nurse to explain the meaning of the word or abbreviation to you. Before long, you will become very comfortable using and understanding the language of the health care profession!

Medical Terminology

Although the strange-sounding language of the health care profession may seem overwhelming at first, it is really quite easy to pick up. Some medical terms come from the names of people (for example, Down syndrome, Alzheimer's disease, Parkinson's disease). Other terms come from Greek or Latin words, just as many everyday English, Spanish, French, and Italian words do. For example, you know what a rhinoceros looks like, right? A rhinoceros is a large animal with a huge horn growing out of its nose (Fig. B-1). *Rhin-* comes from the Greek word for "nose," and *-ceros* comes from the Greek word *keras*, or "horn." Now where else might you find the Greek word *rhin-*? Well, if the mucous membranes on the inside of your nose are inflamed because you have a cold or allergies, the doctor might say that you have *rhinitis* (*rhin-*, nose, + *-itis*, inflammation). If a movie star has had a "nose job," then her publicist may tell the press that the celebrity has had *rhinoplasty*, the medical term for a nose job (*rhin-*, nose, + *-plasty*, surgical repair).

Perhaps you have noticed a pattern here. Big words can be broken down into smaller parts, and if you know the meaning of the individual parts, you can figure out the meaning of the entire word. There are four types of word parts (Fig. B-2):

- **Roots** contain the essential, basic meaning of the word. For example, *cardi-* means "heart." Common roots are listed in Table B-1.

- **Suffixes** are attached to the end of a root to make the root more specific. For example, *carditis* is "inflammation of the heart" (*cardi-*, heart, + *-itis*, inflammation). Common suffixes are listed in Table B-2.

- **Prefixes** are attached to the beginning of a root to make the root more specific. For example, *pericarditis* is "inflammation of the sac that surrounds the heart" (*peri-*, around, + *cardi-*, heart, + *-itis*, inflammation). Common prefixes are listed in Table B-3.

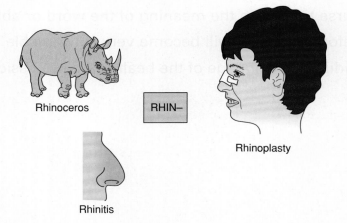

Rhinoceros

RHIN–

Rhinoplasty

Rhinitis

- **FIGURE B-1**

Many of the words you use in everyday conversation have the same Greek or Latin origins as medical words that you may be less familiar with. For example, the Greek word *rhin-* means "nose." You see *rhin-* in words such as *rhinoceros, rhinitis,* and *rhinoplasty.* When you are trying to figure out the meaning of a new medical word, think about similar-sounding words that you may already know!

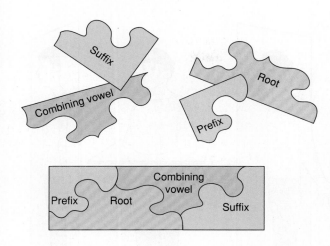

■ **FIGURE B-2**

Big words can be broken down into smaller parts, and if you know the meaning of the individual parts, then you can figure out the meaning of the entire word.

■ **Combining vowels** are often added between the root and the suffix to make the new word easier to pronounce. When a word has more than one root, combining vowels may also be used between the roots. For example, *cardiomyopathy* is "disease of the heart muscle" (*cardi-*, heart, + *o* + *my-*, muscle, + *o* + *-pathy*, disease). The combining vowel is usually "o," but "a" or "i" may also be used sometimes. The combining vowel that is used most often with each root is listed in Table B-1.

You will come across many medical words as you study each chapter in this textbook. When you come across a word in your reading that is new to you, try using what you have learned about the different word parts to guess at the word's meaning. Then look up the word in the glossary and see how well you did!

Anatomical Terms

Anatomy is the study of the structure of the body. To describe the location of one body part in relation to another, health care professionals use specific terms. To ensure that these terms always have the same meaning to everyone, we always imagine the body to be in *normal anatomical position* when we describe it. A person who is in normal anatomical position is standing upright and facing forward with her feet slightly spread apart and arms to the sides and the palms facing forward (Fig. B-3). *Anatomical planes* are used as standard points of reference when describing the body. A plane is a flat surface, like a pane of glass. Health care professionals use three main imaginary planes to divide the body (Fig. B-4):

■ The **sagittal plane** is a vertical plane that divides the body into right and left sides. A sagittal plane that divides the body into exact right and left halves is sometimes referred to as the *mid-sagittal plane.*

■ The **transverse plane** is a horizontal plane that divides the body into upper and lower segments.

■ The **frontal (coronal)** plane is a vertical plane that divides the body into front and back segments.

Directional Terms

When describing the body, health care professionals often need to describe something that is above, under, to the side of, or further away from something else. To

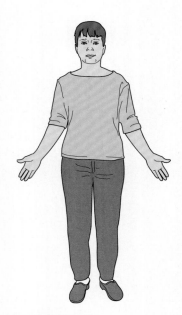

■ **FIGURE B-3**

Normal anatomical position.

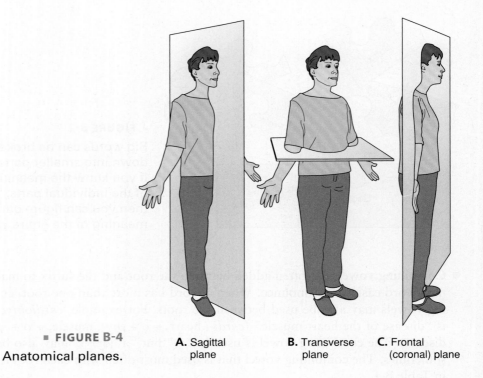

■ **FIGURE B-4**
Anatomical planes.

A. Sagittal plane

B. Transverse plane

C. Frontal (coronal) plane

do this, they use standard directional terms. Directional terms are used to describe the location of one body part in relation to another. When we use directional terms, we need a point of reference that stays the same. If not, just changing a person's body position would change a directional reference. This is where normal anatomical position and the anatomical planes come in.

Using the anatomical planes as reference points gives us the following directional terms (Fig. B-5):

- **Medial:** closer to the mid-sagittal plane of the body (toward the inner side). For example, the nose is medial to the eyes.

- **Lateral:** further away from the mid-sagittal plane of the body (toward the outer side). For example, the ears are lateral to the nose.

- **Superior:** closer to the top of the body (closer to the head). For example, the chin is superior to the breast.

- **Inferior:** further away from the top of the body (closer to the feet). For example, the belly button is inferior to the breast.

- **Anterior:** toward the front, or *ventral surface*, of the body. For example, the abdomen is anterior to the buttocks.

- **Posterior:** toward the back, or *dorsal surface*, of the body. For example, the buttocks are posterior to the abdomen.

Two other directional terms are used to describe the location of one body part in relation to another. These terms describe the relationship between parts of the extremities (the arms and legs) and their points of attachment to the body (the shoulders and hips):

- **Proximal:** closer to the point of origin in relation to something else (for example, the elbow is proximal to the wrist).

- **Distal:** further away from the point of origin in relation to something else (for example, the wrist is distal to the elbow).

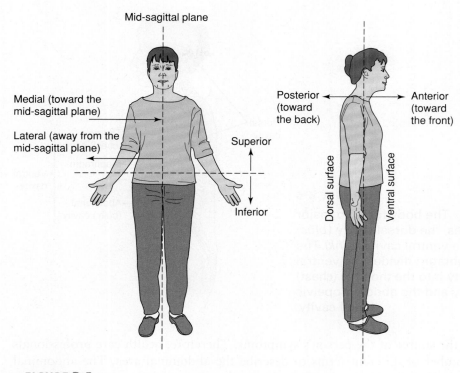

■ **FIGURE B-5**
Directional terms.

Like other terms used in the health care profession, many of these directional terms have similar meanings to words you use every day. For example, *distal* sounds like *distant*, or "further away." Similarly, *proximal* sounds like *proximity*, which means "close by." If you find the terms *ventral* and *dorsal* hard to remember, just think of a shark swimming close to the surface of the water. The shark's dorsal fin, the fin located on the shark's back, is usually visible above the water.

Terms Used to Describe Body Cavities

A *cavity* is a hollow space. In the body, cavities contain organs. There are two major cavities inside the body. The *dorsal cavity*, which contains the brain and spinal cord, is toward the back of the body. The *ventral cavity* is toward the front of the body (Fig. B-6). The ventral cavity is divided by the diaphragm into the *thoracic (chest) cavity* and the *abdominal (belly) cavity*.

■ The thoracic cavity contains the lungs, the heart, and the large blood vessels that enter and leave the heart. Most of the esophagus is also contained in the thoracic cavity.

■ The upper abdominal cavity contains the stomach, liver, pancreas, spleen, large intestine, and small intestine. The lower abdominal cavity contains the urinary bladder, the rectum, and the female reproductive organs. The kidneys lie behind the abdominal cavity. Sometimes the upper and lower abdominal cavity are referred to together as the *abdominopelvic cavity*.

Terms Used to Describe the Abdominal Area

Many patients or residents will experience pain or discomfort in the abdominal area. Often, knowing exactly where the pain or discomfort is occurring can provide

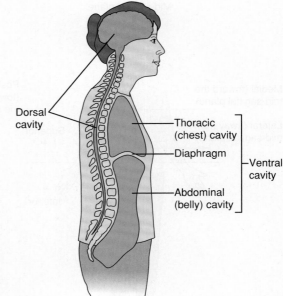

■ **FIGURE B-6**

The body has two major cavities, the dorsal cavity (*blue*) and the ventral cavity (*pink*). The diaphragm divides the ventral cavity into the thoracic (chest) cavity and the abdominopelvic (belly) cavity.

clues to the source of the person's symptoms. Therefore, health care professionals use a number of different terms to describe the abdominal area. The abdominal area can be described in terms of quadrants (fourths) or regions (Fig. B-7). Quadrants are typically used to describe general information, such as where a person is experiencing pain. Regions are used when it is necessary to be very specific (for example, when describing where an incision is located).

Quadrants

Quad means "four." The simplest way to describe the abdominal area is to divide it into fourths, or quadrants. The quadrants are named according to their location: right upper quadrant (RUQ), left upper quadrant (LUQ), right lower quadrant (RLQ), and left lower quadrant (LLQ). By using these quadrants as reference, you can describe where your patient or resident is experiencing pain by saying, for example, "Mrs. Jones is complaining of a sharp pain in her RUQ."

Regions

The abdomen can also be divided into smaller sections, called regions, for the purpose of description. There are nine regions (three rows of three):

■ The upper row consists of the right and left hypochondriac regions and the epigastric region. The hypochondriac regions are named for their relationship to the ribs: *hypo-* means "below" and *chondr/o-* means "cartilage" (of the ribs). The epigastric region is named for its relation to the stomach: *epi-* means "above" and *gastric* means "stomach."

■ The middle row consists of the right and left lumbar regions and the umbilical region. The right and left lumbar regions are named for the region of the spinal column in that area. The umbilical region is named for the umbilicus, or belly button.

■ The lower row consists of the right and left iliac regions and the hypogastric region. The iliac regions are named after the iliac crest, the bone that forms the hip bones. The iliac regions are also sometimes called the inguinal (groin) regions. The hypogastric region is named for its relation to the stomach: *hypo-* means "below" and *gastric* means "stomach."

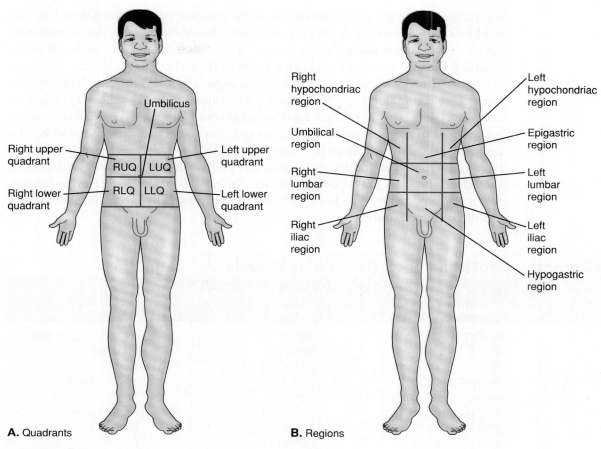

A. Quadrants   **B.** Regions

■ **FIGURE B-7**

The abdominal area can be described in terms of **(A)** quadrants or **(B)** regions. (Remember that when you are using the terms *right* and *left*, these terms are used in relation to the patient's or resident's right or left, not your right or left.)

Abbreviations

Abbreviations are shortened versions of words or phrases. Health care professionals use abbreviations to make recording more efficient. Some abbreviations come from English words. For example, you just learned that *RUQ* means "right upper quadrant." Other abbreviations come from Latin or Greek words, and therefore may seem foreign at first. For example, bid is the abbreviation for "twice daily," from the Latin words *bis* (twice) *in* (a) *die* (day). And NPO, which means "nothing by mouth," comes from the Latin words *nils* (nothing) *per* (by) *os* (mouth). As with other terms used in health care, you can often remember the meaning of a new abbreviation by relating it to an everyday word that you already know. For example, *bid*, *tid*, and *qid* are abbreviations that describe how many times a day an action is to be carried out. The abbreviation *bid* means "twice daily." Now think of how many wheels a *bicycle* has: two, right? Similarly, the abbreviation *tid* means "three times daily." How many wheels does a *tricycle* have?

Abbreviations that are commonly used in health care settings are listed in Table B-4. Although abbreviations can help us to save time and space when recording, it is very important to use only abbreviations that are approved for use in your facility. Otherwise, other members of the health care team may be confused by your meaning. In addition, if you are unsure of the meaning of an abbreviation that you read in a patient's or resident's care plan, you should either look the abbreviation up or ask the nurse to explain it to you. It is important not to just guess at the meaning because guessing could cause harm to the patient or resident.

Some abbreviations are easy to confuse, especially when they are handwritten. For example, *qd* (daily), *qid* (four times a day), and *qod* (every other day) might be easily mistaken for one another. Imagine what could happen if a patient or resident is supposed to receive a medication daily (*qd*) but someone misreads the abbreviation and gives the medication four times a day (*qid*)! To help prevent errors like this from occurring, The Joint Commission has published a list of abbreviations that should not be used (Table B-5A; also see Table B-5B). Health care organizations that are accredited by The Joint Commission or are seeking accreditation will not use these abbreviations.

TABLE B-1   Common Roots and Their Combining Vowels

Root / Combining Vowel	Meaning	Root / Combining Vowel	Meaning
abdomin / o	abdomen	femor / o	femur (thigh bone)
aden / o	gland	gastr / o	stomach
adip / o	fat	gingiv / o	gum
adren / o	adrenal glands	gluc / o	sugar, glucose
angi / o	vessel (usually blood or lymph)	glyc / o	sugar, glucose
		gynec / o	woman, female
arteri / o	artery	hemangi / o	blood vessel
arthr / o	joint	hemat / o	blood
blephar / o	eyelid	hepat / o	liver
bronchi / o	bronchus	hydr / o	water
calc / o	calcium	hyster / o	uterus
carcin / o	cancer	irid / o	iris
cardi / o	heart	lapar / o	abdomen
cephal / o	head	laryng / o	larynx (voice box)
cerebr / o	cerebrum (brain)	leuk / o	white
chol / e	bile, gall	lingu / o	tongue
cholecyst / o	gallbladder	lip / o	fat
choledoch / o	bile duct	lith / o	stone, calculus
chondr / o	cartilage	lumb / o	lower back
col / o	colon	lymphangi / o	lymph vessel
cost / o	ribs	lymph / o	lymph
crani / o	cranium (skull)	mamm / o	breast
cutane / o	skin	mast / o	breast
cyan / o	blue	megal / o	enlargement
cyst / o	bladder	melan / o	black
dent / o	teeth	mening / o	meninges
dermat / o	skin	men / o	menses, menstruation
dipl / o	double		
electr / o	electric	muc / o	mucus
encephal / o	brain	myel / o	spinal cord, bone marrow
enter / o	intestine (usually the small intestine)	my / o	muscle
erythr / o	red	myring / o	tympanic membrane (eardrum)
esophag / o	esophagus		

Root / Combining Vowel	Meaning	Root / Combining Vowel	Meaning
nas / o	nose	sigmoid / o	sigmoid colon
necr / o	death	spermat / o	sperm
nephr / o	kidney	spin / o	spine
neur / o	nerve	spondyl / o	vertebra (backbone)
noct / o	night	stern / o	sternum (breastbone)
odont / o	teeth	stomat / o	mouth
oophor / o	ovary	tend / o	tendon
ophthalm / o	eye	therm / o	heat
orchi / o	testis	thorac / o	chest
os / o	mouth	thromb / o	blood clot
oste / o	bone	thyr / o	thyroid gland
ot / o	ear	toxic, tox / o	poison
pancreat / o	pancreas	trache / o	trachea (windpipe)
pelv / i / o	pelvis	tympan / o	tympanic membrane (eardrum)
pharyng / o	pharynx (throat)		
phleb / o	vein	ureter / o	ureter
pleur / o	pleura	urethr / o	urethra
pneum / o	lung, air	ur / o	urine
proct / o	anus, rectum	uter / o	uterus
pyel / o	renal pelvis	vagin / o	vagina
radi / o	X-rays, radiation	vascul / o	blood vessel
ren / o	kidney	vas / o	vas deferens, vessel
retin / o	retina	ven / o	vein
rhin / o	nose	ventricul / o	ventricle (of brain or heart)
salping / o	fallopian tube		
scler / o	hardening, sclera (white of the eye)	vesic / o	bladder
		vertebr / o	vertebra (backbone)

TABLE B-2 · Common Suffixes

Suffix	Meaning	Suffix	Meaning
-al	pertaining to	-oid	resembling
-algia	pain	-oma	tumor
-ar, -ary	pertaining to	-opia	vision
-cele	hernia, swelling	-osis	abnormal condition
-centesis	surgical puncture	-pathy	disease
-cyte	cell	-pause	cessation
-derma	skin	-penia	decrease
-dipsia	thirst	-pepsia	digestion
-ectomy	excision, removal of	-pexy	fixation
-edema	swelling	-phagia	swallow, eat
-emesis	vomiting	-phasia	speech
-emia	blood	-phobia	fear
-gram	record	-plasty	surgical repair
-graphy	process of recording	-plegia	paralysis
-ia	condition	-pnea	breathing
-ic	pertaining to	-rrhaphy	suture
-ism	condition	-rrhea	flow, discharge
-ist	specialist	-scope	instrument to view
-itis	inflammation	-scopy	visual examination
-lith	stone, calculus	-stenosis	structure, narrowing
-logist	specialist in the study of	-stomy	forming a new opening
-logy	study of	-therapy	treatment
-lysis	separation, destruction, loosening	-tome	instrument to cut
-malacia	softening	-tomy	incision, cut into
-megaly	enlargement	-tripsy	crushing
-meter	measure, instrument for measuring	-uria	urine, urination

TABLE B-3 · Common Prefixes

Prefix	Meaning	Prefix	Meaning
a-, an-	without, not, absent	macro-	large
ab	away from	micro-	small
amb-, ambi-	both, on two sides	neo-	new
auto-	self	para-	near, beside, around
bi-	two, double	peri-	around
brady-	slow	poly-	many, much
dys-	bad, painful, difficult	post-	after, behind
epi-	above, upon	pre-	before
hemi-	half, partly	quadri-	four
hyper-	excessive	sub-	under, below
hypo-	under, below	supra-	above
inter-	between	tachy-	rapid
intra-	within	tri-	three

TABLE B-4   Common Medical Abbreviations

Abbreviation	Meaning	Abbreviation	Meaning
abd	abdomen	CNA	certified nursing assistant
ac	before a meal	CNS	central nervous system
AD	Alzheimer's disease	c/o	complains of
ADA	Americans with Disabilities Act of 1990	COPD	chronic obstructive pulmonary disease
ADL	activities of daily living	CP	cerebral palsy
ad lib	as desired	CPR	cardiopulmonary resuscitation
Adm (adm)	admitted or admission	CVA	cerebrovascular accident (stroke)
AED	automated external defibrillator		
		dc (d/c)	discontinue
AIDS	acquired immunodeficiency syndrome	DD	developmental disability
		disch	discharge
AIIR	airborne infection isolation room	DJD	degenerative joint disease
		DNR	do not resuscitate
AKA	above-the-knee amputation	DOA	dead on arrival
ALS	amyotrophic lateral sclerosis	DOB	date of birth
AM (am)	morning	DON	director of nursing
amb	ambulate, ambulatory	drsg	dressing
amt	amount	DS	Down syndrome
ap	apical	DV	Daily Value
approx	approximately	Dx	diagnosis
ASAP	as soon as possible	ECG (EKG)	electrocardiogram
as tol	as tolerated	EEG	electroencephalogram
ax	axillary	EMS	emergency medical services
bid	twice a day	ePHI	electronic protected health information
BKA	below-the-knee amputation		
BLS	basic life support	ER	emergency room
BM (bm)	bowel movement	F	Fahrenheit
BP, B/P	blood pressure	FBAO	foreign body airway obstruction
B.R.	bed rest		
BRP	bathroom privileges	FBS	fasting blood sugar
BSC	bedside commode	FF	force fluids
C	centigrade, Celsius	fl (fld)	fluid
c̄	with	ft	foot or feet
CA	cancer	Fx	fracture
CAD	coronary artery disease	gal	gallon
cath	catheter, catheterize	GB	gallbladder
CBC	complete blood count	GERD	gastroesophageal reflux disease
CBR	complete bed rest		
CCRC	continuing care retirement community	GI	gastrointestinal
		GSW	gunshot wound
CCU	coronary care unit	gtt	drops
CDC	Centers for Disease Control and Prevention	GU	genitourinary
		h (hr)	hour
CHD	coronary heart disease	HAI	healthcare-associated infection
CHF	congestive heart failure	H_2O	water
cl liq	clear liquids	HBV	hepatitis B virus
CMS	Centers for Medicare & Medicaid Services	Hg	mercury

(table continues on page 726)

TABLE B-4   Common Medical Abbreviations (continued)

Abbreviation	Meaning	Abbreviation	Meaning
HIPAA	Health Insurance Portability and Accountability Act of 1996	N&V	nausea and vomiting
		O_2	oxygen
HIV	human immunodeficiency virus	OB	obstetrics
		OCD	obsessive-compulsive disorder
HOB	head of bed	OJ	orange juice
HS (hs)	hour of sleep (bedtime)	OOB	out of bed
ht	height	O	oral
HTN	hypertension	OR	operating room
ICU	intensive care unit	OSHA	Occupational Safety and Health Administration
ID	identification		
IDDM	insulin-dependent diabetes mellitus	OT	occupational therapy
		oz (Oz)	ounce
in	inch	PACU	post anesthesia care unit
I&O	intake and output	pc	after a meal
IQ	intelligence quotient	Peds	pediatrics
IV	intravenous	PEG	percutaneous endoscopic gastrostomy
L	left, liter		
lab	laboratory	PHI	protected health information
lb	pound	per	by, through
lg	large	PM (pm)	afternoon or evening
liq	liquid	PPE	personal protective equipment
LLQ	left lower quadrant	po (per os)	by mouth
LMP	last menstrual period	post op	postoperative
LPN	licensed practical nurse	pre op	preoperative
lt	left	prep	preparation
LVN	licensed vocational nurse	prn	as necessary
LUQ	left upper quadrant	Pt (pt)	patient
MDRO	multidrug-resistant organism	PT	physical therapy
MDS	Minimum Data Set	PTSD	post-traumatic stress disorder
meds	medications	PVS	persistent vegetative state
mg	milligram	q	every
MI	myocardial infarction (heart attack)	qd	every day
		qh	every hour
min	minute	q2h, q3h, q4h, etc.	every 2 hours, every 3 hours, every 4 hours, etc.
mL	milliliter		
mm	millimeter	qhs	every night at bedtime
MRSA	Methicillin-resistant *Staphylococcus aureus*	qid	four times a day
		qod	every other day
MS	multiple sclerosis	qs	sufficient quantity
MSD	musculoskeletal disorder	qt	quiet
NA	nursing assistant	R	rectal
NB	newborn	RA	rheumatoid arthritis
neg	negative	RBC	red blood cell, red blood cell count
NG	nasogastric		
NIDDM	non-insulin–dependent diabetes mellitus	rehab	rehabilitation
		resp	respiration
nil	none	RLQ	right lower quadrant
no	number	RN	registered nurse
noc, noct	night	ROM	range of motion
NPO (npo)	nothing per mouth (nils per os)	rt (R)	right

Abbreviation	Meaning	Abbreviation	Meaning
RT	respiratory therapy	TLC	tender loving care
RUQ	right upper quadrant	TPN	total parenteral nutrition
Rx	treatment	TPR	temperature, pulse, and respirations
s̄	without		
s̄s̄	half	tsp	teaspoon
SCD	sequential compression device	Tx	treatment
SNF	skilled nursing facility	ty	tympanic
SOB	shortness of breath	UA (u/a)	urinalysis
Spec (spec)	specimen	UK	unknown
SSE	soapsuds enema	URI	upper respiratory infection
ST	speech therapy	UTI	urinary tract infection
STAT, stat	at once, immediately	VRE	Vancomycin-resistant *Enterococci*
STI	sexually transmitted infection		
Surg	surgery	VS (vs)	vital signs
Sx	symptoms	WA	while awake
TB	tuberculosis	WBC	white blood cell, white blood cell count
TBI	traumatic brain injury		
tbsp	tablespoon	w/c	wheelchair
tid	three times a day	WNL	within normal limits
TIA	transient ischemic attack	wt	weight
TJC	The Joint Commission		

TABLE B-5A — The Joint Commission's Official "Do Not Use" List

Do Not Use	Potential Problem	Use Instead
U (unit)	Mistaken for "0" (zero), the number "4" (four), or "cc"	Write "unit"
IU (International Unit)	Mistaken for IV (intravenous) or the number 10 (ten)	Write "International Unit"
Q.D., QD, q.d., qd (daily)	Mistaken for each other	Write "daily"
Q.O.D., QOD, q.o.d, qod (every other day)	Period after the Q mistaken for "I" and the "O" mistaken for "I"	Write "every other day"
Trailing zero (X.0 mg)*	Decimal point is missed	Write X mg
Lack of leading zero (.X mg)		Write 0.X mg
MS	Can mean morphine sulfate or magnesium sulfate	Write "morphine sulfate"
MSO$_4$ and MgSO$_4$	Confused for one another	Write "magnesium sulfate"

This list applies to all orders and all medication-related documentation that is handwritten (including free-text computer entry) or on pre-printed forms.

*Exception: A "trailing zero" may be used only where required to demonstrate the level of precision of the value being reported, such as for laboratory results, imaging studies of lesions, or catheter/tube sizes. It may not be used in medication orders or other medication-related documentation.

Source: The Joint Commission (updated 2009).

TABLE B-5B — Additional Abbreviations, Acronyms, and Symbols for Possible Future Inclusion in the Official "Do Not Use" List

Do Not Use	Potential Problem	Use Instead
> (greater than)	Misinterpreted as the number "7" (seven) or the letter "L"	Write "greater than"
< (less than)	Confused for one another	Write "less than"
Abbreviations for drug names	Misinterpreted due to similar abbreviations for multiple drugs	Write drug names in full
Apothecary units	Unfamiliar to many practitioners Confused with metric units	Use metric units
@	Mistaken for the number "2" (two)	Write "at"
cc	Mistaken for U (units) when poorly written	Write "ml" or "milliliters"
μg	Mistaken for mg (milligrams), resulting in one thousand-fold overdose	Write "mcg" or "micrograms"

Source: The Joint Commission (updated 2009).

GLOSSARY

A

Abandonment: to withdraw one's support or help from another person, in spite of duty or responsibility

Absorption: transfer of nutrients from the digestive tract into the bloodstream

Accreditation: official recognition that the organization meets certain standards of quality

Acquired immunodeficiency syndrome (AIDS): a disease caused by human immunodeficiency virus (HIV), a bloodborne virus that attacks the body's immune system; death usually results when the body becomes unable to recognize and fight off infections

Activities of daily living (ADLs): routine tasks of daily life, such as bathing, eating, and grooming

Acute: a word used to describe a disorder with a rapid onset and a relatively short recovery time, usually unexpected

Acute pain: sharp, sudden pain

Addiction: a physical need for a substance that results in withdrawal signs and symptoms if the substance is withheld

Advance directive: a document that allows a person to make his wishes regarding health care known to family members and health care workers

Afterlife: a state of being where the dead meet again with loved ones who have passed on before them

Agnosia: difficulty recognizing information obtained using the five senses

Airborne pathogens: pathogens that can be transmitted through the air

Alignment: good posture

Alopecia: baldness, loss of hair

Amnesia: difficulty remembering

Amputation: the surgical removal of all or part of an extremity

Anesthesia: loss of the ability to feel pain, caused by administration of a medication

Angina pectoris: the classic chest pain that is felt as a result of the heart muscle being deprived of oxygen

Anorexia: loss of appetite

Antibodies: specialized proteins produced by the immune system that help our bodies to fight off specific microbes, preventing infection

Anuria: the state of voiding less than 100 mL of urine over the course of 24 hours

Anxiety: feeling of uneasiness, dread, apprehension, or worry

Aphasia: a general term for a group of disorders that affect a person's ability to communicate with others; may be expressive (an inability to form words) or receptive (an inability to understand words); often occurs following a stroke

Appetite: the desire for food

Apraxia: difficulty coordinating the steps needed to complete a task

Arteriosclerosis: "hardening of the arteries"; occurs when atherosclerotic plaque interferes with the elasticity of the arterial walls, making them brittle and prone to breaking

Arthritis: inflammation of the joints, usually associated with pain and stiffness

Aspiration: the accidental inhalation of foreign material (such as food, liquids, or vomitus) into the airway

Assistive devices: devices that make certain tasks (such as walking, eating, or dressing) easier for a person with a disability

Asthma: a condition that affects the bronchi and bronchioles of the lungs; triggers (such as cold weather, allergies, respiratory infections, stress, smoke, and exercise) cause the bronchi and bronchioles to become narrower, making breathing difficult

Atherosclerosis: blocking of the arteries, caused by the buildup of fatty deposits called plaque on the inside of the vessel wall

Atrophy: the loss of muscle size and strength

Attitude: the side of ourselves that we display to the world, communicating outwardly how we feel about things

Autopsy: examination of a person's organs and tissues after the person has died, done to confirm or identify the cause of the person's death

B

Bag technique: an infection control procedure used in the home health care setting to keep the home health aide's tote bag free from contamination

Balance: stability produced by even distribution of weight

Basic life support (BLS): basic emergency care techniques, such as rescue breathing and cardiopulmonary resuscitation (CPR)

Bath blanket: a lightweight cotton blanket used to cover a person during a bed bath or linen change to help provide modesty and warmth

Bed protector: a square of quilted absorbent fabric backed with waterproof material that measures approximately 3 feet by 3 feet; used to prevent soiling of the bottom linens; sometimes called an incontinence pad

Bedpan: a device used for elimination when a person is unable to get out of bed

Bedside commode: a device used for elimination when a person is able to get out of bed, but unable to walk to the bathroom; it consists of a chair-like frame with a toilet seat and a removable collection bucket

Benefit period: a unit of time used by the Medicare program to track how many days of skilled health care services a person uses, and how many are still available; begins with hospitalization and ends when a person has not received any skilled health care services, either in the hospital or in nursing home

Benign: "good" or "kind"; adjective used to describe a non-cancerous tumor (that is, one that grows slowly and does not spread)

Biopsy: a diagnostic procedure that involves obtaining a cell or tissue sample for examination under a microscope

Bloodborne pathogens: pathogens that can be transmitted to another person through blood or other body fluids

Body alignment: positioning of the body so that the spine is not twisted or crooked

Body fluids: liquid or semi-liquid substances produced by the body, such as blood, urine, feces, vomitus, saliva, drainage from wounds, sweat, semen, vaginal secretions, tears, cerebrospinal fluid, amniotic fluid, and breast milk

Body mechanics: the efficient and safe use of the body

Braille: a system that uses letters made from combinations of raised dots that allows a blind person to read

Bronchitis: inflammation of the bronchi

C

Calories: the unit of measure used to describe the energy content of food

Cardiac arrest: the condition where the heart has stopped

Cardiac cycle: the pumping action of the heart in an organized pattern (all of the events associated with one heartbeat)

Cartilage: a tough, fibrous substance found in joints and other parts of the body; in slightly movable joints, the cartilage acts as a "shock absorber"; in freely movable joints; the cartilage provides a smooth surface for the bones of the joint to move against

Cataract: the gradual yellowing and hardening of the lens of the eye

Catheter: a tube that is inserted into the body for the purpose of administering or removing fluids

Catheter care: thorough cleaning of the perineal area (especially around the urethra) and the catheter tubing that extends outside of the body, to prevent infection

Cell: the basic unit of life

Central nervous system (CNS): the brain and spinal cord; responsible for receiving information, processing it, and issuing instructions

Cerebrospinal fluid (CSF): a clear fluid that circulates around the brain and spinal cord and acts as a "shock absorber" to protect these structures

Cerumen: a waxy substance that helps to protect the external auditory canal by trapping dirt and other particles; commonly referred to as "earwax"

Chemical restraint: any medication that alters a person's mood or behavior, such as a sedative or tranquilizer

Chronic: a word used to describe a disorder that is ongoing and often needs to be controlled through continuous medication or treatment

Chronic bronchitis: a disorder caused by long-term irritation of the bronchi and bronchioles, such as that caused by inhaling tobacco smoke; one of two forms of chronic obstructive pulmonary disease (COPD)

Chronic condition: a condition that is ongoing and often needs to be controlled through continuous medication or treatment (for example, diabetes, heart failure, or hypertension)

Chronic obstructive pulmonary disease (COPD): a general term used to describe two related lung disorders, emphysema and chronic bronchitis; the leading cause of COPD is smoking

Chronic pain: slow, diffuse, constant pain

Chyme: the liquid substance produced by the digestion of food in the stomach

Circulation: the continuous movement of the blood through the blood vessels; powered by the pumping action of the heart

Civil laws: laws concerned with relationships between individuals

Closed bed: an empty, made bed

Co-existent medical condition: more than one medical condition at the same time in the same person

Cognitive impairment: problems processing, learning, or remembering information

Coma: a deep state of unconsciousness from which a person cannot be aroused

Communication: the exchange of information

Competency evaluation: an exam consisting of a written portion and a skills portion that must be passed at the end of the nursing assistant training course to obtain certification

Conception (fertilization): occurs when the male and female sex cells join, forming a cell that contains the complete number of chromosomes

Condom catheter: a device used to manage urinary incontinence in men; it consists of a soft plastic or rubber sheath, tubing, and a collection bag for the urine

Conflict: discord resulting from differences between people; can occur when one person is unable to understand or accept another's ideas or beliefs

Constipation: a condition that occurs when the feces remain in the intestines for too long, resulting in hard, dry feces that are difficult to pass

Contaminated: adjective used to describe an object that is soiled by pathogens

Continuing care retirement communities (CCRCs): a type of long-term care setting that provides many different levels of care (that is, independent living, assisted living, and nursing home care) and multiple services on the same campus

Continuum of care: the delivery of health care over time as a person moves from being independent to needing assistance with personal care, medical care, or both

Contractures: a condition that occurs when a joint is held in the same position for too long a time; the tendons shorten and become stiff, possibly causing permanent loss of motion in the joint

Coordinated body movement: using the weight of the body to help with movement

Coping mechanisms: conscious and deliberate ways of dealing with stress, such as exercising, praying, or enjoying a hobby

Criminal laws: laws concerned with the relationship between the individual and society

Culture: the beliefs (including religious or spiritual beliefs), values, and traditions that are customary to a group of people; a view of the world that is handed down from generation to generation

D

Decision-making capacity: the ability to make a thoughtful decision based on an understanding of the potential risks and benefits of taking a certain course of action

Defecate: to have a bowel movement

Defense mechanisms: unconscious ways of dealing with stress

Degenerative condition: a condition that gets progressively worse over time (for example, dementia)

Dehydration: too little fluid in the tissues of the body

Delegate: to authorize another person to perform a task on your behalf

Delirium: a temporary state of confusion

Delusions: false ideas or beliefs, especially about oneself

Dementia: the permanent and progressive loss of the ability to think and remember

Depression: an alteration in a person's mood that causes him or her to lose pleasure or interest in all usually pleasurable activities, such as eating, working, or socializing; a feeling of hopelessness

Depth of respiration: the quality of each breath

Dermis: the deepest layer of the skin, where sensory receptors, blood vessels, nerves, glands, and hair follicles are found

Development: changes that occur psychologically or socially as a person passes through life

Developmental disability: a permanent disability that affects a person before he or she reaches adulthood (that is, before 19 to 22 years of age) and interferes with the person's ability to achieve developmental milestones

Diabetes mellitus: an endocrine disorder that results when the pancreas is unable to produce enough insulin

Dialysis: a procedure that is done to remove waste products and fluids from the body when a person's kidneys fail and can no longer perform this task

Diaphragm: the strong, dome-shaped muscle that separates the chest cavity from the abdominal cavity and assists in breathing

Diarrhea: the passage of liquid, unformed feces

Diastole: the resting phase of the cardiac cycle; during which the myocardium relaxes, allowing the chambers to fill with blood

Diastolic pressure: the pressure that the blood exerts against the arterial walls when the heart muscle relaxes; the second blood pressure measurement

Dietitian: a person who has a degree in nutrition

Digestion: the process of breaking food down into simple elements (nutrients)

Disability: impaired physical or emotional function

Disaster: a sudden, unexpected event that causes injury to many people, major damage to property, or both

Disease: a condition that occurs when the structure or function of an organ or organ system is abnormal

Disoriented: the state of being unable to answer basic questions about person, place, or time; a state of confusion

Do not resuscitate (DNR) order: an order written on a person's chart specifying the person's wishes that the usual efforts to save his life will not be made; also called a *no-code order*

Durable power of attorney for health care: a type of advance directive that transfers the responsibility for handling a person's affairs and making medical decisions to a family member

Dyspnea: labored or difficult breathing

Dysuria: painful or difficult urination

E

Edema: too much fluid in the tissues of the body; swelling

Edentulous: without teeth

Ejaculation: the forceful release of semen from the body; method by which sperm cells leave the man's body through the penis

Electronic health record (EHR): a computer information system that stores and saves a person's medical information

Embolus: a blood clot in a vessel that breaks off and moves from one place to another

Emphysema: a disorder caused by long-term exposure of the alveoli to toxins, such as tobacco smoke; one of two forms of chronic obstructive pulmonary disease (COPD)

Enema: a solution that is placed into the large intestine by way of the anus for the purpose of removing feces from the rectum

Enteral nutrition: placing food directly into a person's stomach or intestines

Enzymes: substances that have the ability to break chemical bonds

Epidermis: the outer layer of the skin

Epilepsy: a disorder characterized by chronic seizure activity

Erythrocytes: red blood cells; responsible for carrying oxygen to all of the tissues of the body

F

Fanfolded: adjective used to describe the top sheet, blanket, and bedspread of a closed bed when they have been turned back (toward the foot of the bed)

Fecal (bowel) incontinence: the inability to hold one's feces, or the involuntary loss of feces from the bowel

Fecal impaction: a condition that occurs when constipation is not relieved

Feces: the semisolid waste product of digestion; stool

Fever: a body temperature that is higher than normal

Filtrate: the liquid that forms the basis for urine

Flatulence: the presence of excessive amounts of flatus (gas) in the intestines, causing abdominal distension (swelling) and discomfort

Flatus: gas that is formed as part of the digestive process

Flow meter: a device used to set the rate at which oxygen is delivered to a patient or resident who is receiving oxygen therapy

Fluid balance: a state where the amount of fluid taken into the body equals the amount of fluid that leaves the body

Fracture: a broken bone

Fracture pan: a wedge-shaped bedpan that is used when a person has an injury or disability that makes it too uncomfortable or dangerous to use a regular bedpan

Frequency: urination that occurs more often than usual

Friction: the force created when two surfaces (such as a sheet and a person's skin) rub against each other

G

Gas exchange: the transfer of oxygen into the blood, and carbon dioxide out of it

Gatches: the joints at the hips and knees of the mattresses of most adjustable beds that allow the mattress to "break" so that the person's head can be elevated or his knees bent

Glaucoma: a disorder of the eye that occurs when the pressure within the eye is increased to dangerous levels

Glucose: the body's most basic type of fuel; supplied by carbohydrates and sometimes referred to as "blood sugar"

Graduate: a measuring device used to measure fluids

Grief: mental anguish

Growth: changes that occur physically as a person passes through life

H

Hallucinations: episodes when a person sees, feels, hears, or tastes something that does not really exist

Hangnails: broken pieces of cuticle

Health care-associated infections (HAIs): infections that patients or residents get while receiving treatment in a hospital or other health care facility or that health care workers get while performing their duties within a health care setting

Health care team: group of people with different types of knowledge and skill levels who work together to provide holistic care to the patient or resident

Heart failure: a condition that occurs when the heart is unable to pump enough blood to meet the body's needs

Hematuria: blood in the urine

Hemiplegia: paralysis on one side of the body

Hemoglobin: a protein found in red blood cells that combines with oxygen to carry it to the tissues of the body

Hemorrhage: severe, uncontrolled bleeding

Hepatitis: inflammation of the liver

Heterosexual: a person who is sexually attracted to members of the opposite sex

HIV-positive: the state of being infected with human immunodeficiency virus (HIV)

Holistic: word used to describe care of the whole person, physically and emotionally

Homebound: the person is unable to leave the house without a lot of help from another person

Homeostasis: a state of balance

Homosexual: a person who is sexually attracted to members of the same sex

Hopper: a sink-like fixture that flushes like a toilet and is connected to a sewer line

Hormones: chemicals that act on cells to produce a response

Hospice care: care provided by a health care organization for people who are dying, and their families

Hygiene: personal cleanliness

Hyperglycemia: a state of having too much glucose in the bloodstream

Hypertension: high blood pressure; a blood pressure that is consistently greater than 140 mm Hg (systolic) and/or 90 mm Hg (diastolic)

Hypoglycemia: a dangerous drop in blood glucose levels

Hypotension: low blood pressure; a blood pressure that is consistently lower than 90 mm Hg (systolic) and/or 60 mm Hg (diastolic)

I

Incident (occurrence) report: a preprinted document that is completed following an accident involving a patient or resident

Influenza: an acute respiratory infection caused by the influenza virus; characterized by a sore throat, dry cough, stuffy nose, headache, body aches, weakness, and fever; commonly known as "the flu"

Instrumental activities of daily living (IADLs): more complex tasks that a person must be able to do in order to continue to live independently, such as using the telephone or handling money

Intake and output (I&O) flow sheet: a document used for recording measurements of all of the fluids that enter and leave the body

Interdisciplinary care plan: a specific plan of care for each patient or resident developed with input from all members of the health care team

Interview: a meeting between an employer and a potential employee, during which information is exchanged regarding the organization, the job, and the potential employee's qualifications for the job

Intimacy: a feeling of emotional closeness to another human being

Intra-operative phase: the phase during which the surgery is actually performed

J

Joint: the area where two bones join together

K

Kardex: a card file that contains condensed versions of each patient's or resident's medical record

L

Lactation: the process by which the glandular tissue of the female breast produces milk

Laws: rules that are made by a governing authority, such as the state or federal government, with the intent of preserving basic human rights

Lesion: a general term used to describe any break in the skin

Leukocytes: white blood cells; responsible for fighting infection

Lift (draw) sheet: a small, flat sheet that is placed over the middle of the bottom sheet, covering the area of the bed from above the person's shoulders to below his or her buttocks

Ligaments: very strong bands of fibrous tissue that cross over the joint capsule, attaching one bone to another and stabilizing the joint

Living will: a type of advance directive that states a person's wish that death not be artificially postponed

M

Malignant: "evil"; adjective used to describe a cancerous tumor (that is, one that grows rapidly and spreads)

Masturbation: stimulation of the genitals for sexual pleasure or release, by a means other than sexual intercourse

Medicaid: a federally funded and state-regulated plan designed to help people with low incomes to pay for health care

Medical asepsis: techniques that are used to physically remove or kill pathogens

Medical record: a legal document where information about a patient's or resident's current condition, the measures that have been taken by the medical and nursing staff to diagnose and treat the condition, and the patient's or resident's response to the treatment and care provided is recorded; also called a medical chart

Medicare: a type of insurance plan that is federally funded by Social Security and which all people 65 years and older, and some younger disabled people, are eligible to participate in

Melanin: a dark pigment that gives our skin, hair, and eyes color

Menopause: the cessation of menstruation and fertility that women typically experience in their early 50's

Menstrual period: the monthly loss of blood through the vagina that occurs in the absence of pregnancy

Metabolism: the physical and chemical changes that occur when the cells of the body change the food that we eat into energy

Metastasis: the process by which cancer cells spread from their original location in the body to a new location, which may be quite distant from the first

Microbe: a living thing that cannot be seen with the naked eye; examples include bacteria and viruses

Micturition: urination

Midstream ("clean catch") urine specimen: a method of collecting urine that prevents contamination of the urine by the bacteria that normally exist in and around the urethra

Minimum Data Set (MDS): a report that focuses on the degree of assistance or skilled care that each resident of a long-term care facility needs

Mitered corner: a corner that is made by folding and tucking the sheet so that it lies flat and neat against the mattress

Motor nerves: nerves that carry commands from the brain down the spinal cord and out to the muscles and organs of the body

Mucous membrane: a special type of epithelial tissue that lines many of the organ systems in the body and is coated with mucus

Mucus: a slippery, sticky substance that is secreted by special cells and serves to keep the surfaces of mucous membranes moist

Multiple sclerosis (MS): a disorder of the nervous system in which the myelin sheaths that cover the nerves are damaged, resulting in faulty transmission of nerve impulses

Myelin: a fatty, white substance that protects the axon and helps to speed the conduction of nerve impulses along the axon

Myocardial infarction: a "heart attack"; occurs when one or more of the coronary arteries become completely blocked, preventing blood from reaching the parts of the heart that are fed by the affected arteries

N

Need: something that is essential for a person's physical and mental health

Neuron: a cell that can send and receive information

Nocturia: the need to get up more than once or twice during the night to urinate, to the point where sleep is disrupted

Nonverbal communication: a way of communicating that uses facial expressions, gestures, and body language, instead of written or spoken language

Nosocomial infections: infections that patients or residents get while receiving treatment in a hospital or other health care facility; a type of health care-associated infection (HAI)

NPO status: a doctor's order specifying that a patient or resident is to have "nils per os" (nothing by mouth)

Nursing care plan: a specific plan of care for each patient or resident developed by the nursing team

Nursing process: a process that allows members of the nursing team to communicate with each other regarding the patient's or resident's specific needs (in regard to nursing care), what steps will be taken to meet those needs, and whether or not the steps were effective in meeting the person's needs; consists of five parts: assessment, diagnosis, planning, implementation, and evaluation

Nutrients: substances in food and fluids that the body uses to grow, to repair itself, and to carry out processes essential for living

Nutrition: the process of taking in and using food

Nutritional supplement: a flavored shake or drink that is used to supply extra calories or protein; often served with meals or as a snack in between meals

O

Objective: information that is obtained directly, through measurements or by using one of the five senses (sight, smell, taste, hearing, touch)

Observation: something that you notice about the patient or resident, typically related to a change in the person's physical or mental condition

Occupational Safety and Health Administration (OSHA): an agency within the Department of Labor that establishes safety and health standards for the workplace, to protect the safety and health of employees

Oliguria: the state of voiding a very small amount of urine over a given period of time (for example, voiding only 100 to 400 mL of urine over 24 hours)

Omnibus Budget Reconciliation Act (OBRA): an act passed in 1987 to improve the quality of life for people who live in long-term care facilities by making sure that residents receive a certain standard of care

Open bed: a bed ready to receive a patient or resident

Organ: a group of tissues functioning together for a similar purpose

Organ system: a group of organs that work together to perform a specific function for the body

Orthostatic hypotension: a sudden decrease in blood pressure that occurs when a person stands up from a sitting or lying position

Osteoporosis: a disorder characterized by the excessive loss of bone tissue

Ostomy: an artificial opening in the abdomen for the elimination of feces

Ovulation: the release of a ripe, mature egg from the female ovaries each month

P

Palliative care: care that focuses on relieving uncomfortable symptoms, not on curing the problem that is causing the symptoms; examples include pain medication, chemotherapy or radiation to shrink a tumor, oxygen to make breathing easier, and some surgical procedures

Paraplegia: paralysis from the waist down

Parkinson's disease: a progressive neurologic disorder that is characterized by tremor and weakness in the muscles and a shuffling gait

Pathogen: a microbe that can cause illness

Pension: regular cash payments paid to a person, usually after retirement

Perineal care (pericare): cleaning the perineum and anus, as well as the vulva (in women) and the penis (in men)

Peri-operative period: the term used to describe all three phases of the surgical process as a whole—the pre-operative, intra-operative, and post-operative phases

Peripheral nervous system (PNS): the nerves outside of the brain and spinal cord; receives information from the environment, and carries commands from the brain and spinal cord to the other organs of the body, such as the muscles

Peristalsis: involuntary wavelike muscular movements, such as those that occur in the digestive system to move chyme (partially digested food) through the intestines

Persistent vegetative state: a state of altered consciousness in which the person appears to be awake, but cannot respond in a deliberate or meaningful way to the environment

Personal protective equipment (PPE): barriers that are worn to physically prevent microbes from reaching a health care provider's skin or mucous membranes, such as gloves, gowns, masks, and protective eyewear

Phantom pain: the feeling that a body part is still present, after it has been surgically removed (amputated)

Physical restraint: a device that is attached to or near a person's body to limit a person's freedom of movement or access to his or her body

Plaque: fatty deposits that build up on the inside of the artery wall, blocking blood flow to the tissues and making the artery wall brittle and prone to breaking

Plasma: the liquid part of the blood

Pneumonia: inflammation of the lung tissue, caused by infection with a virus or bacterium, and resulting in impaired gas exchange

Podiatrist: a doctor who specializes in care of the feet

Polyuria (diuresis): excessive urine output

Post-anesthesia care unit (PACU): the recovery room where patients are taken following surgery so that they can be closely monitored by the health care team to make sure that they are recovering without complications from the surgery or the anesthesia

Postmenopausal bleeding: uterine bleeding after menopause

Postmortem care: the care of a person's body after the person's death

Post-operative phase: the phase after the surgery is actually performed

Pre-operative phase: the phase before the surgery is actually performed

Pre-operative teaching: teaching done by members of the health care team to prepare a person and his or her family members for surgery; during pre-operative teaching, the person learns about the surgical procedure, its benefits and possible risks, and what can be expected during the post-operative recovery period

Presbycusis: age-related hearing loss

Presbyopia: age-related loss of the eye's ability to focus on objects that are close

Pressure points: bony areas where pressure ulcers are most likely to form; include the heels, ankles, knees, hips, toes, elbows, shoulder blades, ears, the back of the head, and along the spine

Pressure ulcer: a difficult-to-heal (and possibly even fatal) sore that forms when part of the body presses against a surface (such as a mattress or chair) for a long period of time; also known as *pressure sores* and *decubitus ulcers*

PRN (as-needed) care: personal hygiene care that is provided whenever a patient or resident needs it, throughout the day or night

Procedure: a series of steps followed in a particular order when providing care to a patient or resident that helps to ensure that the care provided is safe and correct

Professional: a person who has credentials, obtained through education and training, that enable him to become licensed or certified to practice a certain profession; also, a person who demonstrates a professional attitude

Prognosis: a doctor's prediction of the course of a person's disease, and his or her estimation of the person's chances for recovery

Prosthetic devices: artificial replacements for legs, feet, arms, or other body parts

Puberty: the period during which the secondary sex characteristics appear and the reproductive organs begin to function

Pulse amplitude: the force or quality of the pulse

Pulse deficit: the difference between the apical pulse rate (the pulse that is measured by listening over the apex of the heart with a stethoscope) and the radial pulse rate (the pulse that is measured by placing the middle two or three fingers over the radial artery, located on the inside of the wrist)

Pulse point: the points where the large arteries run close enough to the surface of the skin to be felt as a pulse

Pulse rate: the number of pulsations that can be felt over an artery in 1 minute; an indication of the heart rate

Pulse rhythm: the pattern of the pulsations and the pauses between them

Q

Quadriplegia: paralysis from the neck down; also known as *tetraplegia*

R

Race: a general characterization that describes skin color, body stature, facial features, and hair texture

Range of motion: the complete extent of movement that a joint is normally capable of without causing pain

Rash: a group of skin lesions

Reciprocity: the principle by which one state recognizes the validity of a license or certification granted by another state

Recording: communicating information about a patient or resident to other health care team members in written form; sometimes called charting or documenting

Reference list: a list of three or four people who would be willing to talk to a potential employer about a job candidate's abilities

Registry: an official record maintained by the state of the people who have successfully completed the nursing assistant training program

Rehabilitation: the process of helping a person with a disability to return to his or her highest level of physical, emotional, or economic function

Reincarnation: the idea that a person's spirit or soul will live again on Earth in the form of an animal or human being yet to be born

Religion: a person's spiritual beliefs

Reminiscence therapy: a technique used for interacting with people who have dementia, in which the person with dementia is encouraged to remember and share experiences from his or her past with others

Reporting: the spoken exchange of information between health care team members

Reproduction: the process by which a living thing makes more living things like itself

Respiration: the process the body uses to obtain oxygen from the environment and remove carbon dioxide (a waste gas) from the body

Respiratory arrest: the condition where breathing has stopped

Respiratory rate: the number of times a person breathes in 1 minute (one breath is both an inhalation and an exhalation)

Respiratory rhythm: the regularity with which a person breathes

Respite care: home care that gives the primary caregiver an opportunity to rest or leave the home for a short period of time

Restorative care: measures that health care workers take to help a person regain health, strength, and function; the means by which rehabilitation is achieved

Résumé: a brief document that gives a possible employer general information about a job candidate's education and work experience

Rigor mortis: the stiffening of the muscles that usually develops within 2 to 4 hours of death

S

Safety Data Sheets (SDSs): a document that summarizes key information about a chemical, its composition, which exposures may be dangerous, what to do if an exposure should occur, and how to clean up spills

Scope of practice: the range of tasks that a nursing assistant is legally permitted to do

Sebum: an oily substance secreted by glands in the skin that lubricates the skin and helps to prevent it from drying out

Sensory nerves: nerves that carry information from the internal organs and the outside world to the spinal cord and up into the brain so that the brain can analyze the information

Sensory receptors: specialized cells or groups of cells associated with a sensory nerve

Sex: the physical activity one engages in to obtain sexual pleasure and reproduce

Sex cell (gamete): special cells contributed by each parent that contain half of the normal number of chromosomes

Sexuality: how a person perceives his or her maleness or femaleness

Sexually transmitted infection (STI): an infection that is most commonly transmitted by sexual contact; also known as venereal disease

Shearing: the force created when something or someone is pulled across a surface that offers resistance

Shroud: a covering used to wrap the body of a person who has died

Signs: objective evidence of disease, based on data that are obtained directly, through measurements or by using one of the five senses

Skeleton: the framework for the body formed by the bones

Social Security Act: an act, signed into law by President Franklin D. Roosevelt in 1935, that established a program designed to provide regular case payments for retired people age 65 years and older

Sphygmomanometer: a device used to measure blood pressure

Sputum: mucus and other respiratory secretions that are coughed up from the lungs, bronchi, and trachea; also known as phlegm

Standard precautions: precautions that a health care worker takes with each patient or resident to prevent contact with bloodborne pathogens; includes the use of barrier methods (such as gloves) as well as certain environmental control methods

Stethoscope: a device that amplifies sound and transfers it to the listener's ears

Stomatitis: inflammation of the mouth, often seen in people who are receiving chemotherapy

Stool: a term used to refer to fecal matter after it has left the body

Stroke: a disorder that occurs when blood flow to a part of the brain is completely blocked, causing the tissue to die; also known as a "brain attack" or cerebrovascular accident (CVA)

Subcutaneous tissue: the layer of fat that supports the dermis (the deepest layer of the skin)

Subjective: information that cannot be objectively measured or assessed

Suicide: the act of taking one's own life intentionally and voluntarily

Supportive care: treatments that will not prolong life, but will make a person more comfortable, such as oxygen therapy, nutritional supplementation, pain medication, range-of-motion exercises, grooming and hygiene, and positioning assistance

Supportive devices: (1) devices that help to stabilize a weak joint or limb; (2) devices used when positioning a person to help the person maintain proper body alignment, such as rolled sheets, towels, or blankets

Surgical bed: a closed bed that has been opened to receive a patient or resident who will be arriving by stretcher; the top sheet, blanket, and bedspread are folded toward the side of the bed, leaving one side open and ready to receive the person

Survey: an inspection of a nursing home carried out by the government to ensure that care is being provided according to standards and regulations

Symptoms: subjective evidence of disease, based on data that cannot be measured or observed first-hand, such as a patient's or resident's complaint of pain

Synapse: the gap between the axon of one neuron and the dendrites of the next

Syncope: fainting

Systole: the active phase of the cardiac cycle, during which the myocardium contracts, sending blood out of the heart

Systolic pressure: the pressure that the blood exerts against the arterial walls when the heart muscle contracts; the first blood pressure measurement that is recorded

T

Tasks: growth and development milestones that must be completed before a person can move on to the next stage of growth and development

Tendons: bands of connective tissue that attach the skeletal muscles to the bones

Terminal illness: an illness or condition from which recovery is not expected

The Joint Commission: an independent, non-profit organization that sets national standards for all types of health care organizations and officially recognizes (accredits) organizations that meet these standards

Thrombocytes: pinched-off pieces of larger cells that are found in the red bone marrow and are responsible for clotting of the blood; also called platelets

Tissue: a group of cells similar in structure and specialized to perform a specific function

Traction: a treatment for fracture in which the ends of the broken bone are placed in the proper alignment and then weight is applied to exert a constant pull and keep the bone in alignment

Transfer: move from one place to another, for example, from the bed to a wheelchair

Transfer (gait) belt: a webbed or woven belt with a buckle that is used to assist a weak or unsteady person with standing, walking, or transferring

Transient flora: microbes that are picked up by touching contaminated objects or people who have an infectious disease

Transient ischemic attack (TIA): a temporary (transient) episode of dysfunction caused by decreased blood flow to the brain

Tuberculosis (TB): an airborne infection caused by a bacterium that usually infects the lungs

Tumor: an abnormal growth of tissue; the cells that form the tumor may be benign or malignant

U

Unintentional tort: a violation of civil law that occurs when someone causes harm or injury to another person or that person's property without the intent to cause harm

Unit: a patient's or resident's room

United States Department of Health and Human Services (DHHS): the primary government agency responsible for protecting this nation's health; includes organizations such as the Food and Drug Administration (FDA), the Centers for Disease Control and Prevention (CDC), the National Institutes of Health (NIH), and the Centers for Medicare and Medicaid Services (CMS)

Unresponsive: a person who is unconscious and cannot be aroused, or conscious but not responsive when spoken to or touched

Urgency: a need to urinate immediately

Urinal: a device used for urination when a man is unable to get out of bed

Urinalysis: examination of the urine under a microscope and by chemical means

Urinary incontinence: the inability to hold one's urine, or the involuntary loss of urine from the bladder

Urinary retention: the inability of the bladder to empty either completely during urination, or at all

Urination: the process of passing urine from the body

Urine: formed by the kidneys; consists of waste products that have been filtered from the bloodstream, along with excess fluid

V

Validation therapy: a technique used for interacting with people who have dementia, in which the caregiver acknowledges the person's reality; rather than correcting the person, the caregiver attempts to distract the person and redirect the conversation whenever possible

Varicose veins: a condition that results from pooling of blood in the veins just underneath the skin, causing them to become swollen and "knotty" in appearance

Verbal communication: a way of communicating that uses written or spoken language

Vital signs: certain key measurements that provide essential information about a person's health

Voiding: urination

Vulnerable adult: a person who is 18 years of age or older who may be in need of community care services because he has a mental or other disability, an illness, or is at an age (elderly) that causes him to be unable to care for or protect himself against significant harm or exploitation

W

Weight-bearing ability: the ability to stand on one or both legs

Will: a legal statement that expresses a person's wishes for the management of his or her affairs after death

Withdrawal: an emotional and physical reaction that occurs when use of the addictive substance is discontinued

Work ethic: a person's attitude toward his or her work

Wound: an injury that results in a break in the skin (and usually the underlying tissues as well)

Note: A t following a page number indicates tabular material, an f indicates a figure, a p indicates procedure material, and a b indicates a boxed feature.